Basic and Applied Aspects of Noise-Induced Hearing Loss

NATO ASI Series

Advanced Science Institutes Series

A series presenting the results of activities sponsored by the NATO Science Committee, which aims at the dissemination of advanced scientific and technological knowledge, with a view to strengthening links between scientific communities.

The series is published by an international board of publishers in conjunction with the NATO Scientific Affairs Division

A	**Life Sciences**	Plenum Publishing Corporation
B	**Physics**	New York and London
C	**Mathematical and Physical Sciences**	D. Reidel Publishing Company Dordrecht, Boston, and Lancaster
D	**Behavioral and Social Sciences**	Martinus Nijhoff Publishers
E	**Engineering and Materials Sciences**	The Hague, Boston, and Lancaster
F	**Computer and Systems Sciences**	Springer-Verlag
G	**Ecological Sciences**	Berlin, Heidelberg, New York, and Tokyo

Recent Volumes in this Series

Volume 105—The Physiology of Thirst and Sodium Appetite
edited by G. de Caro, A. N. Epstein, and M. Massi

Volume 106—The Molecular Biology of *Physarum polycephalum*
edited by William F. Dove, Jennifer Dee, Sadashi Hatano, Finn B. Haugli, and Karl-Ernst Wohlfarth-Bottermann

Volume 107—NMR in the Life Sciences
edited by E. Morton Bradbury and Claudio Nicolini

Volume 108—Grazing Research at Northern Latitudes
edited by Olafur Gudmundsson

Volume 109—Central and Peripheral Mechanisms of Cardiovascular Regulation
edited by A. Magro, W. Osswald, D. Reiss, and P. Vanhoutte

Volume 110—Structure and Dynamics of RNA
edited by P. H. van Knippenberg and C. W. Hilbers

Volume 111—Basic and Applied Aspects of Noise-Induced Hearing Loss
edited by Richard J. Salvi, D. Henderson, R. P. Hamernik, and V. Colletti

Volume 112—Human Apolipoprotein Mutants: Impact on Atherosclerosis and Longevity
edited by C. R. Sirtori, A. V. Nichols, and G. Franceschini

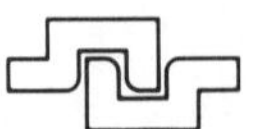

Series A: Life Sciences

Basic and Applied Aspects of Noise-Induced Hearing Loss

Edited by

Richard J. Salvi
D. Henderson and
R. P. Hamernik
University of Texas at Dallas
Dallas, Texas

and

V. Colletti
University of Verona
Verona, Italy

Plenum Press
New York and London
Published in cooperation with NATO Scientific Affairs Division

Proceedings of a NATO Advanced Studies Institute on
Applied and Basic Aspects of Noise-Induced Hearing Loss,
held September 23–29, 1985,
in Lucca, Italy

Library of Congress Cataloging in Publication Data

NATO Advanced Studies Institute on Applied and Basic Aspects of Noise-Induced Hearing Loss (1985: Lucca, Italy)
Basic and applied aspects of noise-induced hearing loss.

(NATO ASI series. Series A. Life sciences; v. 111)
"Proceedings of a NATO Advanced Studies Institute on Applied and Basic Aspects of Noise-Induced Hearing Loss, held September 23–29, 1985, in Lucca, Italy"—T.p. verso.
"Published in cooperation with NATO Scientific Affairs Division."
Abstracts in French.
Includes bibliographies and index.
1. Deafness, Noise induced—Congresses. I. Salvi, Richard. II. North Atlantic Treaty Organization. Scientific Affairs Division. III. Title. IV. Series. [DNLM: 1. Hearing Loss, Noise-Induced—congresses. WV 270 N279 1985b]
RF2935.N38 1985 616.8 86-15109
ISBN 0-306-42369-3

A Division of Plenum Publishing Corporation
233 Spring Street, New York, N.Y. 10013

Printed in the United States of America

PREFACE

In September 1985, NATO sponsored an Advanced Study Workshop entitled, "Noise-Induced Hearing Loss: Basic and Applied Aspects." The meeting was held in a mountain retreat near Lucca, Italy and was attended by scientists, clinicians, and public officials from 12 countries. This was the third in a series of such conferences organized by the authors. The first two were supported by the United States National Institute of Occupational Safety and Health; their proceedings were published as "The Effects of Noise on Hearing" in 1976 and "New Perspectives on Noise-Induced Hearing Loss" in 1982.

The Organizing Committee approached NATO because it was felt that the problem of noise was common to all industrialized countries and was an especially serious problem for the military. Thus, the NATO sponsorship and the Italian site of the meeting were part of the Organizing Committee's plan to obtain an international and thorough representation on the problem of noise-induced hearing loss.

The NATO meeting and proceedings followed the format of the previous two symposia with an initial focus on the anatomical and physiological disturbances resulting from noise-induced hearing loss. This was followed by sections devoted to studies of a more applied nature involving general auditory performance in noise, issues associated with the establishment of noise-exposure criteria, nonauditory effects of noise, and the interaction of noise with other agents.

The proceedings of this symposium will serve as an easily accessible and concise survey of recent advances in the field of noise research from which one can review and reflect upon the gradient of progress made over the past 5 years. The proceedings should help to point out gaps in our knowledge should serve as a useful guide for further research efforts. In reviewing the progress over the last 10 years, it is clear that we have made large strides in understanding the basic "mechanisms" of noise-induced hearing loss. Anatomical studies have advanced from a gross evaluation of sensory structures to assessing the very detailed molecular organization of the hair cell cilia. Physiologists have advanced from recording gross potentials to detecting the physiological changes that occur in individual VIII nerve fibers and hair cells in the cochlea. Substantial progress has also been made in determining how acoustic trauma alters the biomechanical vibration pattern of the cochlea. From the perspectives of the clinicians and psychoacousticians, we have developed more sophisticated means of evaluating complex auditory discrimination abilities, such as frequency selectivity, temporal resolution and speech discrimination. The development of solid state electronic devices and computers has provided powerful new measurement techniques, i.e., monitoring long-term noise exposures or performing rapid spectrum analysis of noise.

In spite of the wealth of information that has been gathered, there are still many unsolved issues and, in fact, significant, new questions have emerged from recent research. The latest symposium helped frame some of these questions and hopefully will provide direction for future research. Some of the issues raised by Dr. von Gierke and others during the discussions were:

The Role of Animal Models: There are a number of interesting findings from experiments using animal models. To capitalize on these results, it is necessary to first explore the generalities of the findings to other species and, second, to develop algorithms for extrapolating the results from animal to man.

Measures of Hearing Loss and the Relationship Between TTS and PTS: In addition to simple threshold testing, psychoacousticians have developed more sophisticated indices of noise-induced hearing loss. These procedures have been applied to human and animal subjects in TTS and PTS experiments. The eventual aim of this work is to develop more sensitive or accurate indices of the degree of hearing impairment and a better understanding of the relationship between TTS and PTS.

Interaction of Ototraumatic Agents: There is a growing awareness that the effects of noise can be exacerbated by ototoxic drugs, vibration, heat, and other noises. The interaction of these agents may be an important, uncontrolled variable in demographic studies. It is clear that ototraumatic interactions will receive further study, especially with the recent formation of the International Society of Complex Environmental Studies (ISCES). A review of progress in this area may be gauged by the upcoming meeting of th ISCES in Kanazawa, Japan in September 1986.

Demographic Studies: The quality and quantity of demographic data is still insufficient to answer many of the questions posed. There is a paucity of information related to levels of noise encountered outside the workplace and what effect "recreational" noise exposures have on hearing over an individual's life span. Another important issue is the validity of the Equal Energy Hypothesis (EEH) as a conceptual framework for developing noise standards. While laboratory support for the EEH is equivocal, the EEH remains a popular conceptual model because of its simplicity. In the future, it would be important to develop models that more accurately represent laboratory and demographic data.

Impulse Noise: This symposium devoted a section to the auditory effects of blast waves and impulse noise. Both the animal data and human demographic data point to different and perhaps more severe effects from impulse noise than from continuous noise. The implications of this research have not yet made an impact on the noise standards. Furthermore, there is a need to develop more realistic damage risk criteria for impulse noise.

Central Effects: Much of auditory theory, and certainly our concern for the effects of noise, has focused on cochlear processes. Several trends of research are showing that damage to the periphery alters the fundamental organization of the central auditory system. A particularly fertile area for exploration is the relationship between (1) peripheral hearing loss and changes in central processes; and (2) how these central changes are manifested in auditory perception.

After organizing three symposia on the deleterious effects of noise and reading other authors' warnings about the levels of noise in the environment, industry and the military, noise continues to be a serious problem for society. Somehow, our warnings about the dangers of noise have yet to reach society's policy makers. While most segments of the health care system are sensitive to the hazards of noise, there is an even larger constituency that needs to be reached. Our information should be put into a format that can be easily understood and disseminated by a broad audience such as architects, engineers, industrial managers and politicians, who, in large measure, control or influence a large segment of our social and work environments.

Richard J. Salvi
D. Henderson
R. P. Hamernik
and
V. Colletti
Editors

ACKNOWLEDGEMENTS

We are honored that NATO decided to support an Advanced Research Workshop on the BASIC AND APPLIED ASPECTS OF NOISE-INDUCED HEARING LOSS. The financial support and organizational guidelines from NATO provided the initial framework for developing the symposium. We are grateful to Dr. di Lullo and his staff for their support and assistance during all stages of the workshop.

In addition to NATO, many other institutions and individuals provided encouragement, advice, technical assistance and financial support. Our sincere thanks go out to all of those who contributed their time and effort in organizing the symposium and publishing the proceedings. The implementation of an international meeting of scientists, clinicians and public officials from 12 separate countries and the publication of the proceedings of the symposium would not have been possible without the generous financial support of the following organizations:

Amplifon S. P. A., MILAN
ASSOCIAZIONE MECCANICI METALLURGICI E AFFINI, TORINO
BRUTON LECTURE FUNDS, TEXAS
BANCO MONTE DEI PASCHI DI SIENA, SIENA
BRUEL & KJAER S. R. L., OPERA, MILANO
COMMISSION OF THE EUROPEAN COMMUNITIES (D. G. V.)
CONFEDERAZIONE GENERALE DELL'INDUSTRIA ITALIANA, ROMA
FEDERAZIONE INDUSTRIALE REGIONALE DELL LOMBARDIA, MILAN
FEDERAZIONE INDUSTRIALE REGIONALE DELLA TOSCANNA, FIRENZE
GROUPEMENT DES ACOUSTICIENS DE LANGUE FRANCAIS
ROYAL NORWEGIAN COUNCIL FOR SCIENTIFIC AND INDUSTRIAL RESEARCH, MINISTRY OF LABOUR, MINISTRY OF THE ENVIRONMENT
UNITED STATES AIR FORCE - EUROPEAN OFFICE OF AEROSPACE RESEARCH AND DEVELOPMENT

We are especially pleased to have received support from the Bruton Lecture Funds administered through the Callier Center for Communication Disorders, University of Texas at Dallas. The Bruton Lecture Fund has supported a series of conferences and reports in the field of communication disorders and the NATO Advanced Study Workshop is clearly within the spirit of that tradition. We would like to acknowledge the support of Dean Tom Tighe and others in the administration for their help with the symposium.

The overall design of the symposium was the responsibility of the Organizing Committee, consisting of Drs. Henderson, Salvi, Hamernik, Axelsson, Borchgrevink, Dancer and Colletti. In addition, Dr. von Gierke helped to organize several of the applied areas of the program and provided a useful update on current trends in noise standards. In Italy, Dr. Rossi helped with many of the important arrangements and we are especially grateful for his cooperation. All the participants appreciated Dr. Rossi's intellectual leadership and were honored to have him as President of the symposium.

Each of us attending the symposium will remember the beautiful setting for the meeting at Il Ciocco and its enthusiastic and professional staff. To a large extent, the friendly ambiance and efficient operation of the symposium was due to the efforts of Mr. Bruno Giannasi and his colleagues.

The publication of the proceedings of the symposium is the product of a number of dedicated people. First, we wish to thank Plenum Press for their cooperation, particularly the help provided by Ms. Pat Van and Ms. Mary Stevenson. A number of individuals should be single out for their efforts during and after the symposium. Sam Saunders operated all of the audio-visual equipment in an efficient and timely manner. We wish to thank the the DEST corporation for loaning us an optical character reader and for Dr. William Ahroon's help in electronically "reading" all the manuscripts into our word processor. Thanks are also due to Karen Switzer and other members of the Technical Services staff who kept the word processing equipment operating efficiently at all times. At the end, it was our able, but underpaid graduate students Rani Shivapuja, Flint Boettcher, Richard Danielson, Michael Anne Gratton and Clyde Byrne who generously helped us prepare the manuscripts. Finally, the manuscripts from the participants were made camera ready after many long hours of proof-reading, editing, formating and typing by Virginia Dottin, Sue Kossey, and Sandra Grace; we are extremely grateful for their help.

CONTENTS

ANATOMICAL BASES OF NOISE INDUCED HEARING LOSS

PHYSIOLOGICAL CHANGES WITH NOISE-INDUCED HEARING LOSS

PSYCHOACOUSTIC PERFORMANCE CHANGES WITH NOISE-INDUCED HEARING LOSS

IMPULSE NOISE/BLAST WAVE EFFECTS

COMPLEX AND INTERACTIN EFFECTS OF NOISE

IMPLICATIONS FOR NOISE STANDARDS

MORPHOLOGY OF STEREOCILIA ON COCHLEAR HAIR CELLS AFTER NOISE EXPOSURE

B. Engstrom,[1] E. Borg[2] and B. Canlon[2]

[1]Dept. of Oto-Rhino-Laryngology
University Hospital
75185 UPPSALA, Sweden

[2]Dept. of Physiology II
Karolinska Institute
10401 STOCKHOLM, Sweden

INTRODUCTION

The stereocilia of the cochlear hair cells are a fragile link in the chain of structures and processes involved in the transduction of acoustic energy into electrical signals. The cilia are the focus of many studies on the normal structure and physiology of the ear. They are also extensively studied in ears with many types of hearing impairment and in the analysis of the effects of noise and toxic agents on the ear. In this paper, a review of different types and patterns of stereocilia damage will be presented with a description of different noise-induced structural alterations such as formation, of blebs, floppy, fused, fractured and giant cilia. Some aspects on species differences, exposure sound intensity and exposure duration are included as well as some functional correlates to cilia alterations.

"Blebbing" on stereocilia is a widening of the stereocilia which can be observed in transmission (TEM) as well as in scanning electron (SEM) microscopy (Fig. 1) [1]. Blebs can occur normally but an increased number of blebs has been found after overstimulation by noise. A somewhat different form has been observed on OHCs after laser irradiation of guinea pig cochleas [2]. Similar modifications have also been seen on stereocilia in the apical and middle turns of cochleas of rats of the AGS strain [3] and on IHCs in the apical part of spontaneously hypertensive rats [4]. The former type of blebbing, after noise, appears to be due to a detachment of the surface membrane of the individual cilia which might occur if the binding between the actin filaments and the surface membrane were broken. The later type of blebbing is situated at the tip of the stereocilia or somewhere along its shaft giving them a drumstick shape (Fig. 1F). This alteration could arise if cross-links between neighboring actin filaments within the stereocilia have been disturbed [5]. An important consideration is to which extent the noise-induced blebbing of the cilia is due to preparation artifacts and/or if it is a consequence of the noise on the hair cell structure and/or function. It has been shown that spontaneously hypertensive rats are more susceptible to noise than rats of the Wistar strain, but it is not known if the increased sensitivity is due to abnormal stereocilia [6].

"Floppy hairs" appear as boiled spaghetti on top of the IHCs in ears during temporary threshold shift (TTS). The floppy hairs have been inter-

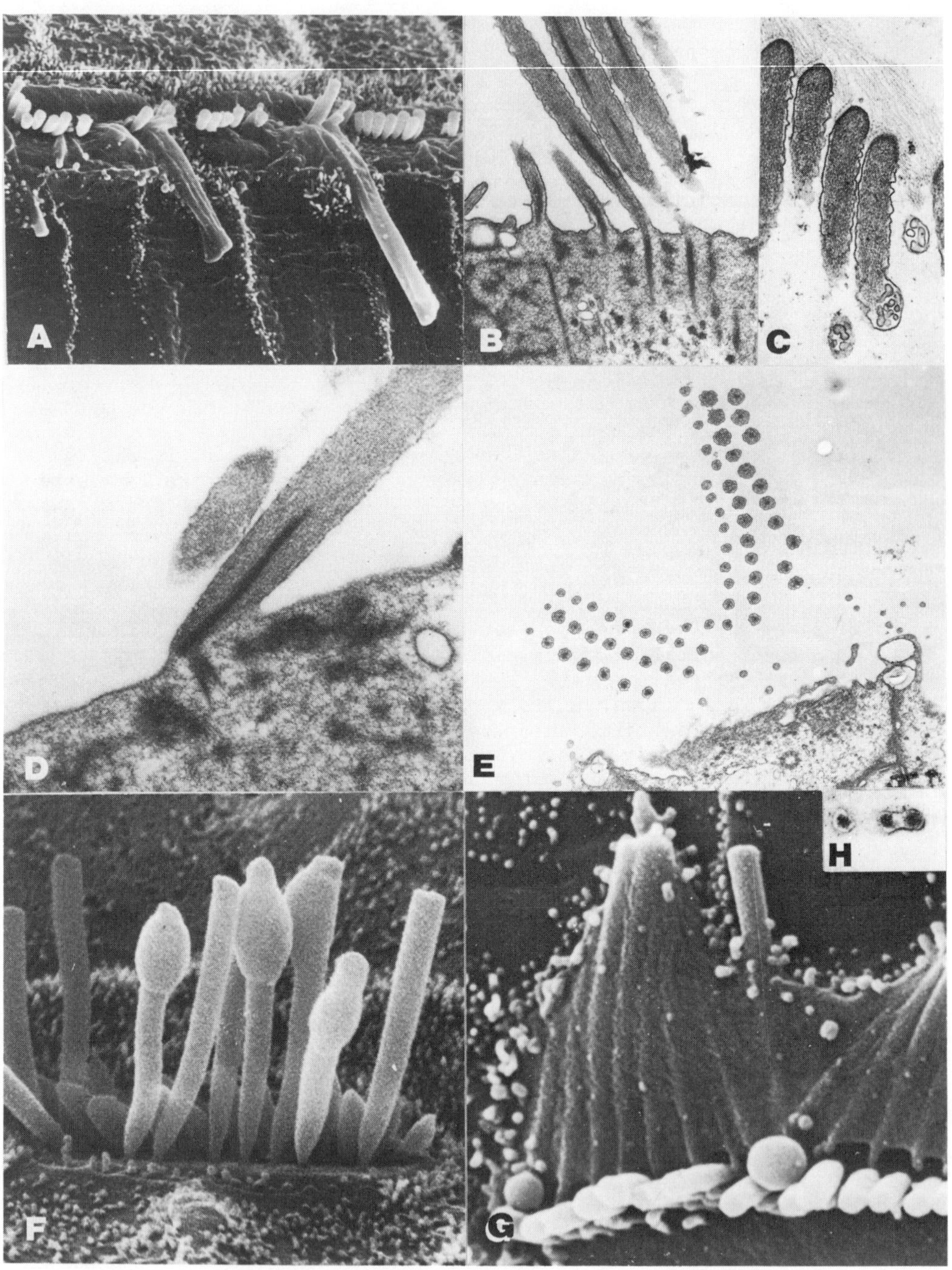

Fig. 1 Illustrations of different types of stereocilia pathologies. A: Giant cilia found on IHCs after two months of recovery from noise exposure (SEM). B: Inclined OHC stereocilia after noise exposure (TEM). C: Blebbing seen on OHC stereocilia after noise exposure (TEM). D: Fractured IHC stereocilia after noise exposure (TEM). E: Missing OHC stereocilia after noise exposure (TEM). F: Blebbing seen on IHC stereocilia of spontaneous hypertensive rats. G: Fusion of IHC stereocilia after noise exposure (SEM). H: Fusion of two cilia on an OHC after noise exposure (TEM).

preted to be a reversible alteration and has not been associated with other cellular changes [7,8]. Floppy hairs have also been described by Tilney et al. [9] who found a loss of the cross linkages between the actin filament in the stereocilia of lizards during TTS. Futhermore, the mild disorder of the cilia described by Liberman et al. [10,11] with light microscopic methods on plastic embedded cat cochleas with noise-induced hearing loss may well correspond to the floppy hairs observed in SEM. We have also frequently observed that the stereocilia sometimes can bend and resemble floppy cilia when struck by the electron beam in the SEM. The observation of floppy cilia is controversial and has been difficult to reproduce systematically. The inconsistent nature of the phenomenon may be due to minor differences during some fixation procedures and not in others. An example of how different technical handling preserve a structure differently was made evident when it was shown that the thin connections between the tips of the stereocilia are seen in SEM only if the specimens are fixed in a particular way [12,13]. Further experiments have, however, to be performed to settle the nature of the "floppy cilia."

Fusion of cilia means that the plasma membrane along the individual cilia have fused with that of its neighbors. Two, a few, or all stereocilia of a cell may be involved in the fusion (Fig. 1G). Fusion has been described in a number of animal species, and in man, after several different types of noise exposures [4,14-18]. Stereocilia fusion also occurs in animals exposed to ototoxic drugs [19]. Fusion of cell membranes is however, not specific for the cilia of the inner ear but it is a common feature in many normal as well as pathological cell functions. If the same mechanism is involved in stereocilia fusion as in other cell fusion processes remains unknown, however it could be speculated that these processes are somewhat different as one never finds fusion between cilia of neighboring hair cells. What is found instead is that two, a few, or all stereocilia on one individual hair cell are involved in the fusion.

In most cases, when cilia on an IHC in the rabbit fuse, they are also inclined, usually towards the OHCs. In other species, such as the guinea pig, the stereocilia of the IHCs are more frequently seen fused without inclination. When two or a few cilia are involved, it is almost always possible to recognize the contour of the original individual cilia within the newly formed one (Fig. 1G and H). When the damage is more pronounced, and most stereocilia are involved in the fusion, the orderly arrangement of the stereocilia on the cell is lost [25] and instead one finds a disorder of the former cilia below the cell surface. This seems to be the case for the IHCs in general, and on the OHCs in the apical turn. The OHCs in the more basal region of noise-exposed cochleas appear to have either only minor cilia damage or the whole cell disappears.

Inclination and Fracture of individual stereocilia is often found in ears with noise damage. A cilium involved in a fusion may be either inclined and still inserted into the cuticular plate (Fig. 1B) or inclined and fractured just above the root (Fig. 1D). A fracture is often difficult to verify in SEM unless the cilia also have been discarded, since the interior of the cilia can not be seen in SEM. In TEM on the other hand, the fracture point of the cilia can be distinctly seen (Fig. 1D). The fracture seems to result from a mechanical stress. The resistance to deformation has been described in terms of a "critical angle" described as the maximum degree of deflection possible for the actin filaments within a stereocilium to undergo before damage occurs in the crystal lattice [20].

Stereocilia of OHCs are often found to be discarded, while the stereocilia on the IHCs remain on the cells fused together with its neighbors [21]. These findings may coincide with the stereocilia of IHCs and OHCs differing considerably in thickness and in the number of actin filaments inserted in the cuticular plate.

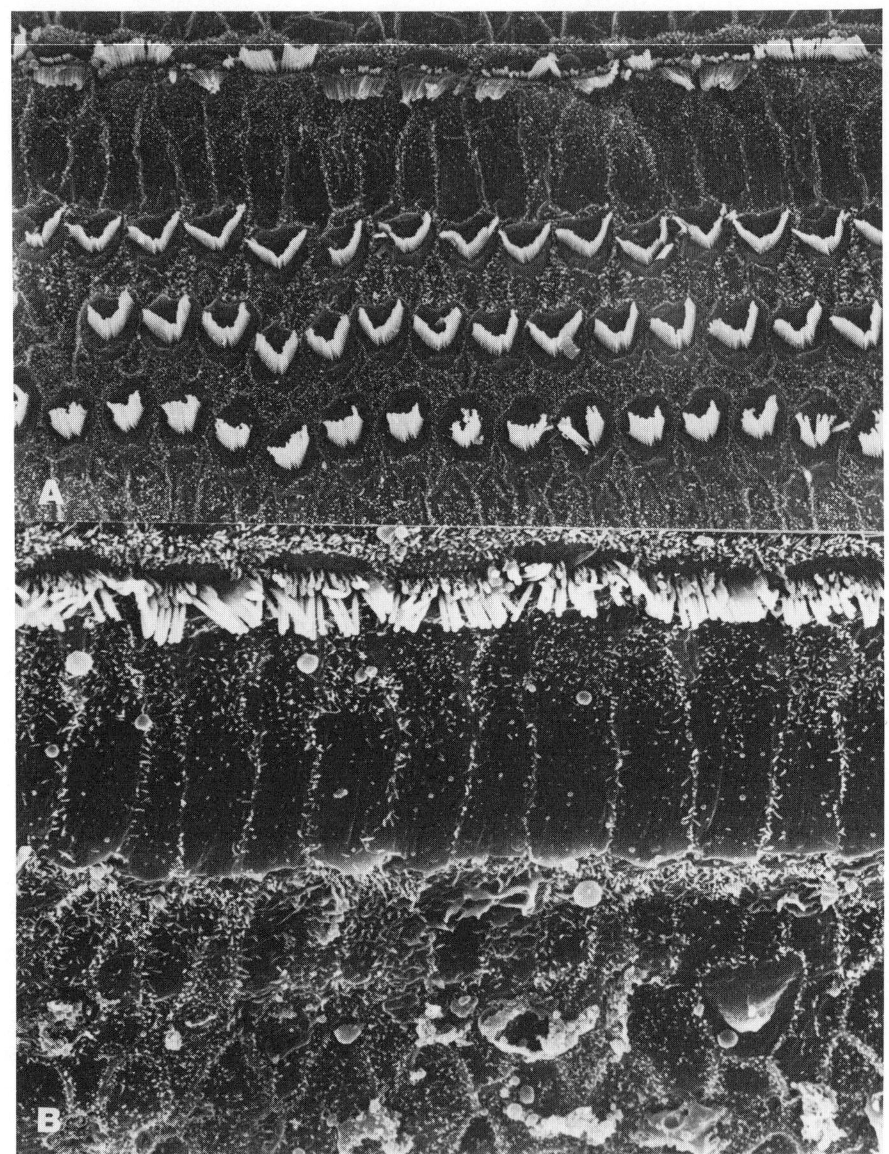

Fig. 2. Illustrations of the morphological differences of hair cell damage and the importance of noise intensity and duration. A: "Rabbit-like" damage of the IHC stereocilia found in the guinea pig 3 weeks after a 146 dB broad-band stimulus for 15 min. B: OHC stereocilia loss seen 3 weeks after a 115 dB exposure to the broad-band noise for 120 min. in the guinea pig.

Giant cilia are predominantly found in ears with severe noise damage. The outgrowth is, at least in the rabbit, not found until two months or more after a noise exposure [22]. The giant cilia are predominantly found in rabbits on OHCs in the apical turn [23,24] and on IHCs in the middle and basal turns of the cochlea [4]. It is not yet known if the actin forming the giant cilia consists of newly formed actin or if it is a reorganization of the actin of the former cilia. A morphometric analysis of the giant cilia is in progress; the primary results available at present indicate that the actin content in a large giant cilium is larger than in the whole array of cilia in a normal IHC from the same region of the cochlea (Viberg and Engstrom, in preparation).

Species differences and importance of noise intensity. The different types of stereocilia alterations described above may be found in several different species and after several different types of noise exposure. The extent and the number of cells with altered cilia may vary much between species and between individuals of the same stock exposed to the same sound (Fig. 2).

The first structures of the rabbit cochlea to show alterations after a broad band noise exposure (115 dB SPL for 15 or 30 min.) are the IHCs in the middle and basal part of the cochlea [23]. In a few of our rabbit ears the only alterations found were fused and inclined stereocilia on the IHCs; all OHCs had a normal appearance. In many ears there was also an area with OHC loss and damage but extending basally of this there was a long distance with only IHC damage [25]. A different pattern of damage may, however, be found if the rabbits are bilaterally exposed to the same total energy of noise (115 dB for 30 min.) but at a sound level of 85 dB SPL for 512 h. These animals exhibited only OHC damage (Engstrom and Borg, in preparation). In contrast to the rabbit, the cat always has OHC damage as well as IHC alterations. In these cochleas of cats the IHC alterations may extend beyond the region of OHC damage [10,26]. On the other hand, it is generally found that the guinea pig stereocilia pathology, induced by noise exposure, can first be observed on the first row of OHCs, then on IHCs and thereafter on the second and third row of OHCs (c.f. Robertson and Johnstone 1979). There was no damage found in the ears of guinea pigs when exposed at 115 dB SPL for 15 min. which would produce IHC fusion and inclination in the rabbit. When prolonging the 115 dB exposure to 60-120 min. to produce a permanent threshold shift (PTS = 30-40 dB), then the classic picture of predominantly OHC loss and damage was found in SEM (Fig. 2B). Some guinea pigs were exposed to the same noise but at a sound level of 146 dB SPL which produced a permanent threshold shift of 30-40 dB with a 15 min. exposure. These guinea pigs showed a different pattern of hair cell damage than those exposed at 115 dB for 60-120 min. The distribution of IHC and OHC stereocilia pathology differed in different parts of the noise lesion. Fig. 3A shows the normally appearing organ of Corti from the basal turn of one of these short duration, high sound level animals. Fig. 3B and C show the alterations seen in the center of the lesion and Fig. 2A shows the "rabbit like" alterations of the IHCs seen for 1/4 - 1/2 of a turn apically of the damage seen in 3B and C (Engstrom et al., in progress).

Functional Correlates

It is not until recently that stereocilia alterations have been studied systematically. It has been shown that even minor cilia damage can be correlated to alterations of ear sensitivity. Inner hair cell stereocilia alterations in the cat have, for instance, been correlated to a shift of the whole tuning curve of single nerve fibers [26]. In the rabbit, alterations of IHC stereocilia have been correlated to a shift of the threshold of the middle ear muscle reflexes in the corresponding frequency range [25]. Alterations of cilia only on OHCs have been shown to correlate to a rise of the threshold of the tip and a hypersensitivity of the "tail" of the tuning curve from single nerve fibers [27]. Furthermore, for example, Slepecky et al. [18] have found that OHC cilia alterations may correlate to a 40 dB hearing loss established with an evoked electrical response measurement.

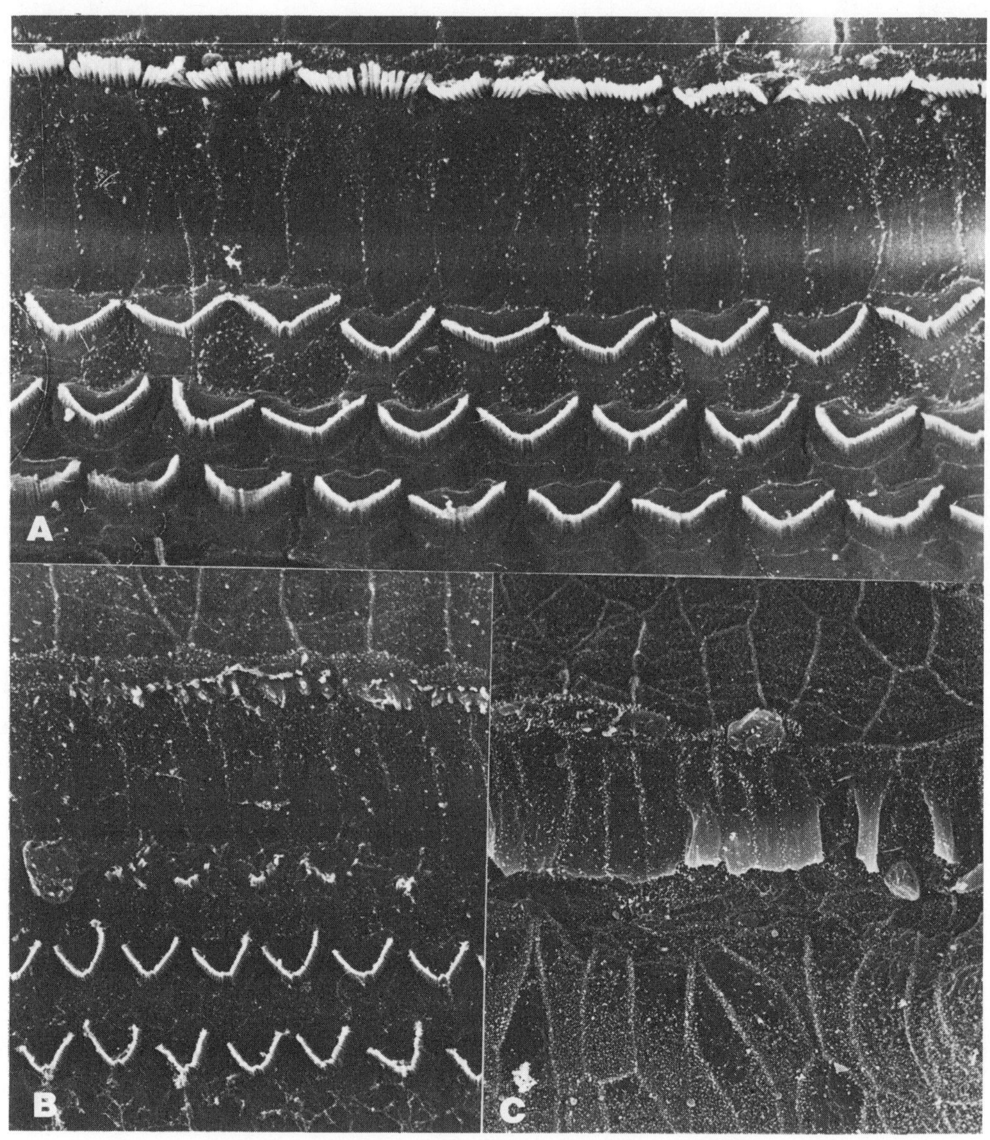

Fig. 3. Normal appearing stereocilia from the basal turn of the noise exposed guinea pig also illustrated in B and C. (SEM). B: Alterations found in the center of the lesion showing IHC stereocilia loss (B) and IHC and OHC-1 loss (C).

The mechanisms of stereocilia fusion and outgrowth are not understood but some relevant information is available. Duvall et al. [28], for example, found fusion of stereocilia a few days and some weeks after mixing cochlear fluids by making a rift in the membrane of Reissner. The fusion was interpreted to be the result of the upper surface of the hair cell being sensitive to the influence of sodium ions from the perilymph. In an attempt to test the role of sodium, we have injected artificial perilymph into the endolymph of guinea pigs. The preliminary results show no stereocilia fusion but extensive OHC loss (Engstrom et al., in progress). Another ion to test for involvement in stereocilia fusion is calcium, since calcium is known to play a role in fusion in other cell systems [29]. It has also been shown that if the calcium concentration is altered in either the perilymph or the endolymph, the cochlear microphonics is affected [30,31]. In an attempt to find out if the fusion needs a normal functioning inner ear, we have exposed rabbits to noise after death. The morphological alterations seen with SEM in these ears do not deviate from what can be seen in an animal terminated the first hours after a noise exposure.

CONCLUSION

All types of stereocilia damage described can be seen in all species commonly used in auditory research. However, the different types of stereocilia alterations are found in different proportions in different species. New results have shown that the proportions of OHC and IHC stereocilia alterations may depend on the exposure level and duration. The different types of stereocilia lesions described cannot at present be tied to specific functional alterations. The most important feature is if the damage occurs on the IHC or the OHC. The degree of cilia damage can roughly be related to the amount of noise delivered and the shift of tuning curve, auditory threshold and threshold of the middle ear muscle reflex.

REFERENCES

1. H. Engstrom and B. Engstrom, Structure of hairs in cochlear sensory cells, Hearing Research, 1:49 (1978).
2. J. Stahle, B. Engstrom, and L. Hogberg, Inner ear microsurgery, using laser, Adv. Oto-Rhino-Laryngol. 19:88 (1973).
3. J. E. Penny, K. B. Hodges, S. A. Kupetz, R. D. Brown, D. W.Glenn and P. C. Jobe, Morphology of the AGS rat organ of Corti. Anat. Rec. 194:199A (1981).
4. B. Engstrom, Stereocilia of sensory cells in normal and hearing impaired ears. Scand. Audiol., Suppl. 19. (1984).
5. J. C. Saunders and N. Coppa, The contribution of stereocilia to rootlet and cuticular plate injury to sensorineural hearing loss, in: "Sensorineural Hearing Loss: Essays Honoring Scott N. Reger," T. Glattke and M. J. Collins, eds., University Park Press Baltimore, MD (1985).
6. E. Borg, Noise-induced hearing loss in normotensive and spontaneously hypertensive rats. Hearing Res. 8:117 (1982).
7. I. M. Hunter-Duvar, M. Suzuki, and R. Mount, Anatomical changes in the organ of Corti after acoustic stimulation, in: "New Perspectives on Noise-Induced Hearing Loss," Hamernik, Henderson and Salvi, eds., Raven Press, New York (1982).
8. D. J. Lim, D. E. Dunn, J. A. Ferraro and B. L. Lempert, Anatomical changes found in the cochleas of animals exposed to typical industrial noise, in: "New Perspectives on Noise-Induced Hearing Loss, Hamernik, Henderson and Salvi, eds., Raven Press, New York (1982).
9. L. G. Tilney, J. C. Saunders, E. Engelman, and D. J. DeRosier, Changes in the organization of actin filaments in the stereocilia of noise-damaged lizard cochlea, Hearing Res. 7:181 (1982).
10. M. C. Liberman and L. W. Dodds, Single-neuron labeling and chronic cochlar pathology. II. Stereocilia damage and alterations of spontaneous discharge rates. Hearing Res. 16:43 (1984).
11. M. C. Liberman and L. W. Dodds, Single-neuron labeling and chronic cochlear pathology. III. Stereocilia damage and alterations of threshold tuning curves, Hearing Res. 16:55 (1984).
12. S. D. Comis, J. O. Pickles, and M. P. Osborne, Osmium tetroxide postfixation in relation to the cross linkage and spatial organization of stereocilia in the guinea-pig cochlea, J. of Neurocytology 14:113 (1985).

13. D. N. Furness and C. M. Hackney, Cross-links between stereocilia in the guinea pig. Hearing Res. 18:177 (1985).

14. H. H. Spoendlin, Primary structural changes in the organ of Corti after acoustic overstimulation. Acta Otolaryngol. (Stockh.) 71:166 (1971).

15. G. Engstrom, B. Engstrom and H. Ades, Effects of noise on Corti's organ, Minerva Med. L'uomo ed il rumore 75 (1976).

16. I. M. Hunter-Duvar, Morphology of the normal and the acoustically damaged cochlea, in: "Scanning Electron Microscopy," vol. 2. ITT Research Institute, Chicago, pp. 421-428 (1977).

17. D. Robertson and B. M. Johnstone, Acoustic trauma in the guinea pig cochlea: Early changes in ultrastructure and neural threshold. Hearing Res. 3:167 (1980).

18. N. Slepecky, R. Hamernik, D. Henderson, and D. Coling, Correlation of audiometric data with changes in cochlear hair cell stereocilia resulting from impulse noise trauma. Acta Otolaryngol. 93:329 (1982).

19. P. A. Leake-Jones, B. F. O'Reilly, and M. C. Vivion, Neomycin ototoxicity: Ultrastructural surface pathology of the organ of Corti, in: "Scanning Electron Microscopy," vol. 3. ITT Research Institute Chicago, pp. 427-434 (1980).

20. J. C. Saunders, M. E. Schneider, and S. P. Dear, The structure and function of actin in hair cells, J. Acoust. Soc. Am. 78:299 (1985).

21. B. Engstrom, A. Flock, and E. Borg, Ultrastructural studies of stereocilia in noise-exposed rabbits. Hearing Res. 12:251 (1983).

22. B. Engstrom and E. Borg, Lesions to cochlear inner hair cells induced by noise. Arch. Otorhinolaryngol. 230:279 (1981).

23. A. Wright, Giant cilia in the human organ of Corti, Clin. Otolaryngol. 7:183 (1982).

24. E. Borg, R. Nilsson, B. Engstrom, Effect of the acoustic reflex on inner ear damage induced by industrial noise. Acta Otolaryngol. 96:361 (1983).

25. B. Engstrom and E. Borg, Cochlear morphology in relation to loss of behavioural, electrophysiological, and middle ear reflex thresholds after exposure to noise. Acta Otolaryngol. Suppl. 402 (1983).

26. M. C. Liberman and M. J. Mulroy, Acute and chronic effects of acoustic trauma cochlear pathology and auditory nerve pathophysiology, in: "New Perspectives on Noise-Induced Hearing Loss," Hamernik, Henderson and Salvi, eds. Raven Press, New York (1982).

27. M. C. Liberman, Single-neuron labeling and chronic cochlear pathology. I. Threshold shift and characteristic frequency shift. Hearing Res. 16:33 (1984).

28. A. J. Duvall and V. T. Rhodes, Ultrastructure of the organ of Corti following intermixing of cochlear fluids. Ann. Otol. Rhinol. Laryngol. 76:688 (1967).

29. E. G. Post and G. L. Nicolson, G.L. eds., Cell Surface Reviews vol. 5: Membrane Fusion, Elsevier North-Holland, Amsterdam (1978).

30. D. H. Moscowitch and R. P. Gannon, Effects of calcium on sound-evoked cochlear potentials in the guinea pig, J. Acoust. Soc. Am. 40:583 (1966).

31. Y. Tanaka, A. Asanuma, and K. Yanagisawa, Potentials of outer hair cells and their membrane properties in cationic environments, Hearing Res. 2:431 (1980).

DISCUSSION

Pfander: Did the location of the cochlear lesion correspond to the frequency of the hearing loss? We have done experiments with animals in which the destruction was near the helicotrema; however, the TTS was at the higher frequency so that the location of the damage did not correspond with the hearing loss. Secondly, what was the percentage of damage of inner hair cells and outer hair cells? It appears that most of your damage is to the inner hair cells. Thirdly, could you describe your exposure?

Engstrom: The exposure was a broad band noise of 115 dB. In the rabbit, location of inner hair cell damage corresponded well with the frequency and range of threshold shift of the stapedius muscle reflex, but not with the threshold shift of the ABR. When there was a shift in the ABR, it corresponded most closely with the combination of inner and outer hair cell loss, but not perfectly. We had mixed damage in the guinea pigs. The damage occurred near the frequency of the exposure, i.e., mainly in the middle part of the cochlea. The area near the helicotrema and near the hook appeared normal.

MECHANICAL CHANGES IN STEREOCILIA FOLLOWING OVERSTIMULATION: OBSERVATIONS AND POSSIBLE MECHANISMS

James C. Saunders, Barbara Canlon and Åke Flock

Department of Otorhinolaryngology and Human Communication
University of Pennsylvania, Philadelphia, PA 19104, and
Department of Physiology II, Karolinska Institute
Stockholm, Sweden

INTRODUCTION

Many experimental observations over the past decade have indicated that the role of stereocilia structure and function in cochlear hair-cell transduction is more complicated than previously thought. Among these recent observations are those that elucidated the cytoskeletal organization of the stereocilia and cuticular plate [21,81], and the extracellular structures that bind individual stereocilia together [6,50,51]. In addition, the kinetics of hair-cell physiology have been well described [7,9, 55] and the directional sensitivity of stereocilia movement on individual hair cells is now known [22,28,75]. Descriptions of static and dynamic stereocilia movement in the mammalian cochlea have recently been presented [23,38,75]; these data are critically important to our understanding of hair-cell function and dysfunction.

Numerous investigations have tried to characterize the effects of intense sound on stereocilia by correlating physiologic responses in the auditory system with structural damage to the sensory hair [41,42]. These reports have provided valuable information about the configurations of stereocilia injury and their possible contribution to auditory function. Unfortunately, the loss of auditory function following exposure to intense sound may arise from the complex interaction of receptor cell and whole organ injuries, and need not be the exclusive result of stereocilia pathology. In order to understand the contribution of stereocilia damage, it is important to isolate the functional injury to the sensory-hair bundle and examine it independent of other cell or organ injuries. The experimental methods to accomplish this have only recently been developed [38, 60-62].

In this report we will briefly summarize what is known about acoustic injuries to stereocilia and the structural damage that might account for these injuries. Finally, we will present data from recent experiments with the isolated guinea pig cochlear coil, which describe micromechanical changes in stereocilia following overstimulation.

ACOUSTIC INJURY TO STEREOCILIA

Stereocilia Pathology Revealed by Scanning Electron Microscopy

Evaluation of the stereocilia by scanning electron microscopy has uncovered numerous pathologies following intense sound exposure. Perhaps the most universal observation following exposure is the presence of hair cells on which part or all of the stereocilia bundle is "missing" [1,17, 33,43,48,53,80].

Another category of acoustic injuries is the so called "floppy," "disarrayed," or "collapsed" sensory hairs. Floppy stereocilia are characterized by curves in the shaft which make it look as though it were built of a compliant (rather than a rigid) material [12,30,31,44,45,73].

"Disarrayed" stereocilia appear straight and rigid [34,40,43], but they are bent at their bases, so that individual members of the bundle appear separated or "splayed-out" [14,15,47,62,68,78,85]. The most severe pathology of this category occurs when the sensory hairs "collapse" onto the cuticular surface of the hair cell [18,32,52,76,80]. When IHCs are affected, the collapse always involves the tallest members of the bundle and is directed away from the modiolus [80].

Another form of stereocilia pathology is "fusion." This injury is characterized by several or all of the hairs on the bundle sharing a common plasma membrane [13,18,54,67,71,79]. Fused sensory hairs have been reported in mammalian [14,16] and non-mammalian ears [62] following noise exposure. Collapsed stereocilia may also fuse with the apical membrane of the hair cell [14,77].

"Giant" stereocilia are hairs that appear abnormally long and thick and are frequently seen collapsed onto the apical surface of the cell [18]. A variation of the giant sensory hairs are the "elongated" stereocilia, which appear longer and thinner than normal [29,57,86]. In the mammalian cochlea, fused, giant, or elongated stereocilia were reported more frequently on IHCs than OHCs [18,48,80].

The stereocilia normally have a conical taper (over the last tenth to quarter of a micron of their length) at their insertion into the top of the hair cell. This tapered base in the "ankle" region of the hair gives the impression that the stereocilia rotate about this point [20,24]. Recent examinations of noise-exposed alligator lizard and chick ears revealed many stereocilia with an "ankle" that appeared "stumpy" rather than conical [8,82,83,84].

More than a decade ago, Spoendlin [70,71] suggested that hair cells expel a damaged cuticular plate into the sub-tectorial space, and this event precipitates hair-cell degeneration. Research since then has identified noise-exposed hair cells on which the cuticular plate appears to "bulge" outward, and still others where the plate is actually being expelled from the cell [2,32,34,80].

The literature suggests that "missing," "disarrayed" and "collapsed" stereocilia are the most frequent forms of sensory hair damage observed after noise exposure. The other forms occur irregularly, though the giant or elongated hairs are frequently seen in the cochlea of noise-exposed rabbits [15]. The floppy condition has been less thoroughly investigated because of its relative rarity. In subsequent sections we will consider the cytoskeletal and extracellular damage in the stereocilia, rootlet region, and cuticular plate that contributes to the abnormalities described above. The reader should realize, however, that the "static" picture developed above has not dealt with the onset and development of these pathologies, their potential for recovery, their correlation with specific sound exposure conditions, their variability from cell to cell, or their contribution to hair-cell function. These issues are significant and at present are basically unresolved.

Steroecilia Damage and Sensorineural Hearing Loss

The relation between stereocilia pathology and the loss of auditory function is only beginning to emerge. Stereocilia damage has been correlated with auditory nerve fiber responses [40,41,42,43,48,52], N1 action potential thresholds [53,54,84], auditory brain stem responses [16], middle-ear muscle reflexes [3], and behaviorally-measured thresholds [4,15, 66,67]. Procedural differences, unfortunately, make it difficult to draw any generalizations from this data. Nevertheless, it is clear that stereocilia pathology is associated with functional alterations in the auditory system. These relations, however, need to be strengthened by describing the functional changes in the stereocilia themselves following exposure to intense sound.

MECHANISMS OF STEREOCILIA, ROOTLET, AND CUTICULAR PLATE DAMAGE

In this section, we plan to briefly describe the cytoskeletal organization of the stereocilia and cuticular plate, and then consider how injuries to this organization might produce the pathological conditions described above. A summary of the sites of damage in stereocilia is presented in Fig. 1; many of the points raised below can be referred to this figure.

The Cytoskletal Framework and Extracellular Morphology of Stereocilia

Flock and his colleagues, in 1977, reported that the microfilaments within stereocilia were composed of the protein actin [20,21]; and subsequent research has identified actin filaments in mammalian, avian, and reptilian species [26,35,58,63,64,65]. The stereocilia actin exhibits three distinct organizational features; a) the actin filaments are oriented vertically, extending along the entire length of the hair shaft; b) the actin filaments are hexagonally packed in the stereocilium; and c) there are protein crossbridges oriented perpendicularly to the filaments which serve, among other functions, as "spacers" to keep the filaments separated. The details of this "crystalline" organization have been presented elsewhere, but one functional role is clear: the actin array imparts enormous rigidity to the stereocilium, allowing each hair to act as a rigid rod pivoting about its base [10,11,64,81,83]. In addition, deflections of a stereocilium cause the filaments to slide past one another, and this shear produces changes in the cross-sectional geometry of the crystal matrix [64, 83]. These changes provide clues to the cytoskeletal structure that might be at risk during overstimulation [57,62].

The extracellular morphology of the stereocilia bundle has become an important region for anatomic evaluation. Two aspects are presently emerging. Iurato [37] first provided some quantitative information from the guinea pig cochlea that stereocilia height varied from the base to the apex. In the high frequency region (the base), the stereocilia were substantially shorter than in the low frequency region (the apex). This observation is the same across all hair-cell rows in the mammalian cochlea [44,87]. In addition, the numbers of stereocilia per hair cell, and their diameter also change with cochlear location [25,82].

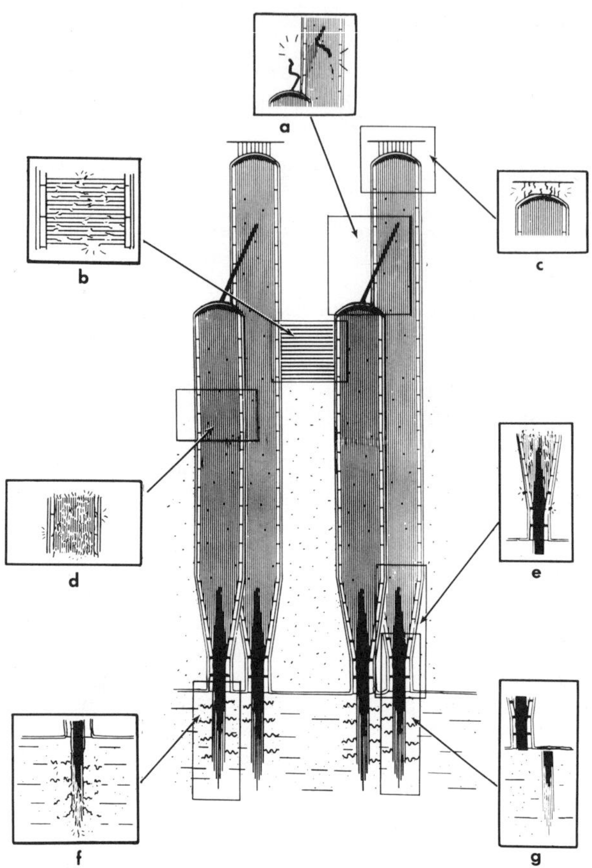

Fig. 1. In the central part of this figure, the normal organization of the stereocilia is presented. The actin filaments, crossbridges, rootlet, cuticular plate and extracellular connections are all represented. Some artistic license has been taken in the representation of these structures for the sake of clarity. The inserts indicate possible damage to the various structures following overstimulation: A) The link between the tip and shaft of adjacent stereocilia has been broken. B) The interconnecting filaments between stereocilia have been broken. This damage may occur to the connections between stereocilia in the same row (as illustrated) and between stereocilia in adjacent rows (not illustrated). C) The connection between the tallest hairs in the bundle and the tectorial membrane has been broken. D) This panel shows disassembly of the actin matrix along the shaft of the stereocilium. Similarly, the filament links between the actin core and the plasma membrane have been broken. Here we see disassembly of the actin matrix at the base of the stereocilium. Also, the filament links between the rootlet structure and the plasma membrane in the tapered base have been broken. F) The fine filaments in the cuticular plate, which interconnect the rootlet with the actin filaments of the plate, have been broken. G) Finally, the rootlet has been severed at the junction point between the stereocilium and the cuticular plate.

The extracellular connections between individual hairs in the stereocilia bundle is another feature that is being studied. These connections were first observed in transmission electron micrographs [20,60] and have now been described for a variety of vertebrate species [26,49,51]. At first it was thought that these links maintained the bundle in an intact condition. This is true, but the recent observations of Pickles and his associates [6,50,51] have raised the importance of these structures. These authors identified crosslinks in guinea pig cochlear hair cells that extended from the tips of the shortest row of stereocilia to the shaft of the middle row of stereocilia. Similarly, the middle row of hairs have a link that extends from their tips to the shafts of the tallest row of stereocilia. The morphology of these crosslinks have subsequently been described in detail [6,50], and there has been speculation concerning their possible role in the micromechanics of hair-cell transduction [27,51].

The Structural Organization of the Rootlet and Cuticular Plate

The cytoskeletal organization of these two regions of the hair cell have recently been summarized [64]. In the core of the hair at the tapered base, an electron-dense material is found which projects down into the cuticular plate and back up into the stereocilium. This rootlet communicates with the fibrous meshwork of the cuticular plate through a population of very fine rootlet fibers about 30 Angstroms in diameter (see Fig. 1). It is not clear how the rootlet communicates with the actin filament within the stereocilium. The rootlet apparently serves to anchor the actin core of the stereocilium to the cuticular plate. Moreover, the rootlet appears to have elastic properties [64].

The cuticular plate contains two populations of microfilaments; the 60 Angstrom actin filaments and a set of smaller 30 Angstrom filaments (for a review see [64]). The organization of these filaments is complex, but they do seem to interact with each other and with the rootlet. It would seem that the principle role of the cuticular plate is to provide a stable platform on which the stereocilia can pivot.

Possible Mechanisms of Cytoskeletal and Extracellular Injury to Stereocilia

Changes in sensory-hair rigidity. Hair cells in the cochlea of noise-exposed alligator lizards have stereocilia so badly damaged that the crystalline array of actin filament crossbridges could not be identified [85]. Tilney and his colleagues [84] argued that these stereocilia would exhibit a great reduction in rigidity, and such a loss could account for the floppy appearance of stereocilia. We should note, however, that an examination of noise-damaged IHC stereocilia in the rabbit failed to replicate these observations [18]. The mechanism that causes the disassembly of the actin array throughout the core of the stereocilium is not known. It is thought that energy absorption at the crossbridge/actin junction, due to the shearing of the actin filaments during deflection, may be one cause [57]. In addition, the idea of a "critical angle" has been proposed [64]. As the filaments slide past one another during a deflection of the hair, there is a reduction in their parallel separation. The amount of shear, however, is limited by the physical dimensions of the actin filaments and crossbridges, and by electrostatic repulsions. When a deflection occurs that exceeds the critical angle, damage to the actin matrix may begin. The shearing action of the filaments may also break the fine filaments connecting the actin array with the inner surface of the plasma membrane (Fig. 1D).

Loss of sensory hair stiffness. The sensory hair is designed to pivot at its base, and during stimulation, the stress on molecular structures in this region will be great. The rootlet is thus the most obvious weak link in the stereocilium, and structural failure here is not surprising. The shearing movements of the actin filaments and crossbridges may produce such stress that disassembly of the actin crystal in the "ankle" region readily occurs. In addition, communication in the tapered base between the plasma membrane and the rootlet (through 30 Angstrom filaments) has been reported [26,35,36,67]. A deflection of the stereocilium will cause the rootlet to bend, producing an alternating compression and stretching of these 30 Angstrom filament. Furthermore, the rootlet has spring properties that resist bending, and during overstimulation, the tolerance limits of this spring may be exceeded. The stress on these structures (the crystalline array, the fine filaments and the rootlet) when the deflections are great and sustained, may lead to structural failure in the form of a rootlet fracture or disassembly of the actin array (see Figs. 1E and G).

Recent investigations have shown that the stereocilia rootlet can indeed be damaged, and thus far two forms of pathology have been identified. One is seen as a depolymerization of the actin core at the base of the hair, while the second is a fracture or break in the rootlet itself [18,67,84].

Another possibility is related to the fact that the rootlet is secured in the cuticular plate by a meshwork of fine filament. Excessive mechanical deflections of the stereocilia will apply stress on these 30 Angstrom "cementing" connections in the plate, and this may cause them to deteriorate (Fig. 1F). Acoustic injury to these fine cuticular plate filaments, however, has yet to be reported.

Injury to the actin crystal, breaks in the rootlet itself, or a reduction in rootlet attachments to the cuticular plate would all serve to decouple the stereocilia from the cuticular plate. The mechanical consequences of this would be a reduction in the stiffness of the sensory hair. Disarrayed" or "collapsed" stereocilia would be expected to arise from structural failure in the region of the rootlet. Finally, damage to the extracellular links between stereocilia (Figs. 1A and B), or to the connections between the distal tips of the OHCs and the tectorial membrane (Fig. 1C), may indirectly contribute to rootlet injury by changing the impedance properties of the hair-cell bundle as a whole. The occurrence of "missing" stereocilia may be the most severe consequence of rootlet damage and in this case the hair is simply torn from the cuticular plate.

In the preceding sections we have made two points. Firstly, the so-called floppy stereocilia are due to changes in sensory-hair rigidity. The loss in rigidity is due to partial or complete damage to the actin crystal along the length of the stereocilium. Secondly, "disarrayed," "collapsed" or "missing" stereocilia are most likely caused by changes in sensory hair stiffness. The loss of stiffness arises from structural failure in the region of the tapered base (Figs. 1E, F and G), and may or may not be accompanied by damage to the extracellular crosslinks between members of the bundle (Figs. 1A, B and C).

Possible Mechanisms of Fused, Giant and Elongated Sensory Hairs

Changes in the electrical properties of the cell membrane during overstimulation may initiate processes that lead to stereocilia fusion. There is evidence that membranes can break down in the presence of excessive intracellular pressure or transmembrane voltage gradients [88]. The voltage gradients and pressures that initiate membrane breakdown and cell fusion are quite high in plant cells [89]. Stimulation of stereocilia may also produce large electrostatic charges on the membrane or increments in intracellular pressure that may contribute to either the dissociation of membrane lipids or disassembly of membrane proteins. Similarly, the membrane surface of the stereocilia is negatively charged, and this is balanced by a layer of positive counter ions derived from the surrounding medium. The repulsive forces of these charges would tend to keep the stereocilia apart. Overstimulation may produce mechanical trauma sufficiently great to overcome the repulsive force between stereocilia and their collapse against each other could result in membrane fusion [24].

It is also possible that the filaments that interconnect the crystalline array with the plasma membrane [26,49,83] denature, and the result might be a more fluid plasma membrane (see Fig. 1D). By these mechanisms, damaged membranes around a sensory hair may fuse with those of a neighboring hair to produce a new structure [45,86].

We understand even less about the formation of giant or elongated stereocilia. In the future, it will be important to learn if the new material in these stereocilia has the same actin organization found in normal hairs, and whether this is constructed from the remains of the old stereocilia or with material transported from the cell cytoplasm or the cuticular plate.

Possible Mechanisms of Cuticular Plate Damage

Damage to this region has not been adequately described, so the underlying mechanisms remain vague. Displacements of the stereocilia will exert stress on the filamentous matrix of the cuticular plate through the rootlet (Fig. 1F); this in turn may cause denaturing of the microfilament structure throughout the plate. Denaturing of the microfilament could "soften" the cuticular plate.

Swelling of the hair cell following noise exposure has been reported [56,72] and was related to changes in the regulation of ionic concentrations or osmolarity [45]. A general edema of the intracellular environment could be the source of pressure that causes the "bulge" seen in noise exposed cuticular plates [19,29,45-47,77]. When the pressure and bulge becomes too great, the softened plate is expelled from the cell [53].

CAN DAMAGED STEREOCILIA BE REPAIRED?

One of the crucial questions is whether or not the injuries described above are reversible. Tilney and his associates [84] were left with the impression that less cytoskeletal damage was apparent in alligator lizard stereocilia following an 11 day recovery period, compared to that seen immediately after exposure. Other authors have also suggested that "floppy" stereocilia seem to recover with the passage of time. However, none of these impressions has been adequately verified [12,30]. Some additional support for this possibility is found in the studies by Stopp [73,74], but her data are also difficult to interpret.

Disarrayed, fused and collapsed stereocilia have been reported in noise-exposed cats, guinea pigs, and rabbits after recovery times ranging from 42 to over 500 days [15,40,43,48,52]. It thus appears that some injuries to the rootlet region do not recover. Nevertheless, further work on this problem is needed.

THE GROWTH AND RECOVERY OF MICROMECHANICAL THRESHOLD SHIFT IN STEREOCILIA FOLLOWING OVERSTIMULATION

In the preceding sections we noted that it was difficult (with conventional acoustic overstimulation studies) to isolate the relation between stereocilia pathology and deficits in auditory function. This is because acoustic injury to the stereocilia may be concurrent with other injuries to the organ of Corti. Moreover, functional changes in stereocilia themselves, following overstimulation, were not identified. Recently, direct measures of stereocilia micromechanics, following exposure to intense stimulation have been used to study the growth and recovery of threshold shift [5,59,61,62]. In addition, the contribution of active cell processes were identified by studying these fatigue processes in metabolically-blocked hair cells. These findings will be summarized below.

The Isolated Cochlea Coil and Stereocilia Stimulation

Following sacrifice, the bulla and temporal bones of pigmented guinea pigs were bilaterally excised. The bones were placed in culture medium [39,61] which partially simulated perilymph. The apical cap and the bony walls of the cochlea (in the apical turns) were dissected away, and the stria vascularis in this region was pulled free. The osseus spiral lamina was removed, and radial cuts in the organ of Corti were made to delineate a region of interest (usually three-quarters of a turn). Beneath these radial cuts, the modiolus was broken to reveal the auditory nerve. The nerve was sectioned and the isolated turn of the cochlea removed and mounted in a miniature vise. Specially designed scoops were used to surround the coil with medium, while it and the vise were transferred to a chamber (also filled with medium) attached to the stage of a differential interference contrast microscope. The preparation was examined with a 40X water-immersion objective (N.A. 0.75) and all measures of sensory hair motion were made at 800X. Testing took place at room temperature (22 degrees C).

The stimulus was an oscillating water jet at 200 Hz, delivered through a glass pipette whose tip diameter was between 8-10 microns. The stimulus could be varied in 1.5 dB steps. The stimulating pipette was attached to a micromanipulator which allowed us to move the tip in the subtectorial space and direct the water jet to selected hair-cell stereocilia bundles. Details of the stimulus system have been described elsewhere [38].

Measurement of Stereocilia Motion

The isolated cochlear coil was placed under the microscope so that the tips of the stereocilia could be viewed while looking down on the reticular lamina. Stereocilia movements produced by the oscillating water jet were made visible by illuminating the coil with stroboscopic light at a frequency slightly offset from that used in the water jet. In this way, the stereocilia appeared to move slowly back and forth with stimulation. All measurements were based on the relative dB value of stimulus needed to produce a visual detection level threshold of stereocilia movement.

Procedure

A pre-exposure detection threshold was measured several times. The sensory hairs were then overstimulated by exposing them to the water jet for various intervals of time at fixed intensity levels above threshold. After the exposure, the stimulus was reduced and the detection level threshold was again measured. The specific procedures for the growth and recovery experiments will be described when the data are presented. The data were converted to threshold shifts by subtracting the post-exposure from the pre-exposure thresholds.

Growth and Recovery of Threshold Shift in Stereocilia Micromechanics

Stereocilia from all four hair-cell rows were examined at each of three exposure levels; 8, 13, and 18 dB above threshold. The hairs were exposed for one minute, and then the stimulus was reduced and a threshold obtained. The exposure then continued for another minute, followed by another threshold estimate. This cycle continued for a total exposure duration of ten minutes. The threshold estimates usually took only 20 seconds. Detailed results have been presented elsewhere [61]; a summary is provided in Fig. 2A. In this figure, the data over all hair cell rows have been averaged for each exposure level. Each data point represents the average threshold shift of 28 hair cells (seven cells from each of the four hair-cell rows). As can be seen, there was a systematic growth in threshold during the first five to six minutes of exposure. This was followed by a plateau in which the amount of threshold shift remained constant. The threshold shift at the plateau differed for each of the three exposure levels with the more intense exposure producing a higher plateau. The relation between threshold shift at the plateau and exposure level is presented in Fig. 2B. Threshold shift grew in a very orderly fashion, and a regression line fitted to these data exhibited a correlation of 0.9. Every dB increase in exposure level (for intensities 5 dB or more above threshold) produced a 0.68 increase in maximum threshold shift.

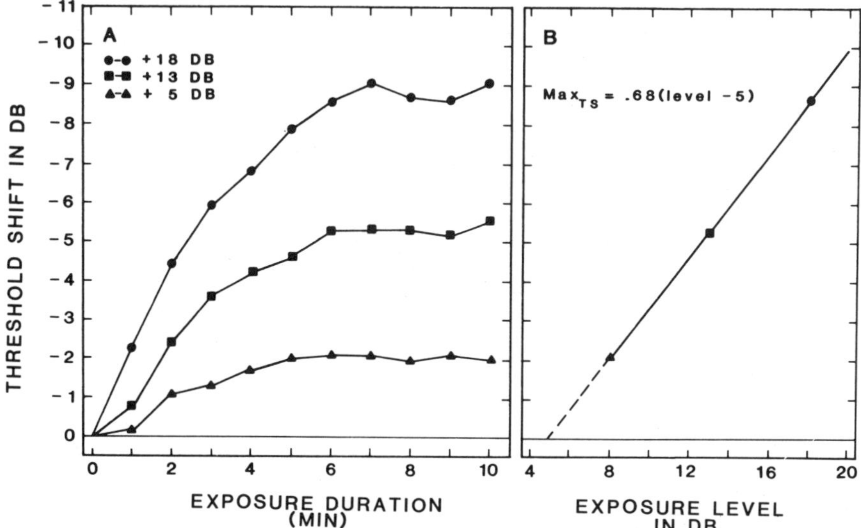

Fig. 2. The growth of threshold shift for three different levels of overstimulation during a 10 minute exposure period is presented in the A panel. Panel B presents the average threshold shift measured between 6 and 10 minutes of exposure at each of the three levels. The regression equation on these data allow a prediction of maximum threshold shift (Max_{ts}) for exposure levels 5 dB or more above threshold.

These results have also been described in terms of hair-cell row and are presented in the left hand portion of Fig. 3. Threshold shift at the plateau was greatest for OHC_1 bundles and this was followed by OHC_2 stereocilia. The IHC and OHC_3 sensory hairs showed about the same level of maximum threshold shift. These data were obtained by summing the results from the three exposure conditions for each hair-cell row.

Stereocilia from hair cells on each row in turns 2-3 and 3-4 (13-14 and 16-17 mm from the base) were stimulated for 5 minutes at an intensity 13 dB above the detection threshold. Following the exposure, detection

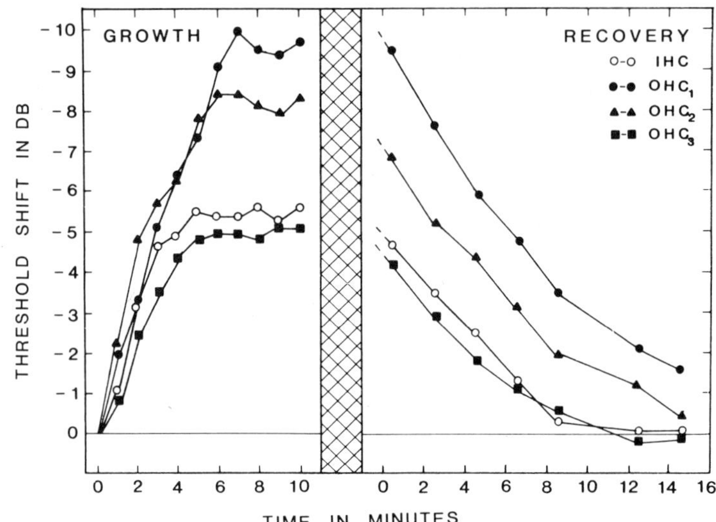

Fig. 3. The left panel indicates the growth of threshold shift for each of the four hair cell rows. The IHC and OHC_3 reached a plateau earlier than the other two OHC rows. The right panel indicates the recovery from threshold shift for each of the four hair cell rows. Regression lines fitted to the recovery data revealed that the recovery slope was the same for each hair cell type.

thresholds were measured at 0.5, 2.5, 4.5, 6.5, 9.5, 12.5 and 14.5 minutes of recovery. The results are presented in the right hand portion of Fig. 3; each point represents stereocilia behavior on about 20 hair cells. Again, the magnitude of threshold shift at 0.5 minutes post-exposure varied among hair-cell rows with OHC showing the greatest shift. During recovery the IHC, OHC_3 and OHC_2 stereocilia returned to the pre-exposure thresholds. The OHC_1 sensory hair bundles recovered to within 1.5 dB of the pre-exposure level. The slope of the recovery curves during the first 8.5 minutes was nearly the same for each hair-cell row, and we have interpreted this to mean that the underlying process was the same [59]. The differences in susceptibility to overstimulation between the four hair-cell rows is not completely clear, but may be related to differences in the height of the sensory hairs. Threshold is defined by a constant deflection (about 0.2 microns) of the stereocilia tips. The angular deflection of taller stereocilia would be less than shorter ones to achieve this 0.2 micron threshold. Since the OHC_1 stereocilia are substantially shorter than the other rows, these hairs would receive a stronger stimulus. If this assumption is correct, then the susceptibility to overstimulation may be more related to stimulus intensity than to some intrinsic property of the stereocilia themselves.

All the threshold shifts were plotted as negative numbers, which indicated that it took less stimulus intensity to achieve a detection threshold following overstimulation. This observation implies that the stereocilia have become "looser" or mechanically less stiff. We have considered three possible explanations for the loss in stiffness. The first of these is damage to the core of the stereocilium similar to that assumed to occur with "floppy" stereocilia (see Fig. 1D). However, the clear impression gained from these experiments was that stereocilia always moved as rigid rods pivoting about their base. A compliant or "rubbery" stereocilia shaft was never observed. The second possibility was that damage occurred to the "ankle" region of the stereocilia (see Figs. 1E, F and G). A third possibility was that the extracellular connections between stereocilia deteriorated and the impedance properties of the bundle as a whole decreased (see Figs. 1 A, B, and C). This would also cause a loss in stiffness. These latter two possibilities seemed most likely, but must await verification by microscopic examination of the stimulated cell.

Threshold Shift in Stereocilia on Metabolically Blocked Hair Cells

A number of procedures were used to metabolically block hair cell activity. These included age, cooling, and poisoning [62]. We will only describe the results from poisoning the hair-cell preparation with NaCN. The isolated coil was prepared as described and detection thresholds were measured in the normal culture medium. Following this, a NaCN solution was injected into the microscope chamber to achieve a 2.0 mM concentration. The preparation was allowed to equilibrate for 30 minutes. The growth and recovery of threshold shift were then studied as described above. Only the results from OHC_1 will be presented, although similar observations were made with the other hair-cell rows. Fig. 4 presents the findings for the growth (left panel) and recovery (right panel) of threshold shift. The variable of interest in these panels is the medium bathing the cochlear coil. The growth of threshold shift in control cells shows the patterns previously described. However, in the poisoned cells, the growth of threshold shift appeared to be delayed by one minute, then increased monotonically during the next nine minutes. The last threshold sampled showed that the poisioned stereocilia had a threshold shift that was 39% larger than the control cells. The recovery from threshold shift is seen in the right hand panel. The initial shifts, following a five minute continuous exposure was different for control and NaCN cells. During recovery the control cells returned to the pre-exposure level, whereas the poisioned cells showed very little recovery.

We have concluded that these observations indicate an active process in the apical region of the cell which is counteracting the loss of stiffness caused by overstimulation. During exposure, the growth of threshold shift reached a plateau, indicating that the injury process had reached some steady state. This may represent a balance between those processes that contribute to a loss in stereocilia stiffness and those that try and maintain stiffness. The poisoning experiments indicated that these processes depend on normal cell metabolism. When the process that maintained stiffness was removed or inhibited, the growth of threshold shift continued unhampered. The same reasoning applies to the recovery curves. The post-exposure improvement in threshold represents a process in the cell repairing damage and restoring stiffness. When this process was removed by poisoning the cell, recovery no longer occurred.

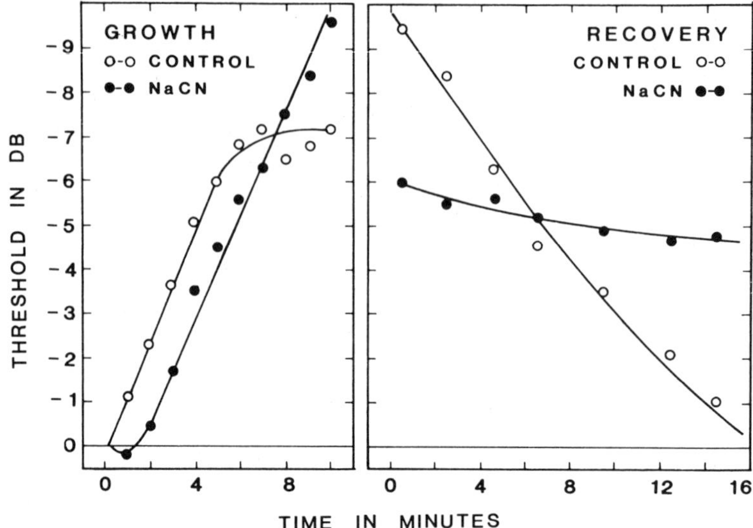

Fig. 4. The growth and recovery of threshold shift is plotted for sensory hair bundles on OHC_1 cells. The behavior of control cells, bathed in normal culture medium, was similar to that seen in the previous two figures. When 2.0 mM NaCN was added to the culture medium, the growth and recovery behavior of the sensory hair bundles changed. The left panel shows that the NaCN-treated stereocilia did not reach a plateau, but continued to show growing threshold shift during the entire 10-minute exposure period. The right panel indicates that the NaCN-treated stereocilia exhibited minimal recovery during the 15 minute test interval.

Since the injury that caused the loss in stiffness has not been identified, it is difficult to speculate on the nature of the repair process. Nevertheless, activity in the protein structure of the stereocilia or cuticular plate is implied. There is a considerable time difference involved in the building of new protein structure or the repairing of damaged structure. Since the recovery process was rapid, we would suggest, as a working hypothesis, that the hair cell is repairing damaged structure rather than synthesizing new material.

CONCLUSION

In this essay, we have described the numerous pathologies that can occur to stereocilia. We have also suggested that knowledge of the cytoskeletal and extracellular organization of the sensory-hair bundle can help us understand the nature of these pathologies. In addition, we demonstrated that it is now possible to isolate stereocilia injury from other forms of overstimulation damage to the hair cells. The data presented indicate that stereocilia can show a loss of stiffness following overstimulation. The growth of threshold shift appeared orderly and was related to the level of the exposure stimulus. Moreover, some sort of restorative process appeared to limit the maximum amount of threshold shift (the plateau) at each exposure level. The recovery data showed that micromechanical stiffness can return to pre-exposure levels following overstimulation. Finally, the presence of an active process controlling and perhaps even modulating the growth and recovery process is intriguing, but needs to be examined further to identify the mechanisms involved. These mechanisms may be fundamental to our understanding of the apical region of the hair cell.

ACKNOWLEDGMENTS

This paper was prepared while the senior author was on study leave from the University of Pennsylvania, partially supported by funds from the Swedish Medical Research Council to Ake Flock, and a study leave award from the American Scandinavian Foundation to James C. Saunders. The contributions of Barbara Canlon were supported by an award from the Swedish Work Environment Fund. The authors appreciate the critical comments of Mats Ulfendahl. The technical assistance of Britta Flock, Katarina Florin and Yvonne Hoppe were also important to the progress of this research.

REFERENCES

1. C. Angelborg and H. Engstrom, The normal organ of Corti. in: "Basic Mechanisms in Hearing," A. R. Moller, ed., Academic Press, New York (1973).
2. B. A. Bohne, Healing of the noise-damaged inner ear, in: "Hearing and Davis: Essays Honoring Hallowell Davis," S. K. Hirsh, D. H. Eldredge, I. J. Hirsh, and S. R. Silverman, eds., Washington University Press, St. Louis (1976).
3. E. Borg and B. Engstrom, Hearing thresholds in the rabbit: A behavioral and electrophysiological study, Acta Otolaryngol., 95:19 (1983).
4. E. Borg and B. Engstrom, Damage to sensory hairs of inner hair cells after exposure to noise in rabbits without outer hair cells, Hear. Res., 10:1 (1983).
5. B. Canlon, J. Miller and A. Flock, High intensity noise effects on stereocilia micromechanics, Abs. Assoc. Res. Otolaryngol., 8:50 (1985).
6. S. D. Comis, J. O. Pickles and M. P. Osborne, Osmium tetroxide post-fixation in relation to the crosslinkage and spatial organization of stereocilia in the guinea pig cochlea. J. Neurocytol., 14:113 (1985).
7. D. P. Corey and A. J. Hudspeth, Kinetics of the receptor current in bullfrog saccular hair cells, J. Neurosci., 5:962 (1983).
8. D. A. Cotanche, L. G. Tilney and J. C. Saunders, SEM analysis of pure-tone overstimulation in the developing avian cochlea. Abs. Assoc. Res. Otolaryngol., 7:55 (1984).
9. P. Dallos, J. Santos-Sacchi and A. Flock, Intracellular recordings from cochlear outer hair cells. Science, 218:582 (1982).
10. D. J. DeRosier, and L. G. Tilney, How actin filaments pack into bundles, Cold Spring Harbor Symp. in Quant. Biol., 46:525 (1982).
11. D. J. DeRosier, L. G. Tilney and E. Egelman, Actin in the inner ear: The remarkable structure of the stereocilium, Nature, (London), 287:291 (1980).
12. D. E. Dunn, J. A. Ferraro and D. Lim, Electrophysiological and morphological correlations of TTS in the chinchilla, Abs. Assoc. Res. Otolaryngol., 4:37 (1979).
13. B. Engstrom, Scanning electron microscopy of the inner structure of the organ of Corti and its neural pathways, Acta Otolarngol. Suppl. 319:57 (1974).
14. B. Engstrom, Fusion of stereocilia on inner hair cells in man and in the rabbit, rat and guinea pig, Scand. Audiol., 27:381 (1983).

15. B. Engstrom, Stereocilia of sensory cells in normal and hearing impaired ears, Scand Audiol., Suppl, 19:1 (1983).
16. B. Engstrom and E. Borg, Cochlear morphology in relation to loss of behavioral, electrophysiological and middle ear reflex thresholds after exposure to noise, Acta Otolaryngol., Suppl. 402:1 (1983).
17. B. Engstrom, A. Flock and E. Borg, Ultrastructural studies of stereocilia in noise-exposed rabbits, Hearing Res, 12:251 (1983).
18. H. Engstrom and B. Engstrom, Structural changes in the cochlea following overstimulation by noise, Acta Otolaryngol. Suppl. 360:75 (1979).
19. S. A. Falk, Combined effects of noise and ototoxic drugs, Environ. Health Perspect, 34:5 (1972).
20. A. Flock, Physiological properties of sensory hairs in the ear, in: "Psychophysics and Physiology of Hearing," E. F. Evans and J. P. Wilson, eds., Academic Press, New York (1977).
21. A. Flock and H. C. Cheung, Actin filaments in sensory hairs of inner ear receptor cells, J. Cell Biol., 75:339 (1977).
22. A. Flock and D. Strelioff, Graded and nonlinear mechanical properties of sensory hairs in the mammalian hearing organ, Nature, 310:597 (1984).
23. A. Flock and D. Strelioff, Studies on hair cells in isolated coils from the guinea pig cochlea, Hearing Res., 15:11 (1984).
24. A. Flock, B. Flock and E. Murrary, Studies on the sensory hairs of receptor cells in the inner ear, Acta Otolaryngol., 83:85 (1977).
25. T. J. Garfinkle and J. C. Saunders, Morphology of inner hair cell stereocilia in C57BL/6J mice as studied by scanning electron microscopy, Otolaryngol., Head and Neck Surg. 91:421 (1983).
26. N. Hirakowa and L. G. Tilney, Interactions between actin filaments and between actin filaments and membranes in quick-frozen and deeply etched hair cells of the chick ear, J. Cell Biol., 95:249 (1982).
27. A. J. Hudspeth, Models for mechanoelectrical transduction by hair cells, in: "Contemporary Sensory Neurobiology," M. J. Correia and A. A. Perachio, eds., Alan R. Liss, Inc, New York (1985).
28. A. J. Hudspeth and D. P. Corey, Sensitivity, polarity, and conductance changes in the response of vertebrate hair cells to controlled mechanical stimuli, Proc. Natl. Acad. Sci. (U.S.A.) 74:2407 (1977).
29. I. Hunter-Duvar, Hearing and hair cells, Canada J. Otolaryngol., 4:152 (1975).
30. I. M. Hunter-Duvar, Morphology of the normal and the acoustically damaged cochlea, Scan. Elect. Micr. 2:421 (1977).
31. I. M. Hunter-Duvar, A scanning study of acoustic lesions of the cochlea, in: "Inner ear biology," M. Portmann and J. M. Aran, eds., INSERM, 68:385 (1977).
32. I. M. Hunter-Duvar, Reissner's membrane and endocytosis of cell debris, Acta Otolaryngol., 351:24 (1978).
33. I. M. Hunter-Duvar and M. Suzuki, Inner ear damage from acoustic trauma, in: "Personal hearing protection in industry," P. M. Alberti, ed., Raven Press, New York (1981).
34. I. M. Hunter-Duvar, M. Suzuki and R. J. Mount, Anatomical changes in the organ of Corti after acoustic stimulation, in: "New perspectives on noise-induced hearing loss," R. P. Hamernik, D. Henderson and R. Salvi, eds., Raven Press, New York (1982).
35. M. Itoh, Preservation and visualization of actin-containing filaments in the apical zone of cochlear sensory cells, Hearing Res, 6:277 (1982).
36. M. Itoh and T. Nakashima, Structure of the hair rootlets on cochlear sensory cells by tannic acid fixation, Acta Otolaryngol., 90:385 (1980).
37. S. Iurato, Submicroscopic structures of the membraneous labyrinth, Z. Zellforsch, 53:259 (1961).

38. K. Karlsson and A. Flock, Sinnesharens i Cortiska organet mikromekanik: In vitro studie med stroboskopiskt ljus, Svensk Otolaryngol. Forening, 2:24 (1983).
39. A. Leibovitz, The growth and maintenance of tissue cell cultures in free gas exchange with the atmosphere, Am. J. Hyg., 78:173 (1963).
40. M. C. Liberman, and D. G. Beil, Hair cell condition and auditory nerve response in normal and noise-damaged cochleas, Acta Otolaryngol., 88:161 (1979).
41. M. C. Liberman and L. W. Dodds, Single neuron labeling and chronic cochlear pathology. II. Stereocilia damage and alterations of spontaneous discharge rates, Hearing Res., 16:43 (1984).
42. M. C. Liberman, and L. W. Dodds, Single neuron labeling and chronic cochlear pathology. III. Stereocilia damage and alterations of threshold tuning curves, Hearing Res., 16:55 (1984).
43. M. C. Liberman and M. J. Mulroy, Acute and chronic effects of acoustic trauma: cochlear pathology and auditory nerve pathophysiology, in: "New perspectives on noise-induced hearing loss," R. P. Hamernik, D. Henderson and R. Salvi, eds., Raven Press, New YorK (1982).
44. D. J. Lim, Cochlear anatomy related to cochlear micromechanics: A review, J. Acoust. Soc. Am., 67:1686 (1980).
45. D. J. Lim and D. E. Dunn, Anatomic correlates of noise-induced hearing loss, Otolaryngol. Clinics North Am., 12:493 (1979).
46. D. J. Lim and W. Melnick, Acoustic damage to the cochlea: A scanning and transmission electron microscopic observation, Arch. Otolaryngol., 94:294 (1971).
47. H. H. Lindeman and G. Bredberg, Scanning elactron microscopy of the organ of Corti after intense auditory stimulation: Effects on stereocilia and cuticular surface of hair cells, Arch. Klin. Exper. Ohren. Nasen, und Kehlkopfheil-Kunde, 203:1 (1972).
48. M. J. Mulroy, and F. J. Curley, Stereociliary pathology and noise-induced threshold shifts: A scanning electron microscopic study, Scan. Elect. Micro., 4:1733 (1982).
49. D.-Ch. Neugebauer and U. Thurm, Interconnections between the stereovilli of the fish inner ear, Cell Tissue Res., 240:449 (1985).
50. M. P. Osborne, S. D. Comis and J. O. Pickles, Morphology and cross-linkage of stereocilia in the guinea pig labyrinth examined without the use of osmium as a fixative, Cell Tissue Res., 237:43 (1984).
51. J. O. Pickles, S. D. Comis and M. P. Osborne, Cross-links between stereocilia in the guinea pig organ of Corti, and their possible relation to sensory transduction, Hearing Res., 15:103 (1984).
52. D. Robertson, Effects of acoutic trauma on stereocilia structure and spinal ganglion cell tuning properties in the guinea pig cochlea, Hearing Res., 7:55 (1982).
53. D. Robertson and B. M. Johnstone, Acoustic trauma in the guinea pig cochlea: Early changes in ultrastructure and neural thresholds, Hearing Res., 3:167 (1980).
54. D. Robertson, B. M. Johnstone and T. J. McGill, Effects of loud tones on the inner ear; A combined electrophysiological and ultrastructural study, Hearing Res. 2:39 (1980).
55. I. J. Russell and P. M. Sellick, Intracellular studies of hair cells in the mammalian cochlea, J. Physiol., 284:261 (1978).
56. R. J. Salvi, R. P. Hamernik and D. Henderson, Auditory nerve activity and cochlear morphology after noise exposure, Arch. Otorhinolaryngol., 224:111 (1979).
57. J. C. Saunders and N. Coppa, The contribution of stereocilia, rootlet, and cuticular plate injury to sensory neural heaing loss, in: "Sensorineural Hearing Loss: Mechanisms, Diagnosis and Treatment," M. J. Collins, T. J. Glattke and L. A. Harker, eds., Univer. Iowa Press, Iowa City, (1986).

58. J. C. Saunders and S. P. Dear, Comparative morphology of stereocilia, in: "Hearing and Other Senses: Presentations in Honor of E. G. Wever," R. R. Fay and G. Gourevitch, eds., The Amphora Press Groton, Connecticut (1983).
59. J. C. Saunders and A. Flock, Recovery of threshold shift in hair-cell stereocilia following exposure to intense stimulation, Hearing Res., (Submitted).
60. J. C. Saunders and L. G. Tilney, Species differences in susceptibility to noise exposure, in: "New Perspectives on Noise-Induced Hearing Loss," R. P. Hamernik, D. Henderson and R. J. Salvi, eds., Raven Press, New York (1982).
61. J. C. Saunders, B. Canlon and A. Flock, Growth of threshold shift in hair-cell stereocilia following overstimulation, Hearing Res. (Submitted).
62. J. C. Saunders, B. Canlon and A. Flock, Recovery of threshold shift in hair-cell stereocilia following exposure to intense stimulation, Hearing Res., (Submitted).
63. J. C. Saunders, S. P. Dear and M. E. Schneider, The anatomical consequences of acoustic injury: A review and tutorial, J. Acoust. Soc Am., 78:833 (1985).
64. J. C. Saunders, M. E. Schneider and S. P. Dear, The structure and function of actin in hair cells, J. Acoust. Soc. Am., 78:299 (1985).
65. N. Slepecky and S. C. Chamberlain, Distribution and polarity of actin in the sensory hair cells of the chinchilla cochlea, Cell Tissue Res., 224:15 (1982).
66. N. Slepecky, R. P. Hamernik D. Henderson and D. Coling, Ultrastructural changes to the cochlea resulting from impulse noise, Arch. Otorhinolaryngol., 230:273 (1981).
67. N. Slepecky, R. P. Hamernik, D. Henderson, and D. Cooling, Correlation of audiometric data with changes in cochlear hair cell stereocilia resulting from impulse noise trauma, Acta Otolaryngol., 93:329 (1982).
68. E. R. Soudijn, Scanning electron microscopic study of the organ of Corti in normal and sound-damaged guinea pigs, Ann. Otol. Rhinol. Laryngol., Suppl. 29:1 (1976).
69. H. Spoendlin, Ultrastructure and peripheral innervation pattern of the receptor in relation to the first coding of the acoustic message, in: "Hearing Mechanisms in Vertebrates," A. V. S. DeReuck and J. Knight, eds., J. A. Churchill, London (1968).
70. H. Spoendlin, Auditory, vestibular, olfactory and gustatory organs. in: "Ultrastructure of the Peripheral Nervous System and Sense Organs: An Atlas of Normal and Pathologic Anatomy," Bischoff, ed., Thieme, Stuttgart (1970).
71. H. Spoendlin, Primary structural changes in the organ of Corti after acoustic overstimulation, Acta Otolaryngol., 71:166 (1971).
72. H. Spoendlin, Anatomical changes following various noise exposures, in: "Effects of Noise on Hearing," D. Henderson, R. P. Hamernik, S. Dosanjh and J. H. Mills, eds., Raven Press, New York (1976).
73. P. E. Stopp, The effect of moderate-intensity noise on cochlear potentials and structure, in: "New Perspectives on Noise-Induced Hearing Loss," R. P. Hamernik, D. Henderson and R. Salvi, eds., Raven Press, New York (1982).
74. P. E. Stopp, Effects on guinea pig cochlea from exposure to moderately intense broad-band noise, Hearing Res., 11:55 (1983).
75. D. Strelioff and A. Flock, Stiffness of sensory-cell hair bundles in the isolated guinea pig cochlea, Hearing Res., 15:19 (1984).
76. H. M. Theopold, Das akustische trauma im tierexperimen. I. morphologische veranderungen der meerschweinchen cochlea nach knalltrauma, Laryngol. Rhinol., 57:706 (1978).

77. H. M. Theopold, Das akustische trauma im tierexperiment. II. morphologische veranderungen der meerschweinchen cochlea nach sinustonstimulation und rosa rauschen, Laryngol. Rhinol., 57:892 (1978).
78. H. M. Theopold, The acoustic trauma in animal experiment. II. morphological reaction in the guinea pig cochlea after traumatisation by pure tones and octave band noise (a SEM-and TEM-Study), Laryngol. Rhinol., 57:892 (1978).
79. P. R. Thorne and J. B. Gavin, Changing relationships between structure and function in the cochlea during recovery from intense sound exposure, Ann. Otol. Rhinol. Laryngol., 94:81 (1985).
80. P. R. Thorne, J. B. Gavin and P. B. Herdson, A quantitative study of the sequence of topographical changes in the organ of Corti following acoustic trauma, Acta Otolaryngol., 97:69 (1984).
81. L. G. Tilney, D. J. DeRosier and M. J. Mulroy, The organization of actin filaments in the stereocilia of cochlear hair cell, Cell Biol. 86:244 (1980).
82. L. C. Tilney and J. C. Saunders, Actin filaments, stereocilia, and hair cells of the bird cochlea. I. Length, number, width, and distribution of stereocilia of each hair cell are related to the position of the hair cell on the cochlea, J. Cell Biol., 96:807 (1983).
83. L. C. Tilney, E. H. Egelman, E. H. DeRosier and J. C. Saunders, Actin filaments, stereocilia, and hair cells of the bird cochlea. II. Packing of actin filament in the stereocilia and in the cuticular plate and what happens to the organization when the stereocilia are bent, Cell Biol., 96:882 (1983).
84. L. C. Tilney, J. C. Saunders, E. Engelman and D. J. DeRosier, Changes in the organization of actin filaments in the stereocilia of noise-damaged lizard cochleae, Hearing Res., 7:181 (1982).
85. F. A. Voelker, C. M. Henderson, A. W. Maclin and W. E. Tucker, Evaluating the rat inner ear, Arch Otolaryngol., 106:613 (1980).
86. A. Wright, Giant cilia in the human organ of Corti, Clin. Otolaryngol., 7:193 (1982).
87. A. Wright, Dimensions of the cochlear stereocilia in man and the guinea pig, Hearing Res., 13:89 (1984).
88. U. Zimmerman, G. Pilivat and F. Riemann, Dielectric breakdown of cell membranes, Biophys., 141:881 (1974).
89. U. Zimmerman and P. Scheurich, High frequency fusion of plant protoblasts by eleetric fields, Planta., 151:26 (1981).

DISCUSSION

Shaddock: I'm curious about the splaying effect of the cilia, especially when they come back together. Which of the mechanisms that you proposed might be responsible for this?

Saunders: One possibility is that the interconnecting links are stretched. We do not know if the links are proteinous, but if they are, they conceivably could be stretchd. If they retain their elastic properties, then they may reform themselves during the recovery period.

Pickles: Do your histological methods enable you to pick up minimal changes in the paracrystalline structure which may affect its mechanical strength without causing complete dissolution which you showed in your previous publications?

Saunders: We have replaced our original optical defraction methods with a laser diffraction method which allows you to look at periodicity below the visual detection level for damage to the actin crystal. So we hope to develop that technique during the coming year to look at what would be injuries to the paracrystalline structure way below that which would occur at these high noise level exposures.

Trahiotis: Could you discuss the relation between your kind of stimulation and natural stimulation? What I am interested in is the differential effects of velocity and displacement.

Saunders: This is a cell preparation and it allows us to measure cell events with great precision. I do not want to make any illusions to the real world and noise exposure. What we are doing, however, is describing what possibilities exist for changing the mechanical stiffness of stereocilia and looking at stereocilia changes in an isolated situation. All I am looking at is the mechanical properties of stereocilia. Up to this point, we haven't been able to disassociate ourselves from the rest of the cell. But now it is experimentally possible to manipulate the stereocilia themselves and look at their mechanical properties. I do not know what the transfer function is between basilar membrane displacement, tectorial membrane displacement and stereocilia motion. If I did, I could turn my microns of displacement into something related to sound pressure level at the eardrum. Until that is known, these must remain cell observations and have no real-world counterpart.

Salvi: Did you ever try raising the temperature? In a previous experiment done by Drescher, elevating the temperaure caused the microphonic potential to decrease faster than it normally would.

Saunders: No, we did not do that. In fact, all testing takes place at room temperature. That may be a criticism of these experiments. Nevertheless, it reduces the bacterial growth to the point where you can actually do the experiments.

von Gierke: Can you make any statement about directional sensitivity of the original individual cilia?

Saunders: No. In the observations that I have made where we examined movements of stereocilia at their maximum displacement in both directions, they appeared to be linearly displaced rather than favoring one direction or the other.

von Gierke: What I meant was, what effect does changing the angle of the force on the cilia have?

Saunders: We have not done that. We simply tried to adjust the pipet to move the face of the hair bundle as effectively as possible.

von Gierke: It could well be that the individual variability comes from different sensitivities to different directions of motion.

Saunders: Yes. It gets more complicated than that. The movement of water out from a pipet source is a very complicated stimulus. The eddy currents generated are very complicated.

Flottorp: It seems that the mechanism you have shown us here could explain the recovery from TTS over time. However, the TTS sometimes recovers over three weeks or more from blast waves. Do you have any suggestions on what the mechanisms could be in this situation?

Saunders: Well, I do not have a suggestion for a mechanism. In our experiments, we are looking at isolated stereocilia mechanics. When you look at the recovery for human threshold shift measured in terms of a subject's response, there are many factors intervening between the stereocilia and the decision process. We have to appreciate that noise-induced hearing loss is not due to any one single simple mechanism. Presumably, other cell factors play a very significant role also.

Pfander: Do you think the cilia of the hair cells are bent down during TTS and then slowly come up again?

Saunders: It was occasionally observed following the exposure that the stereocilia would move vigorously. As the recovery process would start, all of a sudden the cilia would fall over. Well, interestingly, by injecting just a little negative or positive D.C. water pressure out of the pipet, you could force the cilia back up again. Some would go on and recover, while others would just flop over again. They did not rise up by themselves. They would have stayed flopped over forever had I not done something. It is an observation on about 10% of 350 cells.

THE MORPHOLOGY OF STEREOCILIA AND THEIR CROSS-LINKS IN RELATION TO NOISE DAMAGE IN THE GUINEA PIG

J. O. Pickles, S. D. Comis and M. P. Osborne

Department of Physiology
University of Birmingham
Birmingham B15 2TJ, UK

INTRODUCTION

We have previously described the morphology of cross-links between stereocilia, as seen by scanning and transmission electron microscopy [1-4]. The links can be divided into two sets. The links of the first set, which have also been described by other authors [e.g. 5-14], run laterally both between the stereocilia of the same row and the stereocilia of the different rows on a hair cell. The links of the second set, which had not been described before, run upwards from the tips of the shorter stereocilia, to join the adjacent taller stereocilia of the next row. If stretch of the links was associated with a reduction in the membrane resistance at one or both of their points of insertion, then many of the findings from electrophysiological experiments on hair cells, including the functional polarization of hair cells, can be accounted for simply and naturally [1,15,16]. We have, therefore, suggested that the tip links are involved in sensory transduction. The lateral links on our hypothesis have a purely mechanical role in bracing the hair bundle [1].

It is therefore of interest to answer the questions: do the lateral cross-links contribute to the mechanical strength of the stereocilia during acoustic overstimulation? Are the links, and in particular the hypothesized transducer links, the more vulnerable elements among the stereocilia, or are they capable of surviving degrees of overstimulation which cause other damage to the stereocilia? We have sought to gain evidence relevant to these questions, firstly by describing further the morphology of the links in normal animals, and, secondly, by looking for changes in the hair bundle, and looking for possible survival of the links after intense acoustic stimulation.

METHODS

Transmission Electron Microscopy

Guinea pigs were anesthetized with urethane (1.5 g/kg, IP). The temporal bones were rapidly removed, and the cochlea perfused with fixative, introduced through the round window and allowed to leak out of a hole cut at the apex. The fixative consisted of 1% glutaraldehyde and 15% saturated picric acid solution in 0.05 M phosphate buffer (pH 7.4). After 24 h, the organ of Corti was dissected out, dehydrated via ethanol and propylene oxide, and embedded in Epon/Araldite. Sections were cut on a Reichert Ultracut E microtome and were picked up on Formvar coated grids. They were stained with uranyl acetate and Reynolds lead citrate, and examined in a JEOL 120 CX2 microscope, using an accelerating voltage of 80 Kv.

Scanning Electron Microscopy

Specimens were fixed in a 2.5% glutaraldehyde in 0.05 M phosphate buffer (pH 7.4) or in the glutaraldehyde/picrate fixative described above. After 24 h the cochlea was removed from the temporal bone and the thin bony wall removed. After dehydration and critical point drying [1], the modiolus was mounted on a stub with Araldite and sputter-coated with platinum or gold/palladium to a depth of 18 nm, as judged by the thickness monitor. Specimens were examined in a JEOL 120 CX 2 EM with an accelerating voltage of 40 kV and images were observed by a secondary electron detector.

Acoustic Stimulation

Guinea pigs were anesthetized (urethane 1.5 g/kg IP), the trachea was cannulated, the external auditory meati were resected from the skull, and the bulla was ventilated to the atmosphere via a small tube. Tonal stimulation of 3 kHz at 120 dB SPL, as measured at the tympanic membrane, was produced with a Bruel and Kjaer 1/2 in driver [17] in an undamped cavity with a resonance at that frequency. After 24 h stimulation, the animal was removed and immediately prepared for scanning electron microscopy.

RESULTS

Normal Animals: Further Observations on the Links

The links were seen as described previously [1-3]. In addition, further observations were made on the points of attachment of the links.

The "tip" links, which we have suggested might be involved in sensory transduction, were preserved as sometimes incomplete fine strands (arrows, Figs. 1 and 2). Figs. 1 and 2 show that the tip links are associated with electron-dense regions underlying both points of attachment. The upper end of the tip link lies in apposition to a dense region some 40 - 60 nm in height (in the direction of the long axis of the stereocilium), and some 15 - 20 nm thick (arrowheads, Figs. 1 and 2). The dense region here forms a bridge between the external surface of the stereocilium and the filamentous core. There is also an increase in the density of the filaments immediately underlying the dense area. In many cases, there seems to be a small dip in the center of this upper dense region (arrowhead, Fig. 2). The lower end of the tip link, which inserts into the tip of the adjacent shorter stereocilium, is also apposed by a dense area. Unlike the upper dense region, this dense region lies under the surface membrane at the tip of the stereocilium. It forms a cap over the ends of the underlying microfilaments (double arrowheads, Figs. 1 and 2). Unlike the dense cap overlying the apical ends of the filaments comprising the tallest stereocilia on the hair cell, the dense region here covers only the ends of the microfilaments immediately underlying the tip link. The dense region here is 10 - 15 nm thick, and, in sections cut as in Figs. 1, 2 and 4, is 30 - 50 nm wide.

The links of the second set which we described run laterally between the stereocilia. They run both between stereocilia of the same row (intra-row links) and between the stereocilia of the different rows (inter-row links). These links are concentrated near the upper ends of the

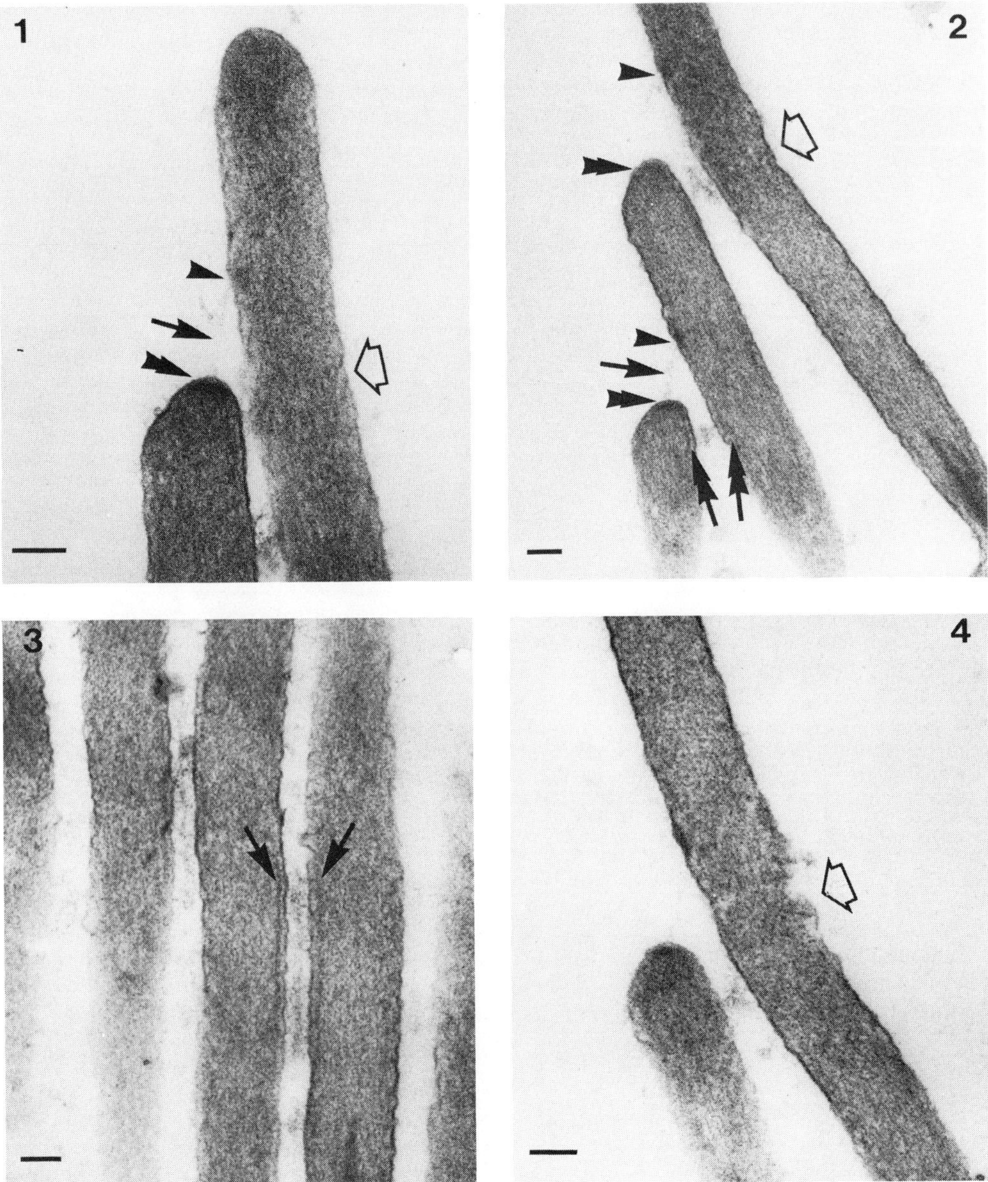

Fig. 1 Transmission micrograph of stereocilia on a guinea pig outer cell, showing tip link (arrow), upper density (arrowhead) and lower density (double arrowhead). Large open arrow: point of flexion of the tallest stereocilium. Scale bar: 100 nm.

Fig. 2 Stereocilia on an outer hair cell. Symbols: as Fig. 1. Double headed arrow: densities underlying lateral inter-row links. Scale bar: 100 nm.

Fig. 3 Stereocilia on an outer hair cell, cut at right angles to the axis of the hair cell. Arrows: densities underlying the lateral intra-row links. Scale bar: 100 nm.

Fig. 4 Stereocilia on an outer hair cell, showing point of flexion of longest stereocilium (large open arrow). Scale bar: 100 nm.

stereocilia, although some can be found nearer the base. The lateral links, too, are faced by dense regions in the stereocilia, though straining rather less densely than the regions underlying the tip links. Fig. 3 (arrows) shows for the intra-row links an increase in density in the filamentous core immediately underlying the links. The surface membrane also often shows an increase in density here, although this must be interpreted with caution, since the apparent density of the membrane is critically dependent upon the angle at which it is cut. Many fine strands running laterally between the membrane and the core can also just be seen in this region. Fig. 2 shows similar findings for the lateral inter-row links (double headed arrows).

When the stereocilia are found to be bent in normal animals, presumably as a result of distortion during preparation, the flexion is commonly found to be concentrated at or just above the most prominent band of lateral inter-row links, but below the point of insertion of the tip link. Figs. 1, 2 and 4 show this for progressively greater degrees of flexion (large open arrows).

Sound-Damaged Animals

The pure-tone stimulus (3 kHz, 120 dB SPL, 24 h) produced a characteristic pattern of damage. Although there was variability in the severity of the damage from guinea pig to guinea pig, the damage fitted into a common pattern. In the center of the lesion there was a region in which all hair cells were damaged. Beyond that there was an area in which the damage was concentrated in OHC1 and the IHC. Furthest from the lesion only IHC were damaged. Stereocilia were analyzed only from regions from which this characteristic pattern of damage was seen. By contrast, in our material, preparation damage tended to affect OHC3 most.

Changes in OHC stereocilia. Many of the OHC showed the changes described by others, with the stereocilia being shrunken and fused. Those cells will not be described further. Rather, the cells which gave indications concerning the role of the cross-links will be described.

Fig. 5 shows OHC3 from a region of damage. The stereocilia are flexed in their apical and basal portions (arrows). However, the portion in between, which is rich in lateral links, remains straight (brackets). The region without links near the roots shows the "ankles" described previously by others. This result suggests that many of the lateral links survived to brace the bundle of stereocilia during degrees of overstimulation that caused flexion of the stereocilia. Nevertheless, the lateral links do seem to be vulnerable, since in general the stereocilia were found to be separated more frequently in sound-damaged cochlea.

Some of the stereocilia are missing in Fig. 5. In the case illustrated, the stereocilia had not been absorbed, but had been pulled off as the tectorial membrane retracted during preparation. Many of these stereocilia could still be seen stuck into the tectorial membrane. Presumably the fracture occurs at the predominant site of weakness. Fig. 6 shows this to be situated where the stereocilium enters the cuticular plate. Fig. 6 and insert, another micrograph of the same area, show that the fractured core of the stereocilium can sometimes be seen in the cuticular plate (arrows).

The tip links can sometimes be seen in spite of severe disarray of the stereocilia bundle (Fig. 7, arrows). Although counts show the number of tip links to be reduced in sound-damaged cochlea, this cannot yet be taken as being reliable, because of the very large degree of variability in the preservation of the tip links from hair cell to hair cell, and from specimen to specimen, even when conditions for preservation seemed optimal.

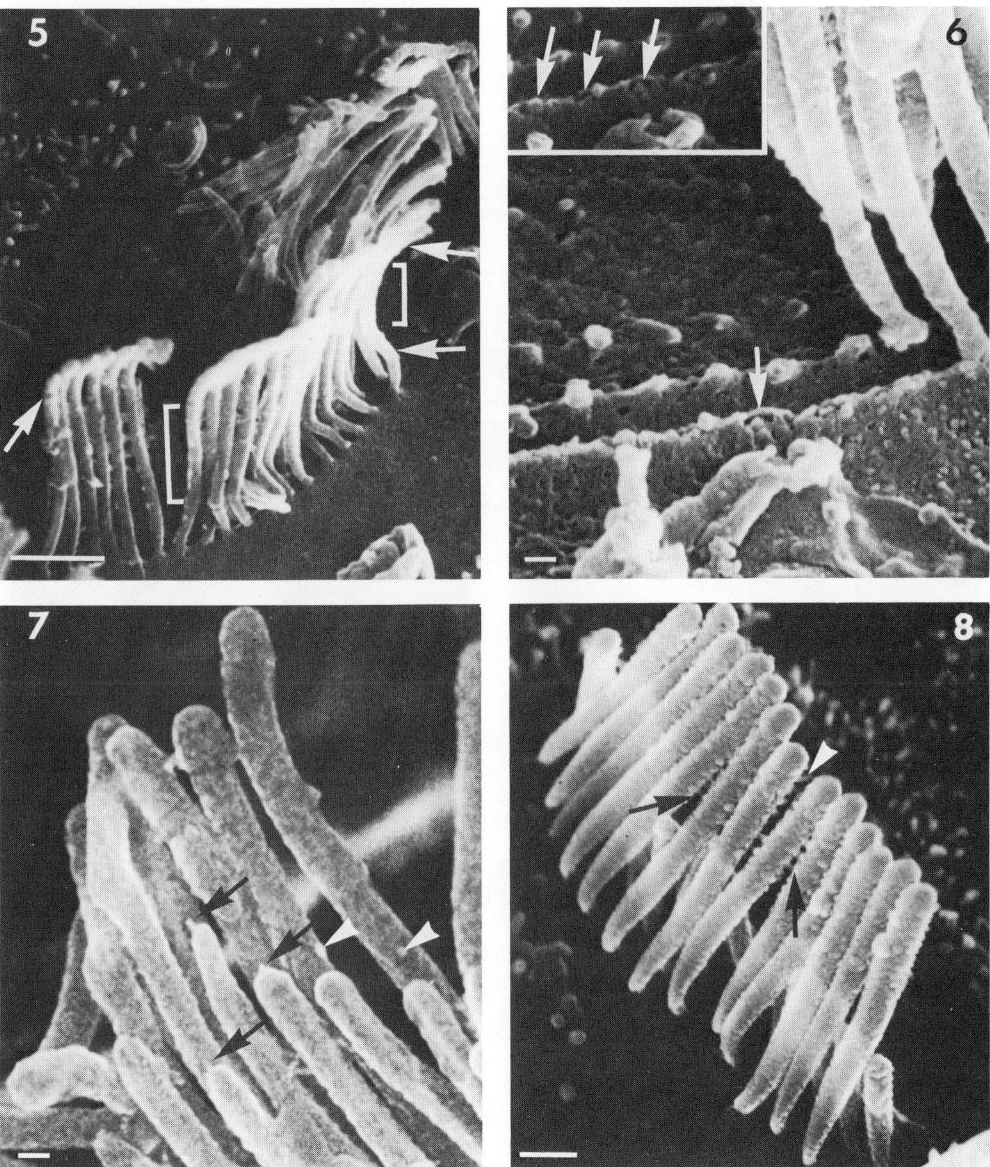

Fig. 5 Stereocilia of the third row of outer hair cells, showing flexions concentrated at the apical and basal regions of the stereocilia (arrows). Bracket: region of stereocilia rich in intra-row and inter-row links. Scale bar: 1 nm.

Fig. 6 Rootlets of outer hair cell, showing points of fracture. The fractured core of the stereocilia can be seen in the cuticular plate (arrows). The inset is another view of the same region. Scale bar: 100 nm.

Fig. 7 Tip links surviving (arrows) in a disrupted outer hair cell. Arrowheads: material associated with upper insertion of (missing) tip links. Scale bar: 100 nm.

Fig. 8 Tallest stereocilia of a guinea pig inner hair cell deflected towards the modiolus. Arrows: intact lateral inter-row links. Arrowhead: broken inter-row link. Scale bar: 500 nm.

Changes in IHC stereocilia. With small degrees of disruption, the tallest stereocilia are found to be deflected either towards or away from the modiolus, often while keeping their normal spatial relations to each other (Fig. 8). In these cases many of the lateral intra-row links are intact (arrows), although, where the stereocilia part slightly, broken links can be seen (arrowhead).

With more severe disruption, the stereocilia separate from each other and can be splayed in all directions. In some hair cells the stereocilia are bizarrely kinked (Fig. 9). However, some of these stereocilia apparently show some lateral links remaining (arrowhead). Other stereocilia seem to be particularly thin, as though they have been stretched (arrow, Fig. 9).

DISCUSSION

In the present paper, where sometimes small degrees of damage have been analyzed, it is important to ensure that the changes result from acoustic trauma, rather than preparation damage. This is particularly important with the fixation techniques used here, since stereocilia tend to be more prone to disorganization after fixation in glutaraldehyde alone than after osmication. The pattern of changes most commonly found around the lesion, with the greatest effects on the IHC and on OHC1, was similar to the changes reported by Hunter-Duvar and colleagues in the chinchilla [18,19] and Robertson and colleagues in the guinea pig [20]. Stereocilia were analyzed only from the region with this characteristic pattern of disruption, which occurred at corresponding distances along the basilar membrane in each specimen. Such a procedure increased our confidence that the changes were the result of sound trauma, rather then preparation damage, which in our material most commonly had its greatest effects on OHC3. Of course, it can never be ruled out that in some specimens preparation damage coincidentally had the same pattern as sound damage.

The studies in normal animals showed that the links between stereocilia are apposed by regions with the classical appearance of desmosomes. This was shown for both the tip links and the lateral links. The densities continue into the actin core of the stereocillium. The morphological basis for strong connections between the stereocilia therefore exists. In the case of the tip links, if the links are indeed involved in sensory transduction, they presumably need to be anchored rigidly, to ensure optimal transfer of stimulus energy to the transducer region. Since on our hypothesis the transducer channels are most likely to be situated at one or both points of insertion of the tip links, further study of these dense regions might be rewarding. These regions are readily visible in the osmium-stained material previously presented by many authors (e.g., Fig. 5 of ref. 21), although they do not draw special attention to them, or to their relations to the tip links, which in their illustrations are usually missing.

Clearly the tip links can survive, albeit perhaps in reduced numbers, those degrees of overstimulation which cause some disruption of the bundle. This suggests that the tip links may not be the most vulnerable elements in the stereocilia. It also suggests the possibility that hair cells might be able to continue transducing after some degree of noise damage, as long as the stimulus can be coupled appropriately.

The lateral links appear to contribute rigidity to the bundle of stereocilia. This is firstly shown in normal material, where flexions, which presumably occur during preparation, are concentrated just above the upper band of inter-row links (Figs. 1, 2 and 4). This result also shows

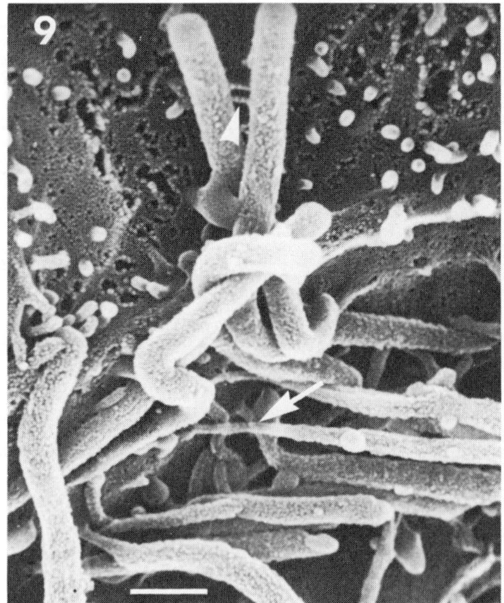

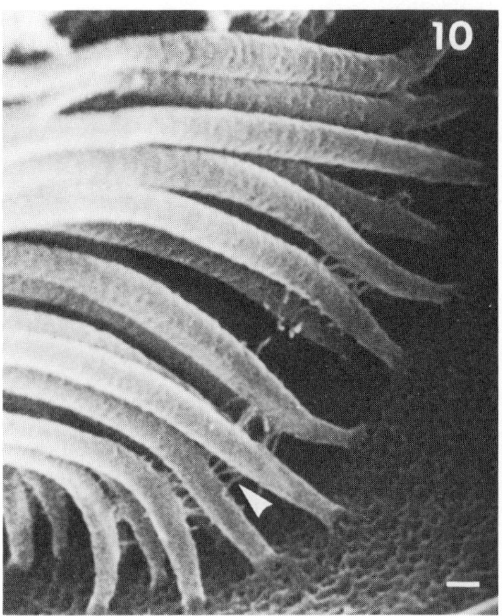

Fig. 9. Kinked stereocilia on an inner hair cell. Arrowhead: two surviving lateral intra-row links. Arrow: abnormally thin stereocilium. Scale bar: 500 nm.

Fig. 10. Lateral links (arrowhead) in a band near the base of the stereocilia of the human ampulla. Twelve week old fetus. Scale bar: 100 nm.

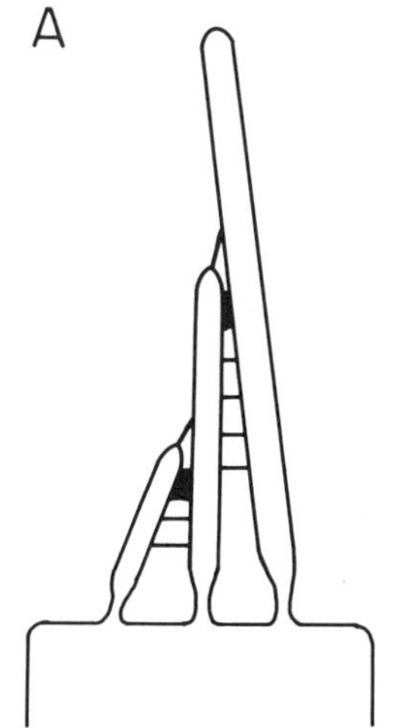

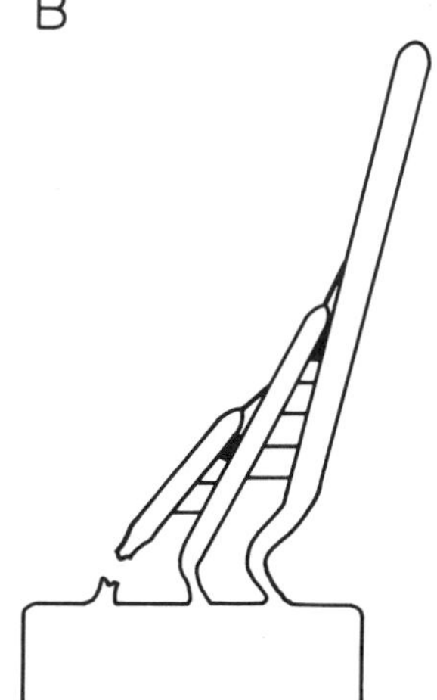

Fig. 11. A. The rows of stereocilia on a hair cell, in lateral view. The stereocilia of the different rows are buttressed against each other. B. If the inter-row links remain intact, deflection of the stereocilia can only be accommodated by lateral kinking of the basal regions of the stereocilia, or by stretching or lifting of the stereocilia from the cuticular plate.

that in the (unknown) fixation state in which this flexion has occurred, the lateral link rather than the tip link has contributed most to the mechanical integrity of the bundle. The importance of the lateral links is also shown in acoustically-traumatized material, where the flexions of the stereocilia are concentrated in regions not supported by the lateral links (e.g., Fig. 5). In the case of IHC, we would expect most of the rigidity to deflections in a direction radial across the cochlear duct to come from the lateral links running between the rows. In the case of the OHC, however, where the rows of stereocilia are arranged in a V-shape, we would expect some of the rigidity to be contributed by the lateral links running along the rows. Our results showing the mechanical importance of the lateral links are in agreement with results from micromanipulation experiments with normal hair cells, which show that if some stereocilia in a bundle are deflected, the adjacent stereocilia tend to move with them [22].

The ankles seen in the traumatized stereocilia of Fig. 5, have also been described by Engstrom and colleagues [23]. However, the pattern of movement will be affected by lateral links between stereocilia. We have shown that the stereocilia of the different rows on a hair cell are braced together to make triangles when seen in lateral view [1], which is presumably a very rigid arrangement (Fig. 11A). Any deflection of the bundle greater than can be accommodated by the lateral links will produce kinking in the root region of some stereocilia (Fig. 11B). This is presumably why, after overstimulation, cracked rootlets are commonly seen to be laterally displaced [23,24]. We might also expect some stereocilia to be broken off or stretched (Fig. 11B, see also Figs. 5 and 9).

In some acousticolateral systems there is an additional band of lateral cross-links in this rootlet region, presumably to brace the stereocilia where the ankles are likely to occur. This was originally shown for the lizard basilar papilla by Bagger-Sjoback [5], and has more recently been shown by ourselves for the human vestibular system (Fig. 10) [25].

The stereocilia of inner hair cells seem more likely to separate after acoustic trauma, perhaps because they seem to be less richly endowed with cross-links [3]. In some cases the separated stereocilia seem to be extensively kinked (Fig. 9). While such bending could have been the result of multiple flexions in different directions, our results with certain ototoxic agents suggest an alternative explanation for this, and for the possible stretching of stereocilia. We have seen similar extensive bending following Cisplatin treatment of guinea pigs [26]. X-ray microanalysis also showed that Cisplatin caused an increase in the calcium content of the apical region of the hair cells [26], and increased calcium is known to cause a dissolution of stereocilia and microvillar actin cores [27-29]. If a similar mechanism is at work here, it is possible that calcium, which can be expected to enter the cell during acoustic stimulation [30,31], acts intracellularly to cause internal dissolution of the actin paracrystal.

SUMMARY

Both the lateral and the "tip" links between stereocilia are apposed by dense regions in the stereocilia, which continue into the central actin core. There is, therefore, a morphological basis for strong connections between the stereocilia. When stereocilia were found to be flexed, whether in preparation or after acoustic trauma, the flexions appeared to be concentrated in the regions not supported by the lateral cross-links. The lateral links, therefore, seemed to brace the bundle of stereocilia during acoustic trauma. Both the tip links, which may well be involved in transduction, and the lateral links [2], sometimes appeared to be capable of surviving degrees of acoustic trauma which otherwise caused disruption to the stereocilia. However, particularly in inner hair cells, the stereocilia were sometimes found to be separated and extensively kinked after acoustic trauma. Here it is suggested that widespread dissolution of the actin core had occurred, perhaps as a result of the influx of calcium during over- stimulation.

ACKNOWLEDGEMENTS

This research was supported by the Medical Research Council and the Endowment Fund Medical Research Committee of the Central Birmingham Health Authority. The expect technical assistance of T. L. Hayward and Mrs. L. M. Tompkins is gratefully acknowledged.

REFERENCES

1. J. O. Pickles, S. D. Comis, and M. P. Osborne, Cross-links between stereocilia in the guinea pig organ of Corti, and their possible relation to sensory transduction, Hearing Res. 15:103 (1984).
2. M. P. Osborne, S. D. Comis, and J. O. Pickles, Morphology and cross-linkage of stereocilia in the guinea pig labyrinth examined without the use of osmium as a fixative, Cell and Tissue Res. 237:43 (1984).
3. S. D. Comis, J. O. Pickles, and M. P. Osborne, Osmium tetroxide post-fixation in relation to the cross-linkage and spatial organization of stereocilia in the guinea pig cochlea, J. Neurocytol. 14:113 (1985).
4. P. H. Rhys-Evans, S. D. Comis, M. P. Osbone, J. O. Pickles, and D. J. R. Jeffries, Cross-links between stereocilia in the human organ of Corti, J. Laryngol. Otol. 99:11 (1985).
5. D. Bagger-Sjoback, The sensory hairs and their attachments in the lizard basilar papilla, Brain Behav. Evol. 10:88 (1974).
6. D. Bagger-Sjoback, and J. Wersall, The sensory hairs and tectorial membrane of the basilar papilla in the lizard Calotes Versicolor, J. Neurocytol. 2:329 (1973).
7. G. Bredberg, H. W. Ades, and H. Engstrom, Scanning electron microscopy of the normal and pathologically altered organ of Corti, Acta Otolor. Suppl. 301:3 (1972).
8. D. E. Hillman, New ultrastructural findings regarding a vestibular ciliary apparatus and its possible functional significance, Brain Res. 13:407 (1969).
9. N. Hirokawa and L. G. Tilney, Interactions between actin filaments and between actin filaments and membranes in quick-frozen and deeply etched hair cells of the chick ear, J. Cell Bio. 95:249 (1982).
10. R. S. Kimura, Hairs of the cochlear sensory cells and their attachment to the tectorial membrane, Acta Otolar. 61:55 (1966).
11. D. J. Lim, Fine morphology of the tectorial membrane, Arch. Otolar. 96:199 (1972).
12. H. Spoendlin, Ultrastructure and peripheral innervation pattern of the receptor in relation to the first coding of the acoustic message, in: Hearing Mechanisms in Vertebrates, A. V. S. de Reuck and J. Knight eds., Churchill, London (1968).
13. N. Slepecky and S. C. Chamberlain, The cell coat of inner ear sensory and supporting cells as demonstrated by ruthenium red, Hearing Res. 17:281 (1985).
14. D. Ch. Neugebauer and U. Thurm, Interconnections between the stereovilli of the fish inner ear, Cell Tissue Res. 240:449 (1985).
15. A. J. Hudspeth, Extracellular current flow and the site of transduction by vertebrate hair cells, J. Neurosci. 2:1 (1982).

16. J. O. Pickles, Recent progress in cochlear physiology, Prog. Neurobiol. 24:1 (1985).
17. J. O. Pickles, Frequency threshold curves and simultaneous masking functions in single fibres of the guinea pig auditory nerve, Hearing Res. 14:245 (1984).
18. I. M. Hunter-Duvar, Morphology of the normal and acoustically damaged cochlea, Scanning Electron Microscopy 1977, 2:421 (1977).
19. I. M. Hunter-Duvar, M. Suzuki and R. J. Mount, Anatomical changes in the organ of Corti after acoustic stimulation, in: New Perspectives in Noise-Induced Hearing Loss, R. P. Hamernik, D. Henderson and R. Salvi eds., Raven Press, New York (1982).
20. D. Robertson, B. M. Johnstone and T. J. McGill, Effects of loud tones on the inner ear: a combined electrophysiological and ultra-structural study, Hearing Res. 2:39 (1980).
21. H. W. Ades and H. Engstrom, Anatomy of the Inner Ear in: Handbook of Sensory Physiology, Vol 5/1, W. D. Keidel and W. D. Neff eds., Springer, Berlin (1974).
22. A. Flock and D. Strelioff, Studies on hair cells in isolated cells from the guinea pig cochlea, Hearing Res. 15:11 (1984).
23. B. Engstrom, A. Flock and E. Borg, Ultrastructural studies of stereocilia in noise-exposed rabbits, Hearing Res. 12:251 (1983).
24. L. G. Tilney, J. C. Saunders, E. Egelman and D. J. DeRosier, Changes in the organization of actin filaments in the stereocilia of noise-damaged lizard cochleae, Hearing Res. 7:181 (1982).
25. D. J. R. Jeffries, J. O. Pickles, M. F. Osborne, P. H. Rhys-Evan and S. D. Comis, Cross-links between stereocilia in hair cells of the human and guinea pig vestibular labyrinth, Journal of Laryngology and Otology, in press (1986).
26. S. D. Comis, P. H. Rhys-Evans, M. P. Osborne, J. O. Pickles, D. J. R. Jeffries and H. A. C. Pearse, Early morphological and chemical changes induced by Cisplatin in the guinea pig organ of Corti, Journal of Laryngology and Otology, in press (1986).
27. D. Ch. Neugebauer and U. Thurm, Chemical dissection of stereovilli from fish inner ear reveals differences from intestinal microvilli, J. Neurocytol. 13:797 (1984).
28. J. R. Glenney, P. Matsudaira and K. Weber, Calcium control of the intestinal microvillus cytoskeleton, in: Calcium and Cell Function, Vol. III, W. Y. Cheung ed., Academic Press, New York (1982).
29. D. R. Burgess and B. E. Prum, Reevaluation of brush border motility; calcium induces core filament solation and microvillar vesiculation, J. Cell Biol. 94:97 (1982).
30. D. P. Corey and A. J. Hunspeth, Ionic basis of the receptor potential in a vertebrate hair cell, Nature 281:675 (1979).
31. H. Ohmori, Studies of ionic currents in the isolated vestibular hair cell of the chick, J. Physiol. 350:561 (1985).

DISCUSSION

Adams: Did your trifloroparazine affect the links?

Pickles: We did not look at that, because that was before we knew about the links.

Adams: In other cells, you can have electron densities near the cell surfaces that are not associated with structural adhesions? I wonder if you would comment on that with regard to what appears to be the lack of any structure that you can see within the links themselves that indicate they are strong.

Pickles: If I understand your question correctly, you are saying why am I emphasizing strength? Right now, I can only see the density at the end, because I have not seen any structures within the link. Thus, I have no answer.

Saunders: I'm a little confused. It looks to me like links are indeed broken following noise exposure. But, can you be sure that the links that are missing were due to the noise exposure or due to the fixation? If you are confident that there is higher incidence of missing links following noise exposure, then that is just the sort of mechanism I am looking for, because even if you only broke a few of them, you would start changing the impedance properties of the bundle.

Pickles: The last slide I showed you quite clearly had very good preservation of links on the very shortest stereocilia, but very poor preservation on the middle to upper rows. The stereocilia on hair cells, immediately adjacent, had good preservation on all rows. Concerning the lateral links, they separate much more obviously after noise exposure than without exposure. That shows that there is some sort of difference in the separation, but it does not talk about cause and effect. It could be that the actin changed, the paracrystal changed or the links changed. So, we can not answer that. The last slide I showed had a kink halfway up at the point at which you would expect the lateral link to be. This suggests to me that there is something making the flexion concentrate in that region. Therefore, at sometime or another, that link must have been intact even though as we see it, it's broken.

D. Nielsen: In your slides, you showed good evidence for strength of the lateral links within a row, yet there were cases when they were broken. They seemed to break into groups of approximately 5. Is there any reason for that in normal morphology?

Pickles: We see that often in many of our normal material. The stereocilia tend to separate off into groups, and obviously, those lateral links do have some sort of strength. When one starts to go between 2 adjacent stereocilia, we get clumps. Now I have actually chosen those latter pictures from regions where clumping was not the case. Thus, there does seem to be variability.

Pujol: I still am a little bit confused by the way you are approaching the problem, because it seems that the outer hair cell and inner hair cell behave the same with respect to links and noise trauma. But, when you try to make a correlation between the links, damage to the cilia, the transduction process and threshold shift, there is a problem because most information comes from the inner hair cell stereocilia. Could you comment on the difference between inner and outer hair cell links?

Pickles: We have no information on the morphology of the link structures on inner and outer hair cells. I think the generally accepted idea is that the outer hair cells are somehow necessary for sharp tuning. They probably feed back into the mechanics, and they certainly look like rather rigid structures. The way they are braced together, inner hair cells look as though they are there to detect the movement. I would just like to mention about TTS. There is an idea that TTS results from the IHC flopping over. If the links reform and the cilia become erect, this would correspond to recovery from TTS. I do not know if that is possible.

SYNAPTOLOGY OF THE COCHLEA: DIFFERENT TYPES OF SYNAPSE, PUTATIVE NEUROTRANSMITTERS AND PHYSIOPATHOLOGICAL IMPLICATIONS

R. Pujol, M. Lenoir, and M. Eybalin

INSERM-U.254, Laboratoire de Neurobiologie de I'Audition
CHR Hopital St. Charles, 34059 Montpellier Cedex, France

INTRODUCTION

This chapter reviews recent neuroanatomical findings concerning the cochlea. First, we outline the general pattern of cochlear innervation; then the different types of synapse within the organ of Corti are briefly described, and morphological indications about putative neurotransmitters are also included, when available. Finally, possible physiopathological implications relevant to noise-induced hearing loss are discussed.

GENERAL PATTERN OF COCHLEAR INNERVATION

The nerve fibers within the organ of Corti are classically divided into two main classes: afferents and efferents. Afferents refer to the dendrites from spiral ganglion neurons which carry messages from hair cells to the brain. Efferents refer to the axonal endings of neurons located in the brain stem which carry messages from the brain to the cochlea.

Two afferent systems are well distinguished. The dendrites of the large myelinated spiral ganglion cells (90 to 95% of the total population; [59,61]) are radially connected to the inner hair cells (IHCs) [27]; each IHC is connected to approximately 20 afferent dendrites [32,59]. The axons from these type I ganglion cells conspicuously terminate within different parts of the ipsilateral cochlear nucleus, mainly its ventral component [37]. The dendrites of the small type II ganglion neurons are spirally connected to the outer hair cells (OHCs); one neuron is in contact with a large number of cells in the three rows of OHCs [27,38]. There is considerable controversy about the termination of axons from these type II ganglion neurons. Spoendlin [61] has postulated that OHCs are not directly connected to the brain; others [37] suggest that there is a dorsal cochlear nucleus projection of fine fibers which may correspond to axons from type II neurons. Thus, the anatomy of the unmyelinated afferent system connected to OHCs is still unclear; and consequently, its physiology is far less understood.

Similarly, efferents have recently been clearly divided into two different systems [63]. The lateral system consists of unmyelinated fibers which essentially originate from small neurons in the lateral superior olive; this system projects either primarily into the ipsilateral cochlea, as in the cat [63], or exclusively, as in the rat [64]. Within the inner spiral bundle, these fibers form synapses with the radial auditory dendrites. The medial efferent system consists of myelinated fibers whose neuronal body is mainly (but not exclusively) in the contralateral trapezoid body [63,64]. These medial efferents course within the inner spiral bundle, cross the tunnel of Corti, and reach the base of OHCs nearly radially where they branch and synapse with numerous OHC's.

In addition to these afferent and efferent systems innervating the organ of Corti, a sympathetic cochlear innervation has been described, which has a clear non-perivascular component [12,62]. Unmyelinated noradrenergic (NA) fibers are distributed within the spiral ganglion and the fibers of spiral lamina [18]; they are abundant at the habenula perforata, but they do not enter the organ of Corti [2,18,62]. It has been proposed [24] that this NA system has a synchronizing effect on auditory fiber discharges.

SYNAPTOLOGY WITHIN THE ORGAN OF CORTI

Four types of morphologically well distinguished synapses are formed at the IHC and OHC levels, namely; synapses between IHCs and radial afferents (auditory dendrites), axo-dendritic synapses between lateral efferent endings and auditory dendrites, synapses between OHCs and spiral afferents, and axo-somatic synapses between medial efferent endings and OHCs.

Afferent Synapses

IHC-afferent synapses. The peripheral process of the type I ganglion neuron is called a dendrite when it loses its myelin sheath on entering the organ of Corti. The afferent dendrites course radially from the habenula perforata to contact the basal pole of IHCs. Liberman [32] distinguishes two types of radial dendrites contacting either the pillar or the modiolar surface of IHCs. A quite constant and typical synaptic junction has been described. This synapse (Fig. 1) is characterized by pre- and postsynaptic membrane densities, and presynaptic specialization, which is generally a synaptic body surrounded by microvesicles, also [4,30,32,40,59]. The shape and size of the synaptic bodies are highly variable; rod-like, ellipsoidal, ovoid, dense-cored and hollowed synaptic bodies have been described. These variations may be only species differences, or related to the functional state of the hair cell; morphological variations have also been observed during ontogenesis [58].

The chemical nature of the IHC-afferent synapse is clearly supported by its morphology. However, the kind of neurotransmitter used by the IHC to initiate auditory messages in afferent fibers is not yet known. Various hypotheses on the matter have been postulated. We restrict ourselves here to offering anatomical arguments in favor of the glutamate hypothesis. We have shown, using autoradiography, that a glutamate-glutamine cycle may exist at the IHC level [15]. This cycle is comparable to the cycle involved in the glutamate turnover at the glutamatergic synapses of the CNS [9]. Another indirect argument comes from the very high sensitivity of auditory dendrites to kainic acid exposure [47]; in adult cochleas, only auditory dendrites connected to IHCs display such a reactivity, which has been related by others [10,11] to glutamate transmission.

OHC-afferent synapses. The type of afferent innervation at the OHC level is considerably different from that at the IHC level. First, the number of afferent neurons reaching the OHCs is very low; 5 to 10% in the cat [59]; 10 to 15% in the guinea pig [38]. Second, the ganglion neurons sending fibers to OHCs appear to be exclusively type 11 unmyelinated cells

[27,43,61]. Furthermore, the dendrites inside the organ of Corti follow a completely different course, spiraling between Deiters' cells after crossing at the base of the tunnel of Corti [59]. Finally, the type of synapse between OHCs and spiral afferents also differs greatly from IHC-afferent synapses [4,51,57,59].

The typical OHC-afferent synapse (Fig. 4) is a small bouton-type ending from a spiral afferent apposed to the OHC membrane; often protuberances from the nerve terminal fit into OHC membrane cavities (Fig. 5). One or two zones of postsynaptic densities can generally be seen. On the OHC presynaptic side, very few specializations appear. There are scarce, clear, irregular vesicles (some coated) which are sometimes attached to the presynaptic membrane to form an endocytotic profile (Fig. 4); a synaptic body is rarely found, at least in the cat and the rat.

The number and morphology of OHC-afferent synapses are subjects of debate within the literature. On the basis of our ontogenetic data [45], we can propose an explanation. Within the OHC of all the species we have studied, we have found only afferents surrounding the OHC base at an early stage of synaptogenesis; at this stage, numerous presynaptic bodies are seen. Subsequently, the number of presynaptic bodies drastically decreases, and many afferents, possibly belonging to the radial system [47], retract when efferents arrive and form large efferent-OHC synapses [30,45, 46,54]. The adult OHC remains connected only to small afferents of the above mentioned type (spiral afferents). This very unusual sequence of synaptogenesis must be related to profound physiological changes in the OHCs, which start from a typical sensory stage and then develop adult properties more closely linked to cochlear micromechanics [6]. This evolution may vary along the cochlear partition and be complete in the basal OHCs, whereas at a more apical level, the OHCs may keep a more "primitive" (i.e., sensory) morphology and properties. The boundary between a "basal" and an "apical" cochlea appears to vary according to the species; in the cat, the rat, and the mouse, the "basal" cochlea appears to extend more towards the apex than in the chinchilla, the guinea pig, and man. This could explain numerous controversies found in the literature concerning OHC synaptology, and even OHC physiological properties.

The putative neurotransmitter of the OHC-afferent synapse is still unknown, but glutamate does not seem to be involved, or at least there is no indication of a glutamate-glutamine cycle as seen at the IHC level [15]. Furthermore, the dendrites of spiral afferents are not affected by kainic acid [47].

Efferent Synapses

Axo-dendritic efferent synapses below IHCs. Below the IHCs, fine fibers (approximately 0.1 um in diameter) belonging to the unmyelinated lateral axons are densely packed to form the inner spiral bundle. Varicose endings (0.8 to 1.5 um in diameter) of these fibers form axo-dendritic synapses with the radial afferent dendrites connected to the IHCs [14,25, 33,57,59]. When they enter the organ of Corti, the axons of these neurons frequently branch, giving rise to varicose collaterals that run underneath the IHCs in an apical and basal direction [33,43]. Liberman [33] has reported that each efferent fiber in the cat synapses with more than one radial afferent dendrite, and that every dendrite has at least one efferent synapse.

The synaptic contact (frequently "en passant") is made between an efferent varicosity and a non-specialized area of the dendrite (Fig. 2). The efferent varicosity is filled with two types of vesicles: clear (20 to 50 nm in diameter) and granular or dense-cored (70 to 120 nm in diameter).

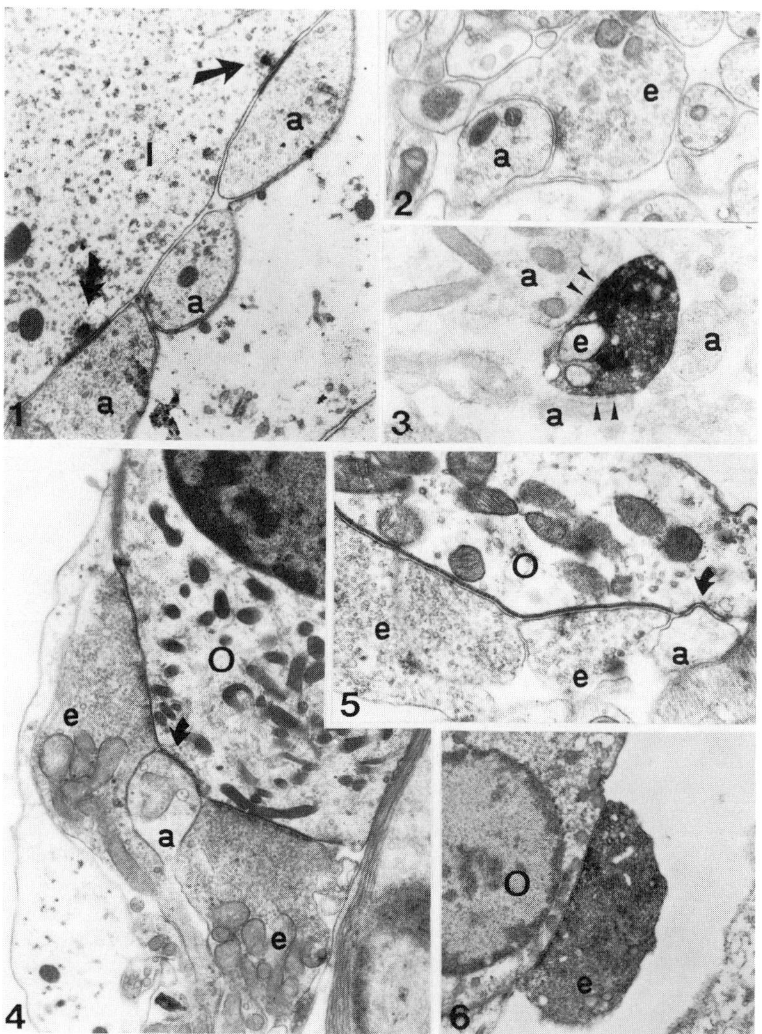

Fig. 1. IHC-afferent synapses. The IHC (I) is contacted by three afferent dendrites (a). Two clear synaptic specializations are seen (Arrows).

Fig. 2. Axo-dendritic synapse in the inner spiral bundle. An efferent varicosity (e) synapses with an auditory afferent dendrite (a).

Fig. 3. A vesiculated efferent varicosity (e) is immunostained with an antiserum against Met-enkephalin. It contacts three efferent dendrites (a) and synapses with two of them (arrowheads).

Figs. 4 and 5. Base of OHC's showing the large efferent (e) synapses and the small afferent boutons (a). Arrows point to an endocytotic profile (4) and to an efferent protuberance into the OHC (5).

Fig. 6. A large efferent varicosity (e) is immunostained with a monoclonal antibody against choline acetyltransferase.

The presynaptic membrane has specializations with a conical spicular shape. On the postsynaptic side, the dendritic membrane generally has an adjacent zone of dense material, sometimes also organized in spicules [44]. Two "atypical" efferent synapses at the IHC level have to be mentioned. First, there are some direct contacts between efferent fibers and IHC soma. They have been reported in the guinea pig [52] and in man [40]; they are an exception in other species [33,59], but are a common feature in young specimens [30,46,54]. Second, Liberman [33] noted some "en passant" efferent-efferent synapses in the cat, also found more recently in the guinea pig [19,20].

Advances have been made in understanding the chemical nature of these synapses. To date, different substances have been localized at the inner spiral bundle level and even within the lateral efferent varicosities. Met-enkephalin (ME) has been immunolocalized by light microscopy in the ISB [16,22,31]. ME-immunostained axo-dendritic synapses have been identified by electron microscopy (Fig. 3 [1,19]). Similarly, we have ultrastructurally immunolocalized two other pro-enkephalin-related peptides, ME-arginine-glycine-leucine [20] and synenkephalin [21], within efferent varicosities at axo-dendritic synapses. Moreover, two pro-dynorphin-related peptides, dynorphin B and neoendorphin, have also been detected at the ISB level [2]. More recently, choline-acetyl-transferase (ChAT) has been immunolocalized by light microscopy within the ISB [3]. Again using immunoelectron microscopy, we were able to localize ChAT in some vesiculated endings forming axodendritic synapses [17] indicating that these synapses probably use acetylcholine (ACh) as a neurotransmitter. Finally, a glutamate-decarboxylase (GAD)-like immunoreactivity has been detected in the ISB, with a predominantly apical distribution [23]; however, without electron microscopic data it is not possible to determine whether GABA is also present in axo-dendritic synapses. More precise anatomical studies together with physiological and pharmacological investigations are now needed to determine which of these substances acts as a neurotransmitter and/or cotransmitter in synapses of the lateral efferent system.

Axo-somatic efferent-OHC synapses. The basal pole of the OHC is directly connected by terminals from efferent fibers forming large axo-somatic synapses. It is almost certain that most of these fibers belong to the medial efferent system as defined by Warr and colleagues [63,64]. The axo-somatic efferent-OHC synapse was classically described in the first EM studies [14,25,51,57,59]. More recently, Nadol [41] has given a precise description of these synapses in the human cochlea.

A typical efferent synapse at the OHC level is shown in Figs. 4 and 5. Presynaptically, a swollen ending is filled with clear microvesicles of regular, spherical size (approximately 30 nm in diameter). Granular vesicles are very rare, in contrast with the efferent endings previously described at the IHC level. Near the presynaptic membrane, the vesicles often form small clusters in areas of low cytoplasmic density. The contact between the nerve ending and the OHC is often very large, as much as 3 or 5 um in some species (such as the cat and the rat). In a given species, the largest synapses are found at the base of the cochlea. The postsynaptic membrane is typically underlaid along its entire length by a subsurface cistern of reticulum closely apposed to the OHC membrane.

For different physiological [28] and morphological [26] reasons, these axo-somatic OHC-synapses have for years been considered to be cholinergic. Recent investigations using immunocytochemistry with a ChAT antibody show a clear labeling at the base of OHCs [3]. At the ultrastructural level, we have demonstrated that this ChAT immunostaining involves most of the vesiculated endings synapsing with OHCs (Fig. 6) [17]. However, the occurrence of ChAT-immunostained and unstained endings at the base of the same OHCs

[17], together with some positive results using GAD [23] and ME [22] antisera, suggests that ACh may not be the only transmitter involved in the efferent OHC-synapses.

A schematic drawing (Fig. 7) can serve as a visual summary of this chapter. The four morphological types of cochlear synapses are represented as well as the neural connections with the brain stem. Indications concerning putative neurotransmitters are given as references to our own findings.

NEUROANATOMICAL ORGANIZATION OF THE COCHLEA AND NIHL

Our understanding of the physiological properties of neural cochlear elements is far from complete. There are no major problems with respect to IHCs and their afferent synapses, but there are still many controversial questions concerning the exact role of the OHC-afferent synapse and the functions of the efferent systems. Consequently, little can be said about their physiopathology. Nevertheless, in light of the latest findings concerning the fine morphology and anatomical aspects of neurotransmitters described here, we can indicate some possible ways of linking the cochlear neurobiological organization with the problem of noise-induced hearing loss.

Direct alteration of neural elements following noise exposure

Although it is difficult to distinguish between direct and indirect (secondary degeneration) damage, some investigators have shown a clear relationship between sound-induced TTS and alteration of the synaptic pole of IHCs [34] and/or swelling of auditory dendrites [50,60]. This type of damage is considered to be reversible and partly responsible for reversible threshold shift.

Some results, which call for further investigation, include alterations of other neural elements such as the OHC synaptic pole [42], and the afferent and efferent endings at the OHC level [29]. Similarly, an increase in the density of efferent synaptic vesicles following exposure to intense sounds has also been suggested by Spoendlin [60].

Neurochemical Correlates of Noise Exposure

Several authors have used noise exposure in an attempt to determine cochlear auditory transmitters [13]. They have used basically the same procedure, i.e., sampling perilymph in silent and noisy periods. Results concerning the recepto-neural transmitter are not conclusive; Sewell et al. [53] refer to an "auditory nerve-activating substance", whereas Drescher et al. [13] propose a "GABA-like component". Moreover, in the same set of experiments, Drescher et al. [13] using high performance liquid chromatography (HPLC), detected an increase in a ME-like component in the perilymph after stimulation (115 dB SPL) on the borderline with respect to the physiological range of exposure. Using a specific radio-immuno autoradiography (RIA), we have recently checked the endogenous level of ME under various noise conditions. Animals that had been exposed to noise for 1 hour at 110 dB SPL showed approximately 50% decrease in ME content relative to controls (Cupo, Rebillard, Eybalin, 1985, unpublished observation). This result strongly indicates that ME, which is probably a lateral efferent neurotransmitter or cotransmitter, plays a role at high intensity levels, perhaps by reducing firing in auditory fibers.

Regardless of the nature of afferent and efferent neurotransmitters, one can postulate that the duration as well as the level of noise exposure

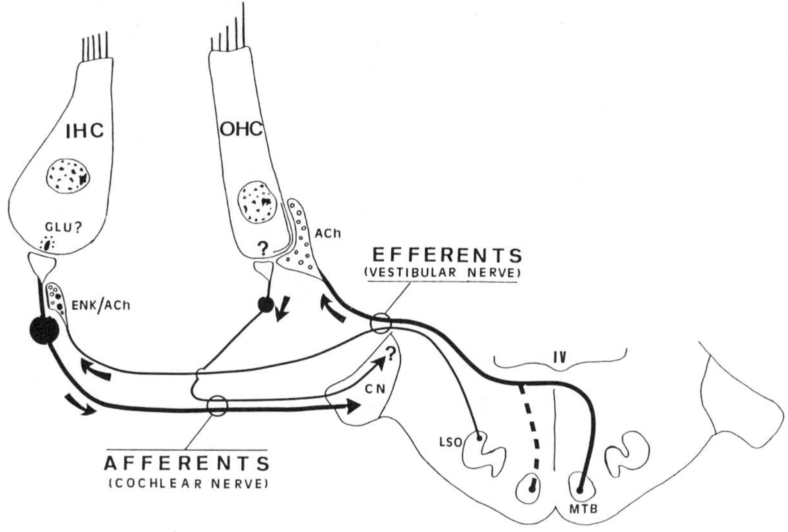

Fig. 7.

are directly related to the quantity of neurotransmitter used at the synapses. This, of course, means that the capacity for recycling, resynthesizing or replenishing presynaptic compartments could be one of the keys to TTS and its recovery. As already reported [65], this could be particularly true at neuropeptidergic synapses, because neuropeptides are only synthesized at the cell body level.

There are also data [8,48] suggesting that contralateral stimulation has a protective effect against TTS; this protection could well occur via an efferent loop [48]. In the case of a protective effect of monaural stimulation, Rajan and Johnstone [49] have considered that there can be no efferent participation because of the ineffectiveness of strychnine. But in fact, the lack of a strychnine effect does not rule out the role of an ipsilateral efferent system working with a non-strychnine-dependent neurotransmitter, such as ME [19].

A last comment can be made concerning synaptic organization at the OHC level. The large efferent cholinergic synapses (from the medial efferent systems) seem to play a role in modulating micromechanics [39,55], thus having an influence on sensitivity [5], frequency selectivity [7,55], and other nonlinear mechanisms [55]. The temporary loss of nonlinearity after noise exposure [36] may well depend on metabolic damage at this synaptic level, which modifies the motion of the cochlear partition [56].

In conclusion, it can be schematically proposed, according to Liberman and Mulroy [35], that whereas it is likely that PTS involves direct mechanical damage, TTS may at least partly depend on direct synaptic or, more generally, neurogenic alterations. Carrying the point further, it is possible to hypothesize that species differences in susceptibility to TTS are in some way related to differences in cochlear synaptology and particularly to differences in the afferent/efferent ratio.

ACKNOWLEDGEMENTS

Thanks are due to S. Ladrech and P. Sibleyras for technical support and to A. Bara for editorial assistance.

REFERENCES

1. R. A. Altschuler, M. H. Parakkal, J. A. Rubio, D. W. Hoffman, and J. Fex, Enkephalin-like immunoreactivity in the guinea pig organ of Corti: ultrastructural and lesion studies, Hearing Res., 16:17 (1984).
2. R. A. Altschuler, D. W. Hoffman, K. A. Reeks, and J. Fex, Localization of dynorphin B-like and alpha-neoendorphin-like immunoreactivities in the guinea pig organ of Corti, Hearing Res., 17:249 (1985).
3. R. A. Altschuler, B. Kachar, J. A. Rubio, M. H. Parakkal, and J. Fex, Immunocytochemical localization of choline acetyltransferase-like immunoreactivity in the guinea pig cochlea, Brain Res., 338:1 (1985).
4. D. Bodian, Electron microscopic atlas of the simian cochlea, Hearing Res., 9:201 (1983).
5. M. C. Brown, A. L. Nuttall, and R. I. Masta, Intracellular recordings from cochlear inner hair cells: effects of stimulation of the crossed olivocochlear efferents, Science, 222:69 (1983).
6. W. E. Brownell, Microscopic observation of cochlear hair cell motility, Scan. Electr. Microsc., III:1401 (1984).
7. E. Carlier and R. Pujol, Sectioning of the efferent bundle decreases cochlear frequency selectivity, Neurosci. Lett., 28:101 (1982).
8. A. R. Cody and B. M. Johnstone, Temporary threshold shift modified by binaural acoustic stimulation, Hearing Res., 6:199 (1982).
9. C. W. Cotman, A. Foster, and T. Lanthorn, An overview of glutamate as a neurotransmitter, in: "Glutamate as a Neurotransmitter," eds., G. di Chiara, and G. L. Gombos, pp. 1-27. Raven Press, New York (1981).
10. J. T. Coyle, Neurotoxic action of kainic acid, J. Neurochem., 41:1 (1983).
11. O. Densert, Adrenergic innervation in the rabbit cochlea, Acta Otolaryngol., 78:345 (1974).
12. O. Densert and A. Flock, An electron-microscopic study of adrenergic innervation in the cochlea, Acta Otolaryngol., 77:185 (1974).
13. M. J. Drescher, D. G. Drescher, and J. E. Medina, Effect of sound stimulation at several levels on concentrations of primary amines, including neurotransmitter candidates, in perilymph of the guinea pig inner ear, J. Neurochem., 41:309 (1983).
14. H. Engstrom, Electron microscopic study of the receptor cells of the organ of Corti, in: "Neural Mechanism of the Auditory and Vestibular System," eds., G. L. Rasmussen and S. F. Windle, pp. C. C. Thomas, Springfield, Illinois (1960).
15. M. Eybalin and R. Pujol, A radioautographic study of ['H]L-glutamate and ['H]L-glutamine uptake in the guinea pig cochlea, Neuroscience, 9:863 (1983).
16. M. Eybalin and R. Pujol, Immunofluorescence with met-enkephalin and leu-enkephalin antibodies in the guinea pig cochlea, Hearing Res., 13:135 (1984).
17. M. Eybalin and R. Pujol, Immunoelectron microscopic localization of choline acetyltransferase in two types of efferent (olivo-cochlear) synapses in the rat organ of Corti, Submitted to Exp. Br. Res., (1985).
18. M. Eybalin, A. Calas, and R. Pujol, Radioautographic study of the sympathetic fibers in the cochlea, Acta Otolaryngol., 96:69 (1983).
19. M. Eybalin, A. Cupo, and R. Pujol, Met-enkephalin characterization in the cochlea: high performance liquid chromatography and immuno-electron microscopy, Brain Res., 305:313 (1984).
20. M. Eybalin, A. Cupo, and R. Pujol, Met-enkephalin-Arg^6-Gly^7-Leu in the organ of Corti: high performance liquid chromatography and immuno-electron microscopy, Brain Res., 331:389 (1985).

21. M. Eybalin, L. Abou-Madi, J. Rossier, and R. Pujol, Electron microscopic localization of N-terminal proenkephalin (synenkephalin) immunostaining in the guinea pig organ of Corti, Brain Res., in press (1985).
22. J. Fex and R. A. Altschuler, Enkephalin-like immunoreactivity of olivocochlear nerve fibers in cochlea of guinea pig and cat, Proc. Natl. Acad. Sci. USA, 78:12b55 (1981).
23. J. Fex and R. A. Altschuler, Glutamic acid decarboxylase immunoreactivity of olivocochlear neurons in the organ of Corti of guinea pig and rat, Hearing Res., 15:123 (1984).
24. E. Hultcrantz, A. L. Nuttall, M. C. Brown, and M. Lawrence, The effect of cervical sympathectomy on cochlear electrophysiology, Acta Otolaryngol., 94:439 (1982).
25. S. Iurato, Efferent fibers to the sensory cells of Corti's organ, Exp. Cell Res., 27:162 (1962).
26. S. Iurato, Efferent innervation of the cochlea, in: "Auditory System, Anatomy-Physiology (Ear), Handbook of Sensory Physiology, Vol. V/1," eds., W. D. Keidel and W. D. Neff, Springer Verlag, Berlin (1974).
27. N. Y. S. Kiang, J. M. Rho, C. C. Nothrop, M. C. Liberman, and D. K. Ryugo, Hair-cell innervation by spiral ganglion cells in adult cats, Science, 217:175 (1982).
28. R. Klinke and N. Galley, Efferent innervation of vestibular and auditory receptors, Physiol. Rev., 54:316 (1974).
29. M. Lenoir and R. Pujol, Sensitive period to acoustic trauma in the rat pup cochlea, Acta Otolaryngol., 89:317 (1980).
30. M. Lenoir, A. Shnerson, and R. Pujol, Cochlear receptor development in the rat with emphasis on synaptogenesis, Anat. Embryol., 160:253 (1980).
31. J. I. Lehtosalo, J. Ylikoski, L. Eranko, O. Eranko, and P. Panula, Immunohistochemical localization of unique enkephalin sequences contained in preproenkephalin A in the guinea pig cochlea, Hearing Res., 16:101 (1984).
32. M. C. Liberman, Morphological differences among radial afferent fibers in the cat cochlea: an electron-microscopic study of serial sections, Hearing Res., 3:45 (1980).
33. M. C. Liberman, Efferent synapses in the inner hair cell area of the cat cochlea: an electron-microscopic study of serial sections. Hearing Res., 3:189 (1980).
34. M. C. Liberman and N. Y. S. Kiang, Acoustic trauma in cats, Cochlear pathology and auditory-nerve activity, Acta Otolaryngol., Suppl. 358 (1978).
35. M. C. Liberman and M. J. Mulroy, Acute and chronic effects of acoustic trauma: cochlear pathology and auditory nerve pathophysiology, in: "New Perspectives on Noise-Induced Hearing Loss," eds., R. P. Hamernik, D. Henderson, and R. Salvi, Raven Press, New York (1982).
36. J. H. Mills, Effects of noise on auditory sensitivity, psychophysical tuning curves, and suppression, in: "New Perspectives on Noise-Induced Hearing Loss," eds., R. P. Hamernik, D. Henderson, and R. Salvi, Raven Press, New York (1982).
37. D. K. Morest and B. A. Bohne, Noise-induced degeneration in the brain and representation of inner and outer hair cells, Hearing Res., 9:145 (1983).
38. D. Morrisson, R. A. Schindler, and J. Wersall, A quantitative analysis of the afferent innervation of the organ of Corti in guinea Pig, Acta Otolaryngol., 79:11 (1975).
39. D. C. Mountain, C. D. Geisler, and A. E. Hubbard, Stimulation of efferents alters the cochlear microphonic and the sound-induced resistance changes measured in scala media of the guinea pig, Hearing Res., 3:231 (1980).

40. J. B. Nadol, Jr., Serial section reconstruction of the neural poles of hair cells in the human organ of Corti, I. Inner hair cells, Laryngoscope, 93:599 (1983).
41. J. B. Nadol, Jr., Serial section reconstruction of the neural poles of hair cells in the human organ of Corti, II. Outer hair cells, Laryngoscope, 93:780 (1983).
42. T. Omata, I. Ohtani, K. Ohtsuki, Y. Ogawa, and J. Ouchi, Electron microscopical and histochemical studies of outer hair cells in acoustically exposed rabbits, Arch. Otorhinolaryngol., 222:127 (1979).
43. R. E. Perkins and D. K. Morest, A study of cochlear innervation patterns in cats and rats with the Golgi method and Nomarski optics, J. Comp. Neurol., 163:129 (1975).
44. R. Pujol and M. Lenoir, The four types of synapse in the organ of Corti, in: "Neurobiology of Hearing: The Cochlea," eds., R. A. Altschuler, D. W. Hoffman, and R. P. Bobbin, Raven Press, New York, in press (1985).
45. R. Pujol and A. Sans, Synaptogenesis in the mammalian inner ear, in: "Advances in Neural and Behavioral Development, V. 2, Auditory Development," ed., R. N. Aslin, Ablex Publ., Norwood, N.J., in press (1985).
46. R. Pujol, E. Carlier, and C. Devigne, Different patterns of cochlear innervation during the development in the kitten, J. Comp. Neurol., 117:529 (1978).
47. R. Pujol, M. Lenoir, D. Robertson, M. Eybalin, and B. M. Johnstone, Kainic acid selectivity alters auditory dendrites connected with cochlear inner hair cells, Hearing Res., 18:145 (1985).
48. R. Rajan and B. M. Johnstone, Crossed cochlear influences on monaural temporary threshold shifts, Hearing Res., 9:279 (1983)
49. R. Rajan and B. M. Johnstone, Residual effects in monaural temporary threshold shifts to pure tones, Hearing Res., 12:185 (1983).
50. D. Robertson, Functional significance of dendritic swelling after loud sounds in the guinea pig cochlea, Hearing Res., 9:263 (1983).
51. E. L. Rodriguez-Echandia, An electron microscopic study on the cochlear innervation. I. The recepto-neural junctions at the outer hair cells, Zeitschift fur Zellforschung, 78:30 (1967).
52. K. Saito, Fine structure of the sensory epithelium of guinea pig organ of Corti: subsurface cisternae and lamellar bodies in outer hair cells, Cell Tissue Res., 229:467 (1980).
53. W. F. Sewell, C. H. Norris, M. Tachibana, and P. S. Guth, Detection of an auditory nerve-activating substance, Science, 202:910 (1978).
54. A. Shnerson, C. Devigne, and R. Pujol, Age-related changes in the C57BL/6J mouse cochlea, II. Ultrastructural findings, Dev. Brain Res., 37:373 (1982).
55. J. H. Siegel and D. O. Kim, Efferent neural control of cochlear mechanics? Olivocochlear bundle stimulation affects cochlear biomechanical nonlinearity, Hearing Res., 6:171 (1982).
56. J. H. Siegel and D. O. Kim, Cochlear biomechanics: vulnerability to acoustic trauma and other alterations as seen in neural responses and ear-canal sound pressure, in: "New Perspectives on Noise-Induced Hearing Loss," eds., R. P. Hamernik, D. Henderson, and R. Salvi, Raven Press, New York (1982).
57. C. A. Smith and F. S. Sjostrand, Structure of the nerve endings on the external hair cells of the guinea pig cochlea as studied by serial sections, J. Ultrastruct. Res., 5:523 (1961).
58. H. M. Sobkowicz, J. L. Rose, G. E. Scott, and S. M. Slapnick, Ribbon synapses in the developing intact and cultured organ of Corti in the mouse, J. Neurosci., 7:942 (1982).
59. H. Spoendlin, The organization of the cochlear receptor, Adv. Oto-Rhino-Laryngol., 13:1 (1966).

60. H. Spoendlin, Primary structural changes in the organ of Corti after acoustic overstimulation, Acta Otolaryngol., 71:166 (1971).
61. H. Spoendlin, Neural connections of the outer hair cell system, Acta Otolaryngol., 87:381 (1979).
62. H. Spoendlin and W. Lichtensteiger, The adrenergic innervation of the labyrinth, Acta Otolaryngol., 61:423 (1966).
63. W. B. Warr and J. J. Guinan, Efferent innervation of the organ of Corti: two separate systems, Brain Res., 173:152 (1979).
64. J. S. White and W. B. Warr, The dual origins of the olivocochlear bundle in the albino rat, J. Comp. Neurol., 219:203 (1983).
65. J. Ylikoski and J. Lehtosalo, Neurochemical basis of auditory fatigue: a new hypothesis, Acta Otolaryngol., 99:353 (1985).

DISCUSSION

Trahiotis: About 1970, Don Elliott and I published a paper in which we measured TTS in some animals in a control group. After having cut the crossed olivocochlear bundle, we measured the amount of TTS and then let the animals recover. We did this four times. Although we did not expect it, we found that the animals that had the bundle cut got the same amount of TTS each of the four times. The normal animals showed a toughening effect like Miller and Watson found. Perhaps there is something in this data that are related to what you are speaking about.

Patuzzi: Ramesh Rajan working in Australia has done a rather elegant series of experiments working the the COCB effects. He has done a series of lesion studies where he has cut the COCB. He has also done a series of destruction experiments where he has destroyed the contralateral ear and a series of strychnine injections looking at the so called protective effect. Both destruction of the contralateral ear and also preexposure on the contralateral ear, the so-called priming effect, toughened the cochlea. It appears as if there is a central priming effect., i.e., a protective effect presumably by the COCB fibers acting on the outer hair cells.

THE MORPHOLOGY OF THE NORMAL AND PATHOLOGICAL CELL MEMBRANE AND JUNCTIONAL COMPLEXES OF THE COCHLEA

Andrew Forge

Institute of Laryngology and Otology,
330-332 Gray's Inn Road, London, WC1X 8EE, U.K.

INTRODUCTION

Examination of the cell membranes in the cochlea is of some importance. Much of the normal functioning in the cochlea is dependent upon cell membrane properties and activities and on the presence of membrane specializations such as intercellular junctions. Further, there is evidence that in some forms of cochlear pathology effects on cell membranes are significant events. For example, the ototoxicity of aminoglycosides is thought to be related to specific interactions of the drugs with particular membrane lipids to produce alterations to membrane structure and function [1,2].

Structural characteristics of membranes may be studied most readily by freeze-fracture [3], a technique for preparing tissue for examination by transmission electron microscopy in which large face views of membranes are exposed. The membrane faces reveal details of membrane structural organization. In non-junctional regions, the faces are covered with particles, "intra membrane particles" (IMP) or show complementary pits. The IMP represent membrane intercalated proteins. Their density and distribution is a reflection of the membrane's function and may vary between different cells and in any particular cell with physiological activity or pathology. Morphometric analysis of particle distribution can be of great value in assessing alterations to membrane structure [4]. Cell junctions also are easily recognizable. Tight junctions, (zonulae occludentes) which act as seals between cells preventing passive diffusion along an intercellular pathway, appear as a series of ridges or grooves (Figs. 1,4,12). There is some correlation between the number of tight junctional strands and the degree of impermeability of the junction [5]. Gap-junctions, which act as sites of direct cell-to-cell communication across the intercellular space, appear as a two-dimensional array of large particles (Figs. 2,14). These particles represent the sites of channels linking the cytoplasms of adjacent cells through which molecules up to the size of small nucleotides may pass [6]. The presence of gap-junctions may enable electrical and ionic coupling between cells.

Further characterization of membrane structural organization is possible by attempting to localize specific membrane components [7]. The most widely employed procedure has been the use of probes, filipin and saponin, which specifically interact with cholesterol to produce visible deformations on membrane fracture faces. With filipin, such "complexes" appear as

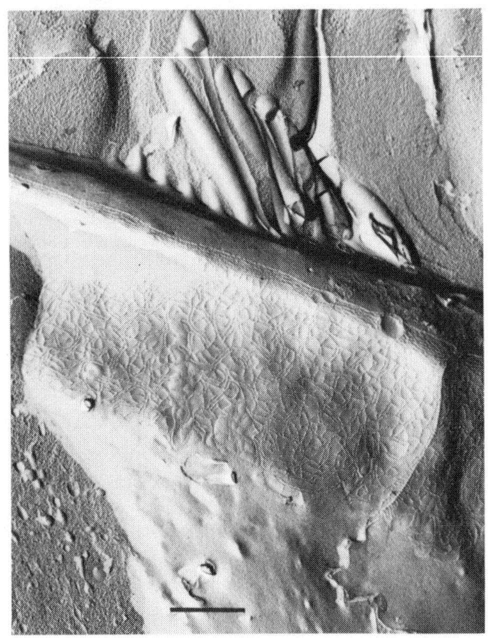

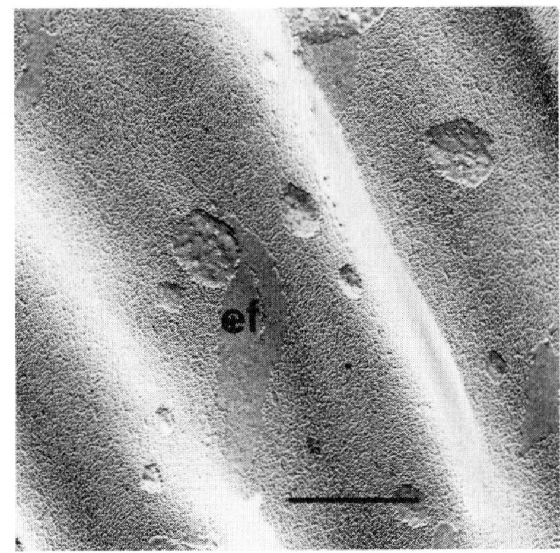

Figs. 1-2. Fig. 1, left: Tight cell junction in the reticular lamina between a supporting cell and an OHC. Note the depth and complexity of the network of strands. Bar = 1.0um. Fig. 2, right: Large gap junction particle array on the membrane of the region of a pillar cell. ef = complementary pits on the membrane face of the adjacent cell. Bar = 0.5 um.

25 nm mounds and depressions (Figs. 4,5). Although detailed interpretation of results requires some caution [7], consistent differences between membranes in their response to filipin or changes in the pattern of response in a particular membrane, indicate structural differences or changes in the membrane.

The purpose of this paper is to illustrate the value of freeze-fracture techniques to studies of the cochlea. Certain features of the membranes in the normal organ of Corti as revealed by standard methods and after filipin treatment are described briefly. It is also shown that various alterations of membranes, identifiable by freeze-fracture, occur in the early stages of the response of the stria vascularis to loop diuretics and to aminoglycoside antibiotics. Several previous reports have presented detailed descriptions of membrane morphology in the normal cochlea following routine freeze-fracture [8-14]. For the work presented here, albino and pigmented guinea pigs and gerbils (Meriones unquiculatus) have been used. Protocols for acute diuretic (ethacrynic acid and furosemide) and chronic gentamicin treatment and for preparation of tissue for filipin labelling and freeze-fracture have been published elsewhere [14-18].

RESULTS AND DISCUSSION

Organ of Corti

i) Tight junctions. Tight junctions are present in the reticular lamina at the apex of the lateral membranes of sensory cells and supporting cells. The system of tight junctional strands is extensive and complex

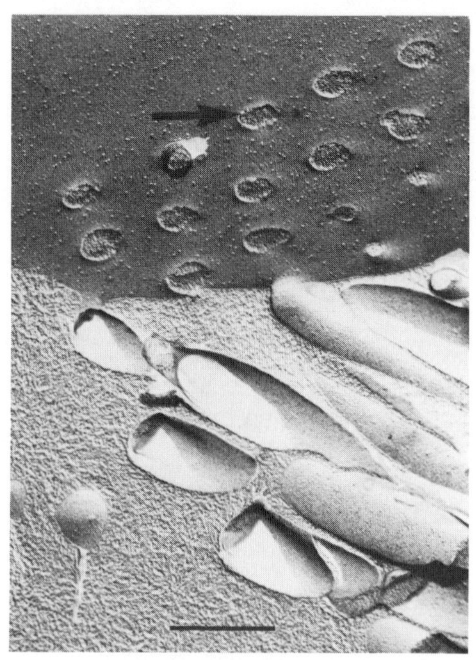

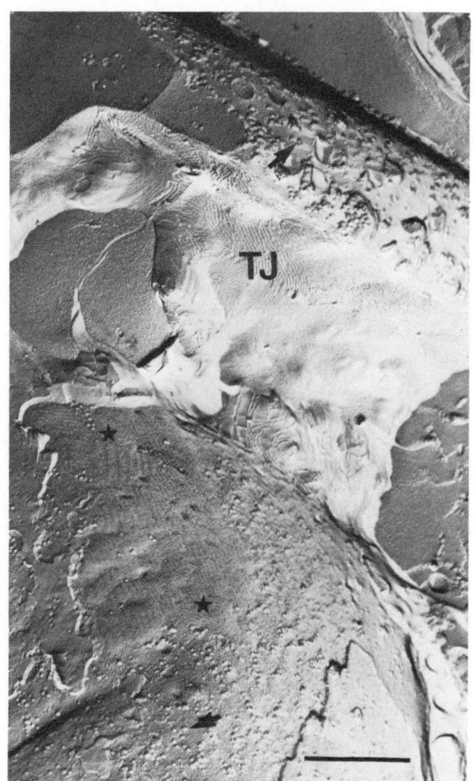

Figs. 3-4. Fig. 3, left: Apical membrane of an OHC with stereocilia. The apical and stereocilial membranes appear similar, displaying dispersed IMP. Internal structure of stereocilia revealed by cross-fracture (arrow). Bar = 0.5 um. Fig. 4, right: IHC after treatment with filipin which produces discrete membrane deformations (arrows). On lateral membranes, tight junction (TJ) and characteristic particle arrays (*) show no visible response. AP = apical membrane. Bar = 1.0 um.

(Fig. 1). The presence of this unusually extensive tight junctional network presumably means that there is extremely effective occlusion of the intercellular space between cells in the organ of Corti preventing passive diffusion of ions between the fluid at the hair cell apex and that around the hair cell body, thereby enabling maintenance of ionic and potential differences between endolymph and perilymph. The loss of a hair cell, either following noise trauma or as a result of the effects of aminoglycosides, potentially will lead to breaches of this barrier. However, recent thin-section and SEM studies of hair cell loss consequent upon chronic gentamicin treatment [18] have suggested that maintenance of tight junctions and formation of new ones may allow for hair cell loss without leaks across the reticular lamina occurring. Further freeze-fracture studies to establish this are currently underway.

ii) Gap-junctions. Gap-junctions in the organ of Corti appear to be exclusively associated with supporting cells. Small junctions infrequently are present on the membranes of the head region of Deiter's cells just below the level of the tight junctions; towards the base of the cell phalanges numerous gap-junctions are observed. On the membrane of the cell body region of pillar cells, the gap-junctions are remarkably extensive, occupying a significant portion of the membrane (Fig. 2). The role of the gap-junctions is not clear. It has been shown that current injections into a supporting cell are able to spread into uninjected supporting cells [19], indicating functional ionic coupling of the cells, presumably via the gap-junctions. It has been suggested that the coupling may provide a nutritive role in the organ of Corti [19].

iii) Outer and inner hair cells. Three distinct membrane regions, apart from the tight junctions, can be identified in both inner and outer hair cells: the apical membrane and stereocilia, the lateral membrane, and the synaptic region. Each of these shows characteristic features, but particularly in relation to the lateral membrane, there are obvious differences between IHC and OHC. The apical membranes of both cell types show relatively few dispersed IMP (Fig. 3), but some workers [12] have reported significantly fewer IMP on the IHC apical membrane than on that of the OHC. The stereocilia membranes appear similar to the respective apical membranes (Fig. 3) and where stereocilia are cross-fractured, the fibrillar nature of the core is recognizable (Fig. 3). The membrane contour of the stereocilium normally appears regular with no blebs or vesiculations. The hair cell apical membranes respond intensely to filipin (Figs. 4,5). However, the stereocilia membranes of the IHC (Fig. 6) consistently show a much higher density of deformations than those of the OHC (Fig. 5). This could indicate some significant difference in structural organization between the stereocilia membranes of inner and outer hair cells.

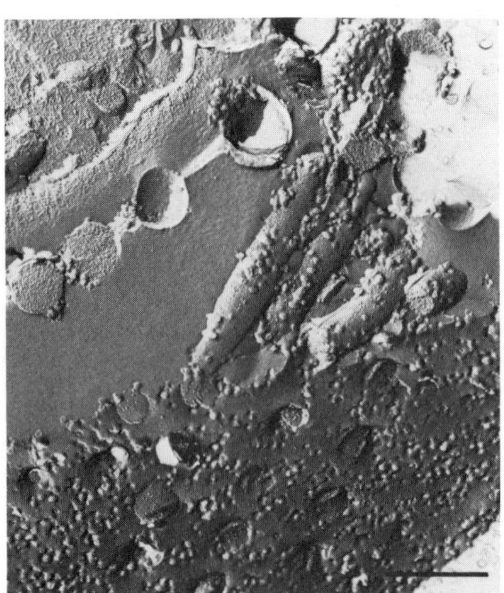

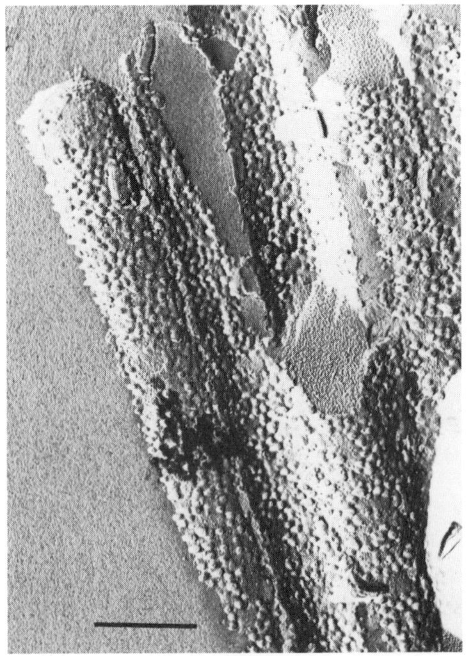

Figs. 5-6. Fig. 5, left: Apical membrane of OHC: the effect of filipin on the stereocilia membrane; deformations are relatively dispersed. Bar = 0.5 um. Fig. 6, right: IHC stereocilia: effect of filipin. Complexes are much more densely packed than on OHC stereocilia membrane (Fig. 5). Bar = 0.5 um.

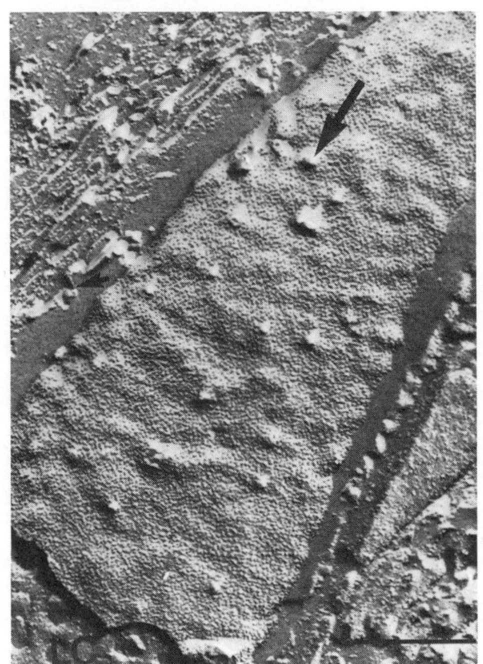

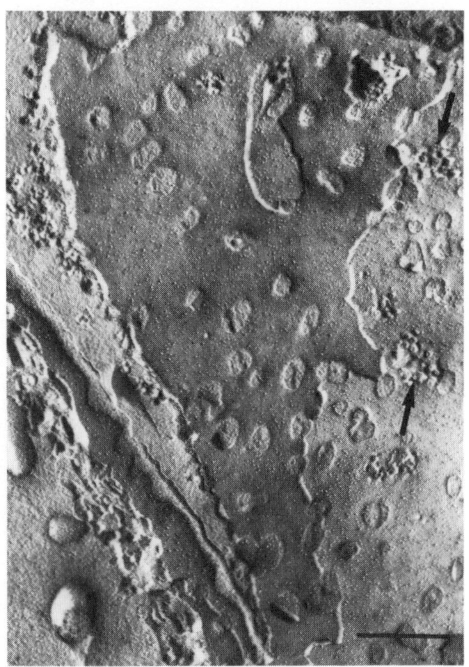

Figs. 7-8. Fig. 7, left: Lateral membrane of OHC. Large IMP are densely distributed and occasional filipin deformations (large arrow) present. Apparent undulation of membrane face correlates with the appearance of the cross-fractured plasma membrane of adjacent OHC (small arrow). LC = lateral cistermal membrane. Bar = 0.5 um. Fig. 8, right: Lateral cisternal membrane of OHC and effects of filipin. Dispersed clusters of deformations (arrows) present of fenestrated membrane sheets. Bar = 0.5 um.

The tight junctions separate the apical membrane from the lateral membrane (Figs. 1,4). On the lateral membrane of the IHC (Fig. 4), IMP are present in much greater numbers than on the apical membrane and are randomly and homogeneously distributed. This membrane, however, is characterized by the presence of plaques of large particles in rectilinear array (Fig. 4). Such plaques are found exclusively in non-junctional and non-synaptic regions (Fig. 4) and their functional significance is not known. The IHC lateral membrane responds to filipin except in the regions of the particle arrays (Fig. 4). The absence of filipin-induced deformations in this region (and also from the tight junction area) is most likely due to structural constraints preventing development of a visible response. In contrast, the lateral membrane of the OHC is characterized by the presence of closely packed large particles (Fig. 7) and filipin-induced deformations are seen only rarely. The membrane appears to undulate, which correlates with the corrugated appearance of the OHC plasma membrane when cross-fractured (Fig. 7) and in thin sections. Fracture of the lateral OHC membrane in the plane of the membrane, as illustrated in Fig. 7, is a rare occurrence. Usually, this membrane is cross-fractured. This fact and the presence of a very high density of large IMP suggests that the membrane is very rich in proteins. Their presence may impair development of a response to filipin. It is possible that some of these proteins have a structural role, perhaps the anchoring of links between the plasma membrane and the underlying lateral cisternae [20]. The lateral cisternae of the OHC themselves are exposed as extensive, fenestrated membrane sheets (Figs. 7,8).

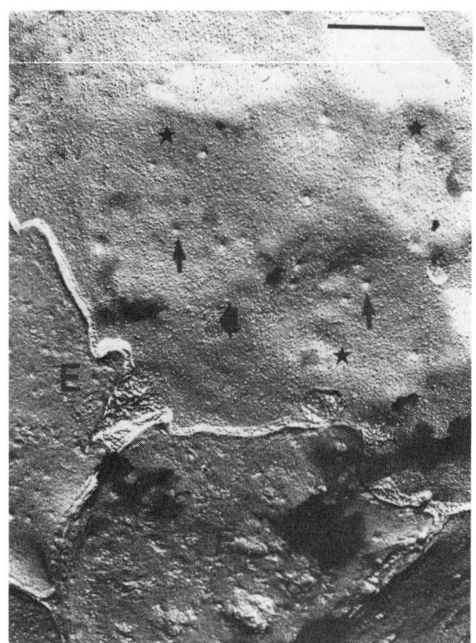

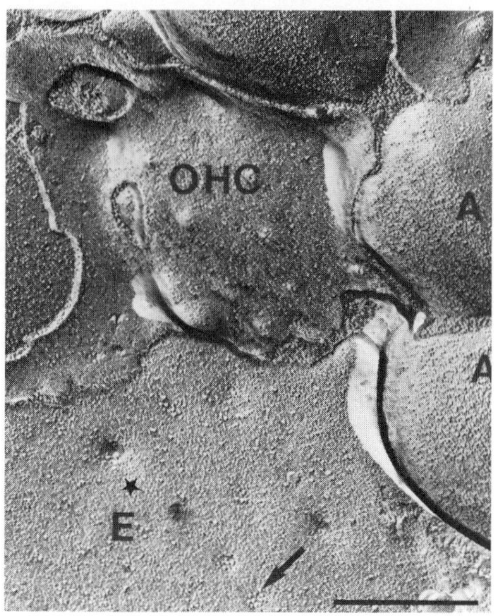

Figs. 9-10. Fig. 9, left: Membrane face of OHC in synaptic region. Impressions of afferent endings induce facets (*) within which are small invaginations (small arrows). Membrane face shows clusters of large particles (large arrows) and smaller IMP. E = efferent endings. Bar = 0.5 um. Fig. 10, right: Afferent and efferent endings. IMP is closely packed in post-synaptic region of afferent ending. OHC membrane overlying afferent ending (OHC) shows invaginations. On membrane of efferent endings (E), large particles clustered especially at sites of invaginations (arrow) and smaller IMP non-homogeneously distributed to leave IMP-free areas (*). Bar = 0.5 um.

There are certain differences in the IMP patterning on the succeeding cisternal sheets which have been described in detail elsewhere [12]. After treatment of cochlear tissue with filipin, the membranes of the lateral cisternae show infrequent clusters of filipin-cholesterol complexes (Fig. 8). Interestingly, a similar pattern of response to filipin has been observed on the membranes of the sarcoplasmic reticulum of muscle cells [7,21].

The synaptic region of the OHC membrane (Fig. 9) may be recognized by the faceting produced by the impressions of the nerve endings. The membrane is clearly different from the lateral membrane. The membrane face (Fig. 9) shows clusters of medium size particles and randomly distributed smaller IMP. Invaginations into the cell, reminiscent of sites of fusion of vesicles with the membrane, are present on the hair cell membrane at the locations of the synapses with afferent nerve endings (Figs. 9,10). The afferent nerve endings appear as mounds at the summit of which the immediate post-synaptic region displays a close clustering of particles (Fig. 10). The larger afferent endings are readily distinguishable, although in some ways resembling the synaptic region of the OHC membrane. Clusters of large particles, sometimes associated with invaginations, and smaller IMP are present. Distinct bare (i.e., IMP-free) regions are also apparent. This latter feature is emphasized in filipin treated tissue (Fig. 11). Deformations are confined to the particle bearing areas, thus defining

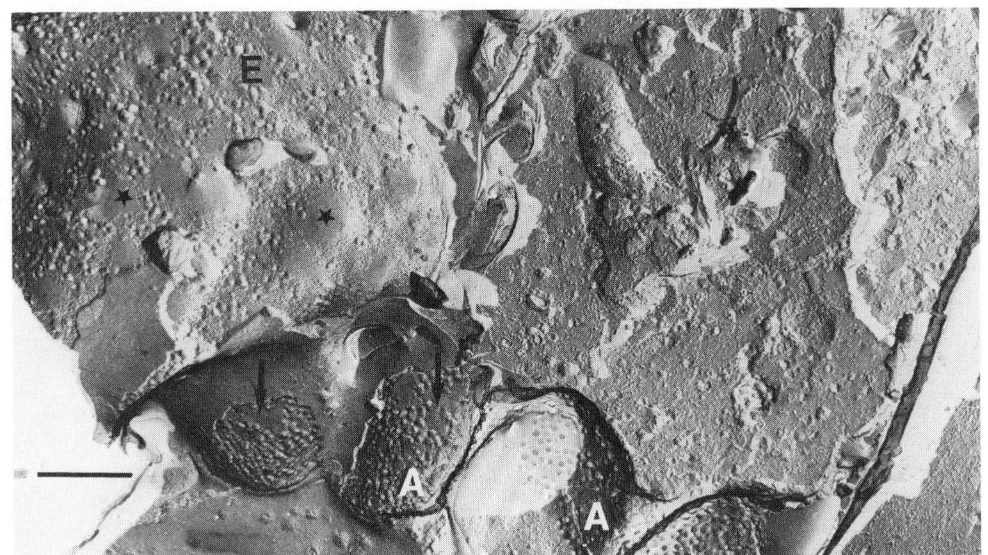

Fig. 11. Filipin-labelling over nerve-endings. On efferent endings (E) complexes are dispersed and areas with neither complexes nor IMP are exposed (*). On afferent endings (A), complexes are closely packed, but bare areas are also revealed (arrow). Bar = 0.5 um.

clear particle- and filipin lesion-deficient patches. On afferent endings, filipin induces closely clustered deformations, but here again patches of membrane not showing a visible response to filipin are revealed (Fig. 11). At present it is not possible to interpret fully the significance of these observations, but the results do show the variety of details of membrane structural organization revealed by freeze-fracture techniques.

Stria Vascularis

i) Tight junctions. Tight junctions are present around the necks of marginal cells towards the endolymphatic aspect of the lateral membrane (Fig. 12). A complex and an unusually extensive tight-junctional network is also present between basal cells. The entire lateral membrane of these cells is covered by an anastomosing system of ridges and grooves (Fig. 13). Studies using electron dense tracers [15] have shown that both marginal cell and basal cell tight junctions prevent passage of tracers, and presumably other materials, into the stria. Thus, the stria is effectively sealed from the rest of the cochlea.

ii) Gap-junctions. Nearly all gap-junctions in the stria appear to be associated with basal cells [16]. They are present between adjacent basal cells, between basal and marginal cells, and basal and intermediate cells. The junctions between adjacent basal cells are present in the islands between the strands of the tight junctional network (Fig. 13). On that membrane of the basal cell which faces the rest of the stria, the junctions are button-like (Fig. 14) and quite numerous; up to 15% of the area of this membrane is occupied by gap-junctions [16]. Gap-junctions are also present between basal cells and cells in the spiral ligament which in turn possess gap-junctions between each other. Cells in the spiral ligament have been shown to possess Na^+-K^+-ATPase [22]. It is also apparent that potassium in endolymph, maintained by activity of the strial marginal cells is derived

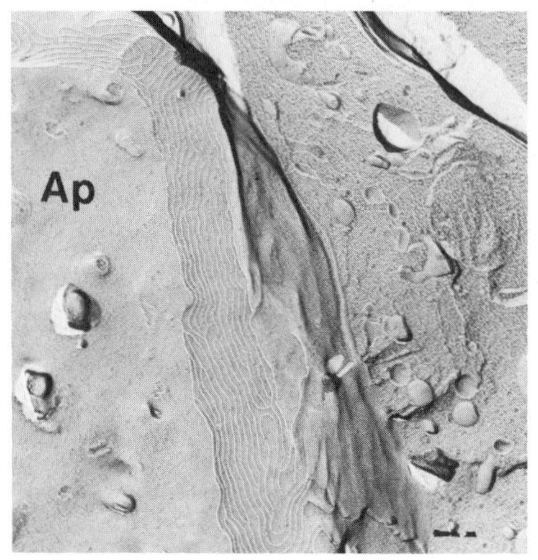

Fig. 12. Tight junction of strial marginal cell. The junction is composed of separate continuous strands parallel to the apical membrane. The lateral membrane below the level of the junction shows few discontinuities. Ap = apical membrane. Bar = 0.1 um.

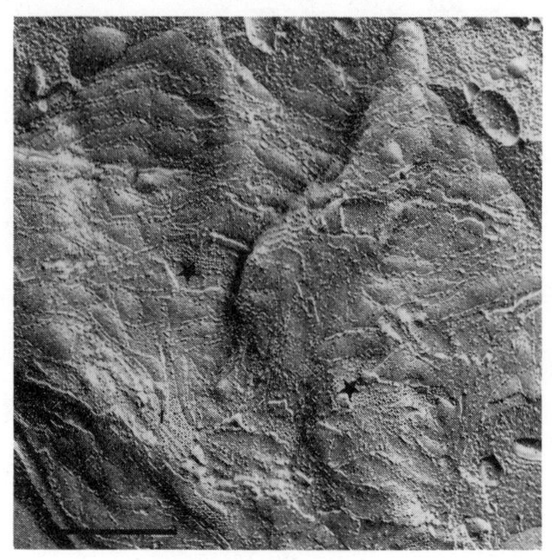

Fig. 13. Strial basal cell lateral membrane shows a complex network of tight junctional strands with gap junctions (*) enclosed in the islands between strands. Bar = 0.1 um.

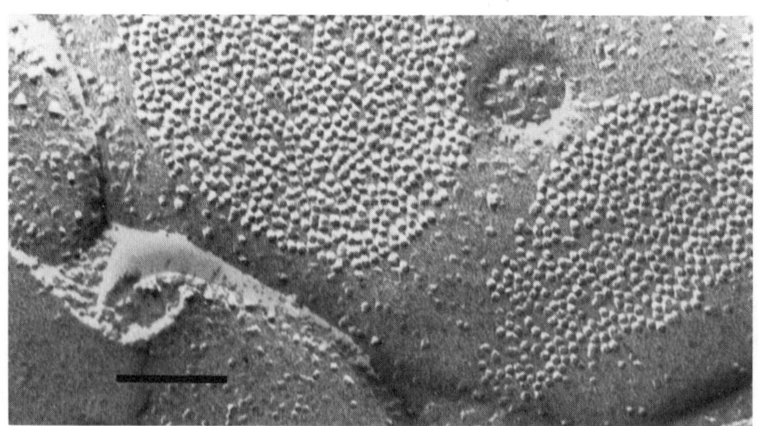

Fig. 14. Gap junctions of basal cell with intermediate or marginal cells are button-like. Junction morphology may be assessed by measuring interparticle spacing (Fig. 20). Bar = 0.1 um.

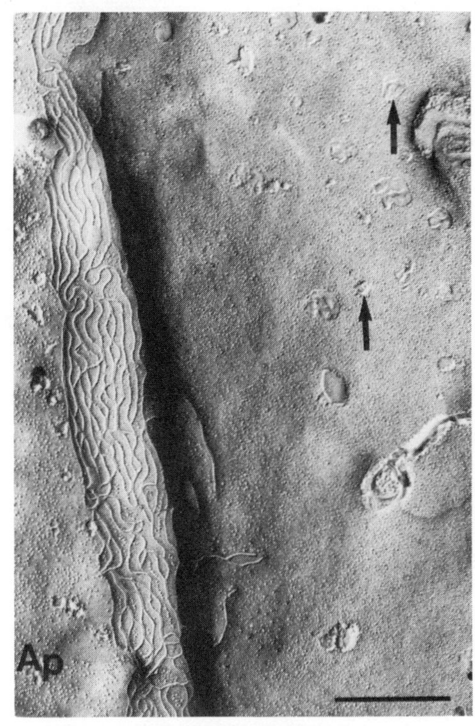

Fig. 15. Lateral membrane of marginal cell following chronic genamicin treatment. Tight junction strands are fused, discontinuous, and disoriented and basally the membrane shows irregular discontinuities (arrows). Ap = apical membrane. Bar = 0.5 um.

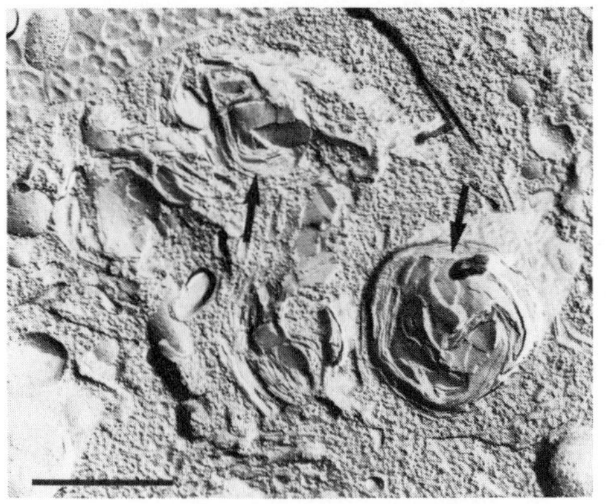

Fig. 16. Apical region of a marginal cell following gentamicin treatment showing presence of lipid bodies (arrows), characterized by stacked, smooth-surfaced fracture-faces. Bar = 0.5 um.

from perilymph [23,24]. It has, therefore, been suggested that the strial gap-junctions may be the route whereby K^+ enters the stria. If this is so, the predominant association of gap-junctions with basal cells and their distribution may indicate that this cell type has some important role in strial functioning.

Effects of aminoglycosides and diuretics on strial membrane structure

i) Aminoglycosides. Aminoglycosides are thought to interact with cell membrane lipids in the cochlea. An initial reversible interaction with anionic phospholipids is followed by a specific irreversible binding to particular lipids polyphosphoinositides (PPI) [2]. These interactions produce alterations to membrane structure and function. PPI's are present at significant levels in both the organ of Corti and stria. On examination of the stria immediately following the end of a course of chronic gentamicin treatment (100 mg/Kg daily for 10 days), abnormalities were found on the membranes of marginal cells. In the tight junction, which normally shows a series of separate strands oriented parallel to each other and to the apical membrane (Fig. 12), the strands were often fused, discontinuous and disoriented (Fig. 15). The lateral membrane of the marginal cell in

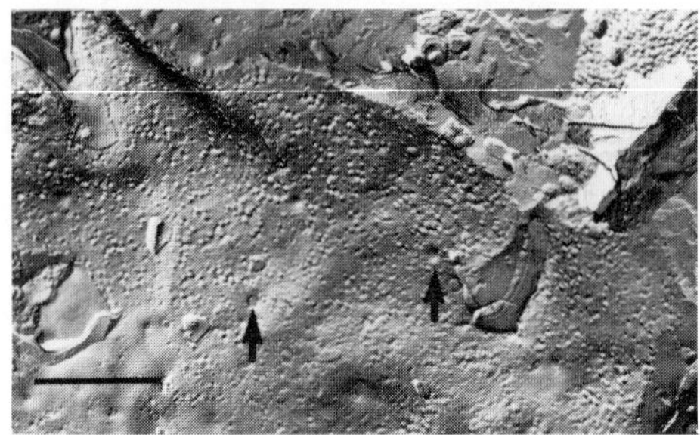

Fig. 17. Effect of filipin on the membrane of a normal intermediate cell. Complexes are dispersed but excluded from the region of pinocytotic vesicle opening (arrow). Bar = 1.0 um.

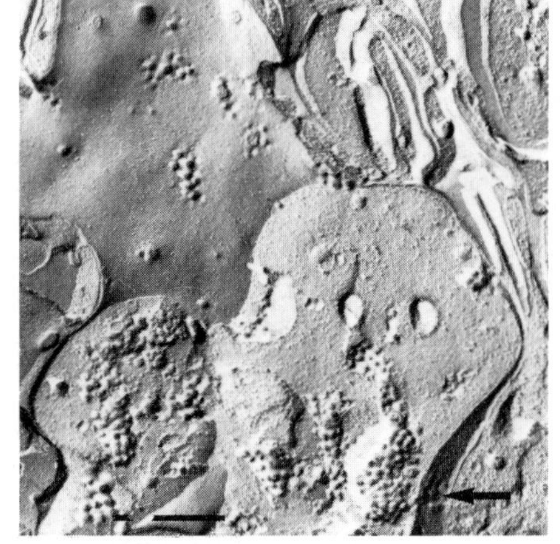

Fig. 18. Effect of filipin on intermediate cell membrane following diuretic treatment. Deformations are clustered on the membrane. Arrow indicates point of continuity between clusters on the plasma membrane and filipin-affected intracellular membranes. Intercellular spaces are not greatly enlarged. (From Ref. 17). Bar = 0.5 um.

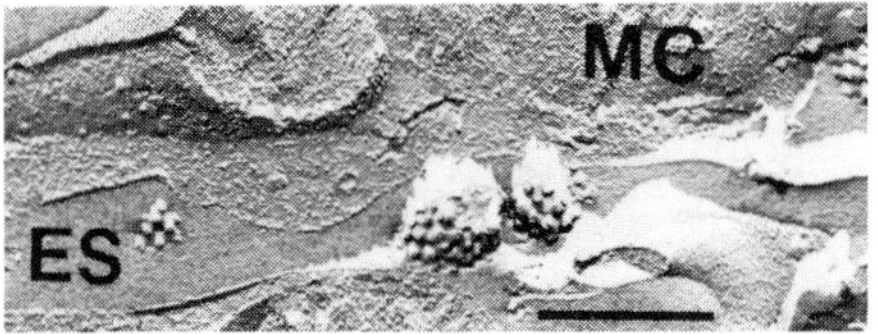

Fig. 19. Ethacrynic acid affected stria in which oedema is present. Membranes of vesicles within extracellular space show an intense response to filipin (arrows). MC = marginal cell, ES = extracellular space. Bar = 0.5 um.

the cell body region also showed alterations. Whereas normally this membrane appears uninterrupted, in the tissue from the treated animals, numerous irregular discontinuities were present (Fig. 15). In some cases, lipid bodies, which appeared in the cytoplasm of marginal cells in tissue from treated animals (Fig. 16), could be seen to be continuous with the plasma membrane. All these features were observed immediately following the end of treatment when there were few other indications of effects of the stria and before any hair cell loss occurred. Thus, they indicate that alterations to marginal cell membranes may be an early consequence of the

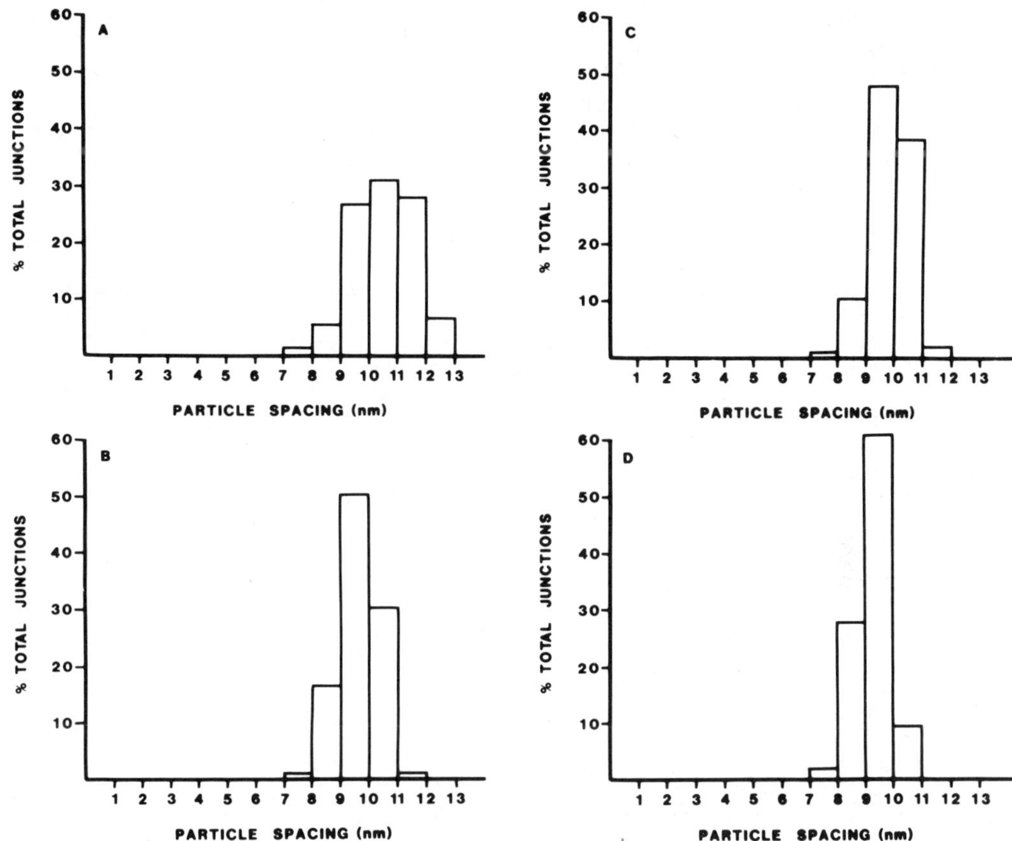

Fig. 20. Histograms of distribution frequency of spacings of gap junction particles in control (A) and ethacrynic acid-affected tissue (B). The EA-affected samples are divisible into two groups: C, in which intercellular spaces had not developed ("early") and D, in which intercellular spaces were enlarged ("late"). There is a distinct shift to smaller spacings in EA-affected tissue (compare A with B). There is a significant change even at the earliest times (C) which becomes greater as intercellular spaces enlarge (D). From Ref. 16.

effects of gentamicin. Several possible interpretations could account for these findings, so at present their significance is not known. However, very recently, freeze-fracture studies of liposomes, model membranes of known composition, in which either an anionic phospholipid or PPI were present, have shown structurally identifiable effects of gentamicin on the lipid bilayers (Forge, Zajic, Schacht and Weiner, unpublished). This indicates that study of the aminoglycoside-damaged cochlea by freeze-fracture may be useful in identifying the initial lesions caused by these agents.

ii) Loop diuretics. The loop diuretics affect the stria, causing a reversible inhibition of active transport processes, decline in endolymphatic potential (EP) and extensive oedema [25,26]. Freeze-fracture has shown a number of alterations to strial membranes many of which appear to be present before functional and structural alterations are well advanced [14,16,17,27]. Quantitation of features of marginal cell tight junctions has been reported [27] to show that the effects of some, but not all, diuretics induce alterations to the number, density and depth of strands. The significance of this is not clear, as the junctions continue to prevent the passage of electron dense tracers even when oedema is well advanced [15]. The alterations to tight-junction morphology may be a reflection of mechanical stresses [28] imposed by the enlargement of intercellular spaces and swelling of the apical cytoplasm of the marginal cell [26].

Effects on intermediate cell membranes also occur. An apparent redistribution of IMP on the membrane resulting in the formation of particle-free areas has been noted [14]. These were observed at times when EP is only minimally depressed and intercellular spaces were not greatly enlarged. When such tissue was treated with filipin, similar indications of alteration to membrane structure were seen. In normal tissue, filipin-cholesterol complexes are relatively homogeneously distributed over intermediate cell membranes (Fig. 17). In the diuretic-affected tissue, these membranes showed clusters of complexes (Fig. 18). Some of the clusters appeared to be continuous with intracellular membranes also showing clusters (Fig. 18). It may well be that the particle-free areas seen by routine freeze-fracture procedures are analagous to the regions showing clusters of complexes. Certainly these results indicate some alteration of intermediate cell membrane structural organization occurring early in the sequence of events consequent upon diuretic-induced inhibition in the stria.

As intercellular spaces in the stria enlarge, intermediate cells undergo a remarkable shrinkage and membranous vesicles appear in the extracellular spaces [14]. Many of these arise from intermediate cells and after routine freeze-fracture appear to possess IMP-deficient membranes indicating a high lipid ratio [14]. In tissue treated with filipin, these vesicle membranes showed an intense reaction to the probe (Fig. 17), suggesting a high cholesterol content. It is possible, therefore, that in response to the effects of diuretics, intermediate cells release cholesterol from the membrane, enabling them rapidly to alter shape and shrink.

A further alteration in the stria as a consequence of acute diuretic treatment is to the morphology of gap-junctions [16]. Significant reduction in the centre-to-centre spacing of the particles which constitute the freeze-fracture image of the gap-junction (Figs. 13,14) have been reported [16]. In unaffected tissue, the mean spacing was 10.4 nm + 0.96 (SD) while in tissue from diuretic-treated animals the mean was 9.5 nm + 0.65. A significant shift to smaller spacings could be discerned even before oedema began to develop (Fig. 20) and this effect became more pronounced as the intercellular spaces enlarged. Reduction of gap-junction interparticle spacing has been correlated with closure of junctional channels and uncoupling of cells in a number of tissues [6,29]. Therefore, these results could indicate that one of the earliest responses to the effects of diuretics in the stria is the uncoupling of cells. If gap-junctions serve to supply K^+ to the stria, then this could be of significance to the development of the functional and structural disturbances produced by diuretics. However, there is some dispute about the significance of morphological peculiarities of gap-junctions [6,29] and the difficulties of drawing functional conclusions from structural data should be emphasized.

CONCLUSIONS

The membranes of the different cells in the stria show a variety of structural characteristics which are easily visualized following freeze-fracture. By attempting to localize cholesterol using filipin, further indications of differences in structural organization may be consistently revealed. These features are of use in assessing early effects of agents which impair cochlear function. Both non-junctional and junctional regions may be examined quantitatively. The features of gap- and tight junctions are easily assessed. Effects in non-junctional regions may be emphasized by the use of procedures which label particular membrane components.

Besides studies of membrane structure, freeze-fracture procedures can also enable investigation of intracellular organization. Recently developed procedures for ultrarapid freezing of tissue allow "etching" of fractured surfaces to expose structures in and around the cell at high resolution. The use of such methods to examine hair cells [30] shows the organization of the structural components of stereocilia in great detail. The further development of the use of such techniques holds out the prospect of the structural examination of relatively subtle changes in cells in relation to hearing impairment.

ACKNOWLEDGEMENT

This work was supported by the Wellcome Trust and the Medical Research Council.

REFERENCES

1. J. Schacht, Biochemistry of neomycin ototoxicity, J. Acoust. Soc. Am. 59:940 (1976).
2. J. Schacht, Molecular mechanisms of drug-induced hearing loss, Abstract, Nobel Symposium 63 (1985).
3. J. E. Rash and C. S. Hudson, eds., "Freeze-Fracture: Methods, Artifacts, and Interpretations", Raven Press, New York, (1979).
4. S. T. Appleyard, J. A. Witkowski, B. D. Ripley, D. M. Shotton and V. Dubowitz, A novel procedure for pattern analysis of features present on freeze-fractured plasma membranes, J. Cell Sci. 74:105 (1985).
5. P. Claude and D. A. Goodenough, Fracture faces of zonulae occludentes from 'tight' and 'leaky' epithelia, J. Cell Biol. 58:390 (1973).
6. C. Peracchia, Structural correlates of gap junction permeation, Int. Rev. Cytol. 66:81 (1980).
7. N. J. Severs and H. Robenek, Detection of Microdomains in biomembranes. An appraisal of recent developments in freeze-fracture cytochemistry, Biochem. Biophys. Acta 737:373 (1983).
8. K. Jahnke, The fine structure of freeze-fractured intercellular junctions in the guinea pig inner ear, Acta Otolaryngol. Suppl. 336 (1975).
9. S. Iurato, K. Franke, L. Luciano, G. Wermbter, E. Pannese and E. Reale, Fracture faces of the junctional complexes in the reticular membrane of the organ of Corti, Acta Otolaryngol. 81:36 (1976).
10. E. Reale, L. Luciano, K. Franke, E. Pannese, G. Wermbter and S. Iurato, Intercellular junctions in the vascular stria and spiral ligament, J. Ultrastruct. Res. 53:284 (1975).
11. R. Gulley and T. S. Reese, Intercellular junctions in the reticular lamina of the organ of Corti, J. Neurocytol. 5:479 (1976).
12. R. L. Gulley and T. S. Reese, Regional specialization of the hair cell plasmalemma in the organ of Corti, Anat. Rec. 189:109 (1977).
13. R. L. Gulley and T. S. Reese, Freeze-fracture studies on the synapses in the organ of Corti, J. Comp. Neur. 171:517 (1977).
14. A. Forge, Freeze-fracture studies of the stria vascularis following administration of ethacrynic acid to guinea pigs, in: "Ototoxic Side-Effects of Diuretics", R. Klinke, W. Lahn, H. Querfurth and J. Scholtholt, eds. Scandinavian Audiology, Suppl. 14:173 (1981).

15. A. Forge, Electron microscopy of the stria vascularis and its response to etacrynic acid. A study using electron dense tracers and extracellular surface markers, Audiol. 20:273 (1981).
16. A. Forge, Gap junctions in the stria vascularis and effects of ethacrynic acid, Hearing Res. 13:189 (1984).
17. A. Forge, Cholesterol distribution in cells of the stria vascularis of the mammalian cochlea and some effects of ototoxic diuretics, J. Cell Sci. (in Press).
18. A. Forge, Outer hair cell loss and supporting cell expansion following chronic gentamicin treatment, Hearing Res. (in press).
19. J. Santos-Sacchi and P. Dallos, Intercellular communication in the supporting cells of the organ of Corti, Hearing Res. 9:317 (1983).
20. A. Flock, Mechanical properties of hair cells, Abstract, Nobel Symposium 63 (1985).
21. J. R. Sommer, P. C. Dolber and I. Taylor, Filipin-serol complexes in the membranes of cardiac muscle, J. Ultrastruct. Res. 80:98 (1982).
22. T. P. Kerr, M. D. Ross and S. A. Ernst, Cellular localization of Na^+, K^+-ATPase in the mammalian cochlear duct: significance for cochlear fluid balance, Am. J. Otolaryngol. 3:332 (1982).
23. T. Konishi, P. E. Hamrick and P. T. Walsh, Ion transport in the guinea pig cochlea. I. Potassium and sodium transport, Acta Otolaryngol. 86:22 (1978).
24. O. Sterkers, G. Saumon, P. Tran Ba Huy, and C. Amiel, K, Cl and H_2O entry in endolymph, perilymph and cerebrospinal fluid of the rat, Am. J. Physiol. 243:F173 (1982).
25. S. K. Bosher, The nature of the ototoxic actions of ethacrynic acid upon the mammalian endolymph system. I. Function aspects, Acta Otolaryngol. 89:407 (1980).
26. S. K. Bosher, The nature of the ototoxic actions of ethacrynic acid on the mammalian endolymph system. II. Structural-functional correlates in the stria vacularis, Acta Otolaryngol. 90:40 (1980).
27. K. E. Rarey and M. D. Ross, A survey of the effects of loop diuretics on the zonulae occludentes of the perilymph-endolymph barrier by freeze fracture, Acta Otolaryngol. 94:307 (1982).
28. D. R. Pitelka and B. N. Taggart, Mechanical tension induces lateral movement of intramembrane components of the tight junction: studies on mouse mammary cells in culture, J. Cell Biol. 96:606 (1983).
29. E. Page and Y. Shibata, Permeable junctions between cardiac cells, Ann. Rev. Physiol. 43:431 (1981).
30. N. Hirokawa and L. G. Tilney, Interactions between actin filaments and between actin filaments and membranes in quick-frozen and deeply etched hair cells of the chick ear, J. Cell Biol. 95:249 (1982).

DISCUSSION

White: How do you measure the spacing between the connections and the number of filaments in the strand, because the strand seems to be a very complex structure.

Forge: I have not measured tight junctional strands. It can be done by putting a grid over the material and measuring where it intersects across the grid. The way I measured connections was to use a bit pad and measure from center to center with the bit pad. A program was written to extract the average. An estimate is obtained of the different centers to centers of paticles across the junction. So we measured all the junctions, all the paticles in a junction and the computer did the rest for us.

MECHANICALLY-INDUCED MORPHOLOGICAL CHANGES IN THE ORGAN OF CORTI

Roger P. Hamernik, George Turrentine and Michele Roberto

University of Texas-Dallas
1966 Inwood Road
Dallas, Texas 75235 USA

Cattedra di Bioacustica
Policlinico
70124 Bari, Italy

INTRODUCTION

Acute exposures to high-level noise impulses damage the cochlea via mechanical mechanisms that are associated with excessive displacements and stresses developed in the delicate epithelial tissues of the organ of Corti. Such damage has been discussed in the literaure a number of times, and an especially clear description was provided by Davis [1]. Davis and his colleagues used continuous noise at levels of nearly 150 dB SPL at the eardrum. They noted that the Hensen cell attachments represent a mechanically weak link in the structural organization of the organ of Corti. This result was confirmed by Beagley [2], who illustrated the separation of cell junctions between the Deiter and Hensen cells following overstimulation. Since then, others (notably Spoendlin [3] and Voldrich [4]), also using high levels of continuous noise, have demonstrated lesions on the basilar membrane of an equivocal mechanical origin, including rupture of the basilar membrane and Reissners membrane. Spoendlin suggested intensities of around 125 dB SPL as the threshold for mechanically-induced lesions as opposed to metabolically-induced damage. However, the dependance of this rms sound pressure on the exposure duration is not clear. Spoendlin is in agreement with Davis and Beagley concerning the susceptibility to acoustic trauma of the Hensen cell attachments, but he further implicates the pillar cells and the medial attachments of the inner hair cell cuticular area as, "weak spots." This paper attempts to provide a clear documentation of the morphological sequence of events which is eventually responsible for producing massive structural damage to the organ of Corti. Using blast waves as a vehicle, we will further attempt to qualitatively illustrate a fundamental difference in the way in which continuous and impulse noise may need to be evaluated when assessing the potential for producing trauma.

METHODS

Thirty-eight binaural chinchillas were used in this study; 6 controls and 32 experimental. From the 32 experimental animals, 6 were prepared for standard surface preparations [3,5] and the remaining 26 experimental and 6 control animals were prepared for Scanning Electron Microscopy (SEM). Each experimental animal was exposed at a normal incidence to 100 blast waves having peak over pressures of 160 dB SPL. The impulses were presented at a

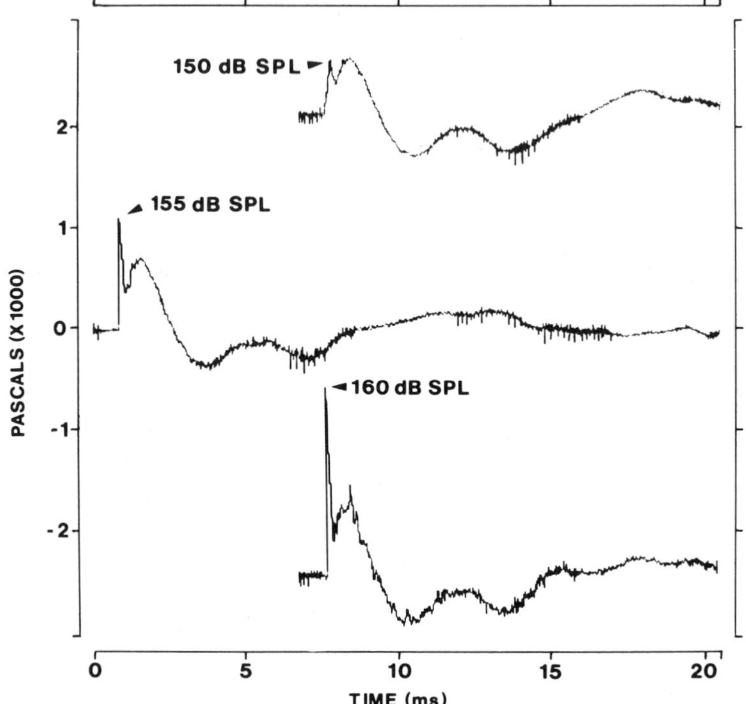

Fig. 1. Examples of three different pressure-time profiles of the blast wave generated by the shock tube.

rate of 2/min. The blast waves were generated using a conventional shock tube (compressed air-driven source) with an expansion section terminating in an exponential horn [6]. The 4 ft. x 4 ft. horn exit was mounted in the wall of an anechoic enclosure to reduce reflections. Pressure-time histories of the typical waves that are generated at different operating pressures are shown in Fig. 1.

All animals were killed by decapitation immediately after exposure or at various postexposure times up to 30 days. The cochleas were perfused through the round window with a cold, 5%, glutaraldehyde in veronal acetate buffer at pH 7.3 (630 Mosm). Following overnight fixation at 4 degrees C, the cochleas were postfixed for 5 min. with a 5% glutaraldehyde/2% aqueous osmium mixture in a 5:2 ratio. Following dehydration and dissection of the bony capsule, the specimens of the organ of Corti were either mounted in glycerin on glass slides as surface preparations, or were critical point dried with liquid carbon dioxide and sputtered with gold or gold-palladium using a cold sputtering head. Cochleas prepared for SEM were viewed with a JEOL JS-35 Scanning Electron Microscope (SEM) operating at 10-20 KeV. More complete details concerning histological preparation procedures can be found in Hamernik et al. [7,8].

RESULTS

Figures 2A and B illustrate the gross appearance of the organ of Corti from two different animals immediately following exposure. The low magnification surface preparation view in Fig. 2A illustrates the extensive tearing of the organ of Corti from its basilar membrane attachments for

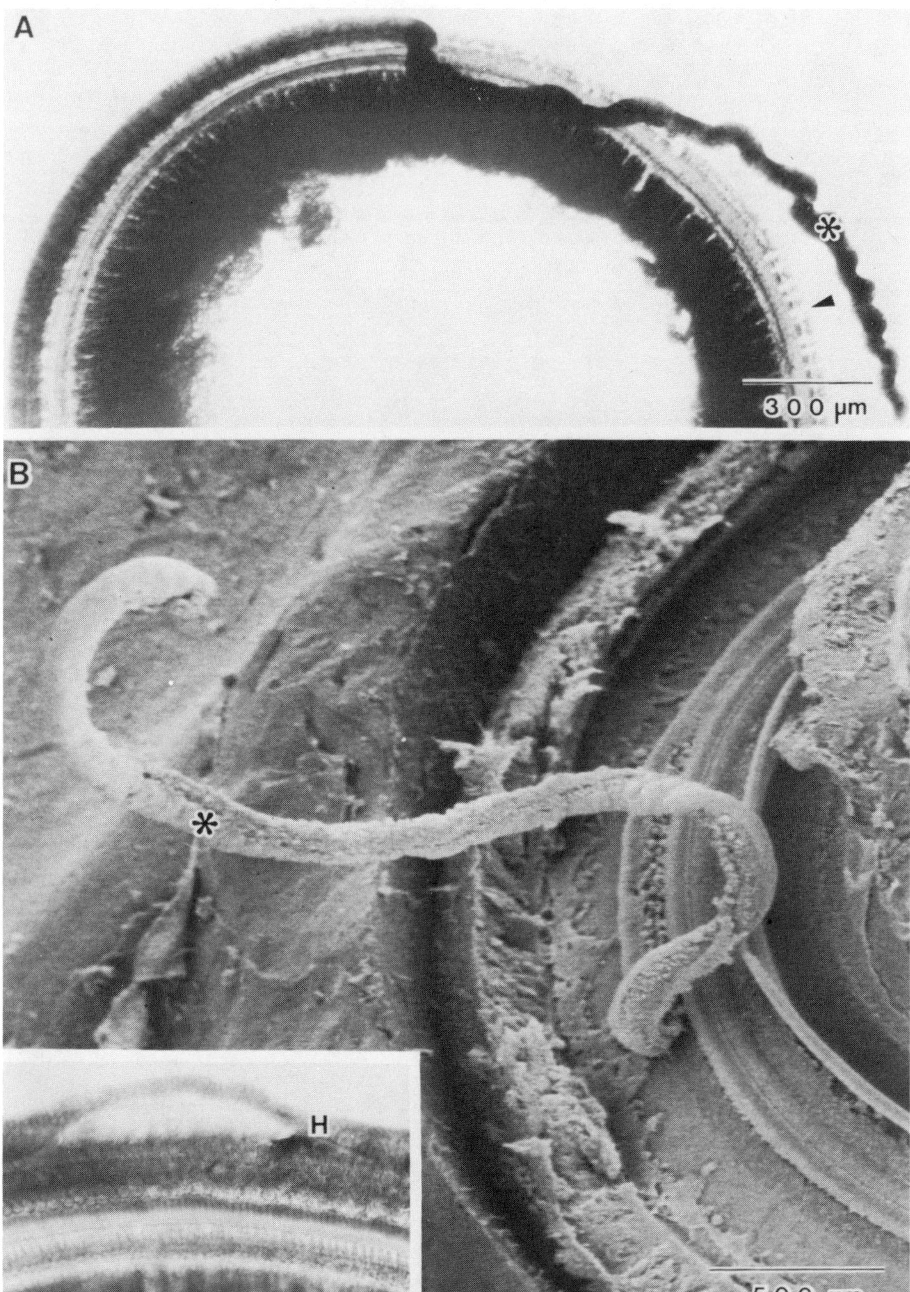

Fig. 2. Immediately following exposure. A) Surface preparation illustrating extensive separation of the organ of Corti (*) in the mid-cochlear region. B) SEM illustrating a similar noise-induced detachment of the organ of Corti (*) Insert - Surface preparation showing the initial separation of the Hensen cells (H) which preceeds the fracture shown in the adjoining micrographs. ► Missing pillar cells.

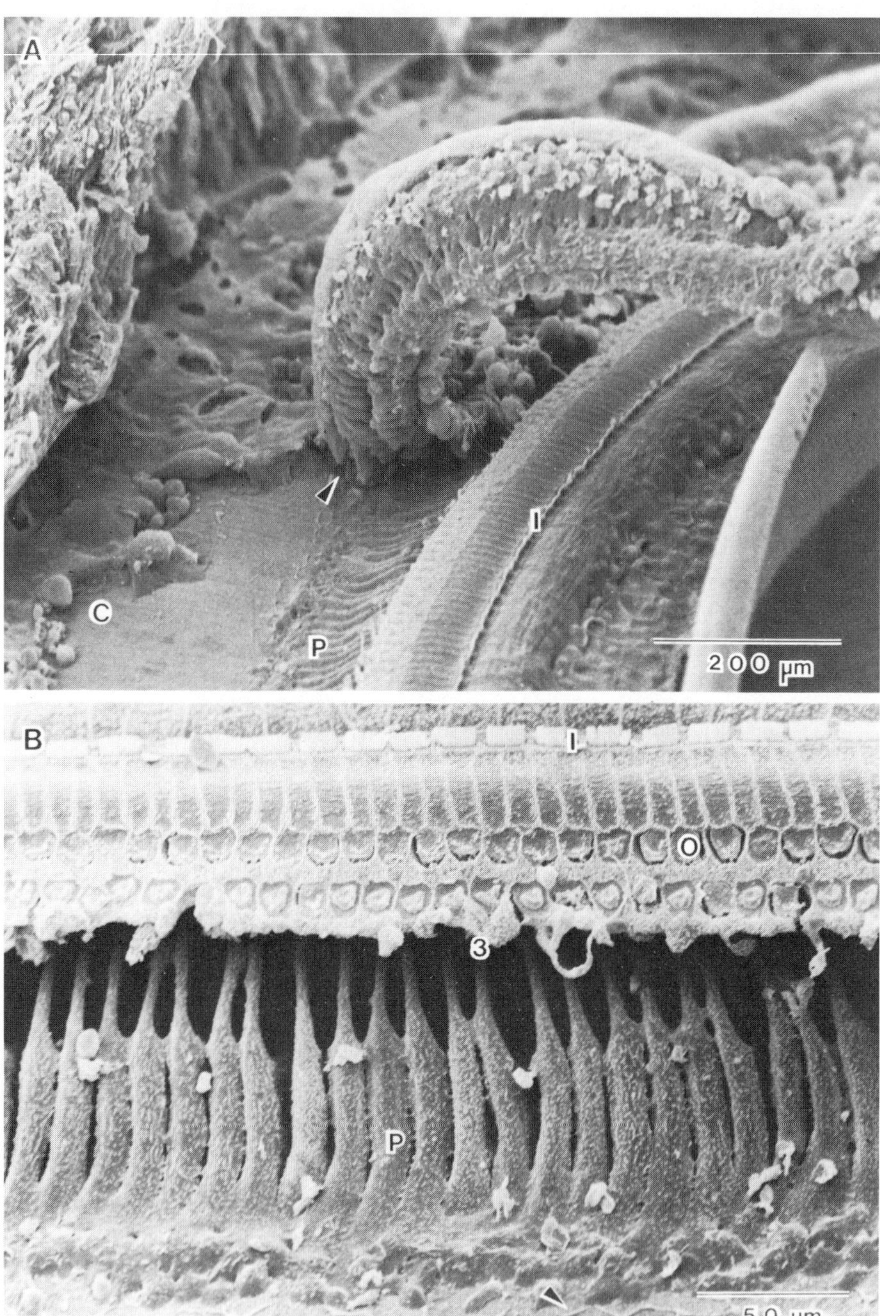

Fig. 3. Immediately following exposure: A) Higher resolution SEM of the fracture ridge. Note missing Claudius cells (C), intact pillar cells (P) and the line of inner hair cell cilia (I). B) Area of the primary lesion showing intact outer pillar processes (P); normal appearing inner hair cell cilia (I) and the cuticular plates of the first two rows of outer hair cells (O) without attached cell bodies. Note Deiter cell attachments at the basilar membrane (►).

over one-third of a mid-cochlear turn. A more graphic view of an even more extensive separation is presented in the SEM of Fig. 2B. The tear can be seen (inset) to originate between the Hensen cells and the reticular lamina of the outer hair cell (OHC) region. At higher resolution (Fig. 3), the line of inner hair cells (IHC), with their cilia that are so readily damaged, appear surprisingly normal in the area of the primary lesion, and the inner and outer pillar cells are structurally intact. The OHC bodies of the first two rows have been torn away just below the tight cell junctions of their attachment into the reticular lamina, leaving the cell's cuticular plate region and the reticular lamina intact (Fig. 3B). Immediately basalward of the main lesion, the organ of Corti is usually structurally intact with relatively normal IHC's. The OHC's, while frequently all present, display irregular cross sections or are greatly swollen. In Fig. 3, the outlines of the Deiter cell base attachments on the basilar membrane can be seen. In this lesion, all the Deiter cells, Hensen cells, OHC's as well as some of the Claudius cells have been torn loose. The outer pillar cells, which are uniformly present, maintain their structural integrity, leaving the tunnel of Corti intact, but open to scala media. While Fig. 3 is typical of the most often observed features of the lesion, variations do occur. Some of the cochleas dissected also displayed a scattered loss of pillar cells as seen in Fig. 2A and in the SEM's of Fig. 4. In Fig. 4, a number of outer pillar processes are completely missing and the tonofibrils of many of the ruptured outer and inner pillar cells have been exposed. Another variant of the structural disintegration of the organ of Corti can be seen in Fig. 4A where the Hensen cells and some of the third row of Deiter cells are left attached to the basilar membrane. Such variations may be important in determining how rapidly epithelial scar tissue forms to seal off the endolymphatic and perilymphatic spaces. Relatively large variations have been noted in the rate of scar formation. Fig. 5 illustrates the lesion from three different cochleas one day after exposure. Fig. 5C shows the denuded basilar membrane covered within one day by a filmy layer of membrane most likely originating from the region of the Claudius cells. This layer of membrane seals the basilar membrane and the fracture ridge created by the dislodged portion of the organ of Corti. In some cases, the seal is incomplete and holes along the ridge of outer pillar cells still connect endolymphatic and perilymphatic spaces (see inset). In other cochleas (Fig. 5B), where the Hensen cells have been left viable, the seal can be complete within the first day post-exposure. However, in other animals (Fig. 5A) with very similar lesions, wide gaps still exist after one day between the tunnel of Corti and the endolymphatic space (note the very normal-appearing IHC cilia). In Fig. 6A, taken from an animal sacrificed 10 days after exposure, the scar formation is still not complete, and large openings into the perilymphatic spaces are common. By 30 days after exposure (Figs. 6B and C), the lesion has usually been sealed and the organ of Corti generally presents a stabilized appearance, but with an extremely variable population of sensory cells. Exceptions to the above are occasionally seen such as in the inset of Fig. 6, where a small defect allowing communication between the scala may still exist. Variability in sensory cell population can be extreme, and virtually every combination of normal and abnormal cilia can be found (i.e., bent, fused, broken or giant cilia). Similarly, no pattern in the OHC cell loss is apparent, and any individual or combination of damaged rows of OHC's can be found, with normal or abnormal populations of IHC.

Other epithelial cell populations in the cochlea are also reacting to the altered milieu of the scala media following trauma. A surprising response was observed in the cells of inner sulcus and the related inner border cells. Figs. 7 and 8 illustrate the surface morphology of the inner sulcus cells (ISC) taken from animals sacrificed 10 days after exposure. A prolific growth of microvilli and pseudopodia has taken place on the surface of these (Fig. 7) cells and various particles are seen entrapped in

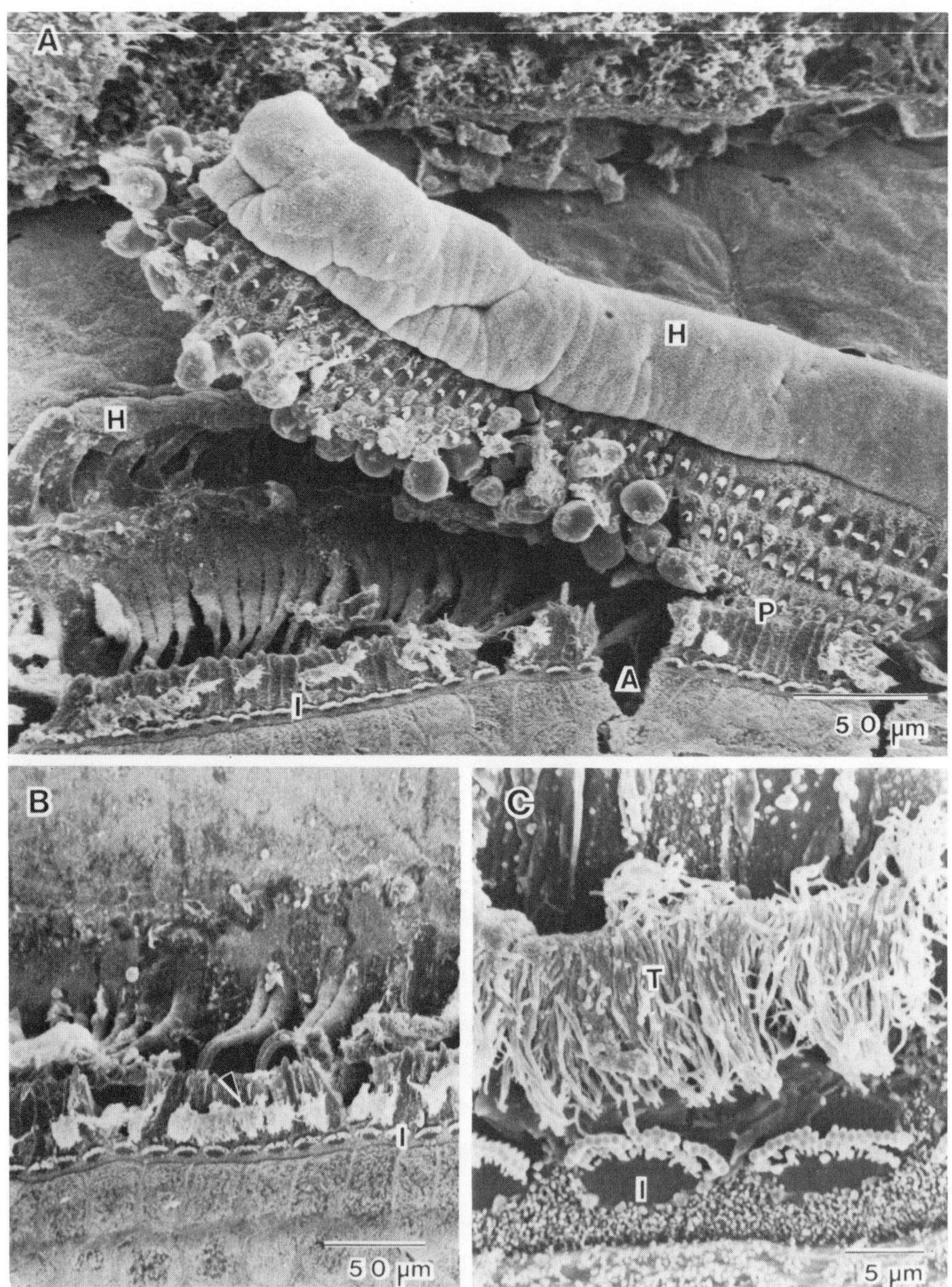

Fig. 4. Immediately following exposure: A) An example of an unusual fracture ridge which follows the line of attachment of the outer pillar heads (P). Note the Hensen cells (H) that remain attached to the basilar membrane. (A) Artifact. B&C) Example of a fracture ridge in which inner and outer pillar cells (P) are ruptured (►) and the tonofibrils (T) are exposed. Note the relatively normal appearing inner hair cell cilia (I) in each plate.

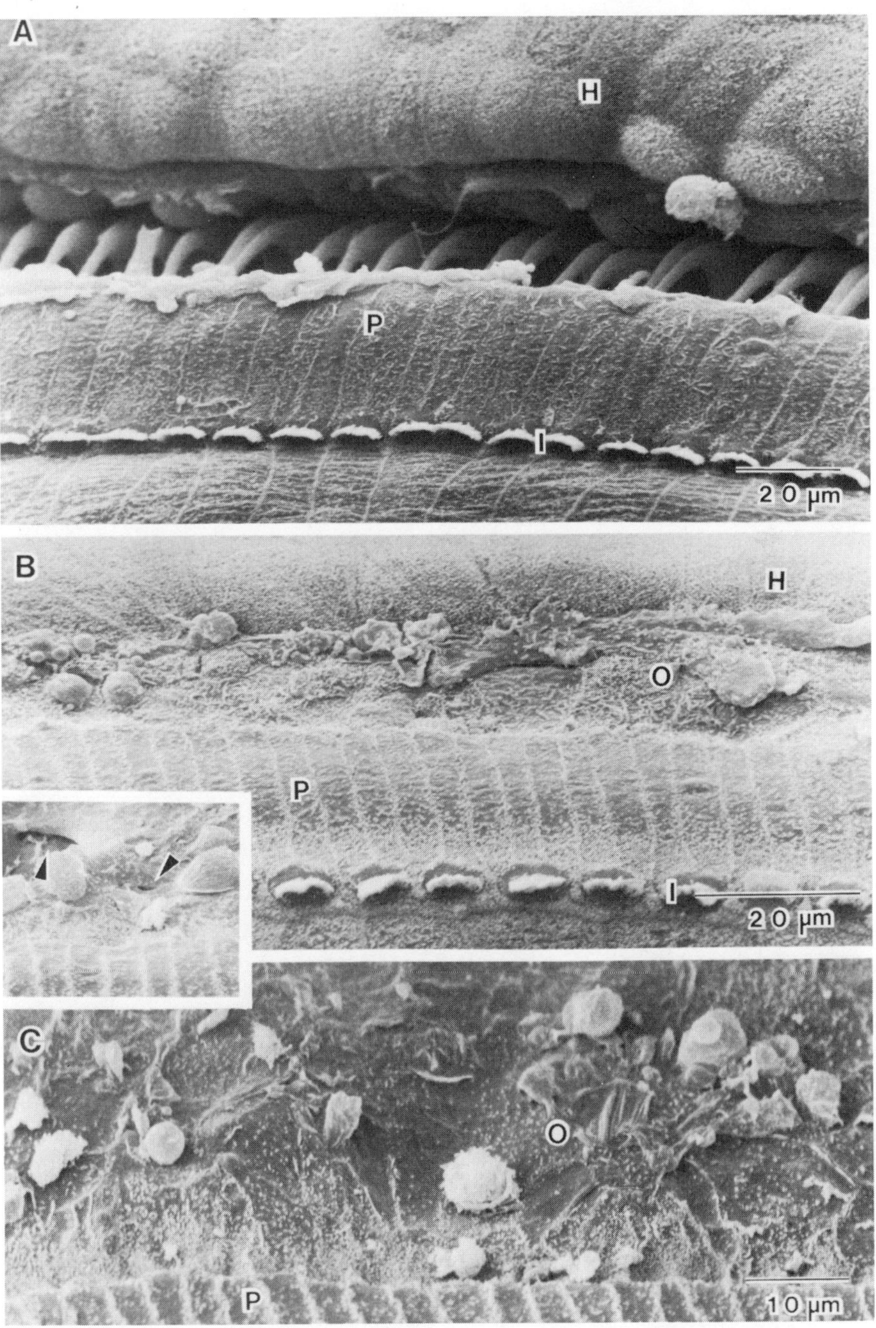

Fig. 5. One day after exposure. A) Scar tissue has not yet sealed off the perilymphatic space. B&C) Region of the outer hair cells (O) from two different animals showing complete scar formation. In plate B the Hensen cell (H) are present just as in plate A, while in plate C the Hensen cells have been torn loose with the bulk of the organ of Corti. Inset - small defects (►) through which cochlear fluids may still intermix. (P) Pillar cells.

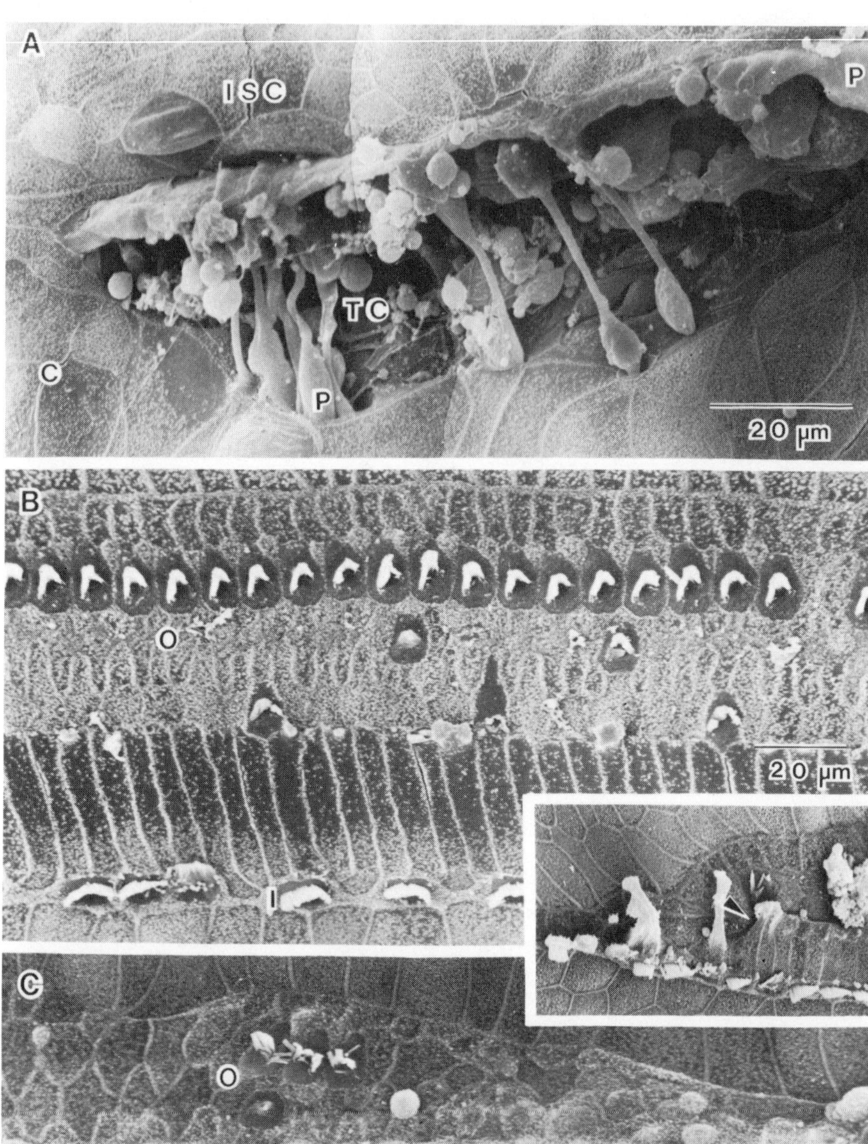

Fig. 6. A) Ten days after exposure the fracture ridge along the pillar cells (P) is often not sealed in some animals and the tunnel of Corti can communicate with the endolymph. (ISC) inner sulcus cells, (C) Claudius cells. B&C) Thirty days after exposure the lesion is usually completely covered by scar tissue: hair cell loss is quite variable. Inset: However even after 30-days in some animals scar formation may be incomplete (►). (O) outer hair cells, (I) inner hair cells.

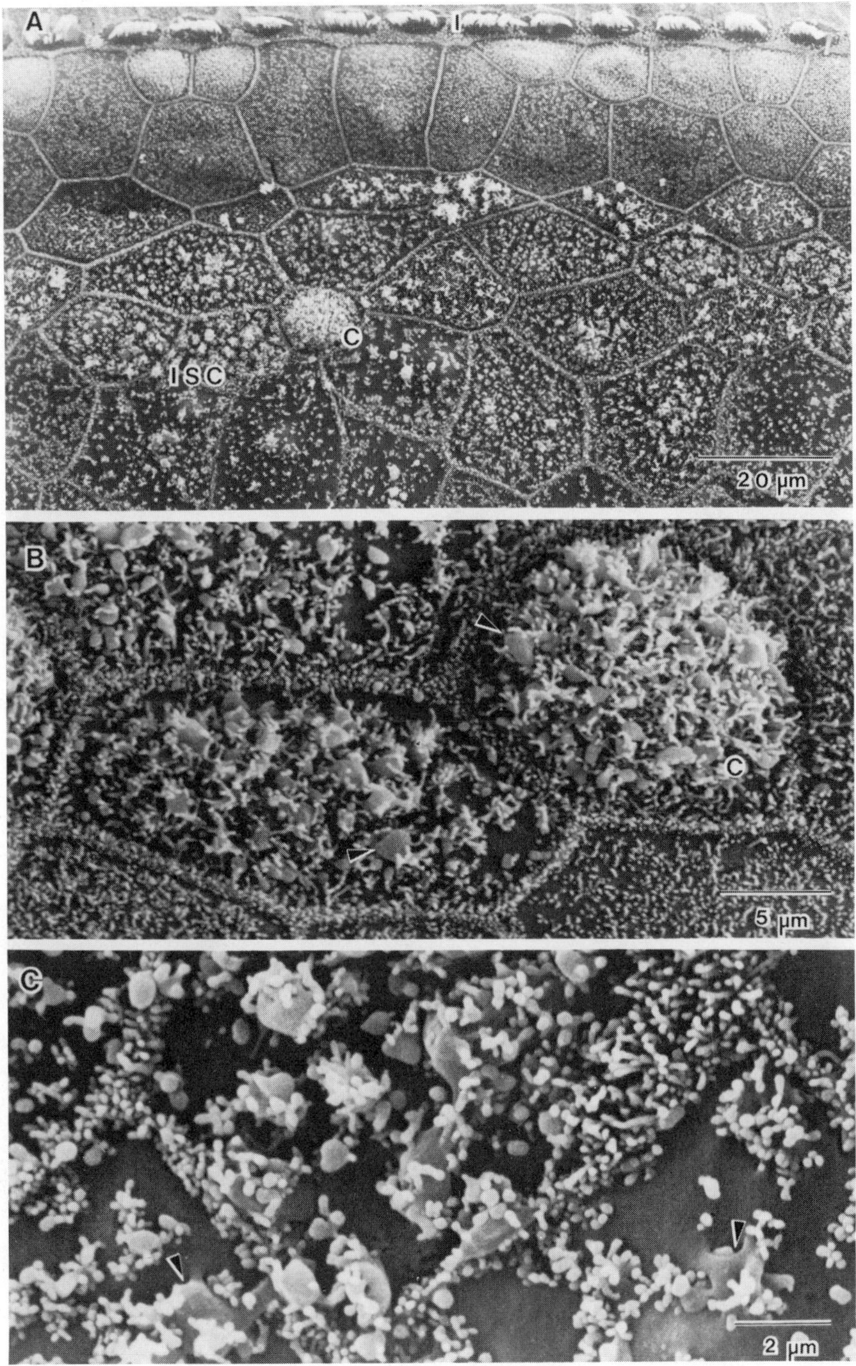

Fig. 7. Surface views of the inner sulcus 10 days after exposure. A) Profuse growth of microvilli on inner sulcus cells (ISC). Note the convex distortion of the surface of cell (C) with a particularily dense growth of villi. B) Higher resolution of ISC surface growth illustrating sac formation (►). C) Surface ISC detail illustrating the formation of extra surface membrane (►) systems.

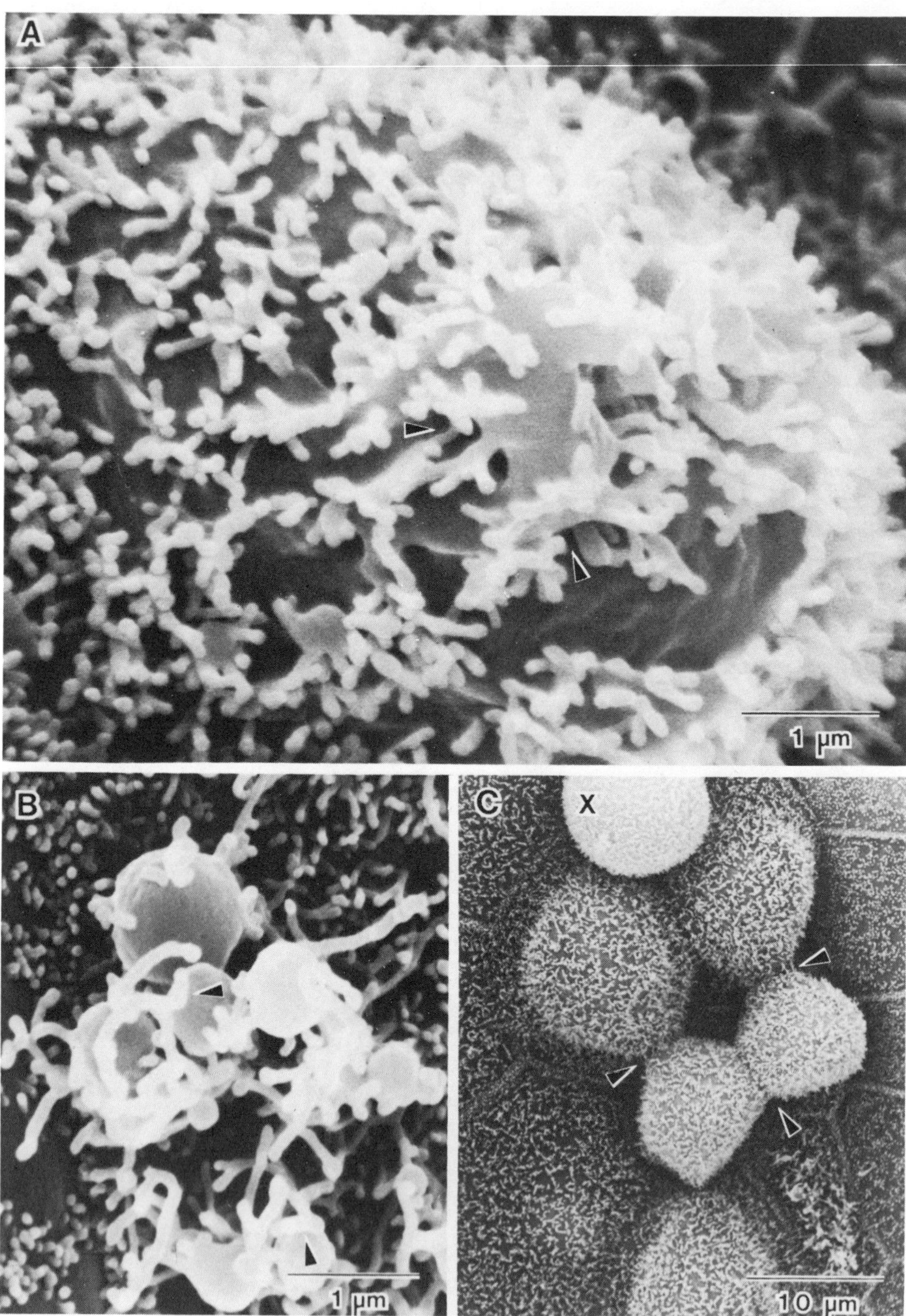

Fig. 8. Ten days after exposure. A) Detail of an ISC with a highly convex surface and an extensive development of extra membrane at the surface (►). B) Example of the relationship between particulate matter and the enveloping pseudopodia (►). C) Low magnification view of several distended ISC surfaces illustrating apparent interactions between cells (►), (X) cell of unknown origin.

the tangle of villi (Figs. 7B and 8B). The cells of the inner sulcus would appear to be extremely active in the endocytosis of debris following trauma to the organ of Corti. Some of the ISC's are greatly distended (Figs. 8A and C) often with extensive sheet-like formations of extra surface membrane studded with irregular and branching villi (Fig. 8C). Other cells of unknown origin are frequently present (Fig. 8C). A further discussion of the ISC's can be found in Hamernik et al. [8].

DISCUSSON

We have shown that an acute exposure to high level blast waves can produce widespread, direct mechanical damage to the organ of Corti. As discussed by other authors, and clearly seen in the inset of Fig. 2, the first structures to fail are the cell junctions associated with the attachments of the Hensen cells to the Deiter cells, the Claudius cells and the reticular lamina. In contrast to the conclusion of Spoendlin [3], our results indicate that the pillar attachments and the first row of Deiter cell heads are relatively tough and resistant to damage. The fracture line most often runs between the second and third rows of OHC's. An appreciation of the strength of the tight cell junctions of the reticular lamina can be obtained from Fig. 3, where it can be seen that the cuticular plates of the outer hair cells remain attached in the matrix of the reticular lamina, while the remainder of the sensory cell body is torn loose from below, along with the strip of Hensen and Deiter cells.

After reviewing the SEM's from animals sacrificed over a 30 day period, we were surprised at the variability in the rate of scar formation. While we cannot explain such variability, the variability associated with scar formation may be important in explaining why animals exposed to the same impulses demonstrate such variable degrees of sensory cell loss. The acceptance of Bohne's [9] fluid-mixing hypothesis would imply that the sooner the fluid compartments are sealed, the less loss there will be to the sensory cell population. While we have no quantitative data, it seems likely that in cochleas that have incomplete scar formation over as much as a 30 day period, the extent of sensory cell loss will be increased. The likely tendency of the lesion to develop over time, especially basalward of the primary lesion, may also have a correlate in hearing threshold measures. A common observation following high-level impulse noise exposure [10] is the growth of TTS over time, i.e., maximum TTS may be reached as much as one day following exposure.

Another surprising feature of these data is the ability of the pillar cells to withstand the mechanical trauma and along with them the inner hair cells. Relatively normal appearing IHC's can be found immediately following exposure as well as at 30 days postexposure, even in the area of the primary lesion. Because of the afferent innervation pattern, the survival of such large numbers of IHC may have implications for hearing function. Impulse noise exposures similar to those described in this paper which produce massive OHC loss over as much as 80% of the cochlea [10,11] are known to produce hearing losses which seldom exceed 40 dB across the 0.5 to 8 kHz test range. Frequently, if the lesion is localized to the middle of the cochlea and does not exceed 10-30% of the entire OHC population, hearing thresholds may be very near normal. In both these situations, the IHC populations, including the integrity of the cilia, can be quite normal.

The extensive growth of villi and pseudopodia on the surface of the inner sulcus cells was also quite unexpected. From the appearance of the surface of these cells, it would appear that they are actively engaged in the endocytosis of substances released during the development of the lesion on the organ of Corti. There is evidence in the literature [12-14] that the prolific growth of villi on the surface of these cells may in fact be triggered by a variety of macromolecules released during trauma. Regardless of the reasons, the extensive growth of extra membrane on the inner sulcus cells may indicate that these cells with their unexciting cytoplasm, may be capable of modifying the composition of the fluids in the inner sulcus and the subtectorial space. The composition of the fluid in this region of the cochlea is still a debatable issue [15].

Approaches to trying to estimate damage threshold levels for the purposes of establishing criteria for exposure are usually based upon a trade-off between intensity and duration of the exposure, i.e., essentially an energy consideration. Considering that a typical acute exposure to impulses or blasts (even large numbers of them) lasts only a fraction of a second, a strict adherence to energy principals may not be completely adequate. Consider the following: We have performed experiments with the 3 waves shown in Fig. 1, i.e., over a dynamic range of from 150 dB to 160 dB peak over pressure (re 0.0002 dynes/cm^2). Using the evoked auditory response as a measure of hearing thresholds and tympanometry as an index of middle ear trauma, we find that exposure to 100 blasts at a rate of 1/min. at 150 dB produces moderate hearing loss (less than 10 dB) and small mid-cochlear OHC loss. At levels of 155 dB, hearing loss can be in excess of 40 dB and losses of sensory cells (especially OHC's) can be extensive over more than 80% of the cochlea; at levels over 160 dB, middle ear problems, including rupture of the tympanic membrane, occur and we find a protective effect on the cochlea. Thus, over a 10 dB range of intensities, we find a wide variety of effects on the cochlea, including the massive structural damage shown in the preceeding micrographs. If we assume the signal to be plane wave, then the energy per unit area transported by the blast wave [16] in the direction of propagation can be approximated by:

$$W = \int_0^t \frac{P^2(t)dt}{Z} \qquad (J/M^2)$$

Where $P(t)$ = instantaneous sound pressure (N/m^2)
Z = specific acoustic impedance ($-S/m^3$)

This relation can be applied to the waveforms shown in Fig. 1. Introducing a level terminology in the sense of the logarithm of a ratio quantity along with a term, 10 log N, to account for the number (N) of blast wave presentations, we find that all the exposures (for N=100) have energy levels (re 1 J/M^2) of between 23 to 24 dB, regardless of their peak intensities (i.e., in the range 150 - 160 dB). Variations of 1 dB occur because of variations in the slow phase of the pressure fluctuations following the shock front. The waves in the traces shown in Fig. 1 were obtained using an 1/8" microphone (B&K 4138) at grazing incidence, and the shock front is represented by the initial pressure spike having an overall duration on the order of 10 usec, essentially a reflection of the time of passage of the wave front across the microphone diaphragm. We are thus faced with three blast wave exposures having similar energies but differing in their peaks and differing substantially in their effects on the hearing mechanism. The question that naturally arises then is what is an adequate characterization of an impulse for the purposes of exposure criteria? In a later paper at this meeting, Patterson et al. will contribute to answering this question by suggesting that both peak pressure and energy need to be considered depending upon the impulse. For the waves shown in Fig. 1, energy is not sufficient to predict the range of observed effects, and in situations where a very high pressure change is instantaneously impressed upon the external canal, impulsive waves may require alternate methods of evaluation.

In the field of structural mechanics, the impulse I of a high intensity transient force is used to evaluate the structural response, where

$$I = \int_0^t F(t)\,dt \qquad \text{(N-S)}$$

and F(t) is the transient force.

Impulse loads on structures are known to produce excessive displacements as well as stresses on structural members that can be very destructive. Thus, depending on the wave form, impulse and energy may be complimentary variables. While this brief discussion is a great oversimplification which ignores a number of important points, it may have some value in stimulating thought on different approaches to evaluating impulse noise exposure.

ACKNOWLEDGEMENTS

This research was partially supported by the U.S. Army Medical Reseach and Development Command DAMD 17-83-G-9555 and the Department of Health, Education and Welfare, National Institute for Occupational Safety and Health, Grant No. 5-R01-OH-01518.

REFERENCES

1. H. Davis, Acoustic trauma in the guinea pig, Wright Air Development Center, WADC TR 53-58 (1953).
2. H. A. Beagley, Acoustic trauma in the guinea pig - Part I, Acta Otolaryngol., 60:437 (1965).
3. H. H. Spoedlin, anatomical changes following various noise exposures, in: "Effects of Noise on Hearing," D. Henderson, R. P. Hamernik. D. S. Dosanjh and J. H. Mills, eds., Raven Press, New York (1976).
4. L. Voldrich, Experimental acoustic trauma - Part I, Acta Otolaryngol., 74:392 (1972).
5. H. Engstron, H. W. Ades and A. Anderson, Structural pattern of the organ of Corti, Almquist and Wiksel, Stockholm (1966).
6. R. P. Hamernik, D. S. Dosanjh and D. Henderson, Shock tube applicatins in bioacoustics research, in: "Recent Developments in Shock Tube Research," D. Bershader and W. Griffith, eds., Stanford University Press, Stanford, CA, (1973).
7. R. P. Hamernik, G. Turrentine, M. Roberto, R. J. Salvi and D. Henderson, Anatomical correlates of impulse noise-induced mechanical damage in the cochlea, Hearing Res., 13:229 (1984).
8. R. P. Hamernik, G. Turrentine and C. G. Wright, Surface morphology of the inner sulcus and related epithelial cells of the cochlea following acoustic trauma, Hearing Res., 16:143 (1984).
9. B. A. Bohne and K. D. Rabbitt, Holes in the reticular lamina after noise exposure: Implication for continuing damage in the organ of Corti, Hearing Res., 11:41 (1983).
10. J. J. Patterson, I. M. Lomba-Gautier, D. L. Curd, R. P. Hamernik, R. J. Salvi, C. E. Hargett and G. Turrentine, The effect of impulse intensity and the number of impulses on hearing and cochlear pathology in chinchilla, USAARL Report No. 85-3 (1985).
11. D. Henderson, R. P. Hamernik and R. W. Sitler, Audiometric and histological correlates of exposure to 1 msec noise impulses in the chinchilla, J. Acoust. Soc. Am. 56:1210 (1974).

12. L. B. Margolis and L. D. Bergelson, Lipid-cell interactions, Exp. Cell Res., 199:145 (1979).
13. F. J. Martin and R. C. MacDonald, Lipid vesicle-cell interactions, J. Cell Bio., 70:515-526 (1976).
14. J. S. Chen, A. Del Fa, A. Diluzio and P. Calissano, Liposome-induced morphological differentiation of murine neuroblastoma, Nature (London), 263:604-606 (1976).
15. G. A. Manley and A. Kronester-Frei, The electrophysiological profile of the organ of Corti, in: Psychophysical, Physiological and Behavioral Studies in Hearing, G. Van den Brink and F. A. Bilsen, eds., Delft University Press, Netherlands, (1980).
16. R. W. Young, On the energy transported with a sound pulse, J. Acoust. Soc. Am., 47:441 (1970).

DISCUSSION

Per Nilsson: Did you do a frequency analysis of your impulse of 160 dB? If so, where was the energy peak located? Did you see any relationship between the location of the lesion and the frequency of the impulse?

Hamernik: Most of the energy is located below 100 hz. It is a very slow wave. The only thing that looks fast is the rising edge of the shock wave. You would expect the damage to be in the upper turn of the cochlea, not down around the 2 kHz region of the cochlea. The lesions did not spread apically, which was somewhat disturbing.

Pfander: You showed disturbances and fractures in the middle ear of the animals. I haven't seen disturbances of the middle ear in humans after peak pressures of 160 dB. What percent of the middle ears examined were damaged?

Hamernik: It was probably around 50 percent. I think the level which causes damage in people is closer to 180 dB for this type of impulse.

Pfander: During the war, I saw massive destruction of the middle ear after explosions; these were apparently over 200 dB. Do you think 180 dB is the damage level which causes damage to the middle ear in humans?

Hamernik: I don't know, but reading some of the old papers that were done shortly after the war gives the impression that 180 dB is the level which causes damage in humans.

Shaddock: Several times you mentioned that the inner ear sensory cells looked completely normal. I am wondering if you did any sectioning to verify that. I think it is a little dangerous to make such a statement based simply on the condition of the stereocilia.

Hamernik: Terribly dangerous! No, we did not section any of the cells. Basically we were just looking at surface pathology. I certainly would have to qualify my comments.

Engstrom: Thirty days after you have this massive damage, what kind of epithelium remains?

Hamernik: It depends a lot on the nature of the lesion. If the lesion is complete so there are no supporting or sensory cells, then it is just a flat epithelium that seems to unite the inner sulcus and the Claudius cell. Sometimes the epithelium seems to grow from the area of the Claudius cells. It appears to come up and seal off the pillar cells and actually grow over the pillar cells.

Engstrom: But the length would be about the same as the snake?

Hamernik: It is variable.

Engstrom: On the first day after the explosion, do you see any kind of invasion of lymphocytes?

Hamernik: In scanning electron micrographs, I am not quite certain how to precisely identify lymphocytes.

Warren: Your talk concentrated on the focal rupture of the organ of Corti in the 0.3, 0.8, and 0.2 kHz regions. Could you comment on the state of articulation between the tectorial membrane and the organ or Corti?

Hamernik: The tectorial membrane always suffers from typical artifacts. Generally, it is always rolled up towards the modiolus no matter where you look.

Warren: Did you do any light microscopic examination of the cochlea?

Hamernik: No. We are doing that now.

White: I wonder if perhaps you could say if there are any desmosomes between the cells in the inner sulcus region? How many are there and are they likely to be damaged by the kind of blasts you were talking about.

Hamernik: As far as I am aware, there are no desmosomes in the inner sulcus region. That does not mean they are not there, I haven't found any yet. Cells in the inner sulcus have received very, very little attention.

Pujol: About 10 years ago when we started to study the effects of acoustic trauma, we exposed hamsters to noise for days and weeks and found a very strange thing at the inner sulcus. There was an increase in the volume of the cells and a fantastic increase in the length of the stereocilia. Since this area of research was new to us, we just put it aside because we could not interpret it. Your results seem to be very similar to our own and are quite surprising.

Hamernik: Your results are very interesting. The cells in the inner sulcus are described in text books as having clear unexciting cytoplasm. In damaged ears, there seems to be something exciting gong on here.

Patuzzi: Did I understand you correctly in suggesting that the wave shape you measured was limited by the travel time of the shock wave across the micro-phone diaphragm?

Hamernik: Not the wave shape so much as the initial rising front. If you talk about the dimension of the shock wave, it is on the order of the mean free path of the molecules in the medium it is traveling in. So what we are actually measuring is the rise time of the 1/8 inch microphone during the first 10 microseconds. The measurement of the rest of the wave is probably reasonable.

Patuzzi: Taking that into account, what does the spectrum of what you measure mean? I do not think you can do a spectrum analysis of that wave and say it had any significance.

Hamernik: That is true at least for the spectrum of the rising position of the wave front; however, useful information can be abstracted from the remaining position of the wave where most of the energy is contained.

THE APPLICATION OF MORPHOMETRIC AND STEREOLOGICAL PRINCIPLES TO EPITHELIAL TISSUES: THEORETICAL AND PRACTICAL CONSIDERATIONS

F.H. White

Department of Anatomy and Cell Biology
University of Sheffield
Sheffield S10 2TN U.K.

INTRODUCTION

The study of the spatial relationships between cells, their contents and the ways in which they interact with each other and with the extracellular matrix can only be studied by microscopical techniques. Apart from the straightforward methods of light and electron microscopy available for examining normal, diseased and experimentally treated cells and tissues, the experimental biologist now has a variety of additional techniques available for investigating cytological and histological features. These include autoradiography, histochemistry and cytochemistry, immunochemistry and quantitative morphology. These techniques enable us to draw conclusions about the structure and functions of cells in their proper arrangement, and by making comparisons between normal and altered tissue or cellular structure, we can learn and ultimately understand the mechanisms which govern and control normal and diseased tissues.

The evaluation of structural changes in cells and tissues has largely been based on qualitative description which can be and is often liable to serious error since it is essentially subjective. In histopathology, for example, in which evaluation of abnormal tissue features is of paramount importance, the examination of tissue sections is qualitative and the diagnosis is dependent upon a number of variables which include the experience and training of the individual pathologist. Morphometric methods which rely less on qualitative observation and thereby reduce such subjectivity are currently being used in diagnostic pathology [1] and in histological and cell biological studies [2]. Morphometry encompasses techniques which have advantages in increasing objectivity enormously, improving reproducibility, and further, they enable the detection of previously unsuspected changes. These advantages are conferred by the acquisition of quantitative data using microscopical images or their representations.

TYPES OF QUANTITATIVE MICROSCOPY

There are a number of different quantitative morphological techniques in use today. These include morphometry, planimetry, stereology, image processing, image analysis, scanning photometry or densitometry and flow cytometry. Etymological morphometry means "the measurement of form." More specifically, Weibel [2] has defined morphometry as "quantitative morphology; the measurement of structures by any method, including stereology." Thus all the methods in the list above are morphometric methods. Planimetry, or planar geometry, relies on direct measurements of features made on a two-dimensional plane. Stereology involves mathematical relationships to define three-dimensional structures from measurements carried out on two-dimensional images. It is these techniques with which the present paper is concerned, primarily because the techniques can be applied to sectioned biological material with the minimum of equipment and are thus accessible and inexpensive. The other quantitative morphological methods require sophisticated and expensive apparatus, and will not be described further. The reader is referred to reviews on automated image analysis [3] and flow cytometry [4,5].

STEREOLOGY: WHAT IT IS AND HOW TO DO IT

Weibel [2] has defined stereology as a body of mathematical methods relating three-dimensional parameters defining a structure to two-dimensional measurements obtained on sections of a structure. There is thus a sound mathematical and statistical basis for the principles of stereological techniques, which are dealt with in depth elsewhere [2,6-11]. It is a common misconception that a great deal of mathematical knowledge is required before any stereological study is undertaken. Stereological techniques are based on principles of spatial geometry and statistics. However, the application of the principles is relatively straightforward and, providing certain rules are followed, a great deal of very valuable information can be obtained by the novice from sections or micrographs with little knowledge of the theoretical basis for deriving that information.

In stereological analyses, several steps can be identified. First, material has to be prepared for analysis in such a way that the components being quantified are unambiguously identifiable. This involves the preparative steps involved in producing sections for light or electron microscopy, selecting an appropriate magnification, and deciding which histological or ultrastructural features you want to quantify. The next step is to choose a technique for measurement of sectioned components. Stereology can be used to define volumes, surface areas, lengths and numbers; several different methods are available. These measurements generate information known as primary data which, taken as it stands, has limited biological significance. By substitution into stereological formulae, this information is used to generate secondary data, which in essence converts the primary data into density estimates. Thus the volume of a component can be related to a unit volume containing the component. Further, if the actual dimensions of the containing volume are known, it becomes possible to derive estimates of absolute component dimensions related to the average cell or average organ, which enables us to draw more relevant conclusions about biological phenomena. These methods will be clarified in subsequent sections.

THE ACQUISITION OF STEREOLOGICAL INFORMATION

Primary Data

The simplest and cheapest way of acquiring quantitative data from microscopical images is to superimpose a transparent lattice containing a repeating pattern of test probes over a micrograph. A wide variety of lattices are available and many of them are illustrated in Weibel [2]. The most useful for general purposes is the coherent double test lattice which comprises arrays of parallel lines arranged perpendicularly to each other. The intersections of the lines provide an array of points. When the micrograph is randomly confronted with the test lattice, a number of significant relationships can be generated as a result of counting interactions or events which occur between the lattice and the micrograph. Such information is known as primary data and is essentially planar morphometric information. If we obtain a section through a cell which contains a nucleus (Fig. 1), we can count the points which fall in the nucleus (P_N) and the points which fall in the cytoplasm (P_{CYT}) and obtain a simple planar estimate, the nuclearcytoplasmic ratio ($=P_N/P_{CYT}$). We can also count intersections of test lines with the plasma membrane (I_{PM}) and obtain an estimate of nuclear membrane profile boundary length (B). In biological terms, the acquisition of planar morphometric or primary stereological data is limited in terms of its biological usefulness and it is almost always preferable to transform primary data into secondary data. Primary data measurements are accumulated for each animal and these totals substituted into the relevant stereological formulae.

Secondary Data

The information generated by event counting can, with relative ease, be used to provide stereological secondary data, which is in the form of density estimates, the majority of which are ratios. Biological structures can be characterised by a variety of dimensions which are volume (V, cm^3), surface (S, cm^2), length (L, cm^1) and number (N, cm^0). In stereology, the dimension of the component is always related to a reference which must be clearly specified. The reference is usually written as a subscript. Thus V_V refers to the volume of a given component within a unit of specified reference volume; S_V to the surface area of a given component within a unit of specified reference volume; S_S to the surface area of a given component with respect to a unit of specified reference surface area and so on.

Provided that the sample of micrographs is random, most density estimates are completely independent of the shape, size and spatial orientation of the component being measured. An important exception is estimation of numerical density in which we need to know the size and shape of the structure [2].

Volume, Surface and Length Densities

Measurement of these parameters provides us with reliable information which represents the aggregate of a particular component within a given reference.

Volume Density - V_V. This parameter represents the volume of a component of interest V_i within a unit reference volume V_r. On two-dimensional sections, it has been shown [2] that the volume density of i within r ($V_{Vi,r}$) is given by

$$V_{Vi,r} = \frac{A_i}{A_r} = \frac{P_i}{P_r} = \frac{V_i}{V_r} \qquad \text{(Equation 1)}$$

where A represents the areas of the components and P represents the points falling on the components after random superimposition of a lattice containing test points. Point counting is generally the most efficient way of estimating volume densities [12]. The alternative is to measure component areas by planimetry or by tracing round their profiles using a digitizing tablet interfaced with a microcomputer, such as is available with most image analyzers.

Because sections have a finite thickness, and stereological principles depend on making measurements from two dimensional planar views, errors known as overprojection effects may be introduced because components present within, rather than on the surface of, the sections are observed and quantified. This results in overestimation. For approximately spherical particles, a correction factor is available which is derived thus

$$k_t = 1 + \frac{3t}{2d} \qquad \text{(Equation 2)}$$

where t is section thickness and d is mean profile diameter. Volume density is corrected for this effect by dividing it by the correction factor k. The larger the particle, the less is the error for any given section thickness and it is generally accepted that if the profile diameter is more than ten times greater than section thickness, overprojection correction is unnecessary. Weibel [2] provides alternative formulations for particles of different shapes.

Surface Density - S_V, S_S . These parameters generate densities which characterize the surface of a component in relation to a unit containing volume (S_V) or surface (S_S). For estimation of these components, the relevant formulae are

$$S_V = \frac{4}{\pi} B_A = 2I_L \qquad \text{(Equation 3)}$$

and

$$S_{Si,r} = \frac{I_i}{I_r} = I_{Ii,r} \qquad \text{(Equation 4)}$$

B_A represents the boundary trace length B of the component of interest divided by the area A enclosing the component, and this formulation can be used if a digitizing tablet or planimeter is being used. $2I_L$ is the formula of choice when using superimposed test lattices in linear arrays. I is the number of intersections the linear lattice makes with the component of interest which is divided by L, the length of lattice line which overlies the reference component. The parameter S_S is obtained very simply by differential intersection counting, I_i being the number of lattice intersections with the component of interest and I_r , the number of intersections with the reference component.

Length Density - L_V. L_V relates the length of a component to its unit containing volume. It is derived from the following equation

$$L_V = 2N_A \qquad \text{(Equation 5)}$$

where N is the number of profiles of the component contained within the reference area of section A. Reference area may be measured directly using a cursor and digitizing tablet, but point counting can also be used to determine A. If a quadratic lattice is used, each point will represent a given area whose dimensions can be determined according to the magnification being used.

Numerical Density - N_V, N_S . Numerical density can be expressed in terms of number of components per unit reference volume (N_V) or per unit reference area (N_S). These estimates are more difficult to determine than the other density estimates mentioned since inherent in the stereological formulae used to calculate them is a measure of their shape and size.

Numerical density in a volume N_V can be obtained from

$$N_V = \frac{N_A}{\bar{H}} \qquad \text{(Equation 6)}$$

where N is the number of components present in reference area A. $\bar{H}$ is the mean caliper diameter of the component, i.e., averaged over all orientations. In the case of spherical objects of uniform size, the mean caliper diameter, $\bar{H}$ is equal to the mean diameter of the object $\bar{D}$. However, if the section contains two different sized spherical particles, $\bar{H} \neq \bar{D}$. It can be appreciated that H for objects with more complex shapes can be more difficult to determine. Similarly, at first sight N_A seems a simple enough parameter to calculate, but the number of profiles seen in a section does not always accurately reflect the number of particles. A particle which is in the shape of a horseshoe can produce either one or two profiles, according to its orientation with respect to the section plane. One can easily imagine how particle numbers can be overestimated, especially when considering structures with a more complex morphology.

Weibel and Gomez [13] have provided an alternative formulation for numerical density

$$N_V = \frac{1}{B} \cdot \frac{N_A^{(3/2)}}{V_V^{(1/2)}} \qquad \text{(Equation 7)}$$

where B is a shape coefficient defined by the relationship between the component's volume and its mean cross sectional area. Values for B can be consulted in the graph provided by Weibel [7]. This method should be used only for particles of constant shape.

In view of the difficulties of computing N_V, it is a parameter which should be measured and interpreted with caution. Mayhew et al. [14] have evaluated several methods for determining numerical densities of mitochondria and show how a number of systematic errors can be introduced by making erroneous assumptions about particle size. They concluded that the number of mitochondria had little meaning, particularly as the *in vivo* morphological characteristics of this organelle are inconstant. Mitochondria in living cells rapidly change their size and shape, fuse with each other and are generally in a state of flux. If at all possible, alternative approaches to N_V should be sought. Otherwise, attempts should be made to determine the size and shape of the component and, at the very least, any assumptions made regarding their features should be clearly stated.

Certain structures which are found on surfaces are best characterized numerically by relating their number to the surface upon which they are situated, rather than to a containing volume. Such estimates may be applied to investigate frequencies of intercellular junctions [10, 15-17]. The method is based on the N_V formulation and is

$$N_S = \frac{N_B}{\bar{\Delta}} \qquad \text{(Equation 8)}$$

where N_B is the number of components, N, present along a surface profile of length B. $\bar{\Delta}$ is the mean diameter of the component. B is readily determined by intersection counting according to the equation

$$B = \frac{\pi}{2} \times I \times h \qquad \text{(Equation 9)}$$

where I is the number of intersections of the lattice with the component and h is the distance between the lattice lines, corrected according to the magnification being used. This equation can also be used to generate the mean profile boundary trace length $\bar{B}$ of the component since, $\bar{\Delta}$

$$\bar{B} = \frac{B}{N} \qquad \text{(Equation 10)}$$

the mean diameter of the component, can prove very difficult to determine. In our studies of desmosomes and hemidesmosomes [15,17], we have assumed these components to be flat circular discs of similar size. On this basis, $\bar{B} \neq \bar{\Delta}$ since if a randomly orientated number of discs are sectioned, their mean diameter will always be lower than their true diameter. We have resorted to using Abercrombie's method [18] to compensate for diameter underestimations; thus

$$\bar{\Delta} = \bar{B} \times \frac{4}{\pi} \qquad \text{(Equation 11)}$$

The acquisition of these density estimates can provide an enormous amount of information on the structure of cells and tissues. It is necessary to stipulate clearly what the component is as well as the exact nature of its containing component. Counting points in mitochondria (P_{MIT}) and in their containing epithelial cells (P_{CELL}) and cytoplasm (P_{CYT}) can thus provide us with either the cytoplasmic volume density ($=P_{MIT}/P_{CYT}$) or the cellular volume density ($=P_{MIT}/P_{CELL}$), with the latter always being lower in value since P_{CELL} contains points falling in both nucleus and cytoplasm. Hemidesmosomes (HD) which are found in the plasma membranes of epithelial cells at the basal lamina complex of the epithelial-connective tissue junction may have their surface densities quantified in relation to unit volume of epithelial cell ($S_{VHD,CELL}$) or in relation to the plasma membrane within which they are found (S_S). The S_S parameter may be derived for the entire plasma membrane (PM) surface as $S_{SHD,PM}$ or it may be more useful in biological terms to relate the hemidesmosomes only to the regions of membrane upon which they are found, i.e., the basal plasma membrane (BM), i.e., $S_{SHD,PM}$. The reference volume or area will thus vary according to the requirements of a study.

Density data are the most commonly used stereological parameters, but one must be wary in the interpretation of such data. Such pitfalls are illustrated in Fig. 1, Table 1 and in the illustrated example. The next step possible in stereology is to obtain tertiary data or average cell values.

Average Cell Data. If we can in some way quantify accurately some component of our experimental system, we can convert our density data to absolute data. From such estimates we can extract a great deal of relevant information which may tell us, for example, whether a particular organelle is undergoing proliferation or involution. How this can be achieved is best illustrated by using the liver as an example. Let us suppose that we wish to know whether the volume of hepatocyte mitochondria in an experimental group differ from that in a control group. Having carried out our experiment, we obtain two sets of livers from two experimental groups, and we measure their volumes (V_{LIV}), for example by fluid displacement. We then process the livers for electron microscopy and using semi thin sections at the light microscope level, the volume density of hepatocytes in unit volume of liver tissues ($V_{VHEP,LIV}$) is determined from a systematic random sample. These blocks are then sectioned for electron microscopy and the volume density of mitochondria in hepatocytes is calculated ($V_{VMIT,HEP}$). From this information we can calculate (i) the mean volume of hepatocytes in the liver V_{HEP} ($=V_{VHEP,LIV} \times V_{LIV}$) and thence (ii) the mean volume of mitochondria in the liver V_{MIT} ($=V_{VMIT,HEP} \times V_{HEP}$).

Another approach is to measure the dimensions of the cell from sections. If we have a population of cells with spherical nuclei of uniform size, the nuclear diameter can be determined by direct measurement and nuclear volume can be calculated from the formula for the volume of a sphere ($= 4/3\pi r^3$). If the ratio of nucleus to cytoplasm (N/C) is also known, we have a means of obtaining the cytoplasmic volume which is independent of cellular shape, since N/C is the ratio of the nuclear and cytoplasmic volumes. We now have estimates of nuclear volume, V_V, and cytoplasmic volume, V_{CYT}. If we estimate the volume density of mitochondria per unit volume of cytoplasm ($V_{VMIT,CYT}$), we can readily calculate the absolute volume of mitochondria in the average cell (V_{MIT}) from

$$V_{MIT} = V_{VMIT,CYT} \times V_{CYT} \qquad \text{(Equation 12)}$$

By using absolute cell volume estimates, surface densities may similarly be transformed to average cell data if they are related to a unit volume of cell or cytoplasm, i.e., S_V. If related to unit surface of plasma membrane, i.e., S_S, it is possible to obtain absolute estimates of the average cell plasma membrane surface (S_{PM}) by substituting cell volumes into the volume to surface ratio formula which is

$$\frac{V}{S} = \frac{V_{CELL}}{S_{PM}} = \frac{Z \times P}{4 \times I} \qquad \text{(Equation 13) [19]}$$

This method requires additional counting to be performed using a test lattice of interrupted lines (see Weibel [2]) of length Z. The ends of the

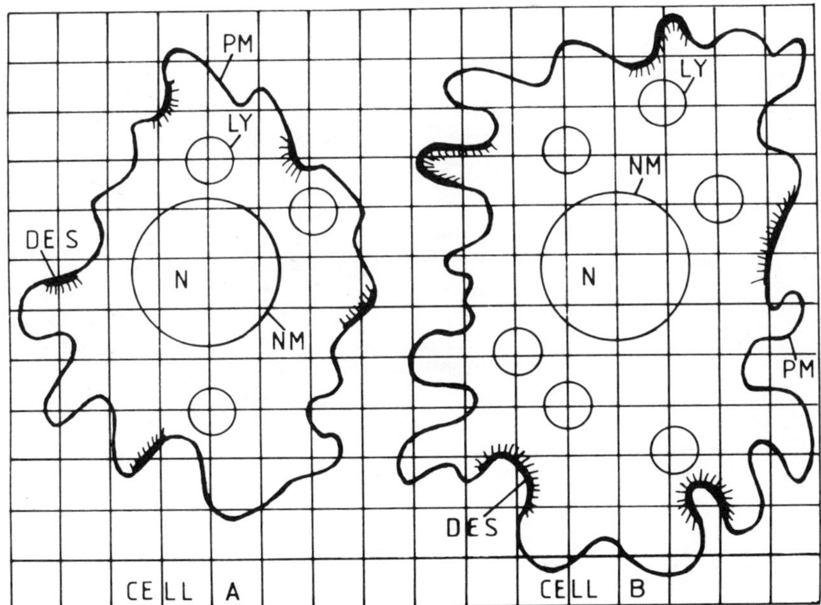

Fig. 1: Diagrammatic illustration of data generation using a double quadratic test lattice of side length 1cm at a magnification of x10,000. N = nucleus; CYT = cytoplasm; LY = lysosomes; MIT = mitochondria; NM = nuclear membrane; PM = plasma membrane; DES = desmosomal contact site. Note: For simplicity, the nuclei and lysosomes are presented as circles of diameters 3cm and 1cm. In random sections of spheres with these diameters, the mean diameters, $\bar{d}$, will be less than the true diameter, D, which is found from the relationship $D = \frac{4}{\pi} \times \bar{d}$. (In originaL 1 grid sq.=1cm).

lines are considered as points. Points falling within the cell are counted (P) as are intersections of the test lines with the plasma membrane (I). If we have a surface density of desmosomes expressed per unit surface of plasma membrane ($S_{SDES,PM}$), then the absolute surface area of desmosomes (S_{DES}) on the average cell is obtained from

$$S_{DES} = S_{SDES,PM} \times S_{PM} \qquad \text{(Equation 14)}$$

An Illustrated Example of Data Generation (Fig. 1 and Table 1)

Let us suppose that we have carried out an experiment on a particular tissue and have acquired a sample of micrographs in group A from control animals and in group B from the experimental animals and that we wish to identify the changes induced by the experimental treatment. In diagrammatic form, Fig. 1 shows a cell from group A and a cell from group B with a quadratic test lattice superimposed over each. The test lattice has a spacing of 1cm, which at a magnification of x10,000, represents an actual length lum. Each point on the lattice thus also represents $1um^2$. By carefully following the worked example, one can appreciate how primary data are obtained and how this can be converted to secondary and tertiary data (Table 1).

In such an example, it is obviously impossible to provide a comprehensive description of all stereological techniques available, but most of the common parameters are described. The data have, of course, been generated from only two cellular representations for simplicity, and are thus purely illustrative, but if we assume that they are derived from representative samples, we can see that several quantitative differences exist between our two hypothetical cell populations. For example, desmosomal surface densities (S_S and S_V) are similar in both populations. However, cell B has a lower frequency of larger desmosomes (compare N_S and $\bar{\Delta}$ data) and the average cell in group B has far more of its plasma membrand differentiated into desmosomal attachment sites (see S_{DES}). Similarly, the lysosomal density estimates V_V and N_V are similar in groups A and B, but their volumes and numbers in the average cell in both instances are actually doubled. These examples clearly show the limitations of the sole acquisition of density data from two samples, from which we might have concluded erroneously that our experimental treatment produced no significant alterations in either desmosomes or lysosomes. In fact, cells from group B were larger by almost $50um^3$, which resulted from cytoplasmic hypertrophy, and this was accompanied by the formation of desmosomes of greater size and by an increase in the volume of the lysosomal population, produced by a doubling of the number of lysosomes in the average cell. It is thus clear that before undertaking stereological analyses, one's aims and objectives should be clearly defined and any interpretations drawn from the study carefully considered.

Sampling Guidelines

Stereology is a science of averages, and depends for its success in terms of reliability and accuracy upon the acquisition of quantitative data from a representative random sample of tissue which is free of selection bias. In practice, this involves a series of steps known as a multilevel, nested or cascade sampling procedur [2]. Ideally, this should not deviate between control and experimental systems. In a simple experiment in which we wish to evaluate ultrastructural morphological changes induced by a particular experimental treatment, our starting point in the stereological analysis would be to obtain a group of animals (matched for strain, age, sex or body weight) which had been subjected to a particular experiment in identical ways and to obtain a control group of similar animals not subjected to such experimentation. From each of these animals in both groups,

Table 1: Acquisition of Stereological Information (derived from Figure 1)

PRIMARY DATA												
	P_N	P_{CYT}	P_{CELL}	P_{LY}	N_{LY}	N_{DES}	I_{DES}	I_{PM}	I_{NM}	I_{LY}	D_N	D_{LY}
Cell A	7	29	36	3	3	5	4	24	6	6	3μm	1μm
Cell B	7	52	59	6	6	5	7	35	6	12	3μm	1μm

SECONDARY DATA				
				Units
$N/C = \frac{P_N}{P_{CYT}}$		$\frac{7}{29} = 0.24$	$\frac{7}{52} = 0.13$	
$V_{V_{N,CELL}} = \frac{P_N}{P_N + P_{CYT}}$	(Eq.1)	$\frac{7}{36} = 0.19$	$\frac{7}{59} = 0.12$	$μm^3/μm^3$
$V_{V_{LY,CYT}} = \frac{P_{LY}}{P_{CYT}}$	(Eq.1)	$\frac{3}{36} = 0.10$	$\frac{6}{52} = 0.11$	$μm^3/μm^3$
$S_{S_{DES,PM}} = \frac{I_{DES}}{I_{PM}}$	(Eq.4)	$\frac{4}{24} = 0.17$	$\frac{7}{35} = 0.20$	$μm^2/μm^2$
$S_{V_{DES,CYT}} = 2 \times (\frac{I_{DES}}{P_{CYT}})$	(Eq.3)	$2 \times \frac{4}{29} = 0.28$	$2 \times \frac{7}{52} = 0.27$	$μm^2/μm^3$
$S_{V_{NM,CELL}} = 2 \times (\frac{I_{NM}}{P_{CELL}})$	(Eq.3)	$2 \times \frac{6}{36} = 0.33$	$2 \times \frac{6}{59} = 0.20$	$μm^2/μm^3$
$S_{V_{LY,CYT}} = 2 \times (\frac{I_{LY}}{P_{CYT}})$	(Eq.3)	$2 \times \frac{6}{29} = 0.41$	$2 \times \frac{12}{52} = 0.46$	$μm^2/μm^3$
$B_{PM} = \frac{\pi}{2} \times I_{PM} \times 1$	(Eq.9)	$\frac{\pi}{2} \times 24 = 37.70$	$\frac{\pi}{2} \times 35 = 54.98$	μm
$B_{DES} = \frac{\pi}{2} \times I_{DES} \times 1$	(Eq.9)	$\frac{\pi}{2} \times 4 = 6.28$	$\frac{\pi}{2} \times 7 = 10.99$	μm
$\bar{B}_{DES} = B_{DES} \div N_{DES}$	(Eq.10)	$\frac{6.28}{1} = 1.26$	$\frac{10.99}{5} = 2.20$	μm
$\bar{A}_{DES} = \bar{B}_{DES} \times \frac{4}{\pi}$	(Eq.11)	$1.26 \times \frac{4}{\pi} = 1.60$	$2.20 \times \frac{4}{\pi} = 2.80$	$μm^2$
$N_{S_{DES,PM}} = \frac{N_{DES} \div B_{PM}}{\bar{A}_{DES}}$	(Eq.8)	$\frac{5 \div 37.7}{1.60} = 0.08$	$\frac{7 \div 54.98}{2.80} = 0.03$	$μm^{-2}$
$N_{V_{LY,CYT}} = \frac{N_{LY} \div A_{CYT}}{\bar{D}_{LY}}$	(Eq.6)	$\frac{3 \div 29}{1} = 0.10$	$\frac{6 \div 52}{1} = 0.11$	$μm^{-3}$

TERTIARY DATA			
	A	B	
$V_N = \frac{4}{3}\pi(\frac{D}{2})^3$	$\frac{4}{3} \times \pi \times (\frac{3}{2})^3 = 14.14$	$\frac{4}{3} \times \pi \times (\frac{3}{2})^3 = 14.14$	$μm^3$
$V_{CYT} = V_N \div N/C$	14.14 ÷ 0.24 = 58.92	14.14 ÷ 0.13 = 108.77	$μm^3$
$V_{CELL} = V_N + V_{CYT}$	14.14 + 58.92 = 73.06	14.14 + 108.77 = 122.91	$μm^3$
$V_{LY} = V_{V_{LY,CT}} \times V_{CYT}$	0.10 x 58.92 = 5.89	0.11 x 108.77 = 11.96	$μm^3$
$S_{DES} = S_{V_{DES,CYT}} \times V_{CYT}$	0.28 x 58.92 = 16.50	0.27 x 108.77 = 29.37	$μm^2$
$S_{NM} = S_{V_{NM,CELL}} \times V_{CELL}$	0.33 x 73.06 = 24.11	0.20 x 122.91 = 24.58	$μm^2$
$N_{LY} = N_{V_{LY,CYT}} \times V_{CYT}$	0.10 x 58.92 = 5.89	0.11 x 108.77 = 11.96	

we would then obtain samples of the tissue or organ, which would then be prepared for electron microscopy. Procedures used for microscopical examination of tissues, such as fixation, dehydration, embedding and sectioning may modify structural dimensions by shrinkage, swelling, compression or extraction of various components. During specimen preparation, carefully controlled, standardized procedures should be used, in order that such procedures affect both groups similarly. Variations in preparative techniques are potential sources of error and can greatly affect the quantitative data obtained [2,20-22].

Having obtained a sample of tissue blocks from each animal, a random sample is obtained, usually by lottery, for sectioning. In theory, such sections should be cut in random planes, but in practice it may be necessary to deviate from this ideal. For example, if studies are directed towards analysis of the different maturation compartments (basal, spinous and granular layers) in a stratified squamous epithelium, random plane sections would pass both perpendicularly and horizontally with respect to the epithelial surface. In horizontal sections, it is impossible to discriminate adequately between the morphology of basal and spinous cells, and for this purpose such sections would be useless. Thus random perpendicular planes are used in which it is assumed that each cellular layer forms a polarized sheet, within which the individual cells are homogeneous [17, 23-26]. In simple columnar epithelia, an analysis of differences between basal and apical portions of the cell would be most efficiently carried out using sections perpendicular to the epithelial surface. Boysen and Reith [27,28] have used such sections for their histological and ultrastructural evaluations of abnormal nasal epithelium in nickel workers. In other cases it may be essential for purposes of cellular identification to obtain cells sectioned through their nuclei or nucleoli [29,30], and such bias can be adjusted by correction procedures [31].

From our random sample of sections, it is then necessary to acquire a random but representative sample of fields from each section. In epithelial organs such as the liver, in which large numbers of hepatocytes are present, a useful randomization procedure is to record photographically only those cells which lie in particular corners of a grid square. This may be highly impractical for tissues with a much smaller volume, for example the stratified epithelium of the epidermis, or columnar epithelium lining the gut or inner ear. In these cases, where less tissue is available for analysis, randomization can be effected by photographing cells adjacent to grid bars, and two or three more between these at equally spaced predetermined intervals.

True randomization at all levels of sampling is of paramount importance and yet does not ensure the representativeness, the other _sine qua non_ of stereology, of our sample. I have already suggested approaches in which sectioning procedures may be biased. In practical terms, randomization is necessary insofar as the final sample of fields which we are to quantify does not in any way include features which we have selected as typical of our sample. If, for example, we wanted to quantify the volume of mitochondria in basal cells in a stratified epithelium, it would be advisable to select perpendicularly sectioned profiles to identify the basal cells, but not to select from those basal cells which appear to have larger or more numerous mitochondria.

The above comments relate to sample quality. However, when conducting a stereological investigation, we also need to know how large each sample should be at each of the levels of our multilevel sampling scheme. In essence, how many animals, blocks, sections and fields should be used to obtain accurate results from a representative sample with the minimum of effort? Obviously, maximal precision is obtained by making the maximum number of measurements. Shay [32] has shown that beyond a certain sample size, the improvement in precision improves only marginally in relation to the extra effort involved in obtaining the measurements. Mayhew [33] has discussed the problems associated with sampling with clarity and in depth recently. In order to carry out efficient stereology, we need to obtain accurate estimates from the smallest sample possible in the shortest time. Optimal sample size is influenced by many factors which include the stereological parameter being measured, the magnitude of the changes we wish to detect and the natural variation between animals and that produced by an experimental treatment, which may induce substantial heterogeneity in the morphology of cells and tissues at all sampling levels.

In order to answer these questions, a statistical approach has been used by several groups to which the reader is referred [32,34-37]. Practically, a pilot study is carried out using a fixed number of animals, blocks per animal, sections per block and fields per section. By using analysis of variance techniques [33-37], it is then possible to assess the contribution to the total experimental variance between animals made by each of the sampling levels. Sampling levels displaying high variances will need to have their sizes increased if this is cost effective [36]. One of the most consistent features of this type of analysis has been to identify the most significant source of variation in experimental studies as that derived from innate biological variation between animals. The implications of this in stereological analyses is that as many animals as is feasible should be used in any given experimental system. The advice offered by Gundersen and Østerby [34] of "Do more less well" is well worth heeding. There is nothing to be gained from measuring tissue or cellular components from each field with great precision when such effort will have little bearing on the overall variation of the experiment.

As we have seen, stereological estimates can be generated most simply by a procedure known as event counting. The number of points or intersections which need to be counted to achieve a given level of precision on a set of micrographs can be determined using the relative standard error (RSE) approach which can be performed to determine test point numbers for volume density [38] or test intersection numbers for surface density [2] estimates. In order to determine an acceptable level of precision, a pilot study is carried out in which approximations of volume or surface densities are determined, preferably from one animal. The relevant formulae are given as

$$RSE = \sqrt{\frac{1-V_V}{P}} \qquad \text{(Equation 15)}$$

for volume density estimates and

$$RSE = S_V \sqrt{\frac{2}{I}} \qquad \text{(Equation 16)}$$

for surface density estimates. The number of points P or intersections I required to provide a defined standard error for a given volume (V_V) or surface density (S_V) can thus be estimated.

Another commonly used approach is that known as the cumulative or progressive mean plot technique. Here a large sample of micrographs from one animal is measured [39,40]. For each micrograph, the desired estimate is derived and then plotted accumulatively against the number of fields. The number of fields required to attain and remain within a specified range of the final mean is then taken to be the minimal sample size for the particular component in one animal within a given experimental group.

The major disadvantage of the relative standard error and accumulative mean approaches is that, while they can provide us with an indication of how many fields or events we need to count for each animal, they do not tell us how many animals, blocks or sections we need. The statistical analysis of variance techniques are thus superior in this respect.

Reductions in intra-animal variation can also be reduced practically by selecting the lowest possible magnification which permits adequate resolution of the component being measured [41]. This will increase the sample size and reduce variation between fields. Sectioning efficiency can be reduced for small organs by dicing the entire organ and randomly embedding the tissue in a single block, which is then sectioned. This technique has been used by Stringer et al. [42] in rat thyroid gland. Counting procedures may be made more efficient by careful design of the test lattice. For volumetric estimates, each point should represent a square which is similar in area to the largest profile of the component being quantified [2]. The use of coherent dual lattices comprising arrays of coarse and light points also improves efficiency enormously, with coarse points being used to evaluate the reference and fine points to quantify the component of interest.

APPLICATIONS OF STEREOLOGY IN EPITHELIAL CARCINOGENESIS

Malignant development is characterised by uncontrolled growth and division of cells which leads to local invasion of the adjacent stroma and eventually to the distant spread, or metastasis, of malignant cells via the blood or lymphatic systems. Epithelial cancers are by far the most prevalent of the malignant diseases, and treatment has more likelihood of success in earlier rather than later stages of the disease. The diagnosis of overt carcinomas is usually straightforward, but many precancerous conditions are difficult to detect and often ambiguous in their histopathological presentation.

The development of cancer in both humans and in experimental animal models is accompanied by a variety of morphological alterations at both tissue and cellular levels. Many of these are quantifiable. Using morphometric and stereological methods, work in our laboratory has been directed towards the identification of structural features in both epithelial lesions and the adjacent connective tissues which are altered during malignant transformation in the hamster cheek pouch mucosa treated with the chemical carcinogen 7,12 dimethylbenz(α)anthracene (DMBA). As an illustration of how stereological methods can be used in experimental pathology, I will summarize some of our recent results obtained from these models using two different experimental approaches.

In the first of these, our intention was to determine whether quantitative changes in the blood vascular system of the lamina propria were induced by carcinogen application as a function of time. DMBA (0.5%) dissolved in liquid paraffin was applied thrice weekly to cheek pouch mucosa for up to 10 weeks and cheek pouches obtained after 6 and 16 weeks. Untreated animals and animals treated thrice weekly with liquid paraffin for 10 weeks were used as controls. Tissue was processed for routine histological examination and five animals were used in each of the groups. Serial sections 5 um in thickness were cut, and one in every ten removed, mounted and stained with Van Gieson. From each section, four equally spaced fields were measured at a final magnification of x104 on each of ten sections obtained from each animal in each group.

Measurements were carried out directly on sections using a Zeiss microscope fitted with a drawing tube attachment arranged over the digitizing tablet of a MOP AM03 semi-automatic image analyzing system. This instrument can be programmed to produce number, length and area measurements automatically from perimeter traces of different components by using a cursor. On each section, the areas of epithelium (A_{EP}), lamina propria (A_{LP}) and blood vessels (A_{BV}) were measured. All blood vessels within the lamina propria were quantified irrespective of morphology. From these primary data, two simple secondary parameters were generated: the ratio of epithelium to lamina propria ($EP/LP = A_{EP}/A_{LP}$) and the volume density of blood vessels in the lamina propria ($V_{VBV,LP} = A_{BV}/A_{LP}$). Primary data were pooled on an individual animal basis and secondary data were generated for each animal. The results are summarized in Table 2.

Qualitatively, the carcinogen induces a variety of changes in the epithelial tissues which results in marked heterogeneity of morphometry at different time intervals. These changes include hyperplasia, dysplasia, carcinoma _in situ_, papilloma and squamous cell carcinoma. Thus, any section obtained from the DMBA-16 group will demonstrate several of these features and random samples from such a section will, upon quantification, reflect this heterogeneity. This is evident in the high deviations in the DMBA-16 group for both parameters in Table 2. Vascularity is increased 10-fold in the DMBA-6 group and more than 25-fold in the DMBA-16 group. This may be a result of induction of vascular proliferation by the transforming epithelial cells, which produce tumor angiogenesis factor [43] by which means malignant cells ensure their survival by providing themselves with an adequate vascular network. The EP/LP ratio is reduced in the DMBA-6 group, but is markedly elevated after 16 weeks. Qualificatively, these changes probably reflect alterations in epithelial volume. Indeed, after 16 weeks, the epithelial component seems to be substantially increased. However, the almost 8-fold increase in vascular volume density following liquid paraffin administration was an entirely unexpected finding. This vehicle is generally believed to be innocuous and to produce no significant histological alterations. However, data in Table 2 suggests that this is not the case and that quantitative morphological changes are induced by the vehicle for the carcinogen.

Malignant invasion by epithelial cells is intimately involved with structural alterations at the epithelial-connective tissue junction. In a second example, a different sampling procedure was used in which ultrastructural quantification of some features of this junction was carried out in histopathologically defined dysplastic, premalignant lesions and compared with normal epithelium. Using the same experimental model as outlined above, cheek pouch lesions were collected for ultrastructural examination and using semi-thin sections, 5 blocks from each of 5 animals were diagnosed as epithelial dysplasia on the basis of their abnormal cytological features [44]. Thin sections were obtained and a systematic random sample of micrographs obtained at two different magnifications. Whole basal cells were recorded at a final magnification of x6,000 for

Table 2: Histological Morphometry of Experimental Cheek Pouch Carcinogenesis

		Normal	liquid Paraffin	DMBA-6	DMBA-16
EP/LP	$\bar{x}$	1.027	0.818	0.649	1.683
	SD	0.220	0.067	0.096	0.630
$V_{V_{BV,LP}}$	$\bar{x}$	0.0042	0.0327	0.0454	0.1085
	SD	0.0012	0.0130	0.0206	0.0733

quantification of average cell features such as cell volume and surface area and a second series of micrographs of the junction recorded at x18,750, from which junctional features such as hemidesmosomes and lamina densa were measured.

Cellular volumes (V_{CELL}) and surface areas (S_{CELL}) were determined using direct nuclear measurements in conjunction with point and intersection counting to estimate nuclear cytoplasmic and cellular volume to surface ratios [17,45,46]. Differential intersection counting was used to calculate the relative surface area of membrane in contact with the junction $S_{SBM,PM}$, [47] and of the relative surface areas of hemidesmosomes, $S_{SHD,BM}$, [48], and lamina densa, $S_{SLD,BM}$, [49], to basal plasma membrane. Following estimation of parameters characterizing the average cell membrane surface, it was possible to obtain tertiary data by multiplying density estimatess by the average area of basal plasma membrane (S_{BM}) i.e., that membrane associated with the epithelial-connective tissue junction. Thus the absolute areas of hemidesmosomes (S_{HD}) and lamina densa (S_{LD}) were derived from the average cell in normal and DMBA-induced dysplastic lesions. Results are presented in Table 3.

Dysplastic basal cells have double the volume and 50% more plasma membrane than normal basal cells. They also have more of their plama membrane in contact with the lamina propria (see $S_{SBM,PM}$) and on this membrane, 40% is differentiated into hemidesmosomal junctions. In dysplastic cells, this proportion is reduced to 27%. 98% of the normal basal plasma membrane is associated with lamina densa, but this is reduced to 77% in dysplastic cells. Average cell data indicate that the absolute surface of hemidesmosomes is similar in both normal and dysplastic cells but that the areas of basal plasma membrane and of lamina densa are significantly higher in dysplastic cells when compared with normal cells. Thus a number of structural alterations are found in pre-neoplastic cells, the most striking finding being an increased surface area of basal plasma membrane in contact with the stromal tissues. Since there is a doubling in S_{BM}, we can conclude that increased plasma membrane synthesis or assembly is occurring. Some of this membrane may be inserted into the basal plasma membrane, producing a dilution of the existing hemidesmosomal junctions which may result in a progressive reduction in adhesion at the epithelial-connective tissue junction. This may be an important prerequisite for malignant invasion.

Morphometric techniques may thus prove to be valuable in the pathogenesis of neoplasia, and if specific morphological descriptors or parameters can be identified, may eventually prove useful as diagnostic aids in the assessment of malignant disease. They also lead one to pose a number of questions. For example, are vascular alterations specific for the carcinogenesis process or are they a result of the accompanying inflammation? Is there any relationship between vascular density and

Table 3: Stereological Analyses of Basal Cell Components in Normal Hamster Cheek Pouch Epithelium and DMBA-induced Dysplasia

		V_{CELL}	S_{CELL}	$S_{SBM,PM}$ (μm²/μm²)	$S_{SHD,BM}$ (μm²/μm²)	$S_{SLD,BM}$ (μm²/μm²)	S_{HD} (μm²)	S_{LD} (μm²)	S_{BM} (μm²)
Normal	$\bar{x}$	352	1088	0.09	0.40	0.98	35	84	86
	SD	85	307	0.02	0.03	0.02	10	19	20
Dysplasia	$\bar{x}$	672	1651	0.12	0.27	0.77	53	149	190
	SD	177	341	0.01	0.06	0.08	18	37	30

epithelial thickness? Are the alterations in vascular volume produced by angiogenesis or neovascularization or by dilatation of existing vessels? Is the quantitative response in carcinogenesis the same or different for the various vascular components, i.e., arteries, veins and capillaries? Can the vascular alterations be modified by anti-neoplastic, anti-inflammatory or vasoactive agents? What is the relationship between vascular volume and the histopathology of the overlying epithelial lesion? Are the density reductions in hemidesmosomes and lamina densa specific for carcinogenesis or are they also present in benign inflammatory and non-neoplastic conditions? Can basal lamina alterations be reversed by specific modulators of epithelial differentiation, such as retinoids? Are any other intercellular junctions, for example desmosomes, reduced in density following carcinogen application? Are there any other quantitative morphological alterations present in intracellular organelles which might prove valuable as indicators of malignant transformation?

The list of questions posed could obviously be extended, but each of these could be answered by the application of stereological methods. Their reliability and objectivity make them very effective techniques for the structural biologist.

MORPHOMETRY IN EPITHELIAL BIOLOGY AND PATHOLOGY

It is obviously impossible to provide an exhaustive list of the possible applications of morphometric and stereological studies to normal and abnormal epithelial tissues within the context of this review. However, some selected examples may serve to stimulate the reader to look more deeply into the subject.

A number of ultrastructural studies of stratified squamous epithelium have been performed. In most of these, different strata have been investigated to determine the maturation pattern of particular features between basal and surface layers [17,23-26,45,46,50-58]. The quantitative histological characteristics of a wide variety of stratified epithelia have also been investigated [59-64] and several studies have incorporated quantification of the supporting connective tissue components [65-69]. Histological and ultrastructural modifications of stratified epithelia following a variety of experimental treatments and in various disease states have been described [70-83] and there is also a significant morphometric interest in the responses of stratified epithelia and their supporting tissues to experimental carcinogenesis [46-49,84-88] and in human neoplasia [89-91]. A variety of other types of epithelia have also been subjected to morphometric and stereological analyses in studies of normal, experimentally-treated or diseased tissues. These include glandular tissues such as the parotid [92-94] liver [95-97] pancreas [98,99] and breast [100-102], endocrine glands such as the adrenals [103] and pancreatic islets [104,105], the columnar cells of the upper respiratory tract [106-110], a variety of components in the lung [111-113] and in the kidney [114-116] and gastrointestinal tract [117-119].

A cursory glance through the above cited references will reveal the rich variety of research problems being tackled in epithelial biology by using quantitative morphological techniques. If the procedures outlined in this paper and described more fully elsewhere [2,7,33,120,121] are adhered to, the novice will be able to exploit these powerful, objective techniques with great benefit in structural studies of comparative morphology, experimental biology and pathology and in the pathogenesis and diagnosis of human disease.

ACKNOWLEDGEMENTS

I gratefully acknowledge the constructive collaboration with Terry Mayhew, Khosro Gohari and Bushra Al-Azzawi during the past decade. My thanks also to Maureen Tune for preparing the illustration and to Jenny Cameron for skillfully producing the manuscript at short notice. Part of this work was funded by the Medical Research Council.

REFERENCES

1. J. P. A. Baak and J. Oort, "A Manual of Morphometry in Diagnostic Pathology," Springer Verlag, Heidelberg (1983).
2. E. R. Weibel, "Stereological Methods, Vol. 1: Practical Methods for Biological Morphometry," Academic Press, London (1979).
3. S. Bradbury, Commercial image analysers and the characterization of microscopical images, J. Microsc., 131:203 (1983).
4. K. Goerttler and M. Stohr, Automated cytology: the state of the art, Archs. Pathol. Lab. Med., 106:657 (1982).
5. R. C. Braylan, Flow cytometry, Archs. Pathol. Lab. Med., 107:1 (1983).
6. R. T. DeHoff and F.N. Rhines, "Quantitative Microscopy," McGraw Hill, New York (1968).
7. E. R. Weibel, Stereologic principles for morphometry in electron microscopic cytology, Int. Rev. Cytol., 26:235 (1969).
8. E. R. Weibel, "Stereological Methods, Vol. 2: Theoretical Foundations," Academic Press, London (1980).
9. E. E. Underwood, "Quantitative Stereology," Addison-Wesley, Reading, Massachusetts (1970).
10. T. M. Mayhew, Basic stereological relationships for quantitative microscopical anatomy - a simple systematic approach, J. Anat., 129:95 (1979).
11. H. J. G. Gundersen, Stereology - or how figures for spatial shape and content are obtained by observation of structures in sections, Microscop. Acta., 83:409 (1980).
12. H. J. G. Gundersen, M. Boysen and A. Reith, Comparison of semi-automatic digitizer tablet and simple point counting performance in morphometry, Virch. Arch. B. Cell Pathol., 37:317 (1981).
13. E. R. Weibel and D. M. Gomez, A principle for counting tissue structures on random sections, J, Appl, Physiol., 17:343 (1962).
14. T. M. Mayhew, A. J. Burgess, C. D. Gregory and M. E. Atkinson, On the problem of counting and sizing mitochondria: a general reappraisal based on ultrastructural studies of mammalian lymphocytes, Cell Tiss. Res., 204:297 (1979).
15. F. H. White, T. M. Mayhew and K. Gohari, Stereological methods for quantifying cell surface specializations in epithelia, including a concept for counting desmosomes and hemidesmosomes, Brit, J, Dermatol., 107:401 (1982).
16. F. H. White and K. Gohari, Hemidesmosomal dimensions and frequency in experimental oral carcinogenesis; a stereological investigation, Virch, Arch, B, Cell Pathol., 45:1 (1984).
17. F. H. White and K. Gohari, Desmosomes in hamster cheek pouch epithelium: their quantitative characterization during epithelial differentiation, J, Cell Sci., 66:411 (1984).
18. M. Abercrombie, Estimation of nuclear population from microtome sections, Anat, Rec., 94:239 (1946).
19. H. W. Chalkley, J. Cornfield and H. Park, A method for estimating volume-surface ratios, Science, 110:295 (1949).
20. A. Reith, T. Barnard and H. Rohr, Stereology of cellular reaction patterns, CRC Crit. Rev. Toxicol., 4:219 (1976).

21. M. A. Williams, Quantitative methods in biology in: "Practical Methods in Electron Microscopy," Vol. 6, A. M. Glauert, ed., Elsevier North Holland Biomedical Press, Amsterdam (1977).
22. M. Lindberg, Variation in epidermal structure as a function of different fixation methods: a stereological and morphological study, J. Submicrosc. Cytol., 15:549 (1983).
23. H. E. Schroeder and S. Munzel-Pedrazzoli, Application of stereologic methods to stratified gingival epithelia, J. Microsc., 92:179 (1970).
24. M. A. Landay and H. E. Schroeder, Quantitative electron microscopic analysis of the stratified epithelium of normal human buccal mucosa, Cell Tiss. Res., 177:383 (1977).
25. F. H. White, D. A. Thompson and K. Gohari, Ultrastructural morphometry of gap junctions during differentiation of stratified squamous epithelium, J. Cell Sci., 69:67 (1984).
26. K. Gohari and F. H. White, A morphometric study of alterations in rough endoplasmic reticulum during differentiation in stratified squamous epithelium, Arch. Dermatol. Res., 276:303 (1984).
27. M. Boysen and A. Reith, Stereological analysis of nasal mucosa III. Stepwise alterations in cellular and subcellular components of pseudo-stratified metaplastic and dysplastic epithelium in nickel workers, Virch. Arch. B. Cell Pathol., 40:311 (1982).
28. M. Boysen and A. Reith, Discrimination of various epithelia by simple morphometric evaluation of the basal cell layer. A light microscopical analysis of pseudostratified, metaplastic and dysplastic nasal epithelium in nickel workers, Virch. Arch. B. Cell Pathol., 42:173 (1983).
29. T. M. Mayhew and M. A. Williams, A comparison of two sampling procedures for stereological analysis of cell pellets, J. Microsc., 94:195 (1971).
30. T. M. Mayhew and L. M. Cruz-Orive, Some stereological correction formulae with particular applications in quantitative neuro-histology, J. Neurol. Sci., 26:503 (1975).
31. T. M. Mayhew and L. M. Cruz-Orive, Stereological correction procedures for estimating true volume proportions from biased samples, J. Microsc., 9:287 (1973).
32. J. Shay, Economy of effort in electron microscope morphometry, Amer. J. Pathol., 81:503 (1975)
33. T. M. Mayhew, Stereology: progress in quantitative microscopical anatomy in: "Progress in Anatomy," V. Navaratnam and R. J. Harrison, eds., 3:81 (1983).
34. H. J. G. Gundersen and R. Osterby, Optimizing sampling efficiency of stereological studies in biology or "Do more less well!", J. Microsc., 121:65 (1981).
35. M. Gupta, T. M. Mayhew, K. S. Bedi, A. K. Sharma and F. H. White, Interanimal variation and its influence on the overall precision of morphometric estimates based on nested sampling designs, J. Microsc., 131:147 (1983).
36. T. M. Mayhew, F. H. White and K. Gohari, Towards economy of effort in quantitative ultrastructural pathology; efficient sampling schemes for studying experimental carcinogenesis, J. Pathol. 138:179 (1982).
37. J. P. Kroustrup and H. J. G. Gundersen, Sampling problems in an heterogeneous organ; quantitation of relative and total volume of pancreatic islets by light microscopy, J. Microsc., 132:43 (1983).
38. A. D. Hally, A counting method for measuring the volumes of tissue components in microscopical sections, Quart. J. Microsc. Sci., 105:503 (1964).
39. H. W. Chalkley, Methods for quantitative morphological analysis of tissue, J. Nat. Cancer Inst., 4:47 (1943).

40. M. S. Dunnill, Quantitative Methods in Histology in: "Recent Advances in Clinical Pathology Series V," S. C. Dyke, ed., 401-416, Churchill, London (1968).
41. L. M. Cruz-Orive and E. R. Weibel, Sampling designs for stereology, J. Microsc., 122:235 (1981).
42. B. M. J. Stringer, D. Wynford-Thomas and E. D. Williams, Physical randomization of tissue architecture: an alternative to systematic sampling, J. Microsc., 126:179 (1982).
43. J. Folkman and R. Cotran, Relation of vascular proliferation to tumor growth, Int. Rev. Exp. Pathol., 26:206 (1976).
44. I. R. H. Kramer, Basic histopathological features of oral premalignant lesions in: "Oral Premalignancy: Proceedings of the First Dows Symposium," I. C. Mackenzie, E. Dabelsteen and C. A. Squier, eds., 23-24, University of Iowa Press (1980).
45. F. H. White and K. Gohari, Cellular and nuclear volumetric alterations during differentiation of normal hamster cheek pouch epithelium, Archs. Dermatol. Res., 273:307 (1982).
46. F. H. White, R. M. Codd and K. Gohari, An ultrastructural morphometric study of cellular and nuclear volume alterations during experimental oral carcinogenesis, J. Submicrosc. Cytol. In press.
47. F. H. White and K. Gohari, A quantitative ultrastructural study of alterations in the area of the basal cell-stromal interface during experimental oral carcinogenesis, J. Oral Pathol., 14:227 (1985).
48. F. H. White and K. Gohari, Quantitative studies of hemidesmosomes during progressive DMBA carcinogenesis in hamster cheek pouch mucosa, Brit. J. Cancer, 44:440 (1981b).
49. F. H. White and K. Gohari, A quantitative study of lamina densa alterations in hamster cheek pouch carcinogenesis, J. Pathol., 135:277 (1981c).
50. H. E. Schroeder and S. Munzel-Pedrazzoli, Morphometric analysis comparing junctional and oral epithelium of normal human gingiva, Heav. Odontol. Acta., 14:53 (1970).
51. G. Rowden, Ultrastructural studies of keratinized epithelia of the mouse III: Determination of the volumes of nuclei and cytoplasm of cells in murine epidermis, J. Invest. Dermatol., 64:1 (1975).
52. G. Rowden, Ultrastructural studies of keratinised epithelia in the mouse IV: Quantitative studies of lysosomes, J. Invest. Dermatol., 64:4 (1975).
53. M. Meyer and H. E. Schroeder, A quantitative electron microscopic analysis of the keratinizing epithelium of normal human hard palate, Cell Tiss. Res., 158:177 (1975).
54. J. P. Bernimoulin and H.E. Schroeder, Quantitative electron microscopic analysis of the epithelium of normal human alveolar mucosa, Cell Tiss. Res., 180:383 (1977).
55. L. Andersen and H. E. Schroeder, Quantitative analysis of squamous epithelium of normal palatal mucosa in guinea pigs, Cell Tiss. Res., 190:223 (1978).
56. A. J. P. Klein-Szanto, Stereologic baseline data of normal human epidermis, J. Invest. Dermatol., 68:73 (1977).
57. F. H. White and K. Gohari, Volumetric alterations in tonofibrils during epithelial differentiation in hamster cheek pouch mucosa, J. Anat., 137:489 (1983).
58. F. H. White and K. Gohari, Stereological studies of differentiation in hamster cheek pouch epithelium: variations in the volume and frequency of mitochondria, J. Anat., 136:801 (1983).
59. T. D. Allen and C. S. Potten, Ultrastructural site variations in mouse epidermal organization, J. Cell Sci., 21:341 (1976).
60. C. D. Franklin and G. T. Craig, Stereological quantification of histological parameters in normal hamster cheek pouch epithelium, Archs. Oral Biol., 23:337 (1978).
61. L. Fleisch, P. Cleaton-Jones and J. C. Austin, Oral mucosa of the vervet monkey, J. Periodont. Res., 15:444 (1980).

62. M. W. Hill, J. H. Berg and I. C. Mackenzie, Quantitative evaluation of regional differences between epithelia in the adult moose, Archs. Oral Biol., 26:1063 (1981).
63. J. Scott, J. A. Valentine, C. A. St. Hill and B. A. W. Balasooriya, A quantitative histological analysis of the effects of age and sex on human lingual epithelium, J. Biol. Bucc., 11:303 (1983).
64. L. S. Sauter and E. R. Weibel, Morphometric evaluation of skin. structure by stereologic methods, Dermatologica, 143:174 (1971).
65. H. E. Schroeder and S. Munzel-Pedrazzoli, Correlated morphometric and biochemical analysis on gingival tissues: Morphometric model, tissue sampling and test of stereologic procedures, J. Microsc., 99:301 (1973).
66. A. J. P. Klein-Szanto and H. E. Schroeder, Architecture and density of the connective tissue papillae of the human oral mucosa, J. Anat., 123:93 (1977).
67. P. B. Klein, W. A. Weilenmann and H. E. Schroeder, Structure of the soft palate and composition of the oral mucous membrane in monkeys, Anat. Embryol., 156:197 (1979).
68. H. E. Schroeder and A. Dorig-Schwartzenbach, Structure and composition of the oral mucous membrane on the lips and cheeks of the monkey, Macaca fascicularis, Cell Tiss. Res., 224:89 (1982).
69. M. J. Stablein, J. Meyer and J. P. Waterhouse, Epithelial dimensions and capillary supply in the oral mucosa of the rat, Archs. Oral Biol., 27:243 (1982).
70. C. D. Franklin and G. T. Craig, Stereological quantification of histological parameters in turpentine-induced hyperplasia of hamster cheek pouch epithelium, Archs. Oral Biol., 23:347 (1978).
71. N. E. Steidler and P. C. Reade, Histomorphological effects of epidermal growth factor on skin and oral mucosa in neonatal mice, Archs. Oral Biol., 25:37 (1980).
72. J. Meyer, M. Stohle and M. Stablein, Correlation of changes in capillary supply and epithelial dimensions in the hyperplastic buccal mucosa of zinc-deficient rats, J. Oral Pathol., 10:49 (1981).
73. M. W. Hill, R. R. Harris and C. P. Carron, A quantitative ultrastructural analysis of changes in hamster cheek pouch epithelium treated with vitamin A, Cell Tiss. Res., 226:541 (1982).
74. A. J. P. Klein-Szanto and T. J. Slaga, Numerical variation of dark cells in normal and chemically-induced hyperplastic epidermis with age of animal and efficiency of tumor promoter, Cancer Res., 41:4437 (1981).
75. G. P. M. Moore, B. A. Panaretto and D. Robertson, Epidermal growth factor delays the development of the epidermis and hair follicles of mice during growth of the first coat, Anat. Rec., 205:47 (1983).
76. L. Andersen, Quantitative analysis of epithelial changes during wound healing in palatal mucosa of guinea pigs, Cell Tiss. Res., 193:231 (1978).
77. V. Trinkaus-Randall and I. K. Gipson, Role of calcium and calmodulin in hemidesmosome formation in vitro, J. Cell Biol., 98:1565 (1984).
78. J. S. Nennie and D. G. MacDonald, Quantitative histological analysis of the epithelium of the ventral surface of hamster tongue in experimental iron deficiency, Archs. Oral Biol., 27:393 (1982).
79. C. A. Squier and C. R. Kremenak, Quantitation of the healing palatal mucoperiosteal wound in the beagle dog, Brit. J. Exp. Pathol., 63:573 (1982).
80. J. S. Rennie, D.G. MacDonald and J. H. Dagg, Quantitative analysis of human buccal epithelium in iron deficiency anemia, J. Oral Pathol., 11:39 (1982).
81. A. J. P. Klein-Szanto, L. Andersen and H. E. Schroeder, Epithelial differentiation patterns in buccal mucosa affected by lichen planus, Virch. Archiv. B. Cell Pathol., 22:245 (1976).

82. A. J. P. Klein-Szanto, J. Banoczy and H. E. Schroeder, Metaplastic conversion of the differentiation pattern in oral epithelium affected by leukoplakia simplex. A stereologic study, Pathol. Europ., 11:189 (1976).
83. M. Chiba, T. J. Slaga and A. J. P. Klein-Szanto, A morphometric study of dedifferentiated and involutional dark keratinocytes in 12-O-tetradecanoylphorbol-13-acetate-treated mouse epidermis, Cancer Res., 44:2711 (1984).
84. F. H. White, T. M. Mayhew and K. Gohari, The application of morphometric methods to investigations of normal and pathological stratified squamous epithelium, Pathol. Res. Pract., 166:323 (1980).
85. J. W. Eveson and D. G. MacDonald, Quantitative histological changes during early experimental carcinogenesis in the hamster cheek pouch, Brit. J. Dermatol., 98:639 (1978).
86. C. D. Franklin and C. J. Smith, Stereological analysis of histological parameters in experimental premalignant hamster cheek pouch epithelium, J. Pathol., 130:201 (1980).
87. S. G. Tarpey and F. H. White, Ultrastructural morphometry of collagen from lamina propria during experimental oral carcinogenesis and chronic inflammation, J. Cancer Res. Clin. Oncol., 107:183 (1984).
88. F. H. White and K. Gohari, Alterations in the volume of the intercellular space between epithelial cells of the hamster cheek pouch: quantitative studies of normal and carcinogen-treated tissues, J. Oral Path., 13:244 (1984).
89. N. S. McNutt, Ultrastructural comparison of the interface between epithelium and stroma in basal cell carcinoma and control human skin, Lab, Invest., 35:132 (1976).
90. G. Wiernik, S. Bradbury, M. Plant, R. H. Cowdell and E. A. Williams, A quantitative comparison between normal and carcinomatous squamous epithelia of the uterine cervix, Brit. J. Cancer, 28:488 (1973).
91. B. U. Pauli, S. M. Cohen, J. Alroy and R. S. Weinstein, Desmosome ultrastructure and the biological behaviour of chemical carcinogen-induced urinary bladder carcinomas, Cancer Res., 38:3276 (1978).
92. G. H. Cope and M. A. Williams, Exocrine secretion in the parotid gland: a stereological analysis at the electron microscopic level of the zymogen granule content before and after isoprenaline-induced degranulation, J. Anat., 116:269 (1973).
93. G. H. Cope.and M. A. Williams, Quantitative analyses of the constituent membranes of parotid acinar cells and of the changes evident after induced exocytosis, Z. Zellforsch., 145:311 (1973).
94. M. K. Pratten, M. A. Williams and G. H. Cope, Compartmentation of enzymes in the rabbit parotid salivary gland. A study by enzyme histochemical, tissue fractionation and morphometric techniques, Histochem. J., 9:573 (1977).
95. A. V. Loud, A quantitative stereological description of the ultrastructure of normal rat liver parenchymal cells, J. Cell Biol., 37:27 (1968).
96. E. R. Weibel, W. Staubli, H. R. Gnagi and F. A. Hess, Correlated morphometric and biochemical studies on the liver cell. I: Morphometric model, stereologic methods and normal morphometric data for rat liver, J. Cell Biol., 42:68 (1969).
97. G. Borgia, J. Crowell, M. Cocchiarano, N. Abrescia, A. Lambiase, G. D'Alfonso, W. Schreil and M. Piazza, Ultrastructural changes in mouse liver cells: a morphometric study on the influence of morphine, heroin and cardiostenol, J. Ultrastruct. Res., 80:123 (1982).
98. R. P. Bolender, Stereological analysis of guinea pig pancreas 1. Analytical model and quantitative description of non-stimulated exocrine cells, J. Cell Biol., 61:269 (1974).

99. J. R. Imrie, D. G. Fagan and J. M. Sturgess, Quantitative evaluation of the development of the exocrine pancreas in cystic fibrosis and control infants, Amer. J. Pathol., 95:697 (1979).
100. M. E. Boon, P. A. Trott, H. Van Kaam, P. J. H. Kurver, A. Leach and J. P. A. Baak, Morphometry and cytodiagnosis of breast lesions, Virch. Arch. A. Pathol. Anat., 396:9 (1982).
101. J. P. A. Baak, P. H. J. Kurver, J. E. Snoo-Nieuwlaat, S. de Graaf, B. de Makkink and M.E. Boon, Prognostic indicators in breast cancer - morphometric methods, Histopathology, 6:327 (1982).
102. J. V. Frei, Objective measurement of basement membrane abnormalities in human neoplasms of colorectum and of breast, Histopathology, 2:107 (1978).
103. P. Rebuffat, C. Robba, A. S. Belloni, G. Mazzocchi, P. Vassanelli and G. G. Nussdorfer, An electron microscopic stereological study of the compensatory hypertrophy of the rat adrenal zona fasciculata after unilateral adrenalectomy, Cell Tiss. Res., 225:455 (1982).
104. K. Saito, T. Takahashi, N. Yaginuma and N. Iwama, Islet morphometry in the diabetic pancreas, Tohoku J. Exp. Med., 125:185 (1978).
105. K. Saito, N. Iwama and T. Takahashi, Morphometrical analysis of topographical differences in size distribution, number and volume of islets in the human pancreas, Tohoku J. Exp. Med., 124:177 (1978).
106. A. J. P. Klein-Szanto, P. Nettesheim, D. C. Topping and A. C. Olson, Quantitative analysis of disturbed cell maturation in dysplastic lesions of the respiratory tract epithelium, Carcinogenesis, 1:1007 (1980).
107. A. J. P. Klein-Szanto, P. Nettesheim and G. Saccomano, Dark epithelial cells in preneoplastic lesions of the human respiratory tract, Cancer, 50:107 (1982).
108. E. M. McDowell, K. P. Keenan and M. Huang, Effects of vitamin A deprivation on hamster tracheal epithelium. A quantitative morphologic study, Virch. Arch. B. Cell Pathol., 45:197 (1984).
109. E. M. McDowell, K. P. Keenan and M. Huang, Restoration of mucociliary tracheal epithelium following deprivation of vitamin A. A quantitative morphologic study, Virch. Arch. B. Cell Pathol., 45:221 (1984).
110. M. Boysen and A. Reith, Light and electron microscopic studies by manual and semiautomatic morphometric analysis of the basal layer, Meth. Achiev. Exp. Pathol., 11:111 (1984).
111. E. R. Weibel, Morphometry of the human lung: the state of the art after two decades, Bull. Eur. Physiopathol. Respir., 15:999 (1979).
112. J. F. Bertram and A. W. Rogers, The development of squamous cell metaplasia in human bronchial epithelium by light microscopic morphometry, J. Microsc., 123:61 (1980).
113. B. Vidic and P. H. Burri, Morphometric analysis of the remodelling of the rat pulmonary epithelium during early postnatal development, Anat. Rec., 207:317 (1983).
114. H. Elias and A. Hennig, Stereology of the human renal glomerulus in: "Quantitative Methods in Morphology," E. R. Weibel and H. Elias, eds.", 130-166, Springer Verlag, Berlin (1967).
115. K. Kawano, J. McCoy, J. Wenzl, J. Porch, C. Howard, M. Goddard and P. Kimmelstiel, Quantitation of glomerular structure. A study of methodology, Lab. Invest., 25:343 (1971).
116. T. Nomppanen and Y. Collan, Morphometricalmethod foranalysis of kidney biopsies in diagnostic histopathology, Stereol. Jugosl., 3: Suppl. 1, 435 (1981).
117. G. C. Schofield, S. Ito and R. P. Bolender, Changes in membrane surface areas in mouse parietal cells in relation to high levels of acid secretion, J. Anat., 128:669 (1979).

118. R.J. Buschmann and D.J. Manke, Morphometric analysis of the membranes and organelles of small intestine enterocytes. 1: Fasted hamsters, J. Ultrastruct. Res., 76:1 (1981).
119. G. H. Cope, Stereological techniques and their application to the gastrointestinal tract and its glands in: "Techniques in the Life Sciences, Vol. P2, Techniques in Digestive Physiology," D. A. Titchen, ed., 1-33, Elsevier Scientific Publishers Ireland Ltd. (1982),
120. E. R. Weibel and R. P. Bolender, Stereological techniques for electron microscopic morphometry in: "Principles and Techniques of Electron Microscopy," M. A. Hayat, ed., 3:237, Van Rostrand Rheinold Co., New York (1973).
121. H. Haug, The significance of quantitative stereologic experimental procedures in pathology, Pathol. Res. Pract., 166:144 (1980).

DISCUSSION

Patuzzi

Presumably there is an optimum unit length or grid size for evaluating the structures you are interested in. How do you determine this?

White

Absolutely, there are ways to determine that. I showed a grid which had identical sized squares. You can use different size squares and count different components. Ideally, the size of the grid squares should be approximately equivalent to the lagest area of the component you are interested in. Obviously, if you are looking at a cell which has a nucleaus, mitochondria and micotubules, then these are all very different in size and diameter. What we usually do under these conditions is to use a coherent double lattice. Where every 5th line or every 10th line is thicker, use the thickest lines for quantifying the large structures and the thin lines to count the small structures. Since there are 10 fine lines to one large line, the width of the thick line is obviously equivalent to 10 times the small line and the area is going to be equal to 10 squared. So, there are methods for increasing the efficiency above what I have shown.

Saunders

You could be measuring with tremendous precision cell structures where the shrinkage level is not known and I could say, so what? An important issue here is what anatomical changes are due to histological processing itself?

White

Right, I omitted to mention the fact that when you are carrying out one of these studies, one of the most fundamental requirements is to make sure you are processing the experimental and control groups in exactly the same way. Thus, the changes you are quantifying morphologically would be the result of the experimental treatment and not of the fixation. I would not like to suggest that the data you obtain are strictly comparable to which you would find in vivo. Obviously, fixation does produce a variety of effects. But if you use the same fixative in your control groups and in your experimental groups, then we would assume the changes would be the same for both groups. The message that I am trying to give those interested in the histology or in ultrastructure of the auditory system is that it is possible to describe the changes which may have some particular biological significance to you quantitatively, rather than simply qualitatively.

MORPHOMETRIC METHODS FOR THE EVALUATION OF THE COCHLEAR MICROVASCULATURE

Lynn Carlisle

Kresge Hearing Research Institute
University of Michigan
Ann Arbor, MI

INTRODUCTION

Although the vasculature of the cochlea has been implicated in a number of etiologies of deafness, experimental verification for such an involvement has proved to be difficult; part of the reason for this difficulty is that, until recently, studies of the cochlear vasculature have been descriptive rather than quantitative. Descriptive studies have contributed significantly to our understanding of gross vascular pathology in the cochlea; however, it is difficult to document subtle morphological changes without resorting to quantitative methods. Since subtle changes in the blood supply to the cochlea may be involved in such clinical conditions as tinnitus, Meniere's disease and temporary threshold shift following acoustic trauma, there has been considerable interest in developing quantitative methods for the analysis of the cochlear vasculature. Several such techniques are described in this chapter, following a brief review of the vascular anatomy of the cochlea.

The Vascular Anatomy of the Cochlea

Detailed descriptions of the vascular anatomy in commonly used experimental animals and in man have been published by Smith [1], Hawkins [2], and Axelsson [3]. The blood supply to the membranous labyrinth is provided by the internal auditory or labyrinthine artery which is a terminal branch of the anterior inferior cerebellar artery. Once inside the membranous labyrinth, the labyrinthine artery divides and sends branches to the vestibular and cochlear tissue. One of these branches, the common cochlear artery, supplies the entire cochlea via its two branches, the cochlear or spiral modiolar artery, which supplies all of the cochlea except the extreme basal end, and the vestibulocochlear artery, which supplies the extreme basal end.

The spiral modiolar artery enters the modiolus and coils around the cochlear spiral to its apical end. In some species, arteriolar glomeruli are observed in the modiolus. The modiolar vessels are in close proximity to adrenergic and cholinergic nerve fibers [4]. Branching arterioles are given off at regular intervals to supply the spiral ganglion, osseous spiral lamina and the lateral wall tissues, eventually forming terminal capillaries which perform their nutritional function and then drain into the venous system.

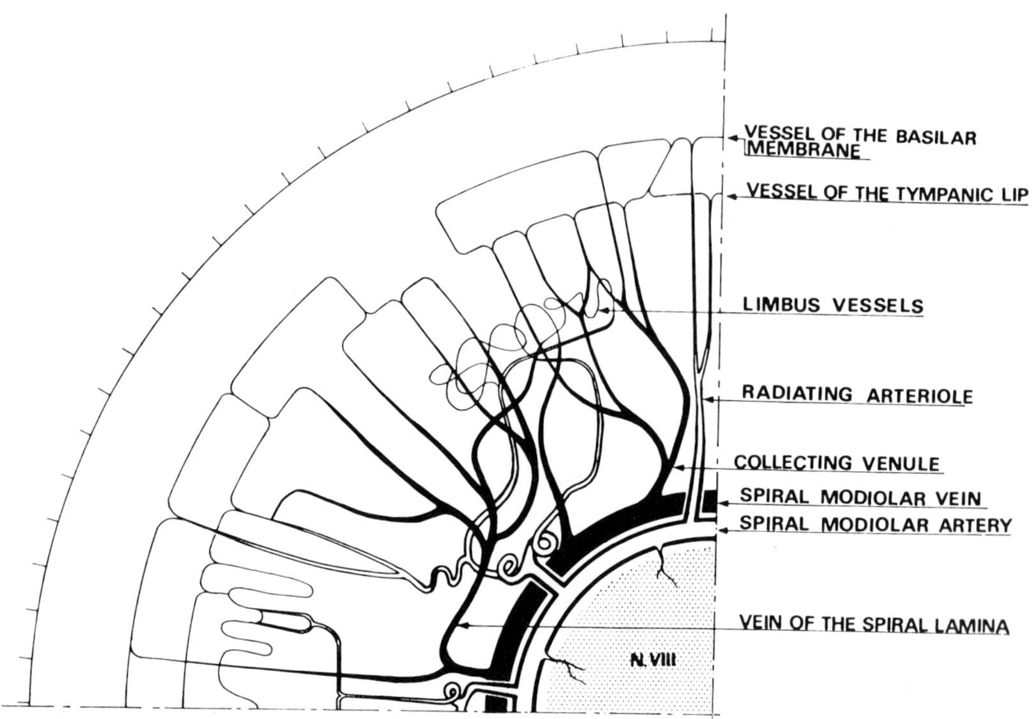

Fig. 1. Schematic representation of the spiral lamina and limbus. The vessel of the basilar membrane is only occasionally present; when present, it is located under the tunnel of Corti. The vessel of the tympanic lip is located in the region of the habenula perforata; it receives most of the radiating vessels. The area peripheral to the tunnel of Corti is avascular (From Axelsson [3]).

The osseous spiral lamina contains two spiral vessels (Fig. 1). The vessel of the tympanic lip, which forms a series of T-shaped loops near the habenula perforata, is the principal vessel of the spiral lamina. Another vessel, the vessel of the basilar membrane, is situated under the tunnel of Corti, but it is not always present. Both vessels are surrounded by numerous pericytes and in some rare instances unmyelinated nerve fibers have been reported terminating on these vessels. These vessels are responsible for the nutritional support of the organ of Corti [5].

A second population of radiating arterioles arch over scala vestibuli and then leave the bony partition to supply the vascular areas of the lateral wall (Fig. 2). All of these vessels are true capillaries, being devoid of nerve fibers and smooth muscle cells. Some of these capillaries pass through the spiral ligament from scala vestibuli to scala tympani, others course through the spiral ligament and then pass into the spiral prominence and still others supply the stria vascularis. The capillaries which supply the stria vascularis ramify extensively to form a complex vascular network. Extensive vascularization of the stria vascularis is necessary to meet the high metabolic demands of this tissue, which is responsible for the maintenance of the high potassium level of endolymph and the endolymphatic potential [6,7].

Due to its vital role in the function of the inner ear, most studies of the inner ear vasculature have focused on the stria vasularis. The stria is composed of three distinct cell layers, the marginal, intermediate

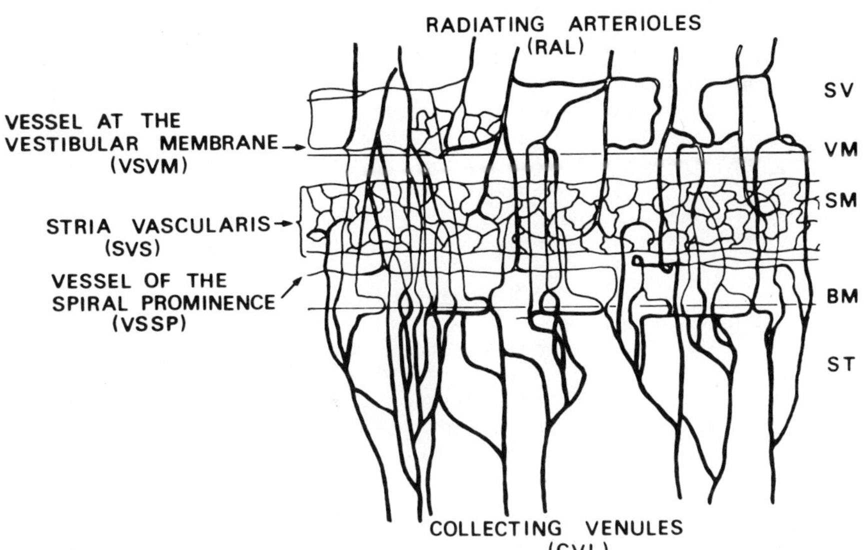

Fig 2. Schematic representation of the cochlear lateral wall. According to Axelsson's nomenclature, vessels are named to reflect their relationship to other anatomical structures and their course through the cochlea; in actuality, all lateral wall vessels are capillaries, based on their size and the absence of smooth muscle (From Axelsson [3]).

and basal cell layers [8]. The marginal cells form the endolymphatic surface of the stria vascularis. These cells are characterized by their dense-staining cytoplasm and their intricate pattern of basal infoldings. The marginal cells are believed to be the ion-transporting cells of the stria [9]. The intermediate cells interdigitate with the marginal cell processes and the capillaries of the stria. The intermediate cells contain a pigment which is believed to be melanin [10]. The capillaries of the stria have a continuous endothelial lining and are occasionally surrounded by pericytes. The border between the stria and the spiral ligament is formed by one or two layers of spindle-shaped basal cells.

MORPHOMETRIC STUDIES OF THE INNER EAR VASCULATURE

The anatomical arrangement of the capillaries in the stria vascularis is such that they lie in a single plane when viewed as a surface preparation. This characteristic enables investigators to study the entire length of the stria and gain a comprehensive picture of its organization. Unfortunately, a surface preparation view of the stria vascularis provides little information regarding the cellular matrix in which the vessels reside, since the three cell layers of the stria lie in a plane orthogonal to that of the vessels and are best illustrated in cross-sectional views of the tissue. For this reason, techniques for the analysis of the stria vascularis have tended to emphasize either the cellular matrix or the vascular component.

Stereology of Stria Vascularis

The technique developed by Santi et al. [9] utilizes the cross-sectional approach to analyze the relative density of the cells and capillaries of the stria. In their first study, epon-embedded cross-sections were taken at four predetermined locations along the cochlear spiral and photomontages were compiled so that an entire cross-sectional profile of the stria was represented. Using a digitizing tablet interfaced to a Terak microcomputer and a stereological technique adapted for analysis of a small, stratified epithelium, the volume density (Vv) of the cells and capillaries of the stria vascularis were quantified. A 2 cm grid was placed over the photo-micrographs (at 7500X magnification) and the relative proportion of the tissue occupied by each component was calculated as:

$$Vv(\text{component}) = \frac{\text{number of point-hits on component}}{\text{total point-hits on stria vascularis}}$$

At each location, the width (measured as the distance along the endolymphatic surface of the stria from the attachment of Reissner's membrane to the edge of the spiral prominence) and the radial area of the stria were also calculated.

The results of this study indicated a 34% increase in the width and a 52% increase in the radial area of the stria from the apical to the basal end of the cochlea. Santi et al. also reported that the relative volume density of each of the components of the stria did not vary among the four regions where measurements were made and concluded that one radial section is sufficient to characterize normal stria volume densities. They reported volume densities of the four components of the normal chinchilla stria vascularis to be: marginal cells = 0.528 (± 0.013); intermediate cells = 0.212 (± 0.026); basal cells = 0.163 (± 0.009); capillaries = 0.097 (± 0.009).

In a subsequent study [11], this technique was used to quantify volume density of strial components in chinchillas dosed with bumetanide and sacrificed at intervals of 10 minutes, 1 hour and 24 hours later. Cross-sections were cut at intervals of 10% for radial area measurements and a single radial section cut at 70% of the distance from the apex was used for the volume density measurements. In addition to quantifying the three cell types and capillaries, the relative volume density of intercellular spaces was also calculated as:

$$Vv(\text{intercellular}) = \frac{\text{point-hits on intercellular spaces}}{\text{total point-hits on stria}}$$

The formula for computing Vv for the other components was modified:

$$Vv(\text{all others}) = \frac{\text{point-hits on component}}{(\text{total hits}) - (\text{hits on intercellular spaces})}$$

Results of the study showed an increase in radial area of the stria vascularis at 10 minutes and at 1 hour, and no change in stria width. The volume density of the marginal cells was significantly decreased and the volume density of the intermediate cells was significantly increased at 10 minutes and at 1 hour after dosage. No significant changes were found for the volume density of basal cells or capillaries in the stria.

Computerized Image Analysis of Stria Vessels

In the first truly morphometric study of cochlear vessels, the morphology of stria vascularis capillaries was studied by Smith et al. [12] using surface preparations of strial tissue from guinea pigs either exposed to noise or treated with quinine and untreated control animals. Optical images of strial tissue were projected onto the monitor screen of a hard-wired image analysis device (Quantimet 720). Areas from each turn of each cochlea were selected at random for measurement. Selected objects were measured by tracing them on the monitor screen with a light pen. Two variables were calculated based on these measurements. They were:

$$\text{Vascular density} = \frac{\text{area of vessel lumen}}{\text{area of total field}}$$

$$\text{RBC distribution} = \frac{\text{area of vessel lumen occupied by RBCs}}{\text{area of total field}}$$

The results were analyzed statistically by location and group using factorial analysis of variance. There was no significant difference in vascular density between control, noise-damaged and quinine-treated animals, but a highly significant difference in vascular density was reported for cochlear location. A significant decrease in RBC distribution was found in both the noise-exposed and quinine-treated groups as compared to controls. The incidence of vessel narrowings was also quantified by averaging the number of vessel narrowings caused by swollen endothelial cells per millimeter of stria length over the sample area from each turn. The results were transformed and submitted to analysis of variance, which indicated a significant increase in both experimental groups as compared to the control group.

The Soft-Surface Specimen Technique

Both methods just described are restricted to an analysis of the stria vascularis and do not consider the other capillary areas of the cochlea. The technique developed by Axelsson and his collaborators [13-15] emphasizes the importance of evaluating all of these capillary areas and the surrounding cellular matrix in order to gain a comprehensive understanding of the cochlear microcirculation. A list of 20 vascular parameters (see Table 1) is used to evaluate all of the regularly occurring vessels in the osseous lamina and lateral wall, and the entire length of the cochlea is analyzed by dividing it into half-turn segments. Each variable is quantified by assigning a numerical rating for each vessel in each half turn.

We used Axelsson's method to study the effect of impulse noise exposure on the vasculature of the chinchilla [16]. Animals were exposed to either 155 or 160 dB peak equivalent SPL (re 20×10^{-6} Pa) blast waves at a rate of 1 per minute for 50 minutes and decapitated without anesthetic after a 45-day recovery period. Axelsson's technique was used to evaluate the vasculature of control and noise-exposed animals, and the results were analyzed using stepwise discriminant analysis, a multivariate statistical technique which produces a hierarchical listing of variables that discriminate between experimental groups. The results of the statistical analysis are shown in Table 2, which lists the parameters which differed significantly from the control group. The decrease in plasma space between the RBCs and the vessel wall and the decrease in columns of RBCs are both suggestive of vessel constriction; the increase in lumen irregularities and in the number of perivascular cells compressing the vessel lumen are consistent with this interpretation. Table 2 indicates a different pattern of vascular change in the strial vessels than in the other vessels analyzed, with the predominant finding being an increase in pigmentation of the strial tissue.

Table 1. Axelsson's Vascular Parameters

	RED BLOOD CORPUSCLES
DENS	Density; frequency and spacing of RBCs in vessel lumen.
COL	Columns; number of rows of RBCs in vessel lumen.
AGGREG	Aggregations and plasma gaps; collections of RBCs and interspaced sections with plasma but without RBCs.
ORIENT	Orientation; manner and plane of RBCs in vessel lumen.
VAR	Variability; in density of RBCs.
PLAS	Plasma space; between RBCs and vessel wall.
	VESSEL LUMEN
LM IRRG	Lumen irregularity; local narrowing and widening of vessel lumen.
PV LUM	Perivascular cell compressing vessel lumen; occurrence of narrow vessel lumen caused by endothelial cell nuclei and/or pericytes.
DIAM	Lumen diameter; width of vessel lumen.
PVS	Perivascular spaces; spaces surrounding vessel lumen.
	STRIA VASCULARIS
GRAN	Granules; pigment formed of fine granulations.
PIGM	Pigment clumps; clusters or collections of pigment granules.
VAC	Vacuoles in stria surface structure.
GAPS	'Gaps' between cells; spaces occurring between stria marginal cells below the tight cell junctions.
	ADDITIONAL VASCULAR PARAMETERS
AVC	Avascular channels.
WBC	White blood cells.
EMB	Emboli in vessel; bound, clear spaces within vessel lumen.
DEP	Deposits; osmiophilic materials surrounding vessels.
MEL	Melanocytes.
SPH	Precapillary sphincters; narrowing of vessel by perivascular elements.

Adapted from Shaddock, Hamernik, and Axelsson [17].

Table 2. Significant Parameters by Vessel

PARAMETER \ VESSEL	RAL	VSVM	SVS	VSSP	CVL	VSTL
PLAS	↓	↓		↓	↓	↓
LM IRRG		↑			↑	↑
COL	↓		↓		↓	
PV LUM		↑			↑	
VAR				↑		
PIGM			↑			
GRAN			↑			
GAPS			↓			
WBC			↑			

Results of statistical analysis showing significant changes (positive or negative) in vascular parameters after 155 or 160 dB SPL impulse noise exposure. RAL-radiating arteriolis, VSVM- vessel of the vestibular membrane, SVS-stria vascularis vessels, VSSP-vessel of the spiral prominence, CVL-collecting venules, VSTL-vessel of the tympanic lip. See Table 1 for definitions of vascular parameters (from Shaddock, Hamernik and Axelsson [16]).

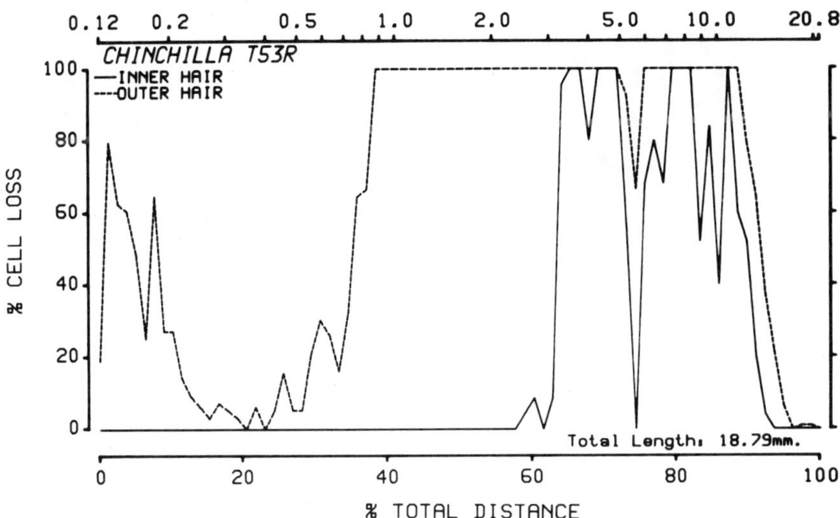

Fig. 3. Example of a cytocochleogram and vasculogram from a chinchilla exposed to 155 dB SPL impulse noise. Vascular pathology was greatest in the basal half of the cochlea, which may be related to the pattern of hair cell loss or may be due to a greater susceptibility of this area to vascular damage. For vasculogram abbreviations, see Table 1. (From Shaddock, Hamernik and Axelsson [16].)

In order to graphically display the relationship between areas of vascular damage and areas of hair cell loss, a "vasculogram" was generated for each cochlea. The numerical value for each parameter identified by the discriminant analysis was compared to the median value of that variable in the control group. The absolute value of the difference was computed and graphed by half turn. Fig. 3 shows the relationship between the cytocochleogram and vasculogram of an animal exposed to 155 dB SPL impulse noise.

In a related study we used the same noise exposure to examine the possible synergism of elevated body temperature and impulse noise exposure [17]; and the results were analyzed using the same statistical methods. Our results indicated no interaction of noise and elevated temperature on

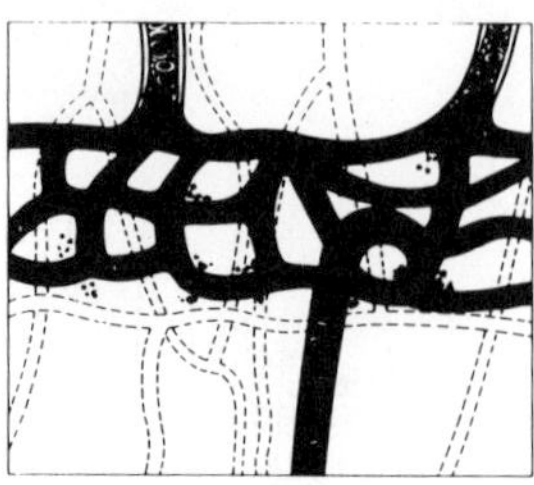

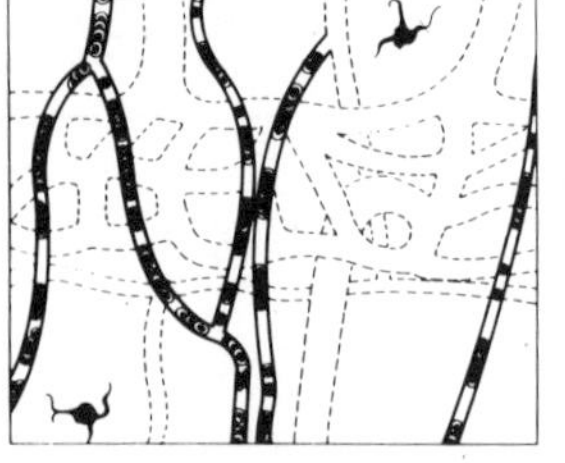

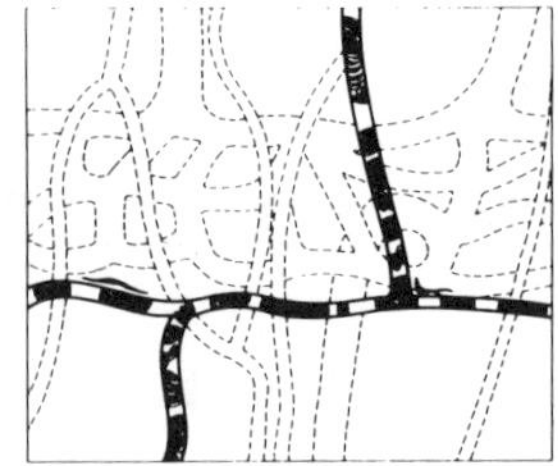

Fig. 4. Schematic representation of the three vessel systems of the cochlear lateral wall vascular variables are quantified in terms of vessel system and location (within system) with respect to scala vestibuli, scala media or scala tympani. (From Shaddock, Hamernik and Wright [19].)

the vasculature; the pattern of vascular changes seen was similar to that reported after impulse noise alone. We did observe that some vasculograms from animals exposed to elevated body temperature, but not exposed to noise, showed the same pattern of increased vascular change in the lower half of the cochlea (see Fig. 3), which might indicate a greater susceptibility to damage unrelated to cause in the lower cochlear turns of the chinchilla.

Axelsson has published a number of studies concerning the effects of noise on the vasculature. In a recent review article, Axelsson and Vertes summarized their conclusions based on these studies [18]. They concluded that noise effects on the vasculature are related to the type, intensity and duration of the exposure and are influenced by individual variability as well. They stressed the importance of evaluating all of the vessels, since which vessels show the most vascular changes is related to exposure parameters. In their experience, certain characteristics of vessel morphology seem to be good indicators of vascular change. These characteristics are RBC parameters (density, columns and aggregations of RBCs); perivascular cell parameters (size and frequency of perivascular cells); and vessel lumen parameters (lumen diameter and lumen irregularities). They also stated that the most common strial pathology involves strial degeneration accompanied by changes in pigment cells. In their studies, vascular changes were not limited to the area corresponding to the greatest sensory cell damage and an overall decrease in the blood supply as a result of noise exposure was observed.

Table 3. Vascular Variables (Shaddock et al.)

VASCULAR DENSITY:	Area occupied by vessels / Area of field.
RBC DENSITY:	Area occupied by RBCs / Area occupied by vessels.
VESSEL WIDTH:	Area occupied by vessels / Length of vessels.
AGGREGATION DENSITY:	Area occupied by aggregations of RBCs / Area occupied by RBCs.
WBC FREQUENCY:	Number of WBCs / Area occupied by vessels.
LUMEN COMPRESSIONS:	Number of lumen compressions / Area occupied by vessels.
PIGMENT DENSITY:	Area occupied by pigment / Area of field.

Vascular variables quantified according to the method developed by Shaddock, Hamernik, and Wright. These measurements were taken for the vessels of the 3 vessel systems described in Fig. 4.

Computerized Image Analysis of the Lateral Wall Vasculature

Our approach has been to classify the vessels of the lateral wall into vessel systems based on specific anatomical structures (the stria vascularis, the spiral prominence and the spiral ligament) and to evaluate these systems independently. These vessel systems (Fig. 4) are evaluated on the basis of location with respect to the specific anatomical structures that they supply.

We developed a set of seven vascular variables (Table 3) based on Axelsson's parameters [13-15] that would be easy to quantify using a system similar to the one used by Smith [12]. Our hardware consisted of a DEC LSI 11/23 microcomputer, an RCA 2000 Ultracon video camera, a Panasonic monitor and a Summagraphics TD 2000 digitizing tablet; the software used for data collection and analysis was written by Drs. William A. Ahroon and Craig M. Allen of the Callier Research Computer Facility, Dallas, Texas.

This method was used to collect normative data on vessel morphology and to compare the vessels of the three systems to see if they were morphologically distinct [19]. Surface preparations of lateral wall tissue from the middle turn of the chinchilla cochlea were analyzed over an area of approximately 1 mm [2]. Results were analyzed statistically using a one-way analysis of variance; the test was performed for data collected in scala vestibuli, scala media and scala tympani. Only four of the seven vascular variables could be analyzed statistically; WBC count and lumen compression count were eliminated from the analysis because no examples of either variable had been found during data collection. The three vessel systems were significantly different ($p < .05$) in terms of vascular density and vessel width in all three scalae, and in terms of RBC density in scala vestibuli and scala media. There was no significant difference between vessel systems for aggregation density. The mean values obtained for vascular density, RBC density, vessel width and aggregation density are contained in Table 4. These results supported the hypothesis that the lateral wall vasculature was composed of three morphologically distinct vessel systems.

The technique was used to analyze the vasculature of the chinchilla at 1 hour, 24 hours, 1 week and 3 weeks after surgical rupture of Reissner's membrane [20]. The results were analyzed in a two-way analysis of variance where the factors were vessel system and survival time; the results are contained in Table 5 and illustrated in Fig. 5, which summarizes the significant trends in the data. The results indicated that the three vessel systems of the lateral wall responded differently to the injury. In the system of stria vascularis vessels, there was a decrease in vascular density over time which reflected the degeneration of some strial vessels, a transient decrease in RBC density at 24 hours post- surgery and an increase in pigmentation in the cellular matrix of the stria. The width of surviving strial vessels, as well as those feeding and draining the stria, was unchanged over the course of the experiment. In the system of spiral ligament vessels, an increase in vascular density due to an increase in vessel width was observed. There was a transient increase in RBC density in the scala vestibuli portion of these vessels at 1 hour post-surgery, and a decrease over time in the number of pigment cells found in scala vestibuli and scala tympani. The system of spiral prominence vessels was least affected. There was an increase in vessel width in the vessels feeding and draining the spiral prominence, and an increase in pigmentation in the cellular matrix of the spiral prominence.

Although each of the four methods just reviewed has taken a slightly different experimental approach, the results of each set of studies have shown that various types of cochlear trauma do result in vascular pathology that can be measured and studied in a systematic way.

TABLE 4

Means (Standard Deviations) by Vessel System and Location for 5 normal chinchillas [19]

System of Stria Vascularis Vessels

S. Vestibuli	0.0516(.0278)	0.5406(.2465)	14.238(2.454)	0.0000(.0000)
S. Media-Str	0.1868(.0487)	0.8711(.2679)	7.447(1.502)	0.0000(.0000)
S. Media-Pro	0.0391(.0198)	0.6877(.0665)	11.829(2.271)	0.0000(.0000)
S. Tympani	0.0299(.0140)	0.6025(.2619)	11.117(2.520)	0.0000(.0000)

System of Sprial Ligament Vessels

S. Vestibuli	0.0622(.0217)	0.3002(.1893)	6.822(1.168)	0.0269(.1041)
S. Media-Str	0.0588(.0159)	0.2902(.0908)	5.485(1.053)	0.0000(.0000)
S. Media-Pro	0.0472(.0169)	0.4697(.1514)	5.846(1.162)	0.0000(.0000)
S. Tympani	0.0553(.0186)	0.4533(.1576)	5.895(1.586)	0.0000(.0000)

System of Spiral Prominence Vessels

S. Vestibuli	0.0276(.0165)	0.5261(.1588)	10.102(2.316)	0.0000(.0000)
S. Media-Str	0.0220(.0165)	0.4866(.0923)	7.088(1.016)	0.0000(.0000)
S. Media-Pro	0.0713(.0265)	0.6520(.1196)	6.733(1.409)	0.0259(.1003)
S. Tympani	0.0282(.0076)	0.4215(.1124)	6.578(1.723)	0.0000(.0000)

Table 5

Results of 2-way ANOVA on system x survival time. (From Shaddock, Wright, and Hamernik [19].)

Results of System X Survival Time 2-Way ANOV

	Vascular Density	RBC Density	Vessel Width	Aggregation Density	Pigment Density
		<u>A. Main effect of vessel system ($p \leq .001$)</u>			
Feeding Vessels	X	X	X	-	CNT*
Target Vessels	X	X	X	-	X
Draining Vessels	X	X	X	-	CNT
		<u>B. Main effect of survival time ($p \leq .01$)</u>			
Feeding Vessels	-	X	-	X	-
Target Vessels	X	X	X	-	X
Draining Vessels	-	-	X	-	-
		<u>C. Interaction effect: system x survival ($p \leq .05$)</u>			
Feeding Vessels	-	-	-	-	-
Target Vessels	X	X	X	-	X
Draining Vessels	-	-	-	-	-

X = statistically significant difference
- = no statistically significant difference
CNT = could not test

PRACTICAL PROBLEMS WITH MORPHOMETRIC STUDIES OF THE MICROVASCULATURE

<u>Sample Size</u>

One common feature of all morphometric techniques is their reliance on statistical analysis of the data for interpretation of the results. Statistical tests require large samples in order for their theoretical assumptions to be valid; on the other hand, because of the intricacy of the vascular pattern of the cochlea, data collection with these techniques is tedious and time-consuming and places practical constraints on sample size. For this reason, most techniques have involved the evaluation of a few restricted areas, since quantification of the entire cochlea would be impractical. The only method which involves the evaluation of the entire cochlear vasculature is the soft-surface specimen technique, but this method is not truly quantitative since the observer must assign a numerical rating which reflects an average value describing an entire half-turn of tissue based on a subjective evaluation of that tissue [15].

Santi [11] found no statistically significant difference in the volume density of the cells and capillaries of the stria vascularis of the chinchilla sampled at four locations along the length of the cochlea and concluded that one complete cross-section was adequate to characterize the normal stria. Smith's results in the guinea pig [12] based on samples taken at six locations along the length of the cochlea, showed a statis-

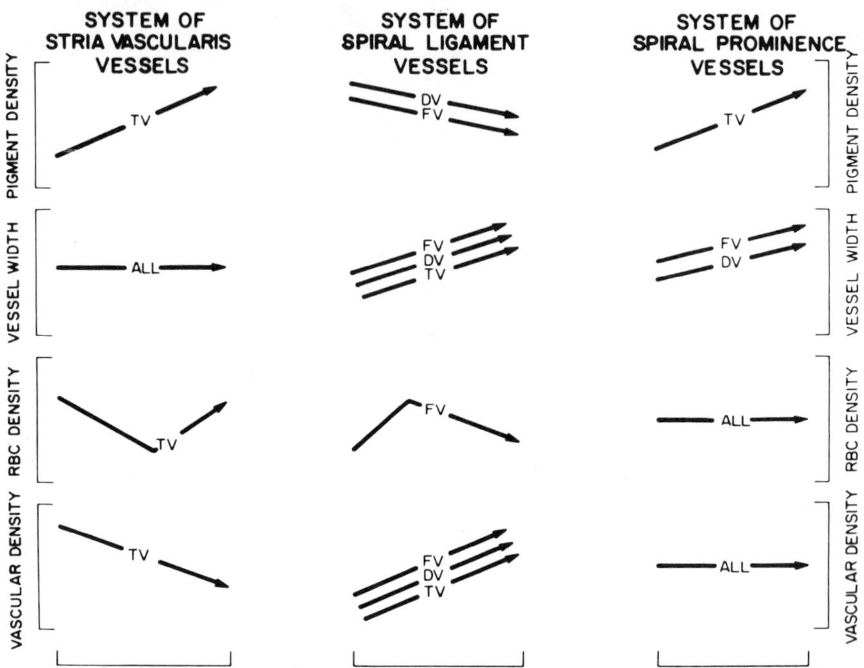

Fig. 5. Results of ANOVA on system X survival time showing vascular pathology after surgical rupture of Reissner's membrane. Arrows indicate significant increase or decrease; horizontal arrows indicate no change over time. For this analysis, vessels were classified as target vessels (TV), feeding vessels (FV) and draining vessels (DV) according to location in scala media, scala vestibuli or scala tympani (From Shaddock, Wright and Hamernik [19].)

tically significant difference for vascular density (which is roughly equivalent to Santi's measurement of volume density of capillaries), indicating that sampling in one area was not sufficient to characterize normal stria. We reported [20] a statistically significant decrease in vascular density 24 hours after rupture of Reissner's membrane [3]; however, Santi et al. [11] found no difference in the volume density of capillaries 24 hours after bumetanide treatment. The disparity between results in these studies could be due to the species difference, the difference in experimental treatment or the different methods used. Even if one sample area is adequate to characterize normal stria, areas from each turn must be sampled when pathological tissue is studied, since different areas of the vasculature may react differently to cochlear trauma.

Method of Sacrifice and Fixation

Due to the susceptibility of the microvasculature to humoral, hormonal and myogenic factors [21], the method of sacrifice used will influence subsequent measurements of vascular parameters. Anesthesia effects on the microcirculation vary, based on the drug used and the period elapsed between administration of the drug and time of sacrifice [22]. The alternative method of sacrifice is decapitation without anesthesia, which may result in vascular changes initiated by the autonomic nervous system. Another factor which could influence vascular measurements is method of fixation. Santi and Duvall [23] reported differences in RBC density and vessel diameter in animals which were perilymphatically perfused either *in vivo* or after decapitation. When animals were perilymphatically perfused after decapitation, vessels were constricted and packed with RBCs, but when animals were perilymphatically perfused *in vivo*, the capillaries of the stria were not constricted or packed with RBCs.

In two of our studies [16,17], we found statistically significant increases in the number of perivascular cells compressing the vessel lumen. The chinchillas used in these studies were sacrificed by decapitation without anesthetic three weeks after the noise exposure. In other studies [19, 20], we found no evidence of perivascular cells compressing vessel lumen in control chinchillas or in chinchillas sacrificed at 1 hr., 24 hrs., 1 wk. or 3 wks. after Reissner's membrane rupture. These animals were sacrificed by decapitation while deeply anesthetized with a mixture of ketamine, acepromazine and xylazine. The effect of anesthesia and/or method of sacrifice on the cochlear vasculature has not been studied in a systematic way. Such studies are needed to begin to understand the function of this vascular system as well as its response to cochlear trauma.

FUTURE TRENDS IN MICROVASCULAR RESEARCH IN THE COCHLEA

At this point, the groundwork has been laid for the development of a comprehensive, quantitative method for the analysis of the cochlear microvasculature. A next important step will be to define the role of anesthesis, method of sacrifice and method of fixation on the morphology of the vessels. Advances in video technology are improving the resolution achievable in images used for data collection, and more efficient computers make data manipulation easier and faster than before. These technological advances should enable researchers to include larger sample areas and to increase sample sizes. Given the work that has been done and the technological advances, morphometric research in the vascular system of the inner ear should be an exciting area of research in the years to come.

ACKNOWLEDGEMENTS

This research was partially supported by National Institute of Occupational Safety and Health grant no. 1 R01 OH1518-01, U.S. Army Medical Research and Development Command grant no. DAMD 17-83-G-9555, and the Swedish Work Environment Fund 81-0792.

REFERENCES

1. C. A. Smith, Capillary areas of the cochlea in the guinea pig, *Laryngoscope* 61:1073 (1951).
2. J. E. Hawkins, Jr., Vascular patterns of the membranous labyrinth, *in*: "Third Symposium on the Vestibular Organs in SPACE Exploration," A. Graybiel, ed., NASA, Washington (1968).
3. A. Axelsson, The vascular anatomy of the cochlea in the guinea pig and in man, *Acta Otolaryngol*. Suppl. 243 (1968).
4. R. S. Kimura and C. Y. Ota, Ultrastructure of the cochlear blood vessels, *Acta Otolaryngol*. 77:231 (1974).
5. M. Lawrence, The function of the spiral capillaries, *Laryngoscope* 81:1314 (1971).
6. S. K. Bosher and R. L. Warren, Observations on the electrochemistry of the cochlear endolymph in the rat: A quantitative study of its electrical potential and ionic composition as determined by means of flame spectrophotometry, *Proc. R. Soc. Lond.* B 171:227 (1968).

7. I. Tasaki and C. S. Spyropoulos, Stria vascularis as source of endocochlear potential, J. Neurophysiol. 22:149 (1959).
8. C. A. Smith, Structure of the stria vascularis and the spiral prominence, Ann. Otol. Rhinol. Laryngol. 66:521 (1957).
9. P. A. Santi, B. Lakhani, and C. Bingham, The volume density of cells and capillaries of the normal stria vascularis, Hearing Res. 11:7 (1983).
10. D. A. Hilding and R. D. Ginzberg, Pigmentation of the stria vascularis, Acta Otolaryngol. 84:24 (1977).
11. P. A. Santi and B. N. Lakhani, The effect of bumetanide on the stria vascularis: A stereological analysis of cell volume density, Hearing Res. 12:151 (1983).
12. D. I. Smith, M. Lawrence and J. E. Hawkins, Jr., Effects of noise and quinine on the vessels of the stria vascularis: An image analysis study, Am. J. Otolaryngol. 6:280 (1985).
13. A. Axelsson, J. Miller, and J. Holmquist, Studies of cochlear vasculature and sensory structures: A modified method, Ann Otol. 83:537 (1974).
14. A. Axelsson, J. Miller, and B. Larsson, A modified "soft surface specimen technique" for examination of the inner ear, Acta Otolarynol. 80:362 (1975).
15. D. Vertes and A. Axelsson, Methodological aspects of some inner ear vascular techniques, Acta Otolaryno1. 88:328 (1979).
16. L. C. Shaddock, R. P. Hamernik and A. Axelsson, Effect of high intensity impulse noise on the vascular system of the chinchilla cochlear, Ann. Otol. Rhinol. Laryngol. 94:87 (1985).
17. L. C. Shaddock, R. P. Hamernik, and A. Axelsson, Cochlear vascular and sensory cell changes induced by elevated temperature and noise, Am. J. Otolarynol. 5:99 (1984).
18. A. Axelsson and D. Vertes, Histological findings in cochlear vessels after noise, in: "New Perspectives on Noise-Induced Hearing Loss" R. P. Hamernik Henderson and R. Salvi, eds. Raven Press, New York (1982).
19. L. C. Shaddock, R. P. Hamernik, and C. G. Wright, A morphometric technique for the analysis of cochlear vessels, Hearing Res. (1985), in press.
20. L. C. Shaddock, C. G. Wright and R. P. Hamernik, A morphometric study of microvascular pathology following experimental rupture of Reissner's membrane, Hearing Res. (1985), in press.
21. B. M. Altura, Humoral, hormonal and myogenic mechanisms in microcirculatory regulation, in: "Microcirculation III," G. Kaley and B. M. Altura, eds., University Park Press (1980).
22. D. Longnecker and P. R. Harris, Anesthesia, in: "Microcirculation III," G. Kaley and B. M. Altura, eds., University Park Press, (1980).
23. P. A. Santi and A. J. Duvall, Morphological alteration of the stria vascularis after administration of the diuretic bumetanide, Acta Otolaryngol. 88:1 (1979).

DISCUSSION

Colletti: I really enjoyed your paper. Being interested in human pathology, I would like to ask you how much of this strategy can be transferred to the study of the vascular system in human temporal bones?

Shaddock: There is no reason why these techniques cannot be applied to human studies. One problem with human temporal bone material, however, is fixing the tissue quickly enough to prevent post mortem artifacts.

McFadden: I missed an important point when you showed the tables of significant differences. Are all those changes in the direction of vessel constriction?

Shaddock: No, they aren't. The direction of change is different for each of the three systems. For instance, you have a decrease over time in vascular density for the strial system and you have an increase over time in vascular density which is related to an increase in vessel width for the vessels in the spiral ligament. I have a table where you see that the three systems are moving in completely different directions for each variable. I think this supports the idea that you mask these changes when you combine the data from different vessels.

McFadden: Are these patterns the same across the length of the cochlea, relative to the exposure point?

Shaddock: My experimental procedure involved the rupture of Reisner's membrane. I was measuring at the area right around the rupture point and have not used noise and have not looked at different locations. This is something that obviously needs to be done.

von Gierke: I may have missed a point in your paper and the first paper. That is, how do you get a stereological 3-dimensional description of volume density or any other parameter from a 2-dimensional section? For that, you really would need the descriptions of the sections in two directions.

White: That's an issue, that to the novice, seems to be very strange. You can actually take a 2-dimensional section and obtain 3-dimensional information, provided that your sections through the tissue are random and hae not been sectioned in any particular way. It is a proven fact that the number of intersections that you count in different parts of the component are equal to the areas of those components, which are also equal to the volumes of those components.

Shaddock: For the vascular system of the lateral wall, the vessels tend to lie within virtually a single plane. We have the luxury of being able to microscopically focus up and down. Consequently, it really isn't very difficult to outline all the strial vessels. The same applies to the spiral ligament, so it's not a volume measurement in the way that Dr. White described, but it's fairly close.

MECHANICAL CORRELATES OF NOISE TRAUMA IN THE MAMMALIAN COCHLEA

Robert Patuzzi

Physiology Department, University of W.A.
Perth, Western Australia, 6009

INTRODUCTION

Recent observations of the vibration of the cochlear partition in the cat [1], the guinea pig [2,3] and the chinchilla [4] have supported and extended the work of Rhode [5] in the squirrel monkey. These studies have shown that in the normal animal many aspects of the electrical responses from inner hair cells (and therefore the primary afferents that innervate them) can be explained in terms of the vibration of the cochlear partition. Futhermore, the changes in vibration observed following surgical trauma and loud sound [2] indicate that at least some portion of noise-induced hearing loss (NIHL) can be attributed to disruption of this vibration. The following paper attempts to summarize what is known of the vibration of the cochlear partition and how this information relates to NIHL.

CHARACTERIZATION OF THE PARTITION VIBRATION

The vibration pattern of the cochlear partition can be characterized in two ways. The vibration of a particular location along the cochlea produced by pure tone stimuli of different frequencies and intensities can be measured, or the variation in vibration amplitude and phase along the length of the cochlea produced by a pure tone of fixed frequency, but variable intensity can be observed. This latter view of the partition vibration is often called the traveling wave envelope. With the exception of the original observations of von Bekesy [6], the mechanical data have always been obtained by observing the vibration at a point and estimating the vibration profile from this data. This is so, since the cochlea is extremely sensitive to trauma of any kind, and the surgical manipulations required to observe a wide expanse of the partition disrupt its function.

The estimation of the vibration profile from the measurements of the vibration at a point can be done by assuming that the shape of the vibration profile does not alter significantly with stimulus frequency, but merely shifts laterally along the length of the partition in accordance with the known logarithmic place-frequency map. In the guinea pig, this produces a 2.5 mm lateral shift with each octave change in frequency. By then measuring the amplitude and phase of the basilar membrane motion relative to the motion of the incus or stapes, we can estimate the vibration amplitude and phase for each point along the length of the partition for an incus vibration of fixed amplitude and frequency.

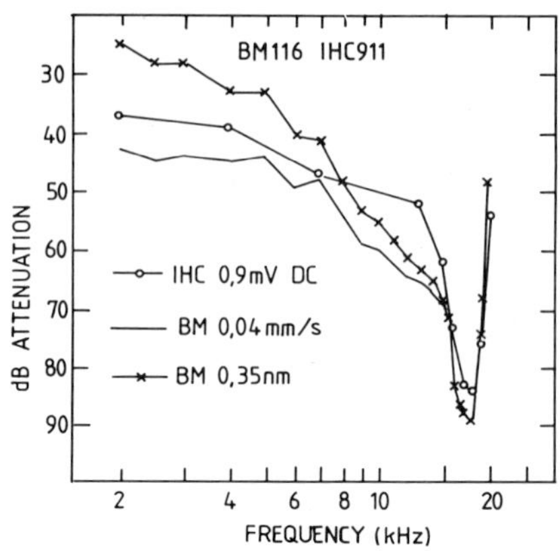

Fig. 1. A comparison of the iso-velocity and iso-displacement tuning curves of basilar membrane motion with a DC receptor potential tuning curve from an inner hair cell. (From Sellick et al. [2].)

Fig. 1 shows the iso-displacement and iso-velocity contours as measured at a particular location in the basal turn of the guinea pig cochlea using the Mossbauer technique [8] and compares them with a DC receptor potential iso-potential tuning curve recorded from an inner hair cell at about the same location. It can be seen that like inner hair cells and primary afferents, the vibration is most sensitive at a particular frequency termed the characteristic frequency, or CF, which in this particular example is 18 kHz. It can also be seen that there can be little difference between the frequency selectivity of inner hair cells and that of the transverse vibration of the cochlear partition. The 10-15 dB discrepancies that do occur may be present in the normal intact cochlea, but it is more likely that they are caused by the loading of the partition by the radioactive speck of metal required to measure the vibration [9].

The data of Fig. 2 show the increase in vibration amplitude with increase in sound level. The stimulus frequency in kHz is the parameter. It can be seen that increases in sound level only produce proportional increases in vibration amplitude for frequencies lower than the CF of the vibration (in this case 18 kHz). At 10 kHz, for example, doubling the vibration amplitude requires a doubling of the sound pressure (that is, a 6 dB increase in the stimulus). For frequencies near CF, however, a larger sound pressure increase is needed to double the vibration amplitude. In the case of the 18 kHz stimulation, up to 12 dB increase in sound level may be required to double the vibration. This disproportionate or nonlinear increase in vibration with elevation in sound level is known as compression. It is most clearly seen in the changes in vibration profile with sound level, as shown in Fig. 3. Here it can be seen that for very low sound levels the vibration is very localized along the length of the partition, but that as the level of pure tone stimulus is raised, the vibration becomes less localized. Not only does the vibration become less localized, but the position of maximum vibration changes with stimulus level, moving in a basal direction as sound level is increased. Measurements obtained using the Mossbauer technique indicate that shifts as large as 2 mm may be possible [2]. The implication for noise trauma is that if the amount of NIHL is simply related to the amount of excessive vibration, then for pure tone exposures, the place most at risk is 2 mm or so more basal than the position of peak vibration at low levels. Since this point normally detects low level sounds with frequencies about half an octave

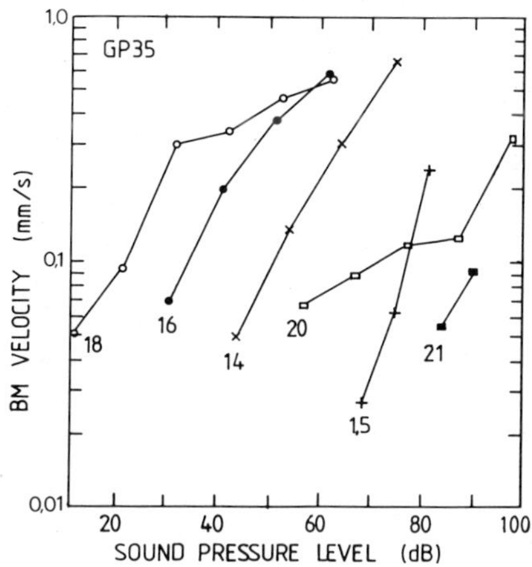

Fig. 2. The nonlinear growth of partition vibration at one location with increase in sound pressure level. The stimulus frequency in kHz is the parameter. (From Sellick et al. [2].)

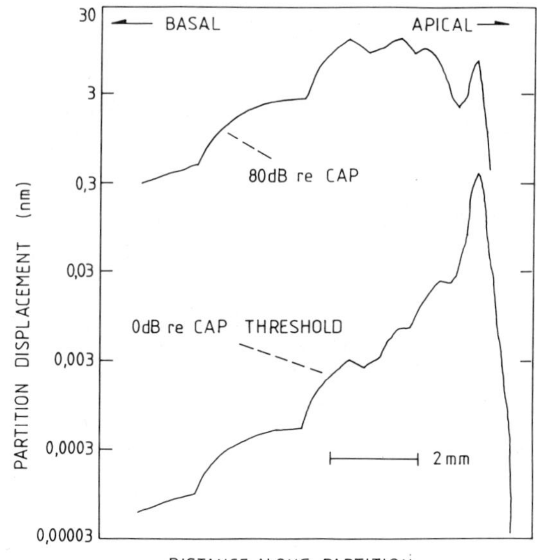

Fig. 3. Estimates of the vibration profile along the cochlear partition for a pure tone stimulus of fixed frequency. The two curves are for pure tones at the compound action potential threshold, and 80 dB above this level. (Corresponding to about 25 and 105 dB SPL).

higher than the exposure frequency, we would expect the maximum threshold elevation or NIHL to occur at this frequency. This difference between the exposure frequency and the frequency of maximum threshold elevation is commonly observed in psycho-acoustic and neuro-physiological investigations of NIHL. It can be seen that this "half-octave shift," as it is called, can safely be explained by a shift in the peak of partition vibration with sound level.

In summary, the fact that inner hair cell receptor potentials, primary afferent firing and basilar membrane vibration share similar tuning and non-linear properties suggests that the inner hair cell response, and therefore the neural response, is determined largely by the transverse vibration of the cochlear partition. This view is supported further by the observation that loss of neural sensitivity correlates well with the loss of mechanical sensitivity over a relatively large range of threshold elevation.

LABILITY OF PARTITION VIBRATION

Following surgical trauma, the vibration of the cochlear partition is reduced in amplitude and becomes less localized along its length. The loss of mechanical sensitivity correlates well with the loss of neural sensitivity, as can be seen from the data of Fig. 4. In the basal turn of the guinea pig, it appears that a transverse vibration of about 0.3 nm is necessary to elicit a gross neural response from the auditory nerve in response to a brief tone burst [2]. This becomes apparent when comparing the sound pressure required to elicit the compound action potential (CAP) and that required to produce the 0.3 nm displacement of the partition with a pure tone with a frequency equal to the CF. It can be seen from Fig. 4 that there is an approximately one-to-one correlation between the mechanical and neural sensitivities at CF. It must be stated, however, that the precise reason for the loss of threshold in these experiments is not known. The threshold elevation occurred progressively during the course of the experiments. The important point still remains, however, that when the mechanical sensitivity is reduced, the neural sensitivity correlates well. Futhermore, it is not simply the neural and mechanical sensitivities at CF that correlate. If we compare the changes that occur in the mechanical iso-response curves with those that occur in the neural tuning curves following cochlear trauma and loud sound, we find that there are similarities in the changes in tuning as well as sensitivity. The changes in the mechanical tuning curves can be seen in Fig. 5. During the course of the experiment, the vibration of the partition became less sensitive and also less frequency selective. The response after death is also shown.

This lability of vibration also explains why the vibration observed in later studies differs from that observed previously. The animal preparations used in the early studies were severely traumatized during surgery or sound calibration, and in some cases the animal's temperature was not maintained. In other cases the measurement technique required drainage of the perilymph, a manipulation now known to alter partition vibration [10]. When adequate precautions are taken to preserve the integrity of the cochlea, and the gross nerve action potential to tone burst stimuli is used to monitor the condition of the preparation, then the relationship between mechanical and neural sensitivities becomes clear.

From the results discussed above, it is reasonable to suggest that at least some portion of NIHL might be due to changes in the vibration of the partition. Indeed, there is now some direct evidence that this is the case. Fig. 6 shows the growth of vibration amplitude with sound level observed in the basal turn of the guinea pig cochlea for 18 kHz (CF)

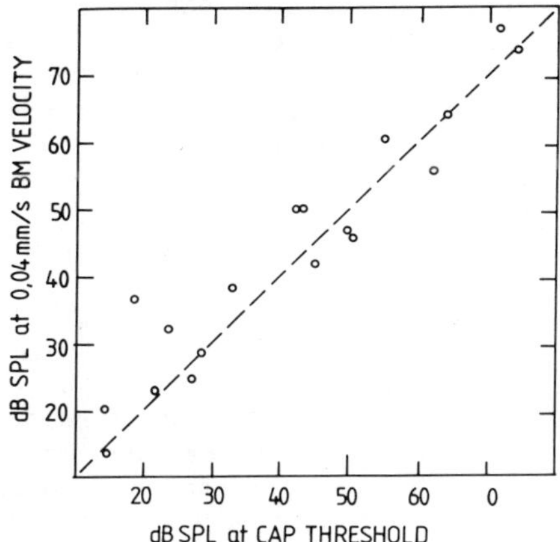

Fig. 4. The correlation between mechanical and neural sensitivities at CF during deterioration of a Mossbauer preparation. The data are from 6 animals. (From Sellick et al. [2].)

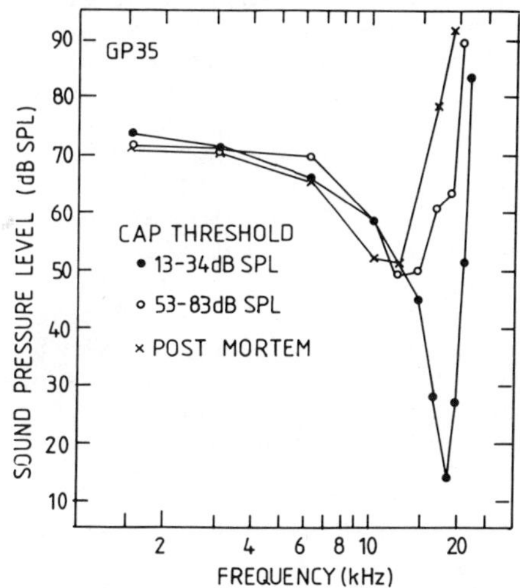

Fig. 5. Changes in the 0.04mm/s iso-velocity contour with deterioration of the Mossbauer preparation, and post mortem. Note the loss of sensitivity and frequency selectivity. (From Sellick et al. [2].)

stimulation. Note the nonlinear growth of curve A, the initial estimate of the mechanical input/output curve. Following this initial estimate, however, a redetermination of the input/output curve (curve B) showed a loss of sensitivity and a loss of the nonlinear growth. Apparently, the accumulated high intensity exposure during the first determination desensitized the preparation at CF. No such desensitization was observed for frequencies lower than CF. It should be noted that the desensitization or NIHL was produced by a sound stimulus equal to the CF of the preparation. As already discussed, we would expect maximum threshold elevation for frequencies half an octave higher that the exposure frequency, and little elevation at the exposure frequency (at least with the exposure intensities and durations used). This apparent inconsistency is probably the result of an increased susceptibility to trauma caused by the presence of the Mossbauer source. For this reason we should treat these data as indicative of the fact that mechanical changes can occur following intense sound.

There are two other important practical points that should be discussed in light of this data. So far, in discussing the variations of the vibration along the length of the cochlear partition, the phrase "traveling wave envelope" has been avoided, and the phrase "vibration profile" has been used in its place. This has been quite intentional. Although the concept of the traveling wave is quite accurate in the context of vibration in the mammalian cochlea, it has lead to many misconceptions about the mechanics of the vibration. The most common misconception, and the one that causes the greatest problems in the long run, is that the vibration energy travels from the oval window end of the cochlea to the apical end through the partition itself, passing from one segment to the next like a long carpet being shaken. Certainly when observed in its entirety, as von Bekesy originally observed it, it would appear very similar. But as von Bekesy emphasized in his original report of his observations, this is not the case. The energy travels through the fluid at the speed of sound (that is to say, very fast compared with the travel of the peak of vibration along the membrane) and is fed to each segment of the cochlear partition in parallel. Von Bekesy emphasized this point by constructing a swinging pendulum model of the partition with no longitudinal coupling between the segments. The model still exhibited a travelling wave. This point is of great practical significance. If it were the case that the vibration traveled through the partition rather than through the fluid, we could not possibly observe a localized loss of partition vibration at the basal end of the cochlea without a loss of vibration at more apical points. That is, we cannot stand on the carpet and expect the vibration to pass! A 50 dB reduction in vibration at the 20 kHz region, for example, would produce a 50 dB reduction for all lower frequencies. If this were so a high frequency hearing loss would be a very rare complaint indeed! The apparent "traveling wave" is the result of the graded phase delay (or sluggishness) between the fluid pressure stimulus and the oscillatory response of the segments. This in turn is due to the fact that each segment is tuned to a different frequency.

The second point to be discussed is the phenomenon of loudness recruitment observed following cochlear trauma. Traditionally, the phenomenon has been explained in terms of the change in neural tuning curve shape. In the normal ear, the tuning curves are very sharp, with steep slopes on either side of the CF. As a result, the recruitment of adjacent fibers is relatively slow as the intensity of a pure tone stimulus is increased. In the pathological cochlea, however, the tuning curves are broad and the slope on the low frequency side of CF is much less. As a result, only small increments of stimulus intensity above neural threshold are required to recruit more basal neurons and cause high frequency recruitment. As we have already seen, the change in neural tuning curve shape is primarily due to changes in the vibration of the partition, but the above explanation is still valid. What should also be considered, however, is the loss of the compression in the growth of vibration amplitude with stimulus level at CF. As can be seen from Fig. 6, cochlear trauma, and loud sound in particular, not only produces desensitization, but also loss of compression. Before exposure to the loud sound, the nonlinear growth of the partition meant that a 70 dB range of sound level could be compressed into a 40 dB range of vibration amplitude. In the normal intact cochlea, this compression is probably greater. In the traumatized ear, however, the linear growth of the vibration means that a 40 dB increase in vibration amplitude requires only a 40 dB increase in sound level. This loss of compression would cause

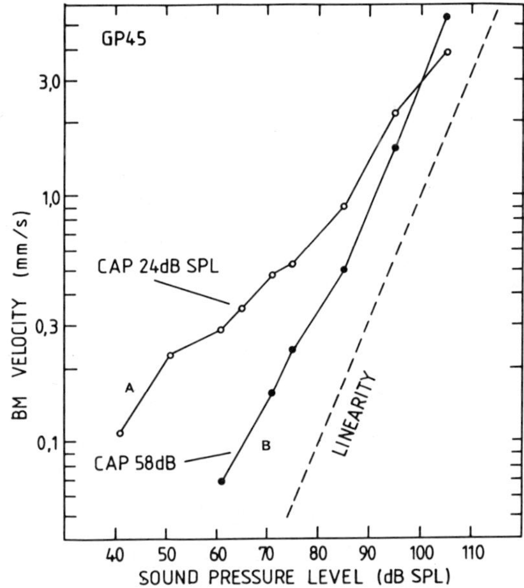

Fig. 6. The loss of mechanical sensitivity and nonlinearity following loud sound. Open circles represent the initial input-output function determination. Closed circles show the input-output function following the high intensity exposures used to determine the initial curve. (From Sellick et al. [2].) Initial CAP is also shown.

loudness recruitment, even without the accompanying change in tuning curve shape. As it is, the combination of the linear growth and the abnormally rapid spread of stimulation means that more fibers are stimulated harder than they would be in a normal ear, and the dramatic loudness recruitment so indicative of cochlear pathology results.

"MIXED" COCHLEAR LOSSES

Lest I give the impression that the cochlear partition vibration can explain all of cochlear physiology, some of the aspects of NIHL that cannot be explained in terms of alterations to the partition vibration should be discussed. In just the same way as we refer to a "mixed" hearing loss to describe a loss consisting of both conductive and sensori-neural components, we must now consider differentiating between different cochlear lesions. This is adviseable since it is entirely likely that different deficiencies in the transduction processes of the cochlea could lead to quite different psychophysical changes. For example, it might be that a particular individual has a deficiency in the neurotransmitter release processes at the base of the inner hair cells. The inner hair cells would presumably receive normal stimuli from the frequency selective and non-linear vibration of the partition, but be unable to communicate this information correctly to the auditory nerve. This kind of deficiency would presumably have a very different affect on auditory perception from a deficiency in partition vibration with normal hair cell transduction and transmitter release. What evidence is there that such mixed cochlear lesions exist.

The most compelling evidence is that of Fig. 5. Even after death, the maximum loss of partition vibration is only 50 to 60 dB. Greater elevations in threshold are commonly seen in neural responses following acoustic overstimulation [11]. Obviously, such NIHL must involve other deficiencies in the transduction process, and future investigations of NIHL should aim at distinguishing between these different components. Since it has been demonstrated that following cochlear trauma, only the vibration at frequencies near CF is altered and that vibration at frequencies much below this frequency remains unchanged, it may prove fruitful to examine in detail the changes that occur in the neural response at these low frequencies, as well as at CF. For example, in investigations of the response of primary afferents to very low frequency stimulation, it has been observed that cochlear trauma, including loud sound, altered the response of the afferents, producing a phase reversal in their response, and producing a hypersensitivity [12]. Similar changes have been observed in chronic experimentation [13]. Hypersensitivity of the tuning curves for frequencies lower than CF but higher than the very low frequencies used in these studies has also been observed [14]. Since we can be reasonably confident that these changes have no correlate in the vibration of the partition, the changes must indicate changes in other processes of transduction. We do not yet know what these changes are.

THEORETICAL CONSIDERATIONS - THE ACTIVE COCHLEA

Although the experimental results summarized so far are useful in helping us understand NIHL, future research will need to be more sophisticated than the descriptive approach taken to date. It will need to rely on a more theoretical framework. For this reason the remainder of this discussion will touch on the more theoretical side of cochlear mechanics.

At its simplest, each segment of the cochlear partition can be modeled as a simple mass which is restored to its rest position by a stiffness restoring force. Any oscillatory movements of the mass are damped by the viscous drag of the fluid and cellular structures of the organ of Corti. The extraordinarily high sensitivity of the vibration of the partition is most easily explained by the action of hypothetical mechanical feedback elements within the organ the Corti that act to reduce the viscous drag [15,16]. This could only be achieved if these elements applied forces to the partition that were synchronous with the viscous forces (i.e., synchronous with partition velocity), but in the opposite direction to the damping forces. For this reason the action of the hypothetical feedback process is often termed "negative damping," and since it would appear that the process requires metabolic energy (see Davis [17] for a review), the negative damping is also called the active process, or even the "cochlear amplifier." In partially cancelling the viscous forces, the feedback elements increase the sensitivity of vibration near the CF for that location only. For frequencies away from CF, the motion of the partition is dominated by stiffness or inertial forces, and the viscous forces (and their reduction by the negative damping) are insignificant. Close to CF and resonance, however, when the stiffness and inertial forces cancel and motion is dominated by the viscous forces, the negative damping process is crucial. The simplest hypothesis to explain the changes observed following trauma to the cochlea and loud sound is that the negative damping process is disrupted, and the viscous damping forces are left uncancelled.

In a similar way, we can understand the nonlinear growth of vibration near CF as a result of the limited dynamic range of the active process. For relatively low level sounds, when vibration is small, the active elements are capable of producing forces sufficiently large to counter the viscous forces. As the sound level increases, however, and vibration amplitude also increases, the active forces are limited in amplitude, and are unable to counter the increased viscous forces. As a result, the partition vibration becomes more and more like the passive vibration observed after death. This can be seen to some degree by comparing the broad tuning of the post mortem results of Fig. 5 with the poorly localized vibration profile at high intensities shown in Fig. 3. For frequencies off CF, where forces are dominated by stiffness or mass, vibration is unaffected by such changes in the viscous forces. As a result, vibration growth is linear for these frequencies (the picture at frequencies higher than CF is complicated by the complex hydro-dynamical interaction between segments of the partition through the fluid). To emphasize this progression from the active and undamped mechanics at low intensities to the passive and damped mechanics at high intensities, and how this progression produces a nonlinear input-output function at CF, Fig. 7 shows a set of four hypothetical input-output functions. Each of these input-output functions is assumed to be the result of a different amount of negative damping. The curve on the far left is assumed to be produced by the action of all damping elements producing the full affect. As a result, sensitivity is high. The curve on the far right, however, is assumed to have no active contribution, and represents the insensitive passive vibration. The intermediate curves are hypothetical curves in which intermediate levels of negative damping are the case. If we could progressively turn the active process on (i.e., reverse a sensori-neural hearing loss), we would move the input-output curve to the left. In increasing the sound level, and we assume progressively saturating the active process, we would move from our most active curve (curve A) to intermediate curves (curves B and C), and finally to the passive curve at very high intensities. The resultant input-output curve would be the dotted curve E, which can be compared with the nonlinear input-output curve of Fig. 2 (18 kHz). The important point is that the nonlinearity is not a hardening spring non-linearity, such as that which may cause distortion in a poor quality Hi-Fi speaker system. It appears to be an adaptive gain amplifier, similar to the Dolby equalization system so ubiquitous in recording equipment.

Since the changes in the mechanical response following cochlear trauma, and loud sound in particular, seem consistent with the loss or disruption of the active mechanical component and a reversion of the cochlea to passive mechanics, the important questions concerning the origin of noise trauma must be:

> "Where is the active process, what is its nature and how is it disrupted by loud sound?"

There is evidence accruing that the active process is intimately associated with the outer hair cells. The crudest indication of this is that the destruction of the outer hair cells using the antibiotic kanamycin produces a loss of neural sensitivity [7,18]. Similarly, noise exposure also causes a selective loss of outer hair cells in chronic experiments [19,20] and similar changes in the neural response, now known to be at least partially the result of changes to partition vibration. Of course, such experiments are open to the criticism that the damage need not be localized to the outer hair cells, and that other more subtle effects may be causing the mechanical changes. This criticism is difficult to counter, even with the most sophisticated studies correlating morphological changes with associated sensori-neural loss.

There are other pieces of evidence, however, that suggest the involvement of outer hair cells in the active process. The efferent fibers of the

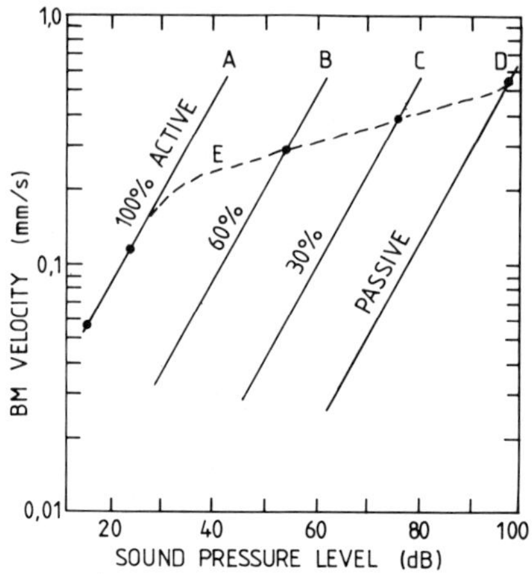

Fig. 7. Hypothetical input-output curves for partition vibration with different active contributions, as indicated. The dashed curve illustrates how the experimentally-observed growth function at CF could be derived from a progression from one hypothetical curve to another as the active process progressively saturates at higher sound levels.

cochlea seem to modulate the mechanical response [21] and these fibers almost exclusively innervate the outer hair cells. Perhaps the more compelling pieces of evidence involve the nonlinearity of the cochlea, and in particular the similarity between the electrical non-linerarity of the outer hair cell transduction process and that of the basilar membrane mechanics. Put at its simplest, it can be shown that the outer hair cell receptor currents begin to saturate for transverse partition displacement at which nonlinear growth of the partition is observed [2,22]. Below this level (about 10 nm), the outer hair cells and cochlear mechanics are predominantly linear. Similarly, low frequency tones that bias the outer hair cell receptor currents into partial saturation also modulate the sensitivity of cochlear mechanics [23,24]. These points suggest that the outer hair cells, and in particular, their receptor currents or the potentials produced by them (or, in fact, the receptor proteins that produce the currents!), are intimately associated with the active process. This association had been suggested previously by Weiss [25].

Whatever the mode of action of the outer hair cells may be, their involvement appears most likely. As a result, we should look to the way in which their function is altered in a sensori-neural loss, and in particular, following loud sound. Crucial steps towards this understanding have already been taken by Cody and Russell [26]. Auditory investigation and the study of noise induced hearing loss cannot remain at the purely descriptive level. An understanding of noise-induced hearing loss will require detailed investigations of the fundamental molecular mechanisms governing the motion of the cochlear partition and the transduction processes that follow it.

ACKNOWLEDGEMENTS

The author wishes to thank Dr. Ute Proschel for her kind assistance in the preparation of this manuscript.

REFERENCES

1. S. M. Khanna and D. G. B. Leonard, Basilar membrane tuning in the cat cochlea, Science, 215:305 (1982).
2. P. M. Sellick, R. Patuzzi and B. M. Johnstone, Measurement of basilar membrane motion in the guinea pig using the Mossbauer technique, J. Acoust. Soc. Am. 72:131 (1982).
3. E. L. Le Page and B. M. Johnstone, Non linear mechanical behaviour of the basilar membrane in the guinea pig cochlea, Hearing Res. 2:183 (1980).
4. L. Robles, M. A. Ruggero and N. C. Rich, Mossbauer measurements of basilar membrane tuning curves in the chinchilla, J. Acoust. Soc. Am. 76:S35 (1984).
5. W. Rhode, Observations of the vibration of the basilar membrane in squirrel monkeys using the Mossbauer technique, J. Acoust. Soc. Am. 49:1218 (1971).
6. G. V. Bekesy, "Experiments in Hearing," McGraw-Hill, New York (1960).
7. D. Robertson and B. M. Johnstone, Aberrant tonotopic organization in the the inner ear damaged by kanamycin, J. Acoust. Soc. Am. 66:466 (1979).
8. P. M. Sellick, R. Patuzzi and B. M. Johnstone, Comparison between the tuning properties of inner hair cells and basilar membrane motion, Hearing Res. 10:93 (1983).
9. P. M. Sellick, G. K. Yates and R. Patuzzi, The influence of Mossbauer source size and position on phase and amplitude measurements of the guinea pig basilar membrane, Hearing Res. 10:101 (1982).
10. R. Patuzzi, P. M. Sellick and B. M. Johnstone, Cochlear drainage and basilar membrane tuning, J. Acoust. Soc. Am. 72:1064 (1982).
11. A. R. Cody and B. M. Johnstone, Single auditory neuron response during acute acoustic trauma. Hearing Res. 3:3 (1980).
12. R. Patuzzi and P. M. Sellick, The alteration of the low frequency response of primary auditory afferents by cochlear trauma, Hearing Res. 11:125 (1983).
13. W. G. Sokolich, R. P. Hamernik, J. J. Zwislocki and R. A. Schmeidt, Inferred response polarities of cochlear hair cells, J. Acoust. Soc. Am. 59:963 (1976).
14. N. Y. S. Kiang and E. K. Moxon, Tails of tuning curves of auditory nerve fibers, J. Acoust. Soc. Am. 55:620 (1974).
15. E. de Boer, No sharpening? A challenge for cochlear mechanics, J. Acoust. Soc. Am. 73:567 (1983).
16. S. J. Neely, and D. O. Kim, An active cochlear model showing sharp tuning and high sensitivity, Hearing Res. 9:123 (1983).
17. D. Davis, An active process in cochlear mechanics, Hearing Res. 9:79. (1983).
18. R. A. Schmeidt, Single and two-tone effects in normal and abnormal cochleas: A study of cochlear microphonics and auditory-nerve units, ISR Special Report, Syracuse University, New York (1977).
19. D. Robertson, Effects of acoustic trauma on stereocilia ultrastructure and spiral ganglion tuning properties in the guinea pig cochlea, Hearing Res. 7:55 (1982).
20. M. C. Liberman and M. J. Mulroy, Acute and chronic effects of acoustic trauma: Cochlear pathology and auditory nerve pathophysiology, in: "New Perspectives on Noise-Induced Hearing Loss," Raven Press, New York, (1982).

21. D. C. Mountain, Changes in endolymphatic potential and crossed olivocochlear bundle stimulation alter cochlear mechanics, Science 210:71 (1980).
22. R. Patuzzi, A simple model of the generation of the cochlear microphonic, (in preparation).
23. R. Patuzzi and P. M. Selliek, The modulation of the sensitivity of the mammalian cochlea by low frequency tones: II. Hair cell receptor potentials, Hearing Res. 13:9 (1983).
24. R. Patuzzi, P. M. Sellick, and B. M. Johnstone, The modulation of sensitivity of the mammalian cochlea by low frequency tones: III. Basilar membrane motion, Hearing Res. 13:19 (1983)
25. T. F. Weiss, Bidirectional transduction in vertebrate hair cells: A mechanism for coupling mechanical and electrical processes, Hearing Res. 7:353 (1982).
26. Cody, A. R. and I. J. Russell, Outer hail cells in the mammalian cochlea and noise-induced hearing loss, Nature 315:662 (1985).

DISCUSSION

Trahiotis: Could you please relate your transverse functions to Kim and Molnar's neural data? Do you remember if they corrected for the effect of the middle ear? As I remember the neural data, they used the first coefficient of the Fourier transform of the neural spike train; so it is hard to relate the relative amount of activity across frequency or place. The point is that they did not get a greater response higher in frequency, whereas you show the potential for a greater response one half octave above the characteristic frequency. If you did not correct for the middle ear, would this still occur?

Patuzzi: It is still evident if you look at the input/output functions that I showed without any corrections. You still get the input/output functions crossing.

Salvi: In normal ears, you also see some auditory nerve fibers with low spontaneous rates which have thresholds that are 60 dB above the units with the best thresholds. Surprisingly, the tuning curves of these fibers are still very sharply tuned, whereas the basilar membrane response becomes less sharply tuned. Could you comment on this discrepancy?

Patuzzi: I obviously have no explanation for that.

Flottrop: It seems to me you said something about the energy going through the fluid and not through the basilar membrane in order to produce that traveling wave. Would you comment on this?

Patuzzi: I think the best model for the basilar membrane is either the swinging pendulem model of von Bekesy or a series of tubes representing the cochlear partition, each filled with a ping-pong ball with a different mass and restoring force. Each one of the sections of the cochlea responds relatively independently of the next. There is no longitudinal coupling within the membrane or relatively little coupling in the membrane as if they were joined by springs. The coupling appears to be via pressure perturbations through the fluids.

Dancer: The cochlea partition is driven by the differential pressure acting on the elements of the membrane. So in the passive case, when the preparation is anoxic after acoustic trauma, what would happen to the phase lag curves?

Patuzzi: Interesting changes in the phase curves pre- and post-mortem. For a good preparation, the phase curve is nearly at a plateau at low frequencies, but then a very fast roll occurs at higher frequencies. But, as the preparation deteriorates, the curve becomes steeper at lower frequencies and then less steep as you go into the steeper part of the curve. If you look at where the points cross, it is roughly at the characteristic frequency. I think that is good evidence that the changes that we observe by elevating sound pressure level or following trauma are where the response is approaching the asymptote of passive mechanics. If you look at the phase versus intensity function for the Mossbauer preparations and also the hair cell and neural data, one sees that as sound pressure level is increased the phase only changes on either side of the characteristic frequency. But at the characteristic frequency, the phase does not change much at all.

McFadden: Two comments. One regards the maximum loss of about 50 dB or so that you see in your preparations. This exists elsewhere. One of the more interesting instances is in salicylate-induced hearing loss. No matter how much salicylate you give, they never get more than about 40 dB of hearing loss. Second comment: I am not sure you really represented von Bekesy's point correctly. Twenty years ago or so, I discovered an article authored by Weaver, Lawrence and von Bekesy.* They indicated that there are two ways in which energy can be delivered to a particular spot along the membrane. It can be delivered through the fluid or it can be delivered to the membrane at a basilar location and the energy can be transmitted through the membrane. The article says that Wever and Lawrence believe that energy is delivered through the fluid; Bekesy believed it is transmitted through the membrane. In Bekesy's pendulum model, if he blocked the wave at a particular basilar membrane location, displacement occurs at an apical location, but it is enormously attenuated. I am not trying to argue facts, but rather to point out Bekesy's position in 1950. Obviously, both factors are operating. The question is which is the more important.

Patuzzi: In answer to that, I think we have demonstrated the energy is transmitted through the fluid.

von Gierke: You showed that the tuning curves became detuned with increasing intensity. Do you think this is still in the range where effects are reversible?

Patuzzi: We have little evidence on this, but I think at 80 dB the effects are reversible. The reason why I believe you can get rather large losses in the mechanics and still recover is the fact that in another series of experiments, we put in very low frequency tones, in addition a tone at the characteristic frequency; we found that as the low frequency tones pushed the partition up or down, it could turn the mechanics off by as much as 20 decibels.

von Gierke: When the sharp tuning disappears, does the phase shift change markedly?

Patuzzi: About 40 degrees at lower frequencies and larger shifts at higher frequencies. I think there is probably some evidence that there is a reversible mechanical loss in that anything that seems to take the tip off a tuning curve would seem to have a correlate in mechanics.

---

* E. G. Wever, M. Lawrence and G. von Bekesy, "A note on recent developments in auditory theory," Proceedings of the national Academy of Sciencs, 40:508 (1954).

D. Nielsen: I just want to make a quick comment in support of Dr. Patuzzi. That is, that the pressure is transmitted all along the basilar membrane stimultanously due to the incompressability of the fluids. Bekesy did two experiments on his models. One was the paradoxical traveling wave where he put the stapes at the apex and still got the traveling wave in the same direction. Second, he put a lesion in the basilar membrane and the wave still traveled across it. If it was transmitted in the membrane, it would not do that.

AUDITORY SENSITIVITY, AUDITORY FATIGUE AND COCHLEAR MECHANICS

A. Dancer,[1] R. Franke[1] and P. Campo[2]

(1) French-German Research Institute of Saint Louis
68301 Saint Louis, France
(2) Institut National de Recherche et de Securite
P.O. Box 27, 54501 Vandoeuvre Cedex, France

INTRODUCTION

Transduction of an acoustic signal into a neural response in the cochlea is generally considered to occur at the level of the organ of Corti via the motion of its structures. Mechanical deformation of the organ of Corti is the starting point of the hearing process.

Our aim was to determine the physical parameter(s) of this motion which is(are) mainly responsible for the detection of the acoustic signal at behavioral threshold and for auditory fatigue. Knowing these parameters would increase our understanding of cochlear physiology. Because no direct measurements of the motion of the various components of the organ of Corti have been reported, we shall examine only the motion of the basilar membrane (BM).

THRESHOLD OF AUDITORY SENSITIVITY

In the cat [1,2] (Fig. 1), the guinea pig [3,4] and to a lesser extent in man [5,6] (only above 3 kHz), the shape of the behavioral threshold curve as a function of frequency is determined by the transfer function which connects the acoustic pressure in the free field to the acoustic pressure at the cochlear input (ACI) (i.e., the acoustic pressure in the basal end of scala vestibuli) [10,11]. Thus, at the threshold of hearing for tones, the sound pressure level at the input to the cochlea (ACI) would be approximately constant for all frequencies.

We now seek a measure of the BM motion whose amplitude is also nearly constant at threshold with the condition that for each frequency the measure is taken close to the site along the cochlea that is most sensitive (making the assumption that the sensory cells have the same sensitivity to the amplitude of this parameter independent of frequency and cochlear location from base to apex).

For a constant amplitude of ACI at any frequency, intracochlear acoustic pressure measurements [7] and cochlear models [8,9] indicate that the amplitude of the differential pressure acting on the cochlear partition is almost constant on the part of BM located close to the CF point (on the basal side).

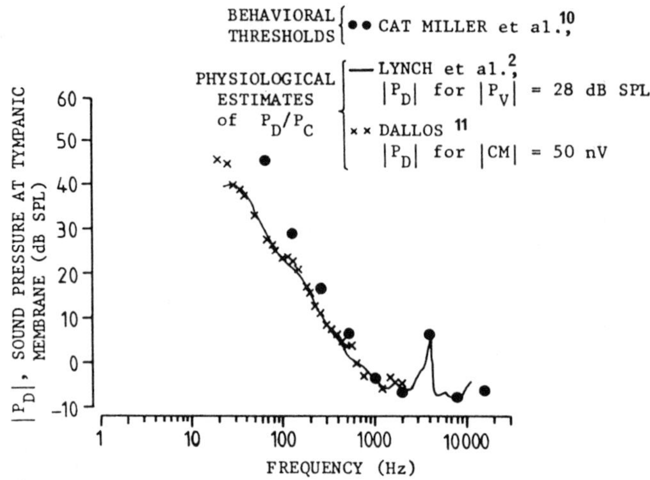

Fig. 1. Comparison of the frequency dependence of behavioral threshold and sound pressure at the input to the cochlea. P_C = pressure across the basal end of the cochlear partition. (From Lynch et al. [2].)

According to Zwislocki [12], the compliance of the BM increases by a factor of about 250 from base to apex in the guinea pig. This indicates that the compliance of BM near CF doubles each time the frequency is halved (i.e., about every 2.5 mm from base to apex) (see Campo et al. [13]). If the force acting on BM remains constant while the compliance doubles when halving the frequency (getting closer and closer to apex), the amplitude of the displacement of BM (close to CF on the basal side) doubles too, and the velocity of BM (always close to CF on the basal side) remains constant all along the cochlea.

No direct proof (measurement) of this assumption exists, but given that cochlear microphonic (CM) amplitude is proportional (in the linear range) to BM displacement [14], then CM amplitude recorded by differential electrodes in each of the first three turns increases in agreement with the above assumption [15] (provided also that a given amplitude of displacement of the cochlear structures gives rise, from base to apex, to the same CM amplitude). Also in support of this position, are plots of BM displacement by Zwislocki [16] (Fig. 2).

From all this it seems logical to think that velocity of the BM could be the parameter of the motion responsible for the auditory system's response. Direct support of this assumption has been given by Johnstone et al. [17], who showed a close correspondence between neural and basilar membrane iso-velocity tuning curves for a given point on BM near the base (Fig. 3). Extending this idea, we hypothesize that neural responses and hence the behavioral threshold occur at a constant velocity all along the cochlea. We shall now consider whether BM velocity is important for the onset of threshold shifts.

SHORT TERM HEARING LOSS (STHL)

Our aim is to study STHL after the application of fatiguing pure tones with a given acoustic level at the input to the cochlea. Indeed, if we want to look at the influence of a measure of BM motion on the resultant

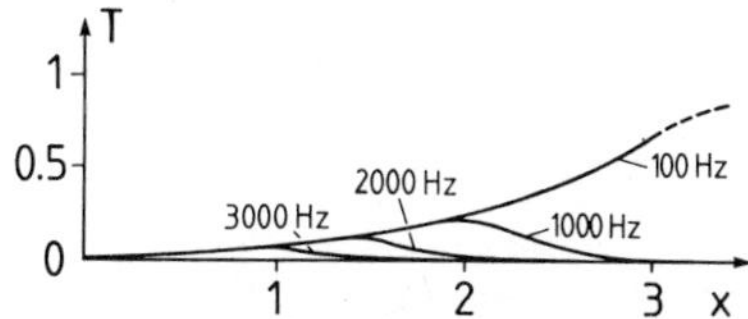

Fig. 2. Ampitude of the BM displacements versus the distance from oval window, with constant pressure amplitude at the entrance to the cochlea (from Zwislocki [16]).

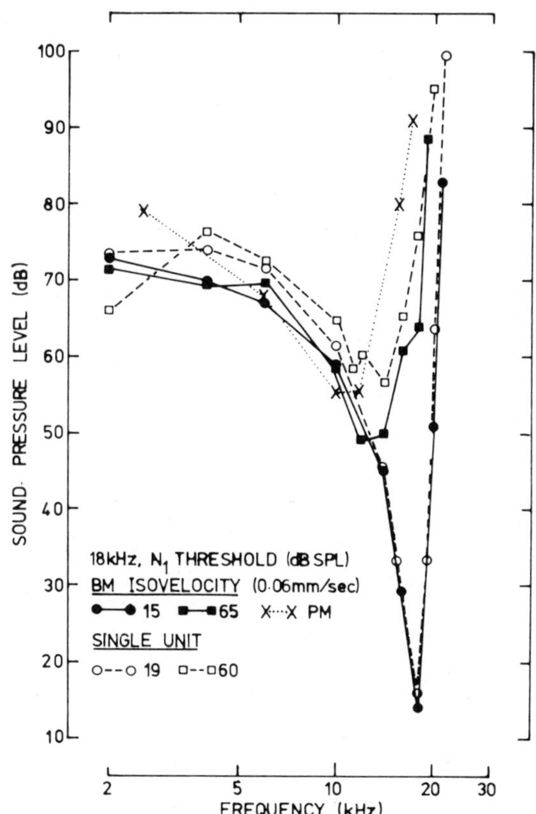

Fig. 3. Comparison of neural and basilar membrane tuning curves. The basilar membrane recording was performed when neural thresholds were 15 dB SPL and later when they were 65 dB SPL. The corresponding neural curves have thresholds of 19 dB SPL and 65 dB SPL (from Johnstone et al. [17]).

STHL, we have to control ACI in order to remove variations arising from the outer and middle ear, so as to be able to restrict the observed results to inner ear mechanisms.

METHOD

Control of the acoustic stimulation. The only way to control ACI directly is to measure the acoustic pressure at the base of the scala vestibuli. Because this measurement can damage the cochlea, it cannot be performed on each animal. Consequently, for the purpose of the present experiment, the acoustic stimulus has to be controlled indirectly. We know that in the first cochlear turn, the shape of the curve representing the amplitude of the differential CM as a function of frequency is almost identical to the differential pressure acting on BM (i.e., acoustic pressure in scala vestibuli minus acoustic pressure in scala tympani) [7] and that the differential pressure recorded at the extreme base of the cochlea would be equal to the pressure in scala vestibuli [9,18]. Therefore, at frequencies up to its cut-off, CM amplitude (recorded in the linear range) is a good representation of the relative amplitude of ACI.

To avoid any modification of the physiological state of the cochlea during our experiments, we recorded the CM with a round window electrode. If CM is recorded with differential electrodes and a round window electrode in the same animals [19], the results are quite comparable, at least from 1 to 10 kHz. For higher frequencies, the round window electrode recording probably represents ACI amplitude even better than differential recording, due to its lack of cut-off. Hence, the round window electrode gives us a good estimate of the relative amplitude of ACI as a function of frequency. For reference, we used CM output at 8 kHz (measured in the linear range). At this frequency the 0 dB stimulation level corresponds to a given voltage applied to the amplifier input (corresponding to 103 dB SPL in front of the tympanic membrane at 8 kHz and about 135 dB SPL for ACI [20]). To use the same reference during all the other experiments (stimulus frequency from 2 to 11.3 kHz by half octave steps), the level of the stimulus was adjusted, with the help of the round window CM, by comparing the level of the CM at the stimulus frequency versus the level at 8 kHz (always in the linear range) and adjusting the input to the amplifier to produce a CM response equal in amplitude to the response at 8 kHz. In this manner we were able to refer ACI for all frequencies to the 0 dB value at 8 kHz.

Animal preparation and audiometry. Pigmented guinea pigs of 300 to 350 g were used. For anesthesia we used a premedication of levopromazine (2.5 mg/kg) and atropine sulfate (0.1 mg); half an hour later we injected a dose of 150 mg/kg of ketamine. During the experiment, the body temperature of the animal was monitored and controlled by a heating pad. The pinna was removed, the bulla opened and an electrode (Ni-Cr) was placed upon the round window (bulla was left open). The animals were stimulated with closed-tube system using a condenser microphone as a loudspeaker [13]. With the round window electrode we established pre-exposure sensitivity by measuring the amplitude of the N1 component of the compound action potential elicited by tone bursts of frequencies from 2 to 32 kHz (half octave steps, 9 frequencies). From these responses we determined an "audiogram." An amplitude of 1 to 2 uV of 200 averaged responses was considered as the threshold. The time required for a complete audiometric procedure was about 10 minutes.

Experiment. After the first audiometric test, the animal was exposed to a pure tone (2, 2.8, 4, 5.6, 8 or 11.3 kHz) of a given pressure for 20 minutes. Twenty minutes after the end of the exposure, sensitivity was remeasured. The threshold shifts are the differences between pre- and post-exposure thresholds. These results have been called STHL because it is not

Figs. 4 to 9: STHL as a function of the tone burst frequency for various levels of the 20 minutes fatiguing tone. The standard deviations (SD) of the STHL measurements at one level (SL) are also shown just above the abscissa.

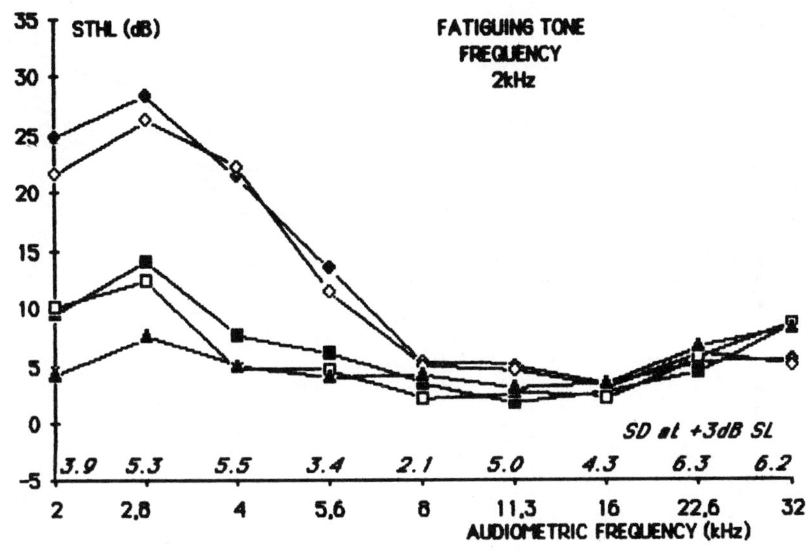

Fig. 4

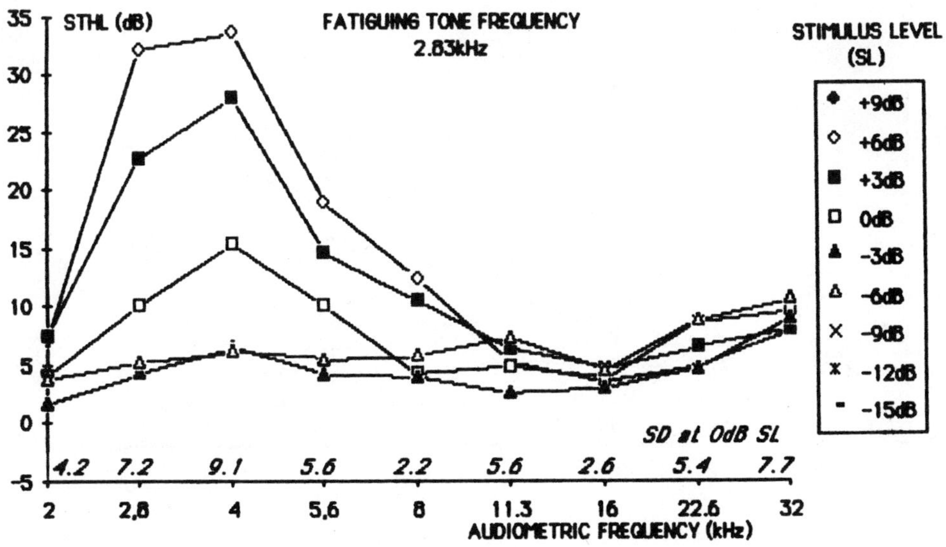

Fig. 5

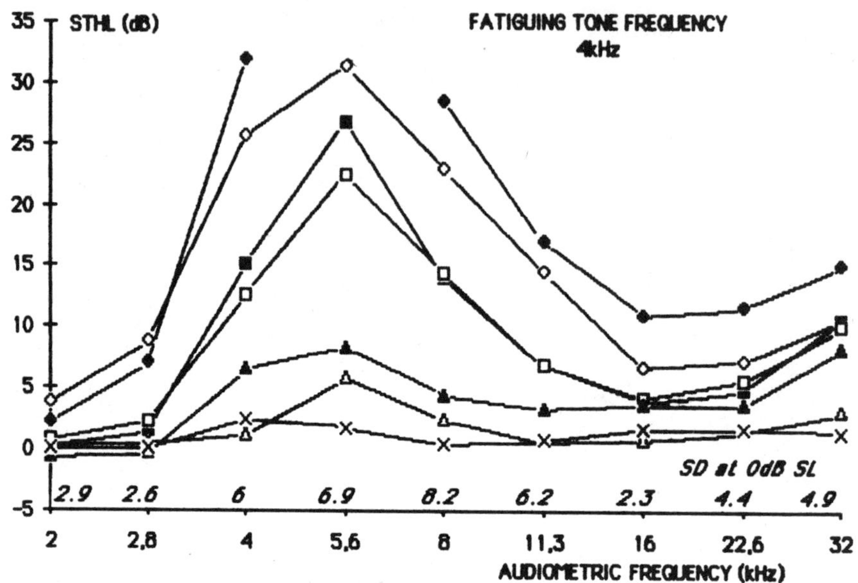

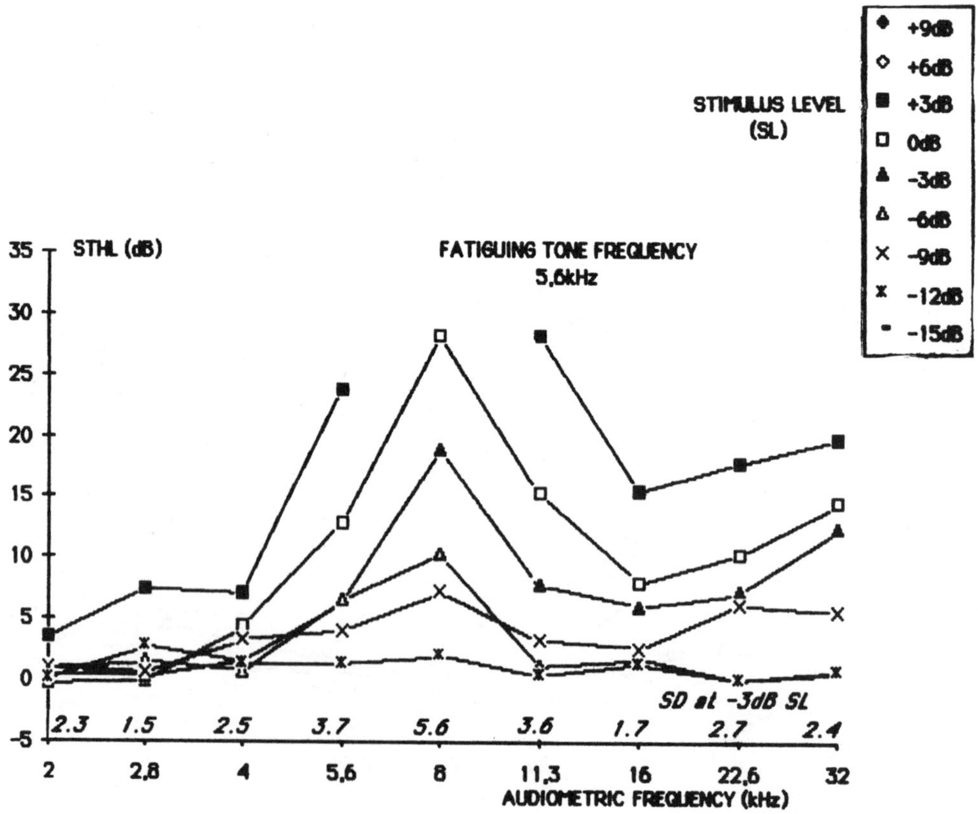

STHL (dB)
FATIGUING TONE FREQUENCY
4kHz
35
30
25
20
15
10
5
0
-5
SD at 0dB SL
2.9
2.6
6
6.9
8.2
6.2
2.3
4.4
4.9
2
2,8
4
5,6
8
11,3
16
22,6
32
AUDIOMETRIC FREQUENCY (kHz)

Fig. 6

+9dB
+6dB
+3dB
0dB
-3dB
-6dB
-9dB
-12dB
-15dB
STIMULUS LEVEL
(SL)
STHL (dB)
FATIGUING TONE FREQUENCY
5,6kHz
35
30
25
20
15
10
5
0
-5
SD at -3dB SL
2.3
1.5
2.5
3.7
5.6
3.6
1.7
2.7
2.4
2
2,8
4
5,6
8
11,3
16
22,6
32
AUDIOMETRIC FREQUENCY (kHz)

Fig. 7

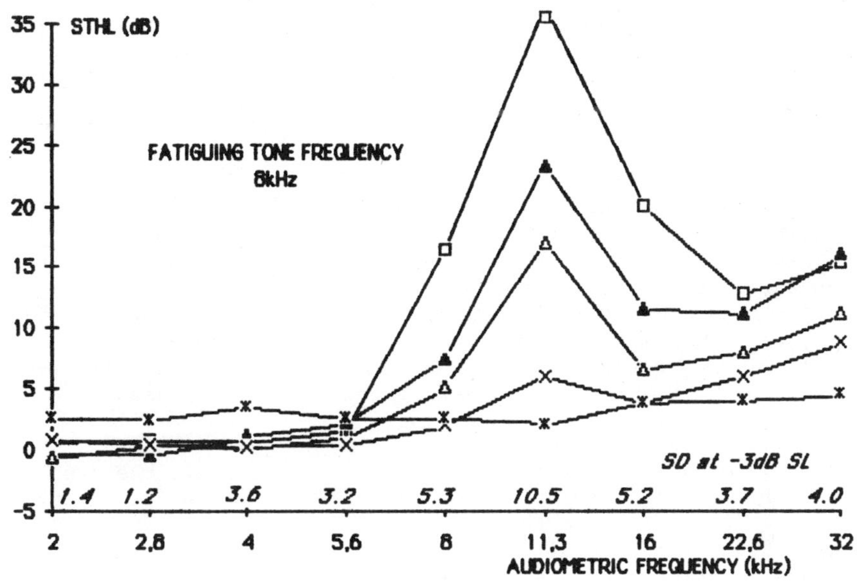

STHL (dB)
FATIGUING TONE FREQUENCY
8kHz
SD at -3dB SL
1.4 1.2 3.6 3.2 5.3 10.5 5.2 3.7 4.0
AUDIOMETRIC FREQUENCY (kHz)

Fig. 8

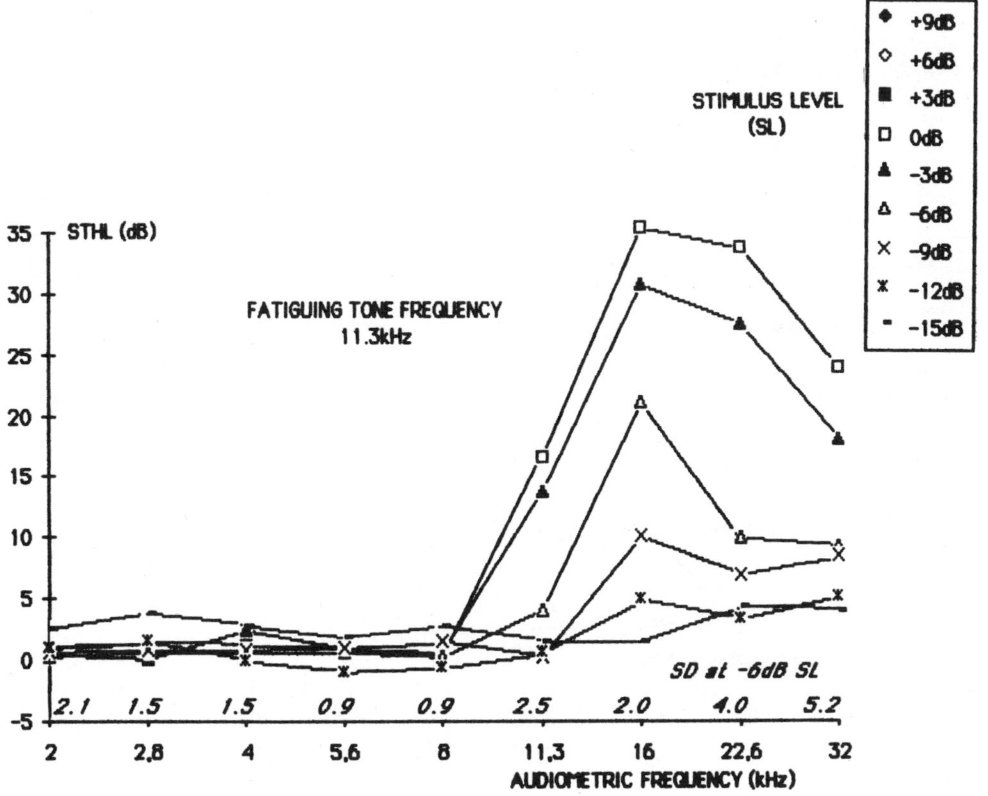

STHL (dB)
FATIGUING TONE FREQUENCY
11.3kHz
STIMULUS LEVEL
(SL)
+9dB
+6dB
+3dB
0dB
-3dB
-6dB
-9dB
-12dB
-15dB
SD at -6dB SL
2.1 1.5 1.5 0.9 0.9 2.5 2.0 4.0 5.2
AUDIOMETRIC FREQUENCY (kHz)

Fig. 9

possible to determine whether this difference corresponds to a pure auditory fatigue or to a mixing of temporary and permanent losses. For each exposure condition, measurements were made in 5 to 10 animals. The influence of the time required for the experiment and of the order of presentation of the stimulus frequencies during the audiometric test had a negligible effect on the results [13].

Results

In Figs. 4 to 9, measurements of STHL are presented for each pure tone exposure as a function of the audiometric frequency and of the exposure level. Dispersion of individual results was small (to avoid overcrowding the figures, standard deviations are presented for only one curve corresponding to mean STHL; all results are reported in Campo et al. [13]). Generally the maximum STHLs occurred half an octave above the exposure frequency even for the lowest exposure. We are, of course, limited in specifying the exact maximum and its exact location by our use of half octave steps in audiometry.

For a given ACI, the higher the stimulus frequency, the greater the STHLs (Fig. 10). Significant amounts of STHL were observed at high frequencies (F > 16 kHz), even for low frequencies exposures. Because the body temperature was controlled and care was taken to keep the cochlear temperature constant, at least for up to 22.6 kHz [21], these STHLs cannot be related to the cooling of the cochlea.

From these results we determined the exposure levels required for each exposure frequency to produce STHLs of 10 +/- 6 dB and 25 +/- 6 dB half an octave over the stimulus frequency (Fig. 11a). The higher the stimulus frequency, the lower the intensity required (the slopes of the regression lines are respectively -4.2 and -4.6 dB/octave with correlation coefficients of 0.77 and 0.90).

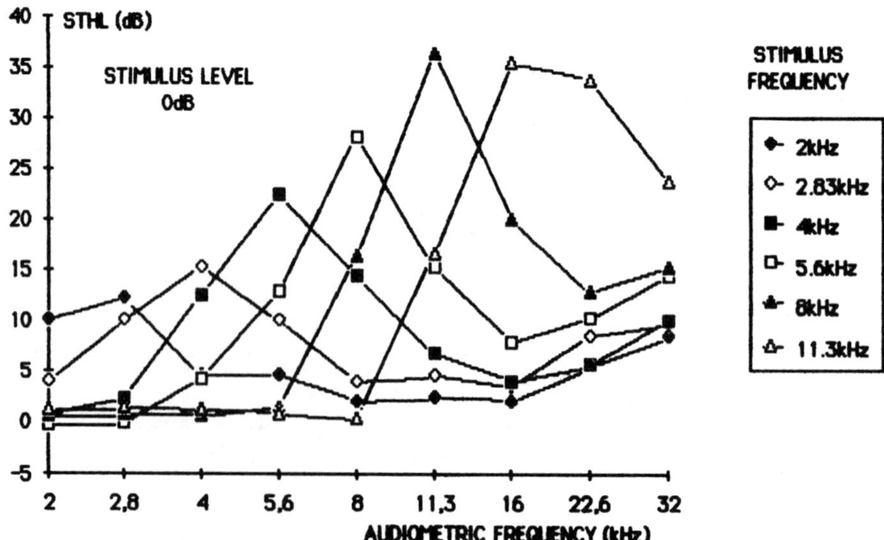

Fig. 10. STHL as a function of the tone burst frequency for different fatiguing tone frequencies of the same level (0 dB).

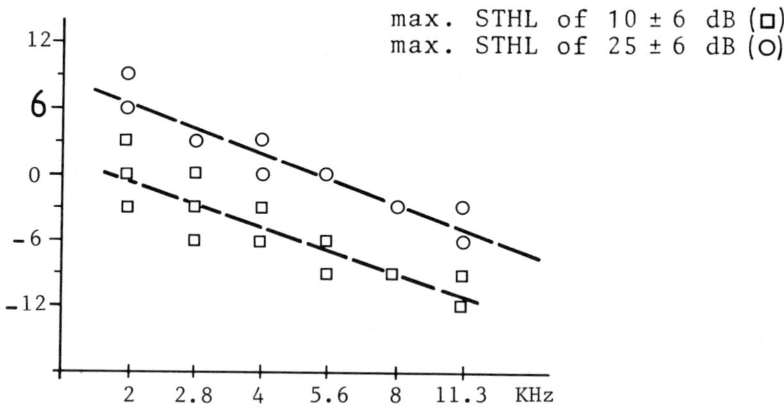

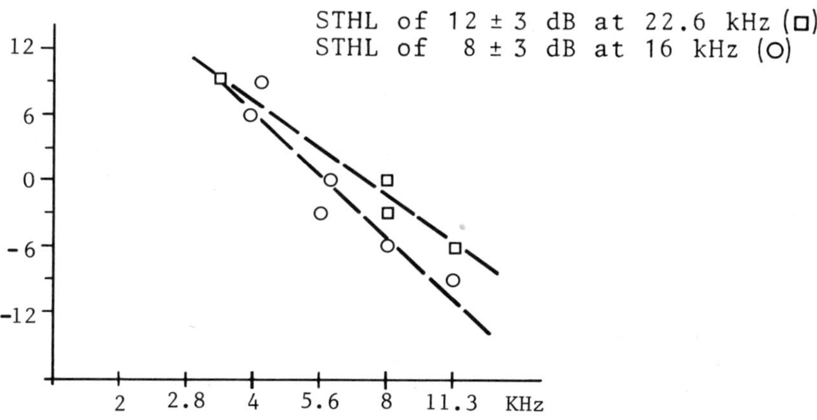

Fig. 11. Iso-STHL curves as a function of the frequency and the level of the fatiguing tone:

a) iso-maximum STHL
b) iso-high-frequency STHL

In Fig. 11b we plotted the relative pressure required for each exposure frequency to obtain STHL of 8 +/- 3 dB at 16 kHz and 12 +/- 3 dB at 22.6 kHz. The higher the exposure frequency, the lower the pressure required (the slopes of the regression lines are -11.3 and -9.2 dB/octave respectively with correlation coefficients 0.90 and 0.88).

CONCLUSION

For a given ACI and within a large frequency range, the velocity of the BM near CF is nearly constant from base to apex. For the same conditions, the velocity of a BM element near the base is proportional to the frequency (for frequencies lower than the CF of this element). Indeed, for a constant ACI, the amplitude of BM displacement near the base is constant for stimulus frequencies below CF. If we suppose that, for a given exposure duration, the threshold shifts are directly correlated with the local velocity of BM, there must be, as a function of the stimulus frequency, a difference between the maximum STHL (half an octave higher than the stimulus frequency) and the STHL at high frequencies (corresponding to the response of the cochlear base). From Fig. 11 we can see that there is a difference in the slopes between the sound pressures inducing iso-maximum STHL and the sound pressures producing iso-high frequency STHL. This difference is about -6 dB/octave which corresponds to the difference of the velocity of BM as a function of the stimulus frequency between a CF region and the basal part of the cochlea.

On the other hand, the -4 dB/octave slope of the maximum STHL as a function of the stimulus frequency and a constant ACI is not consistent with the simple velocity hypothesis. Indeed, if this parameter were the only one responsible for the threshold shifts, this slope should be equal to zero because of the constant velocity of BM near CF. Many possibilities exist: (1) other parameters could be involved or (2) the velocity of the BM increases near CF from the apex to the base of the cochlea for a constant ACI, or (3) even though the velocity remains constant all along the cochlea the sensory cells are not equally sensitive to velocity from base to apex (due to the modification of the relative displacement of BM, of the tectorial membrane, of the stereocilia, etc). This point remains unanswered at present.

ACKNOWLEDGMENTS

We are very grateful for the help provided by Professor W. T. Peake and G. R. Price who made corrections of the manuscript and gave us useful comments.

REFERENCES

1. P. Dallos, "The Auditory Periphery," Academic Press, New York (1973).
2. T. J. Lynch, V. Nedzelnitsky and W. T. Peake, Input impedance of the cochlea in cat, J. Acoust. Soc. Am. 72:108 (1982).
3. A. Dancer, R. Franke, K. Buck and G. Evrard, Etude de la transmission du stimulus acoustique au niveau du recepteur auditif chez le cobaye, ISL Rpt. R113/79 (1979).
4. A. Dancer, Etude experimentale des traumatismes acoustiques, in: "Physiologie et physiopathologie des recepteurs auditifs," GALF ed., Paris (1983).
5. J. Zwislocki, Analysis of some auditory characteristics, in: "Handbook of Mathematical Psychology," R. D. Luce, R. R. Bush and E. Galanter, ed., John Wiley and Sons, Inc., (1965).

6. J. Zwislocki, The role of external and middle ear in sound transmission, in: "The Nervous System," D. B. Tower, ed., Raven Press, New York (1975).
7. A. Dancer and R. Franke, Intracochlear sound pressure measurements in guinea pigs, Hearing Res. 2:19 (1980).
8. L. P. Peterson and B. P. Bogert, A dynamical theory of the cochlea, J. Acoust. Soc. Am. 22:368 (1950).
9. A. Dancer and R. Franke, Pression acoustique intracochleaire: mesures directes et modeles, Acustica 51:18 (1982).
10. J. D. Miller, C. S. Watson and W. P. Covell, Deafening effects of noise on the cat, Acta Otolaryngol. Suppl. 176 (1963).
11. P. Dallos, Low-frequency auditory characteristics: Species dependence, J. Acoust. Soc. Am. 48:489 (1970).
12. J. Zwislocki, Cochlear waves: interaction between theory and experiments, J. Acoust. Soc. Am. 55:578 (1974).
13. P. Campo, A. Dancer and R. Franke, Mecanismes cochleaires impliques dans le seuil de sensibilite auditive et la fatigue auditive, ISL Rpt. R119/84 (1984).
14. J. P. Wilson, Basilar membrane vibration data and their relation to theories of frequency analysis, in: "Facts and Models in Hearing," E. Zwicker and E. Terhardt, eds., Springer Verlag, Berlin, (1974).
15. P. Dallos, M. A. Cheatham and J. Ferraro, Cochlear mechanics, non linearities and cochlear potentials, J. Acoust. Soc. Am. 55:597 (1974).
16. J. Zwislocki, Theorie der Schneckenmechanik, Acta Oto-Laryngol. Suppl. 72 (1948).
17. B. M. Johnstone, D. Robertson and A. R. Cody, Basilar membrane motion and hearing loss, in: "Hearing and Hearing Prophylaxis," Scandinavian Audiology, Suppl. 16:89 (1982).
18. V. Nedzelnitsky, Sound pressure in the basal turn of the cat cochlea, J. Acoust. Soc. Am. 68:1676 (1980).
19. R. Franke and A. Dancer, Etude du potentiel microphonique cochleaire chez le cobaye en fonction des conditions experimentales, Acustica 52:160 (1983).
20. A. Dancer, R. Franke and G. Evrard, Stimulation acoustique en circuit ferme chez le cobaye, mesure de quelques parametres, ISL Rpt. N608/84 (1984).
21. M. C. Brown, I. Smith and A. L. Nuttall, Anesthesia and surgical trauma: their influence on the guinea pig compound action potential, Hearing Res. 10:345 (1983).

DISCUSSION

Patuzzi: The way you normalized your exposure intensity was by measuring the microphonic. Was that the round window microphonic?

Dancer: Yes. We compared in the same animals differential cochlear microphonic in the first turn with the round window microphonic and in the range we used here, from 1 kHz to 10 kHz, the curves have the same shape for the differential microphonic and the round window microphonic.

Patuzzi: What was the best frequency of the tuning curve shape for the round window microphonic?

Dancer: The best frequency was about 11 kHz.

Patuzzi: If you are going to create constant CM at the round window, isn't it possible that you are just moving up the tuning curve of the microphonic at the round window and in doing so actually reducing the intensity of the sound at a higher frequency?

Dancer: We think that the round window microphonic is a better estimate than the differential microphonic because there is less or perhaps no high frequency cut off as with differential electrodes. So for high frequencies, we have greater confidence in the round window microphonic than with differential microphonics.

THE RESPONSE OF MAMMALIAN COCHLEAR HAIR CELLS TO ACOUSTIC OVERSTIMULATION

A. R. Cody and I. J. Russell

M. R. C. Neurophysiology
Group School of Biological Sciences
University of Sussex, Brighton, BN1 9QG

INTRODUCTION

The distinct morphological division of the inner and outer hair cells (IHC, OHC) within the organ of Corti, and their respective innervation, suggest two separate roles for these receptors in normal auditory function. The IHCs receive a massive afferent innervation while the afferent innervation of the OHCs is comparatively sparse with a large number of efferent synapses on their baso-lateral surfaces [1,2]. This has contributed to speculation that there is a division of labour in the cochlea, with the IHCs playing a sensory role and the OHCs fulfilling a motor role, controlling the mechanical stimulus delivered to the IHCs. As primary receptors, the IHC and the OHC appear to be vulnerable links in the auditory pathway during acoustic overstimulation and therefore prime targets for the site and origin of noise-induced hearing losses (NIHL). We have attempted to substantiate this hypothesis in a series of experiments by recording directly from the IHCs and OHCs during conditions of acoustic overstimulation. The results suggest that functional differences in the behavior of these two cell groups to overstimulation may underlie the cellular basis for NIHL. These cellular changes probably account for the altered activity of the afferent fibers we have monitored in the spiral ganglion of the cochlea in previous studies, at least for temporary losses of auditory sensitivity and possibly, the more significant, permanent losses.

PERIPHERAL STUDIES IN NOISE-INDUCED HEARING LOSS

The recording techniques for both intracellular hair cell experiments and extracellular afferent fiber recording in the spiral ganglion have been extensively described [3-5]. Basically, both techniques require careful removal of the bone just above the spiral ligament, which is easily visualized with back illumination of the cochlea. In the guinea pig this produces a view of the basilar membrane (BM) in the region 2.4 to 3.5 mm from the basal end of the cochlea. Best or characteristic frequencies (CF) of the mechanical vibration of the cochlea partition, sensory receptors or afferent fibers in this area of the cochlea are in the range 23-17 kHz. Although this is a rather restricted range with regard to the functional bandwidth of the cochlea, this is the only location where a direct comparison can be made between location, the tuning properties of afferent fibers,

IHCs and the vibration of the basilar membrane. That is, the complete description of the transduction pathway from the vibration of the cochlear partition up to, but not including, the first processing stage in the cochlear nucleus. The advantage of recording the activity of afferent neurons in the spiral ganglion lies in the fact that the dendrites run radially from the ganglion and innervate IHCs in the basal coil that are accessible for intracellular recording [1]. This enables a direct comparison between the activity of the primary afferent neuron and the receptors they innervate in terms of their respective sensitivity and filter properties. These two components of sensory transduction are considered vital in the interpretation of responses to acoustic stimuli.

HAIR CELL RESPONSE TO ACOUSTIC STIMULI

The resting potentials of IHCs are always more positive than -50mV and they always produce predominantly depolarizing receptor potentials regardless of the stimulus frequency (Fig. 1). At low frequencies, during the rarefaction phase of the sound pressure, the amplitude of the depolarizing phase (with respect to the resting membrane potential) can be up to three times larger than the hyperpolarizing phase [4]. At frequencies less than about 1 kHz, the receptor potential is usually seen as a phasic voltage modulation of the resting potential with peak-peak receptor potentials reaching 30mV in the sensitive cochlea. As the stimulus frequency increases the phasic, a.c. component of the receptor potential decreases at a rate of approximately 6 dB/octave for stimulus frequencies above 750 Hz until at or near the CF of the cell, the a.c. component is below the noise level of the recording electrode and only a d.c. component is obvious (Fig. 1). The decrease in the phasic component of the receptor potential is thought to result from the electrical properties of the cell membrane acting as a single pole, low pass filter [4]. The d.c. component recorded at high stimulus frequencies can be substantial with levels of 15 mV not uncommon. Both the a.c. and the d.c. component of the IHC show identical tuning properties in the same cell, which in turn match those recorded for afferent neurons. However, because of a combination of the hair cell time constant and an asymmetrical transducer conductance, the d.c. component is thought to dominate the excitation of the afferent synapse at high stimulus frequencies [4].

Recent intracellular studies of OHCs in the basal coil of the guinea pig cochlea [6] show that these cells differ from IHCs in their responses to acoustic stimuli (Fig. 1). Their resting potentials are typically more

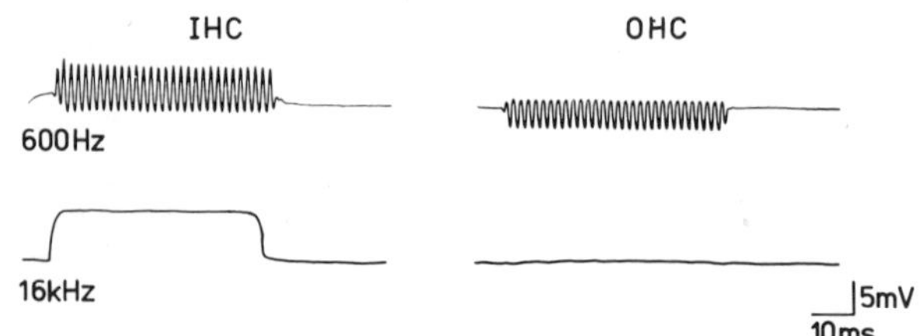

Fig. 1. IHC receptor potentials to a 600Hz tone (80dB SPL) and a 16kHz tone (65dB SPL) recorded in the basal turn of the cochlea together with the OHC intracellular record for the same acoustic stimuli and for a similar location in the cochlea.

polarized than IHCs (-70 to -95mV) and, in the presence of low frequency tones, receptor potentials are symmetrical at low intensities, increasingly asymmetric in the hyperpolarizing phase at moderate levels, and depolarizing when stimulus levels approach or exceed 90 dB SPL (re 20u Pa). The OHCs do not produce d.c. potentials at high frequencies delivered at moderate levels and, because the a.c. component is attenuated by the hair cell time constant, this means that no modulation of the membrane potential is observed until the SPL approaches levels that may temporarily decrease the sensitivity of the cochlea (90 - 100 dB SPL). The amplitude of the receptor potential is also significantly less than that of the IHC and only reaches 3-5 mV at stimulus levels of 100-110 dB SPL. The absence of a d.c. component at high stimulus frequencies or, for that matter, any measurable modulation of the resting membrane potential at physiological stimulus levels, argues against a sensory role for this group of cells. The limited a.c. tuning data from the OHCs in the basal coil suggests that they are as sharply tuned as the IHC and therefore the filter properties of the BM, the hair cells and the afferent neurons at any one location along the cochlear partition are coincident.

ACOUSTIC OVERSTIMULATION AND COCHLEA HAIR CELLS

Exposure of the animal to short (225 ms), high intensity pure tones (12.5 kHz, 110 dB SPL) results in significant changes in the response of the IHC to low frequency test tones. The intracellular record of a IHC to a 600 Hz (85 dB SPL) test tone (solid line, Fig. 2) demonstrates three points. Immediately following a loud tone (dotted line), there is a loss of peak-peak amplitude, an increase in the symmetry of the receptor potential and a phase delay of about 60 . Largest loss of amplitude is seen for the depolarizing phase of the voltage response of the hair cell which gives rise to the increase in symmetry. The amplitude of the receptor potential gradually recovers following the loud tone, and the phase of the waveform reverts to its pre-exposure value within 10-15 cycles; at this frequency this represents a time span of 16-25 ms. Multiple presentations of the loud tone result in additional loss in amplitude of the a.c. receptor potential, while the recovery of the voltage responses of the IHC appears to depend on the duration and intensity of the exposure.

In the case of the OHC the loss of receptor potential peak-peak sensitivity to low frequency stimulation (dotted line, Fig. 2) is difficult to assign to the depolarizing or hyperpolarizing phase because of a shift in the postexposure membrane potential. However, other experiments where short tones were used as control stimuli show that the largest loss is restricted to the hyperpolarizing phase. This is in direct contrast to the responses of IHCs where the largest loss is in the depolarizing phase. Some evidence of this is seen in Fig. 2 in the receptor potential recorded one minute after the end of the loud tone. In this case the hyperpolarizing phase has not yet recovered to pre-exposure amplitudes. Fig. 3 demonstrates another characteristic of the OHC. When a train of five 225 ms, 110 dB SPL tones is presented to the animal, the OHC membrane potential demonstrates a cumulative depolarization that is not seen in the intracellular records from the IHC. For the duration of the loud tone, the OHC membrane continues to depolarize to more positive potentials, while the IHC intracellular potential adapts after the onset of the loud tone and plateaus at levels 10-15 mV more positive than the resting membrane potential. At the offset, normal pre-exposure resting potentials are almost instantaneously established in the IHC, while in the OHC, the recovery time constant is substantially greater. If the loud tone is repeated, then the OHC membrane potential demonstrates a cumulative depolarization. Given a sufficient recovery period, the OHC repolarizes over a similar time course to that recorded for the recovery in amplitude of the a.c. component of the

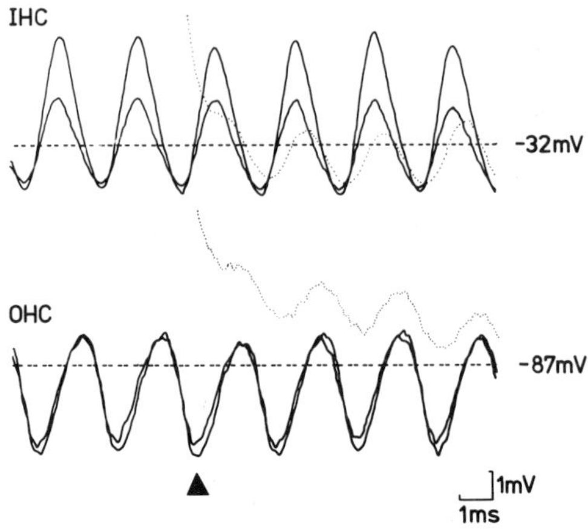

Fig. 2. IHC and OHC receptor potentials to a 85 dB SPL 600 Hz continuous tone before (solid line), immediately following (dotted line) and after exposure of the cochlea to a 225 ms, 100 dB SPL, 12.5 kHz tone. Dashed line is the resting membrane potential of the cell. The arrow denotes when the loud tone finished.

receptor potential and significantly, the a.c. and d.c. component of the IHC receptor potential. This suggests a common mechanism is operating in the recovery of sensitivity of the receptor potentials for both groups of hair cells.

When the test tone is delivered at or near the CF of the IHC together with a series of loud, short tones, then the loss of the d.c. receptor potential demonstrates similar characteristics to that recorded for the a.c. receptor potential, inasmuch as sensitivity is lost; this is additive with each loud tone. An intracellular record for an IHC presented with gated tones near the CF (16 kHz, 60 dB SPL) is shown in Fig. 4. For this hair cell, the recovery time constant after exposure to the first and fifth loud tone in a series of exposures is similar, at around 200 ms. The recovery time constant in this particular case is probably a function of the intensity and duration of the loud tone, as other studies [7] have suggested.

One of the characteristic responses of the IHC to tones of increasing intensity at the CF is a compressive saturation of the d.c. receptor potential. The non-linear behavior is only recorded for stimulus frequencies at or around the CF and is believed to derive from the non-linear vibration of the cochlear partition [3,8]. Fig. 5 shows the input-output functions for a stimulus frequency at the CF (20 kHz) of an IHC and for a stimulus frequency 0.8 octaves below the CF (12kHz). In the sensitive cochlea, the receptor potential demonstrates typical non-linear growth, but when a series of short duration, high intensity exposures (30 sec, 110 dB SPL, 12.5 kHz) are presented to the cochlea, the compressive saturation is progressively lost until the growth of the transfer function is essentially linear with a slope that approaches unity (dashed line). In contrast, the loud tones have virtually no effect on the 12 kHz transfer function. Thus it would appear that the non-linear properties of the hair cell at CF are

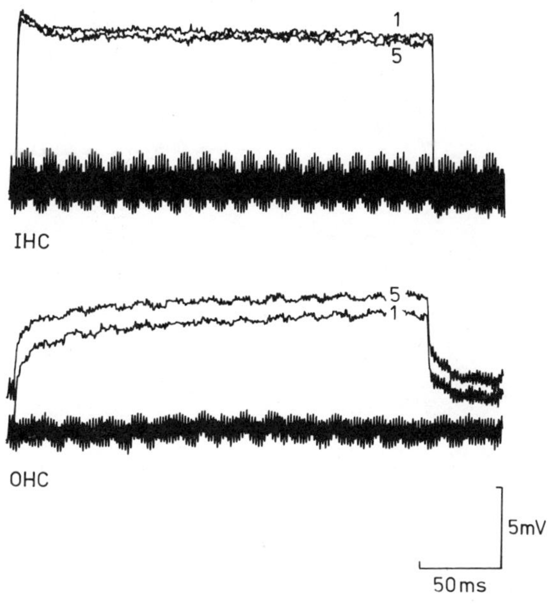

Fig. 3. Intracellular records from an IHC and OHC before and during exposure of the cochlea to a train of 225 ms, 12.5 kHz, 100 dB SPL tones. A continuous 600 Hz 70 dB SPL was delivered as a test stimuli. The receptor potential to this tone was suppressed during the exposure and was reduced in amplitude at the offset. The numbers 1 and 5 represent the response of the cell to the first and the fifth loud tone. In addition to the loss of receptor potential amplitude to the 600 Hz tone in both cells, the OHC demonstrates a cumulative elevation of its membrane potential. The low frequency modulation of the 600 Hz receptor potential is due to sampling aliasing.

vulnerable to acoustic overstimulation, as has already been demonstrated for cochlear asphyxia studies [9]. The loss of the hair cell non-linear properties mimics those seen in the vibration of the BM where there are large losses of cochlear sensitivity, which suggests that the hair cell changes derive from mechanical changes in the cochlea partition [8]. Long term exposures have not been attempted for the OHC mainly because of the extreme instability of the recordings when loud tones are presented to the cochlea. This is presumably due to the motion of the cochlea partition during the presentation of acoustic stimuli.

In summary, both the IHC and the OHC demonstrate sensitivity losses in the receptor potentials generated in response to test tones; these responses become more linear, as evidenced by the loss of the asymmetry of the receptor potential and linearization of their transfer functions. Finally, the recovery of the a.c. and d.c. components of the receptor potential for OHCs and IHCs parallels the repolarization of the OHC membrane

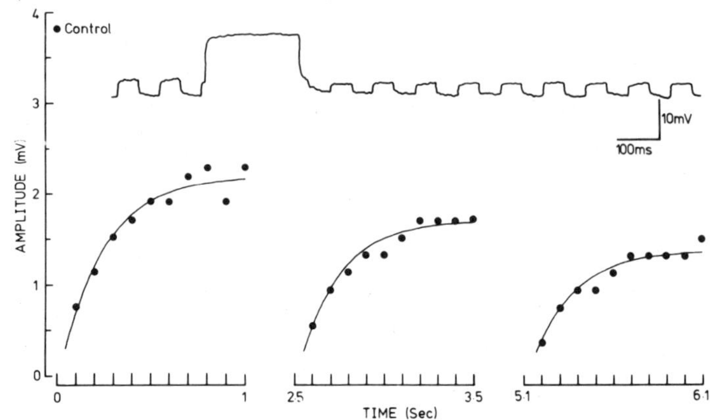

Fig. 4 Loss and recovery of the d.c. component of the IHC receptor potential after exposure to three sequential 12.5 kHz 110 dB SPL tones. The control amplitude of the receptor potential to the 16 kHz 60 dB SPL test tone was 3.8 mV. The recovery time constant is about 220 ms. The top part of the figure is a record of the IHC d.c. response before and after one loud tone. [From Cody & Russell, J. Physol. 345:150P (1983)].

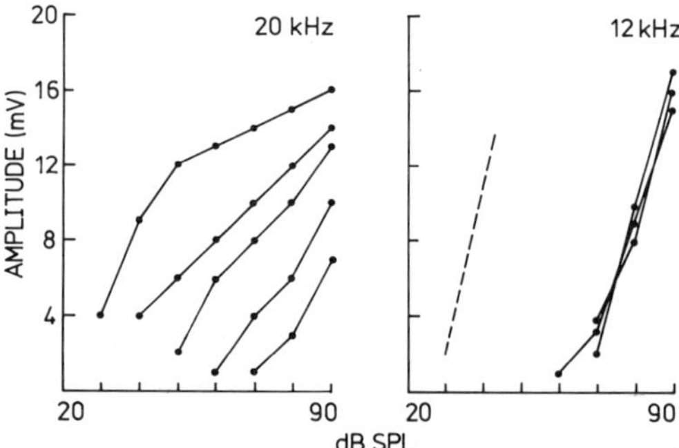

Fig. 5. IHC input-output functions for stimulus frequencies of 20 and 12 kHz before and following five exposures of the cochlea to 30 sec, 110 dB SPL, 12.5 kHz loud tones. The compressive saturation of the 20 kHz transfer function is progressively lost and the IHC requires higher SPLs to produce iso-voltage receptor potentials. The 12 kHz transfer function shows little change. The dashed line indicates linearity.

potential. The intracellular potential changes may have a mechanical correlate in the vibration of the cochlear partition.

ACOUSTIC OVERSTIMULATION AND AFFERENT NEURON RESPONSES

Recording from spiral ganglion neurons in the basal coil of the guinea pig cochlea enables a direct comparison between the sensitivity and tuning properties of the afferent neuron and the sensory receptor on which their dendrites form functional synapses. Although this type of comparative recording has not been attempted in the same cochlea, the use of the first negative component (NI) of the eighth nerve compound action potential (CAP) serves as the common link between the different experiments. With pure gated tones, this physiological probe provides an accurate measure of the functional status of discrete locations in the cochlea in terms of the threshold sensitivity of the afferent fibers. Cochleas showing similar absolute sensitivity of the CAP always show similar tuning properties and sensitivity for the afferent neurons and IHCs recorded at the same location. This is seen in Fig. 6, where the location of cochlea pathology induced by a high intensity pure tone is compared with the frequency specific loss of threshold sensitivity of the CAP. The close agreement between hair cell damage and the loss of threshold sensitivity is typical of the relationship between cochlea pathology and the physiological status of the afferent fibers. This tight relationship is not restricted to lesions induced by pure tone exposures but, is also seen for impulse noise studies [10], mechanical traumas [11] and cell damage resulting from the administration of ototoxic aminoglycosides [12]. The correlations of single cell activity with the CAP shown in Fig. 6 show that afferent neurons innervating IHCs located outside the lesion (sites 1, 3) demonstrate normal levels of sensitivity and tuning, while neurons innervating IHCs located within the lesion are detuned and have lost sensitivity (site 2). Thus, absolute losses of single cell sensitivity appear to accord with that measured in the CAP, given that the CAP will only monitor the most sensitive units at threshold levels of acoustic stimulation. One point to note in this figure is that the lesion of the receptors in the organ of Corti resulting from the pure tone is restricted to the OHC stereocilia of the first row (OHC1). This type of damage is typical for a pure tone exposure that produces a permanent loss of threshold sensitivity (PTS) in the basal coil of the guinea pig cochlea. The other rows of the OHCs, and in particular the IHCs, are not obviously affected until the intensity of the exposure is raised to levels exceeding 115 dB SPL[13]. The damage produced by the pure tone is usually seen as a fusion or loss of the individual stereocilia on the arms of the stereocillary bundle, or in some cases a complete loss of the cell body. The IHC shows no obvious pathology of the stereocilia and would appear to be morphologically normal in cochleas showing this type of restricted lesion. Although cochlear surface pathology of the receptors is a rather limited method of assessing acoustically-induced lesions, the fact that these changes in the OHCs coincide with the first visible signs of permanent losses of threshold sensitivity would suggest that this group of receptors is the most vulnerable and therefore a prime candidate for the site and origin of NIHL.

THE ORIGIN OF NOISE-INDUCED HEARING LOSS

Along with the present series of hair cell intracellular studies, previous afferent fiber and cochlear morphological studies, lead us to the inevitable conclusion that NIHL is a phenomen of the cochlea and more specifically the OHCs. This is the only site that demonstrates a persistant elevation of the membrane potential which recovers at a similar rate to receptor cell and general cochlea sensitivity. The OHC is the first

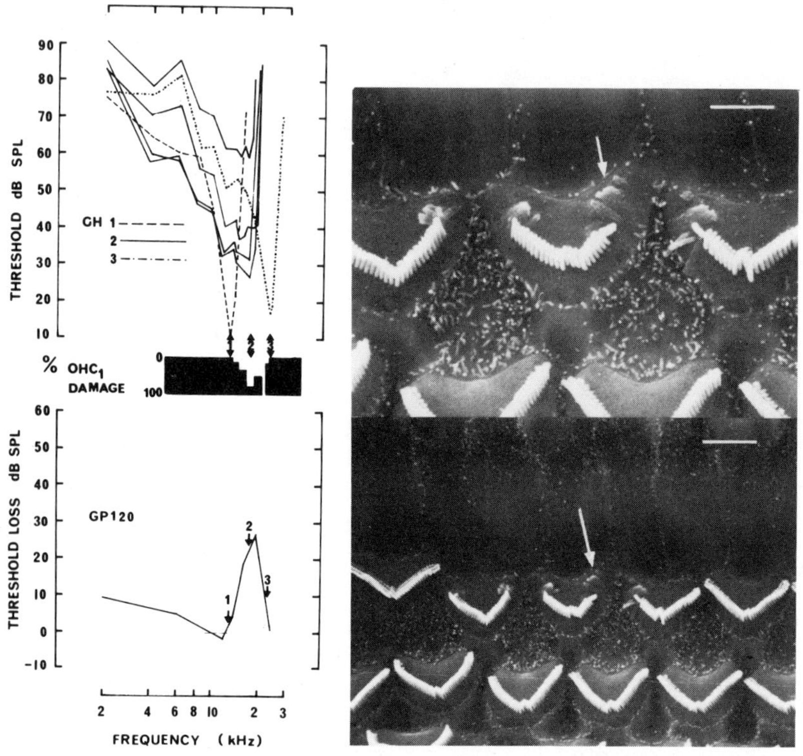

Fig. 6. Spiral ganglion afferent fiber threshold tuning curves, CAP thresholds and cochlear morphology of the guinea pig showing a permanent threshold loss after exposure to a 13 kHz, 112 dB SPL tone for one hour. The numbers 1-3 represent recording sites across the lesion. The plates are scanning electron micrographs of the stereocilia of the OHCs. Arrows indicate specific damage to the stereocilia. Calibration bars, 7 um.

mechano-receptor in the auditory transduction chain. Based on present theories of cochlear transduction, any change in the functional status of the OHCs will alter both the mechanical motion of the cochlear partition and also the sensitivity of the IHCs on which the majority of the afferent fibers synapse. The similarities in the tuning properties of the mechanoreceptive hair cells and the mechanical motion of the BM strongly suggest that the OHCs and BM are intimately related by a common, single tuning mechanism. Any trauma that acts directly on this mechanism should manifest itself in a similar manner in the tuning of the hair cells and the BM. Fig. 7 demonstrates these changes for an IHC, for an afferent fiber and in the vibration of the BM following acoustically-induced desensitization. In all cases the loss in sensitivity is accompanied by decrease in the tuning properties of the cell and shifts of the CF to lower frequencies. With large sensitivity losses, the BM mechanical tuning reverts to a broadly tuned base line little different to that measured post mortem [4]. Although the afferent fiber can demonstrate further losses of sensitivity and tuning [14], these are believed to be the result of a progressive dysfunction of the afferent terminal [15] rather than the IHC. The interesting point is that regardless of the iso-voltage levels used to derive the IHC tuning curve from its input-output functions, this cell is much more vulnerable than the BM or the afferent fiber. Since the afferent

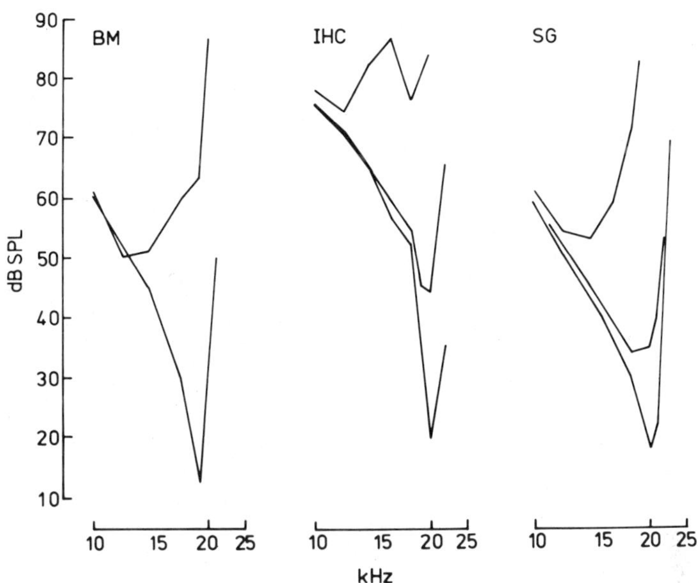

Fig. 7. Tuning curves for the basilar membrane (BM), inner hair (IHC) and afferent neuron recorded in the spiral ganglion of the guinea pig cochlea (SG). The IHC and SG tuning curves show progressive detuning and loss of threshold with loud tones which accord with the loss of tuning of the BM. (BM tuning redrawn from Sellick et al. [8].)

fiber almost certainly derives its normal filter properties from the IHC, this at first sight would appear as an anomaly. However, there is evidence that the afferent synapse can be directly depolarized by extracellular current at low frequencies [16] and more recently, that at high SPLs the OHCs dominate the extracellular potentials in the form of a +ve summating potential [17]. If this is the case, then the anomaly may be explained in terms of the receptor currents developed by the OHCs directly exciting the afferent fiber when the IHC is no longer able to produce excitatory intracellular potentials.

The loss of the tuning properties of the BM is probably the crux of the mechanism of NIHL. Since the discovery that sound may be emitted from the ear, interest has focused on the idea that there must be a metabolically dependant active process in the cochlea capable of injecting energy back into the vibration of the cochlear partition as part of a "negative damping" feedback loop [18]. This so-called active component has been modeled as located in the OHCs and is a prerequisite for the high degree of tuning that is associated with the vibration of the BM in a sensitive cochlea. In functional terms, "negative damping" is manifest at or close to the CF of a mechanical tuning curve by a non-linear, compressional saturation of the input-output function [4,19,20]. This type of curve is also measured in the IHC receptor potentials (Fig. 5) and the afferent fiber response. As already discussed, the loss of this compressional saturation at the CF in the IHC receptor potential and the BM vibration is a classical response to loud sound. Although not yet recorded for the OHC, the increased symmetry of the response to low frequency tones following the loud tone (Fig. 2) suggests a similar behavior for this cell. That is, a loss of the frequency dependant non-linear responses of the cell to acoustic stimuli. Loud sound may abolish the action of the active process, leading to detuning and desensitization of the cochlear elements. What evidence do we have for this?

Mountain [21] has shown that electrical stimulation of the crossed olivo-cochlear bundle (COCB) can modify acoustic distortion products recorded in the ear canal. These distortion products are thought to originate in the mechanical motion of the cochlear partition. Since COCB fibers predominantly innervate OHCs [1,2], this suggests an active, mechanical role for this group of receptors feeding back into the vibration of the cochlear partition. A similar finding has also been shown by Siegal and Kim [22]. As shown in Fig. 6, pure tone damage is generally restricted to the first row of the OHCs and relatively minor damage to the stereocilia of these receptors results in substantial losses in cochlea sensitivity and frequency selectivity. The first row of the OHCs also show the most extensive distribution of COCB terminals, thus suggesting that this row of hair cells may exert the greatest influence on cochlear function. Possible acoustically-evoked activity of the COCB has been shown to modify the cochlear desensitization produced when the ear is exposed to loud sound for both temporary and permanent threshold losses, again suggesting an active role for the OHCs [23,24]. Intracellular recordings from cochlear hair cells in this study show that the non-linear properties of IHCs and more importantly OHCs are modified during acoustic overstimulation in a similar manner to that recorded for the BM. It has also been shown that the OHC membrane potential is intimately linked with the loss and recovery of cochlear sensitivity, as monitored in the IHC receptor potentials and the gross response of the eighth nerve.

We propose that the intracellular changes in the OHC potentials are electrical analogs of micromechanical changes in this cell that give rise to the loss of cochlear frequency selectivity and sensitivity. To that extent, the decrease in the BM tuning properties is an epiphenomenon, simply because the BM probably derives its filter properties from the electro-mechanical properties of the OHC-tectorial membrane complex. The elevation of the OHC membrane potential and its subsequent repolarization may mirror the loss and recovery of the theoretical active process. An exact location for the site of NIHL may be extremely difficult to pinpoint until a mechanism and site for this process is finally described. In this respect the OHC stereocilliary complex is a prime candidate. The evidence to date, however, points to the OHCs as the site and origin for NIHL.

ACKNOWLEDGEMENTS

This work was supported by the M.R.C. The authors would like to thank Dr. A. Palmer for his constructive criticisms of this manuscript. A.R.C. is a N.H. and M.R.C. (Australia). C. J. Martin is a traveling fellow.

REFERENCES

1. H. Spoendlin, The innervation of the cochlear receptor, in: "Basic Mechanisms in Hearing," A. Moller, ed., Academic Press, New York (1973).
2. W. B. Warr, The olivocochlear bundle: its origins and terminations in the cat in: "Evoked Electrical Activity in the Auditory Nervous System," R. F. Nauton and R. Fernandez, eds., Academic Press, New York (1978).

3. I. J. Russell and P. M. Sellick, Intracellular studies of hair cells in the mammalian cochlea, J. Physiol., 284:261 (1978).
4. I. J. Russell and P. M. Sellick, Low frequency characteristics of intracellularly recorded receptor potentials in mammalian hair cells, J. Physiol., 338:179 (1983).
5. D. Robertson and G. A. Manley, Manipulation of frequency analysis in the cochlear ganglion of the guinea pig, J. Comp. Physiol., 91:363 (1974).
6. A. R. Cody and I. J. Russell, Outer hair cells in the mammalian cochlea and noise-induced hearing loss, Nature, 313:662 (1985).
7. G. K. Yates, A. R. Cody and B. M. Johnstone, Recovery of eighth nerve action potentials after exposure to short, intense pure tones: similarities with temporary threshold shift, Hearing Res., 12:305 (1983).
8. P. M. Sellick, R. Patuzzi and B. M. Johnstone, Measurement of basilar membrane motion in the guinea pig using the Mossbauer technique, J. Acoust. Soc. Am., 72:131 (1982).
9. I. J. Russell and E. M. Cowley, The influence of transient asphyxia on receptor potentials in inner hair cells in the guinea pig cochlea, Hearing Res., 11:373 (1983).
10. A. R. Cody and B. M. Johnstone, Electrophysiological and morphological correlates in the guinea pig cochlea after exposure to "impulsive noise", Scand. Audiol., Suppl. 12:121 (1980).
11. D. Robertson, A. R. Cody, G. Bredberg and B. M. Johnstone, Response properties of spiral ganglion neurons in cochleas damaged by direct mechanical trauma, J. Acoust. Soc. Am., 67:1295 (1980).
12. D. Robertson and B. M. Johnstone, Aberrant tonotopic organization in the inner ear damaged by kanamycin, J. Acoust. Soc. Am., 66:466 (1979).
13. A. R. Cody and D. Robertson, Variability of noise-induced damage in the guinea pig cochlea: Electrophysiological and morphological correlates after strictly controlled exposures, Hearing Res., 9:55 (1983).
14. A. R. Cody and B. M. Johnstone, Single auditory neuron response during acute acoustic trauma, Hearing Res., 3:3 (1980).
15. D. Robertson, Reversible structural abnormalities in the organ of Corti of guinea pigs with reversible hearing loss, Proc. Aust. Physiol. Pharmacol. Soc. 12:31P (1981).
16. P. M. Sellick, R. Patuzzi and B. M. Johnstone, Modulation of responses of spiral ganglion cells in the guinea pig cochlea by low frequency sound, Hearing Res., 7:199 (1982).
17. I. J. Russell and A. R. Cody, Transduction in cochlear hair cells, Mechanics of Hearing Workshop (in press).
18. S. J. Neely and D. O. Kim, An active cochlear model showing sharp tuning and high sensitivity, Hearing Res., 9:123 (1983).
19. W. S. Rhode, Observations of the vibration of the basilar membrane in squirrel monkeys using the Mossbauer technique, J. Acoust. Soc. Am., 49:1218 (1971).
20. S. M. Khanna and D. G. Leonard, Basilar membrane tuning in the cat cochlea, Science, 215:305 (1982).
21. D. C. Mountain, Changes in endolyphatic potential and crossed olivocochlear bundle stimulation alter cochlear mechanics, Science, 210:71 (1980).
22. J. H. Siegal and D. O. Kim, Efferent neural control of cochlear mechanics? Olivocochlear bundle stimulation affects cochlear biomechanical non-linearity, Hearing Res., 6:171 (1982).
23. A. R. Cody and Johnstone, B. M., Temporary threshold shift modified by binaural acoustic stimulation, Hearing Res. 6:199 (1982).

24. A. R. Cody, Temporary and permanent threshold shifts: An electrophysiological and histological study of the effects of acoustic overstimulation in the guinea pig, Ph. D. Thesis, University of Western Australia (1982).

DISCUSSION

Pickles: How can you be sure you were recording from outer hair cells?

Cody: One of the easiest ways to identify hair cells is to dye inject while you are recording. Unfortunately, when you dye inject cells, it means you have to use electrodes which are filled with something like Lucifer Yellow and that has to be in distilled water. So, that means the impedance of your electrodes is on the order 600-700 Mohms. Now, when you are recording in hair cells with such high impedances, it is difficult to look at the electrical properties of hair cells. So it is very difficult to say for sure we are recording from OHC. We therefore rely on a number of physiological pointers to identify response from outer hair cells. One, the resting membrane potentials of these cells are much lower than we would record from any other hair cells. Now if you go through the basilar membrane from scala tympani to scala media, you actually go first through supporting cells, then usually through extracellular space, then you have another cell which we presume is in an outer hair cell, then it is directly into scala media after that. So, position is one important criteria. The second is characteristic responses. The responses of these cells in terms of intracellular receptor potentials is larger than what you record in the extracellular space. They show a hyperpolarizing depolarizing phase which you do not record extracellularly. Third, supporting cell responses are usually much smaller, about 1/3 of the size of response from outer hair cells.

Hamernik: In some species such as Gerbils, the inner hair cells sit right over the boney limbus. How do you reconcile the responses of inner hair cells with basilar membrane mechanics when the boney limbus probably does not vibrate very much.

Cody: It is simple, because we consider the inner hair cells as rather passive sensory elements. They are just sitting there waiting for mechanical stimulation which is derived from the vibration of the cochleas partition. We think they are under the control of outer hair cells so therefore you are talking about a radial stimulus to the stereocilia of those inner hair cells. They are actually transducing stimuli delivered to them via that radial mechanical coupling.

Trahiotis: Do you have any comments on the possible role of the afferent fibers from the outer hair cells that Bohne and Morest suggest project to the central nervous system?

Cody: The d.c. component comes out of the outer hair cells at about 80-90 db SPL. Then it grows to about 5 mV. Now it is possible that somehow the outer hair cells are acting as null detectors. They are actually looking at their intracellular voltages. When they detect a d.c. component, that is signalled by the apparent fiber, but only at high intensities, that signal may form part of the negative feedback loop with the efferent system. That changes the intracellular potentials of the hair cells and in most cases this causes a hyperpolarization which you have seen in most other cellular systems with efferents being stimulated. That somehow, re-adjusts the set point of the basilar membrane so that the basilar membrane is operating in the linear portion of its input/output transfer curve so the outer hair cell afferents and outer hair cells efferents may only operate at high intensities.

Patuzzi: Since we know that low frequency displacement of the partition can turn the mechanics on and off, I suspect that it is a good correlate of the depolarization you get following TTS in outer hair cells. The question is, which comes first? Do hair cells become depolarized and does that cause a change in mechanics or is there a change in mechanics following TTS, like a d.c. shift, that turns the outer hair cells off. One clue might be how large these depolarizations are compared to the largest AC responses you can get from your outer hair cells.

Cody: Right. We cannot yet separate the two possibilities. We do not know whether the electrical events we record intracellular are responsible for mechanical changes or the mechanical changes are responsible for the electrical. We cannot tell.

Patuzzi: Do you have a feel for how large a depolarization you can get?

Cody: The maximum is about 5 mV out of these cells at around 110-115 dB SPL.

Patuzzi: That is the largest change in the membrane potential you can get?

Cody: The change in the membrane potential is less. With those types of exposures, the changes is on the order of 2-3 mV which we think is significant.

STRUCTURE-FUNCTION CORRELATION IN NOISE-DAMAGED EARS: A LIGHT AND ELECTRON-MICROSCOPIC STUDY

M. Charles Liberman[1], L.W. Dodds and D.A. Learson

Eaton-Peabody Laboratory
Massachusetts Eye and Ear Infirmary
243 Charles St., Boston, MA 02114

[1]Department of Physiology
Harvard Medical School
Boston, MA 02115

INTRODUCTION

Of the roughly 50,000 afferent fibers in the cat's auditory nerve, approximately 95% terminate peripherally on inner hair cells (IHCs), as the so-called "radial fibers" (RFs) [24,25]. RFs comprise the population of neurons sampled when the auditory nerve is impaled with glass microelectrodes [9]. In the cat, the great majority of RFs is unbranched, terminating on a single IHC via a single terminal swelling [24,8]. Thus, by sampling the activity of a single RF we have a window onto the functional state of a very restricted region of the organ of Corti. By sampling the activity of different single fibers, with different characteristic frequencies (CFs), we can assess the functional state of the entire cochlea, from base to apex.

Over the last 10 years, we have studied the responses of single, auditory-nerve fibers in cats with drug- or noise-induced damage of the inner ear [11-17]. The abnormalities seen in the responses of these neurons have been correlated with the structural changes in the cochlear duct, both at the light- and electron-microscopic levels. These correlations have been useful in at least two different contexts. First, they have allowed us to infer something about the normal function of those structures which have been damaged, and second, they have suggested differences between the structural bases for temporary vs. permanent hearing loss.

Using noise exposures, or treatment with ototoxic drugs, we have produced a variety of lesion types. In some cases, the IHCs are damaged while the OHCs remain nearly normal, while in other cases the OHCs can be eliminated, leaving the IHCs apparently intact. The changes in the single-unit tuning curves associated with each of these conditions tell us something about the normal mechanisms underlying the generation of frequency selectivity in the auditory nerve.

Application of single-neuron labeling techniques to these studies has greatly increased the precision with which we are able to make correlations between structure and function [13,14,16]. In both normal and abnormal ears it is possible to inject a single RF with horseradish peroxidase (HRP) after studying its discharge properties [9,10]. After suitable histological preparation, the labeled terminal can be followed to the IHC of origin

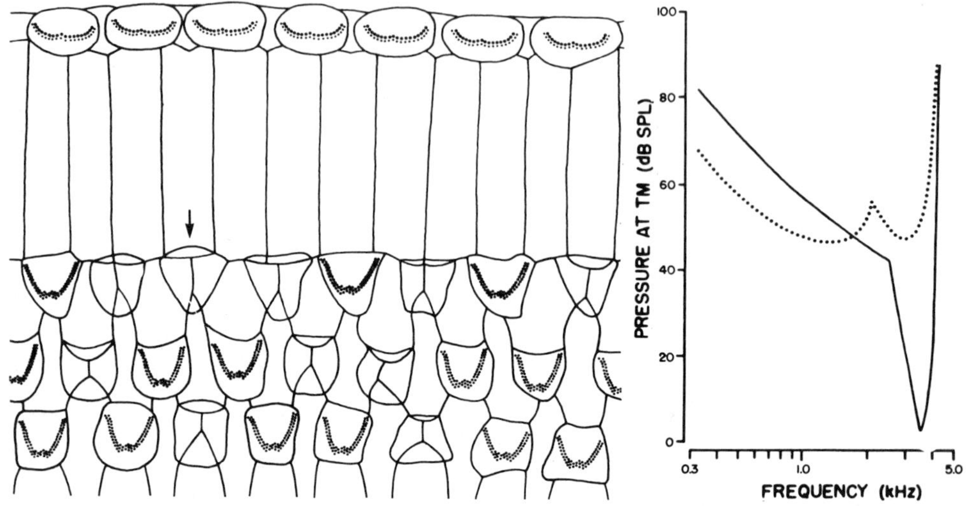

Fig. 1: Functional effects of subtotal loss of OHCs with intact IHCs. At the right, a normal tuning curve (solid) is compared with the type of abnormal curve (dotted) associated with this lesion pattern. In this and all subsequent Figs., the tuning curves have been smoothed and adjusted to represent a distillation of data from many normal and abnormal ears. The organ of Corti is schematized as it appears in a LM analysis of a surface preparation (one row of IHCs at the top, three rows of OHCs at the bottom). Each missing OHC is marked by a scar (see arrow). Since the viewing angle is perpendicular to the endolymphatic surface of the hair cells, each stereocilium appears as a small dot. Only two rows of stereocilia are clearly visible in each tuft at the LM level. On each OHC, the stereocilia are arrayed in a "W". On each IHC, they form a broader arc.

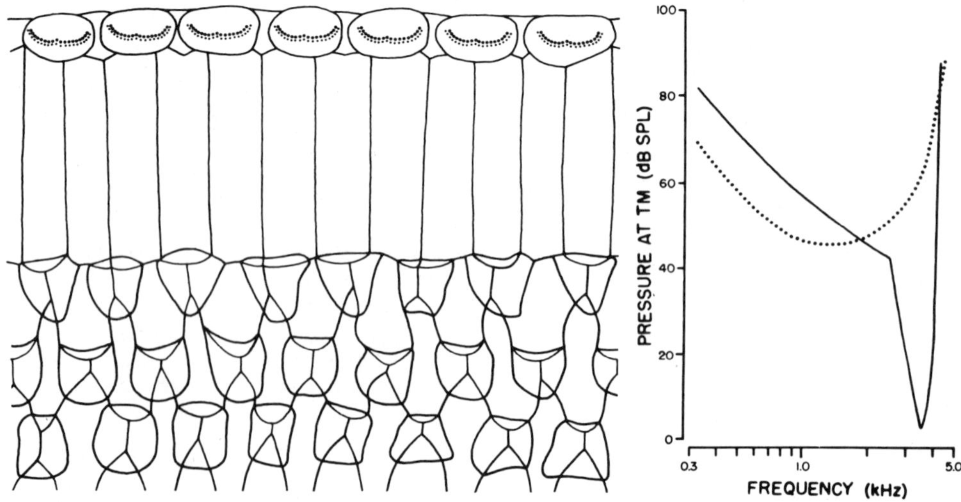

Fig. 2: Functional effects of total loss of OHCs with intact IHCs. All conventions are as described in the caption for Fig. 1.

in the organ of Corti, and the abnormalities in the response properties directly compared with the structural changes in the IHC which generated them and in the surrounding cells of the organ of Corti.

The present report summarizes some of the results obtained in the study of single-unit responses from damaged ears. Since most of the results correlating function and light-microscopic (LM) structure have been published elsewhere, only an overview is presented. Much of the electron microscopic (EM) data is previously unpublished; thus it is treated here in somewhat disproportionate detail.

GENERAL METHODOLOGY

To study permanent threshold shift (PTS), we have exposed anesthetized cats to narrow bands of noise at levels of 100 to 115 dB SPL for two hours. After survival of at least four weeks (to allow temporary components of the threshold shift to disappear [19]), recordings were made from the auditory nerve. Our strategy was to create restricted lesions, both in extent and severity. By restricting the cochlear extent of the lesion, we provide an internal control by leaving regions with normal structure and function for comparison within the same ear. We restrict the severity of the lesion, since it is difficult to assess the effect of one structural change if several other abnormalities coincide with it.

To study temporary threshold shift (TTS), we have exposed anesthetized cats to narrow-band noise at intensities between 105 and 120 dB SPL for durations under 20 minutes [17]. Single-unit activity is recorded prior to, as well as after, the exposure. Thus, the abnormal responses can be compared to those from a similar population of units from the same animal before the exposure. Roughly 18 hours after the exposure, the ear is fixed. By this time, the threshold shifts (roughly 40 dB) are changing slowly enough with time that the minutes which elapse between the last recording and the fixation of the ear are not significant. The assumption that the threshold shifts are fully reversible in these cases is based on comparisons to behavioral thresholds of noise-exposed cats collected by Miller et al.[19].

In our early experiments on ears with PTS, histological assessment was performed using serial sectioning of celloidin-embedded, decalcified temporal bones [15]. These techniques allowed LM evaluation of all structures of the middle and inner ears. Such evaluations indicated that, of all the structures in the inner ear, the hair cells themselves were apparently the most vulnerable to acoustic trauma. Thus, damage was only seen in the accessory structures of the cochlear duct (e.g., stria vascularis, spiral prominence, limbus, etc.) in cases in which there was extensive hair cell loss.

In later studies, we have avoided producing extensive lesions and have studied the cochleas as epon-embedded surface preparations. With this technique we can evaluate the condition of all the sensory cells and their stereocilia at the LM level [12-14], locate a single intracellularly-labeled fiber terminal, and, finally, remove selected regions of the organ of Corti for study in the transmission electron microscope.

STRUCTURE-FUNCTION CORRELATIONS AT THE LM LEVEL

PTS Ears

In acoustically-traumatized ears, we have found that clear-cut morphological change in the organ of Corti is always associated with dramatic threshold elevation in single auditory nerve fibers, whereas threshold shifts of less than 20 or 30 dB can be seen in cochleas which appear to be perfectly normal. Apart from the loss of sensory cells, the most important determinant of threshold shift is the degree of damage to the stereocilia. Thus, by evaluating the presence or absence of sensory cells as well as the condition of their stereocilia, we can "account for" most of the threshold shift in the auditory nerve. Similar conclusions have been reached by other authors [2,20,23].

Our studies of the functional changes associated with noise exposure have concentrated on spontaneous discharge rates (SRs) and the threshold tuning curve, since many other aspects of auditory-nerve activity are at least qualitatively predictable given these two measures. In normal ears, the tuning curve provides a measure of the CF and, thus, the position of innervation along the cochlear spiral. The SR is important, because in normal animals there is a strict correlation between SR and fiber threshold (defined as the intensity required to produce a 10 spikes/second increase over SR [7]).

The normal tuning curve of an auditory nerve fiber can consist of a sharply tuned "tip" and a broadly tuned "tail" [6]. The observation that a wide variety of cochlear insults can selectively affect the tip and leave the tail apparently intact [4,5,15], has long suggested that the tip and tail may be generated by different mechanisms, perhaps one involving the OHCs and the other involving IHCs. In our studies of cochleas damaged by noise or drugs, there are many examples of selective elevation of the tuning-curve tip, but we have also found cases in which both the tip and tail were elevated and other cases in which tip elevation was associated with tuning-curve tails which were hypersensitive by as much as 30 dB [15].

A tuning curve with an attenuated tip and a hypersensitive tail, as illustrated in Fig. 1, can be seen when there is subtotal OHC loss in a cochlear region in which the IHCs remain normal. This type of structural change is typical of that seen with ototoxic drugs, but is less typical of noise trauma. In our hands, such lesions have only been produced with high-frequency exposures (> 9 kHz). Similar lesions have been produced by Robertson [20] using a 10-kHz pure tone.

As schematized in Fig. 2, total loss of the OHCs in a region in which the IHCs remain normal results in bowl-shaped tuning curves which appear to completely lack a sharp tip. These bowl-shaped curves can be apparently hypersensitive in comparison to normal tuning-curve tails. This lesion type is most easily produced with ototoxic drugs.

Results such as those summarized in Figs. 1 and 2 provide evidence that the OHCs are required for the sharp tip of the tuning curve. In addition to providing the IHC and its RFs with increased sensitivity at the CF, the OHCs may also decrease the sensitivity of the IHC to frequencies below the CF.

Other evidence from noise-exposed animals suggests that the OHCs in the first row are more important to the generation of the tuning-curve tip than the OHCs in the other two rows. Thus, as is schematized in Fig. 3, severe disarray and loss of stereocilia on first-row OHCs apparently eliminates tuning-curve tips, even though nearly normal OHCs are present in the other two rows. The tuning curve schematized in Fig. 3 not only lacks a sharp tip, but the "tail" that remains is extremely hyposensitive, in contrast to the situation in Fig. 2. Our data suggest that this tail hyposensitivity arises because of the damage to the IHC stereocilia.

Significant damage to the IHC stereocilia is always associated with significant threshold shift on the tail of the tuning curve. If the associated damage to the OHC is not severe, the result can be a tuning curve with nearly normal shape but elevated thresholds at all frequency regions. Combined damage to IHCs and OHCs is typical of the lesions seen in our material following noise exposures at middle and low frequencies.

We don't yet know what type of tuning curve is associated with pure IHC stereocilia damage, since IHC damage (in our material) is always associated with at least some disarray of OHC stereocilia. However, a case which most closely approximates that ideal is schematized in Fig. 4. A fiber contacting an IHC missing the entire tall row of stereocilia (at arrow) in a region with only modest disarray of OHC stereocilia showed a tuning curve with a normal Q_{10}, although thresholds were elevated by roughly 40 dB. From a case such as this, it would appear that the tall IHC stereocilia are not necessary for sharp tuning in auditory nerve fibers.

One simple summation of all the data from pathological ears is that threshold elevation on the tail is proportional to IHC damage, while the ratio of tip to tail thresholds is indicative of the condition of the OHCs. Although oversimplified, this summary allows general prediction of the nature and extent of cochlear damage from a population of abnormal tuning curves. The main problem with this oversimplification is that factors other than the condition of the sensory cells can affect thresholds. For example, a total focal loss of the organ of Corti (including all hair cells and supporting cells) can apparently raise thresholds at remote locations with seemingly normal structure more than one mm from the lesion [14]. Furthermore, factors outside of the organ of Corti, e.g., strial function and associated values of endolymphatic potential, also have a significant effect on both tip and tail thresholds [21]. Obviously, the correlations between hair cell damage and auditory-nerve dysfunction are clearest when the damage is restricted to the hair cells themselves.

TTS Ears

Ears with temporary threshold shifts can show functional changes similar to those seen in the PTS ears. In some cases, the tips of the tuning curves are elevated, while the tails become hypersensitive. In other cases, both tip and tail are elevated. In the TTS paradigm, these tuning changes are directly demonstrable by recording from the same unit before and after noise exposure.

The structural picture in the TTS ear is very different from the PTS ear. Up to 60 dB of reversible threshold shift can be produced without any visible structural change at the LM level, while, in our material, 60 dB of PTS is always associated with significant hair cell loss or stereocilia damage. In some TTS ears, the afferent dendrites under the IHCs appear grossly swollen [17]. However, this phenomenon has only been seen when the exposure stimulus was a pure tone (three out of three cases) and never in the six cases when the exposures were bands of noise. In some cases of narrow-band exposure, we have seen apparent alterations in the refractile properties of the cuticular plate, visible in the light microscope as a frothy cloud in the apical portion of the hair cell. However, we have not seen significant alterations in the LM appearance of the stereocilia themselves in any case of apparently reversible threshold shift.

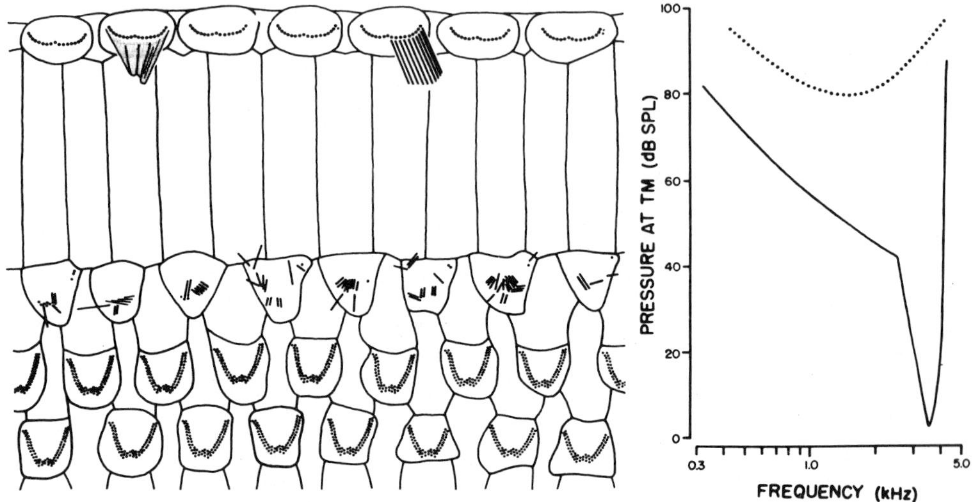

Fig. 3: Functional effects of severe damage to IHC and OHC stereocilia. Most of the tall IHC stereocilia (the row closer to the OHCs) are missing. On the second IHC from the left, a fused bundle of tall stereocilia is depicted. On the fifth IHC from the left the remaining tall stereocilia are bent at 90 degrees from their normal orientation. Other conventions are described in the caption to Fig. 1.

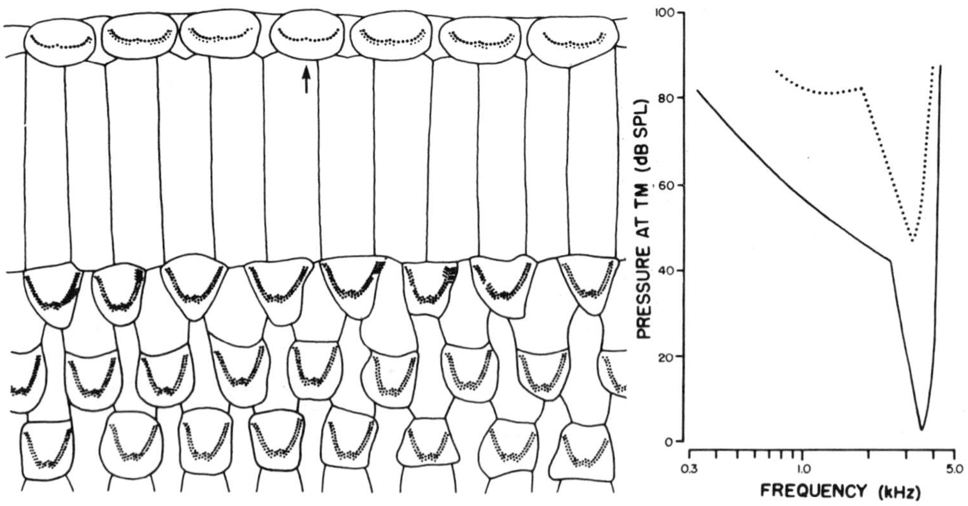

Fig. 4: Functional effects of moderate damage to IHC stereocilia and minimal damage to OHC stereocilia. Many of the tall row of IHC stereocilia are missing. All tall stereocilia are missing on the IHC above the arrow. OHC stereocilia disarray is confined to the first-row cells.

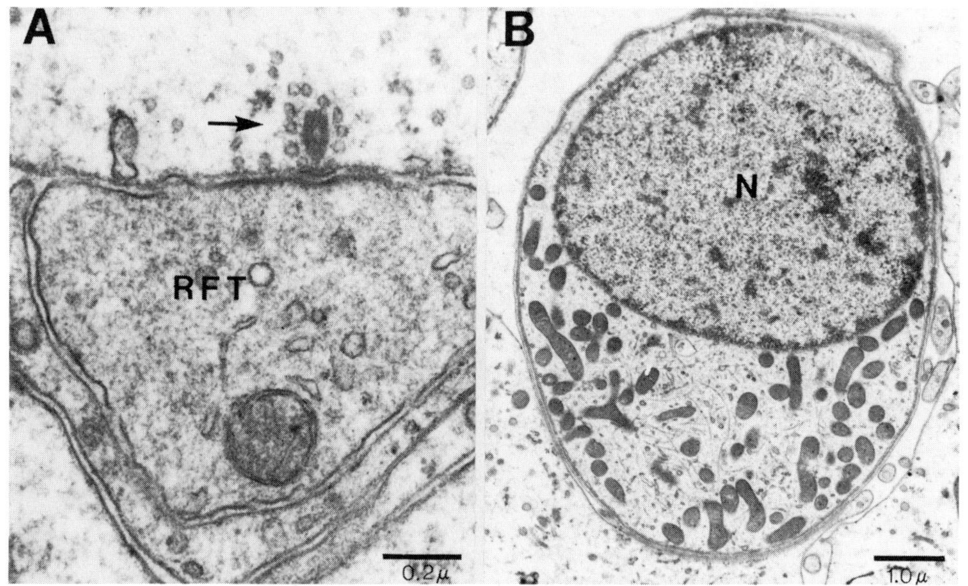

Fig. 5: Electron micrographs from a cochlear region with 40 to 50 dB of PTS. For this and all subsequent micrographs, the plane of section was parallel to the endolymphatic surface of the hair cells. Panel A depicts the synapse (at arrow) between an IHC and a radial fiber terminal (RFT). Panel B shows a cross section through an OHC at the level of the nucleus (N).

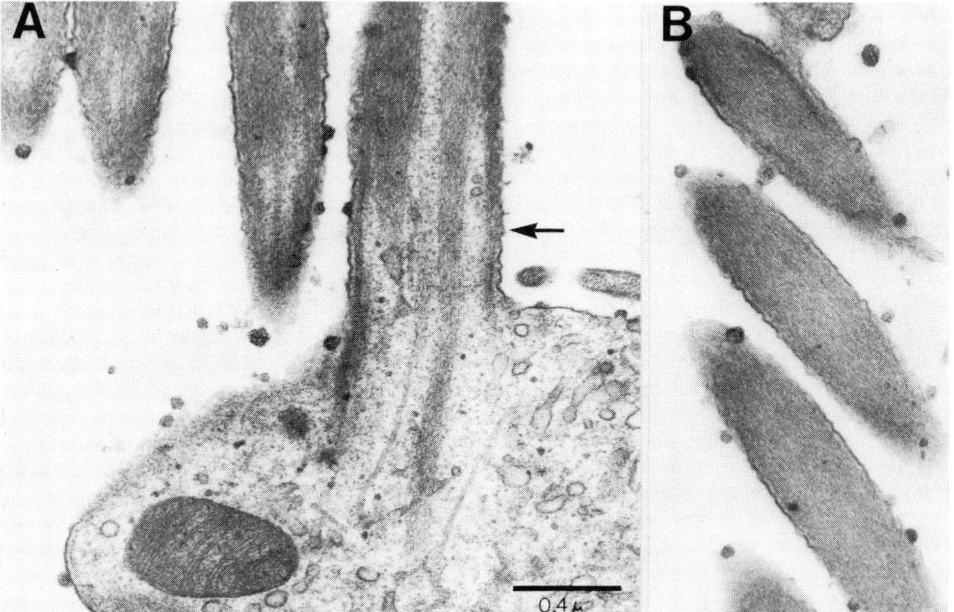

Fig. 6: Electron micrographs of tall IHC stereocilia from a case with PTS. Those in panel A were partially fused and bent at roughly 90 degrees to their normal orientation. Those in panel B were bent at roughly 45 degrees. Scale for panel B is the same as for panel A.

STRUCTURE-FUNCTION CORRELATIONS AT THE EM LEVEL

PTS Ears

Our EM data suggest that most of the important structural changes in PTS ears are actually visible at the LM level. Figs. 5 through 9 illustrate some of the ultrastructural features of sensory cells from a region of the organ of Corti with 40 to 60 dB of PTS. These micrographs are of tissue taken from the 1.1 to 1.8 kHz region of case MCL125; the single-unit physiology and LM histology for this case were summarized in Figs. 4 and 5 of a previous publication [17]. The IHC damage in this area (as seen at the LM level) was similar to that schematized in Fig. 3 of this report, while the OHC damage was intermediate between that illustrated in Figs. 3 and 4. Hair cell loss in this region was minimal.

The ultrastructure in MCL125 is representative of all our PTS cases. As shown in Fig. 5, the cell bodies of IHCs and OHCs appear normal, even in regions in which there is significant damage to the stereocilia, as reported by Cody and Robertson [2]. Others have reported ultrastructural pathology in the organelles of noise-damaged sensory cells (e.g., [1,18]). However, it may be that intracellular pathology only appears in hair cells for which the stereocilia damage is so severe as to render the region of the organ of Corti non-responsive to acoustic stimulation. Thus far, all of our EM data are from acoustically responsive regions.

The stereociliary tufts on both IHCs and OHCs from MCL125 were analyzed via serial EM sections to assess whether there was additional damage not visible at the LM level. Normally, each stereocilium is densely packed with a regular latticework of actin filaments [26]. Tilney et al. [27] have reported that disorganization of this actin network is common within stereocilia from noise-exposed lizards. However, we found little evidence for disorganization of the actin filaments within the stereocilia themselves, except when several stereocilia were fused (see arrow in Fig. 6a). Even when only one or two tall stereocilia remained on a cell, the actin filaments within those remaining hairs appeared to be normally distributed (see Fig. 7a), even if the stereocilia were bent as well (Fig. 6b). Rarely, we saw a stereocilium (arrow in Fig. 7b) in which all the actin appeared depolymerized. In such cases, the plasma membrane was also severely disrupted. We never saw swelling of the bases of the stereocilia, reported to occur in cochleas from noise-exposed lizards [27].

By far the most prevalent ultrastructural change was seen within the cuticular plate, in and around the rootlets of the stereocilia. A normal rootlet consists of a tubular matrix of electron dense material, extending roughly one micron into the cuticular plate beneath each stereocilium and somewhat less than one micron above the cuticular plate, through the center of each stereocilium. In the lizard cochlea, the rootlet appears to be made of actin filaments [26]. However, in the mammalian ear, rootlet composition is less clear [22]. Within the cuticular plate, normal rootlets of the tallest row of stereocilia appear as dark circles (see rootlet "1" in Fig. 8a) when sections are cut parallel to the endolymphatic surface of the hair cell. In sections roughly 0.5 microns above the cuticular plate, the rootlet appears as a dark dot at the center of each stereocilium (Fig. 9).

In MCL125, ultrastructural damage to the rootlets on the first-row OHCs was much worse than that to the third row tufts, mirroring the greater disarray of the OHC1 stereocilia seen in the light microscope (Fig. 4, reference [17]). Some rootlets on the first-row OHC appeared to be partially destroyed (rootlet "2" in Fig. 8a), while others were completely missing in several sections (rootlet "3" in Fig. 8a). Many rootlets

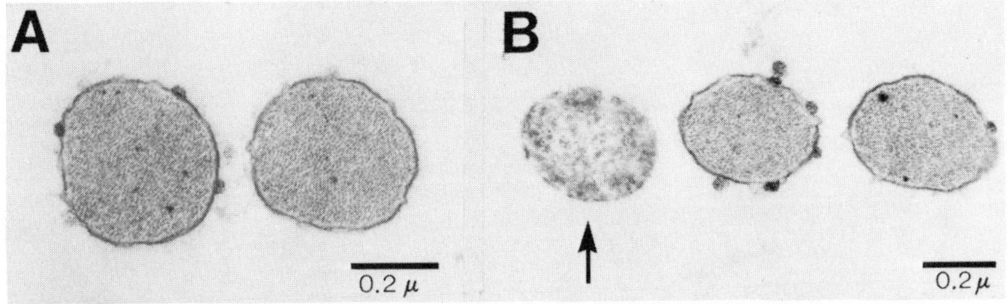

Fig. 7. Micrographs of tall IHC stereocilia from a case with PTS.

appeared to have been broken just at the surface of the cuticular plate, as described in ears from acoustically-traumatized lizards [27] and rabbits [3]. The upper portion of these broken rootlets is often displaced such that, in one cross section, the rootlet can appear to be doubled (rootlet "4" in Fig. 8b). Broken rootlets were always associated with obvious lateral displacement of the stereocilium (arrows in Fig. 9), which corresponds to the disarray visible at the LM level. However, damaged or missing rootlets could be seen on stereocilia which did not appear to be displaced or bent, and missing stereocilia (see bracket in Fig. 9) often had normal rootlets within the cuticular plate. Thus, the relation between stereocilia posture and rootlet condition is not a simple one.

The ultrastructural damage to the stereocilia in the IHC region was somewhat different and, in general, more severe in appearance. In many cells it appeared that the matrix of the cuticular plate had broken into numerous pieces, allowing whole groups of stereocilia and rootlets to fall over. The apparent breakup of the cuticular plate seemingly had allowed cytoplasm to flow up around the bases of the stereocilia. All cases of IHC stereocilia fusion we saw were associated with cytoplasm pools at the bases of the stereocilia, where normally only the dense matrix of the cuticular plate substance should be seen (Fig. 6a).

In the context of the structure-function correlations discussed above, the importance of the EM observations on PTS ears is to support the contention that the most important structural changes in noise-induced hearing loss are in the stereocilia tuft, and that these changes have manifestations which are visible at the LM level. Nevertheless, rootlet abnormalities which are not reflected in obvious displacement of the corresponding stereocilium may explain moderate threshold shifts not associated with recognizable stereocilia disarray.

TTS Ears

Ears with TTS have shown no consistent pathology at either the LM or EM levels. Four of the TTS ears have been examined at the EM level, but one particular case of broad-band exposure was chosen for serial-section EM study (MCL124). The physiology and LM histology for this case have been summarized in Figs. 17 and 18 of Liberman and Mulroy [17]. This case showed roughly 40 to 50 dB of acute threshold shift over a wide frequency range (CFs from 1.0 to 20 kHz). Thus we can be absolutely sure that the regions selected for serial-section analysis (3.5 and 8.0 kHz) did indeed have significant threshold shift. The LM analysis had revealed no stereocilia abnormalities.

At the EM level in this case, we saw no abnormalities in the cell bodies of either IHCs or OHCs (Fig. 10) including the synaptic apparati

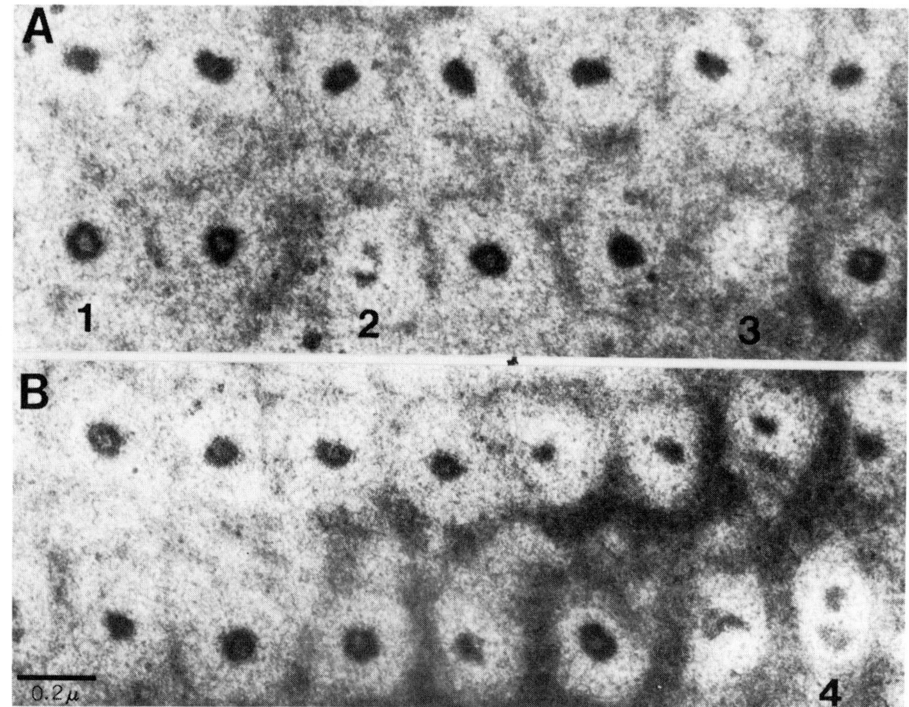

Fig. 8: Electron micrographs of stereocilia rootlets from the first row OHCs from a case with PTS. Panels A and B each show two rows of rootlets. In each panel, the lower row shows 7 of the roughly 33 rootlets from the outermost (and tallest) row of stereocilia. (A micrograph of an entire set of rootlets on an OHC is shown in Fig. 11.)

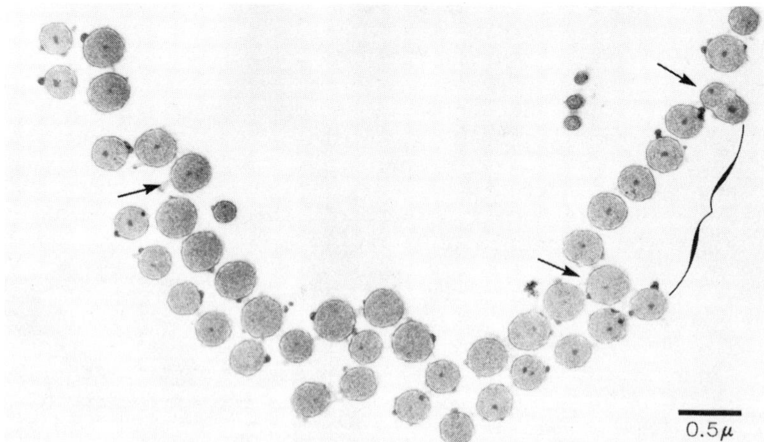

Fig. 9: Electron micrograph through an abnormal stereociliary tuft on a first-row OHC at a level roughly 0.7 microns above the cuticular plate. Stereocilia indicated by the arrows showed fracture of the rootlet at the surface of the cuticular plate. In the region of the bracket at the upper right, five stereocilia from the outer row are missing.

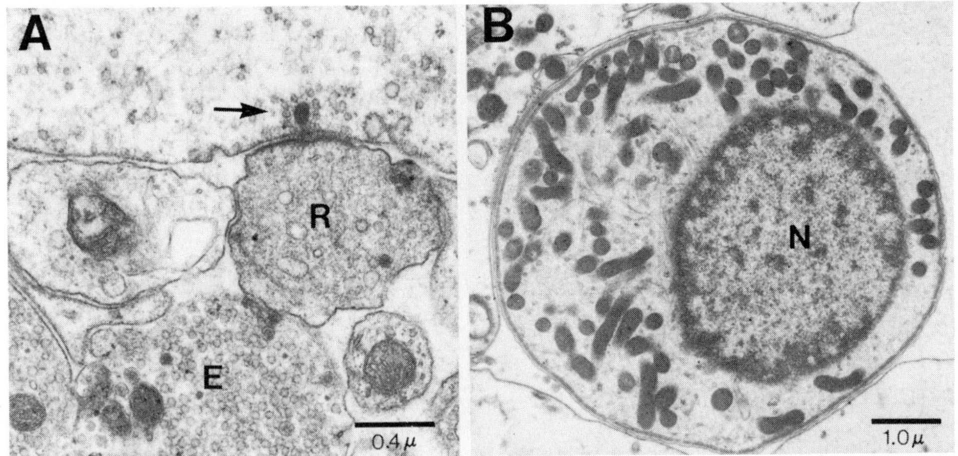

Fig. 10: Electron micrographs from a region with 40 to 50 dB of TTS. Panel A shows the synapse (arrow) between an IHC and a radial fiber (R). Panel B shows a section through the an OHC at the level of the nucleus (N).

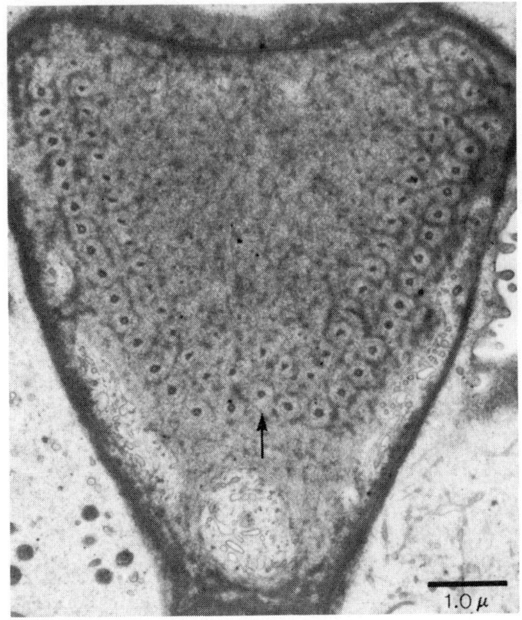

Fig. 11: Electron micrograph of a section through the cuticular plate of a first-row OHC from the same TTS case illustrated in Fig. 10.

on both cell types. Serial sections through the cuticular plates and stereocilia revealed no depolymerization of actin or fracture of rootlets as was seen in the PTS ears (see Fig. 11). The only potential pathology was that the rootlets of the OHC stereocilia appeared shorter than normal. This suggestion is based on comparison of six OHCs from two cochlear locations in one TTS ear with three OHCs from a similar cochlear region of a normal animal. Based on the physiological changes in this TTS ear, elevated tuning-curve tips and hypersensitive tuning-curve tails, we would expect, by analogy to the PTS ears, to see selective damage to the OHCs. The apparent reduction in length of the OHC stereocilia rootlets may constitute that damage and may be reversible. However, the structural data are too preliminary to draw any firm conclusions.

SUMMARY AND CONCLUSIONS

Our data suggest that virtually all of the threshold shift seen in cases of permanent noise-induced threshold shift can be correlated with loss of sensory cells or damage to their stereocilia. Stereocilia damage alone can apparently account for at least 80 dB of threshold shift. The disarray of OHC stereocilia seen in the light microscope apparently arises from loss and/or fracture of the stereocilia rootlets within the cuticular plates. Following rootlet damage, the entire stereocilium begins to bend at its point of insertion in the cuticular plate. The bending and/or fusion of IHC stereocilia appears to arise in association with a break-up of the cuticular-plate matrix.

In cases with acute and probably reversible threshold shift, the only definitive structural changes seen have been dendritic swelling in the IHC area. However, since that phenomenon was not seen when the exposure was not a pure-tone, this condition cannot be the underlying explanation for all TTS. The finding that OHC stereocilia rootlets are shorter than normal in one case of TTS following broad-band noise suggests one avenue for further study. The possibility exists that TTS is caused by disruption (reversible) in the cuticular plate which is not serious enough to cause obvious bending of the stereocilia.

In ears with permanent threshold shifts, caused either by acoustic trauma or drug damage, we find extremely regular correlations between structural changes and functional changes. These correlations are consistent with the idea that the OHCs modify cochlear micro-mechanics in such a way as to provide sharp tuning and sensitivity. This mechanical modification is presumably transmitted to the RFs via the IHCs and their stereocilia. The presence of the OHCs, especially the first-row OHCs, appears to modify the normally broadly tuned response of the organ of Corti by adding sensitivity at the CF and decreasing sensitivity off CF. Loss of IHC stereocilia appears to decrease sensitivity both on and off CF, possibly by reducing the number of ion channels available to transduce the mechanical motion.

Although damage to both sensory cell types causes threshold elevation, the total set of functional changes is apparently very different depending on the ratio of IHC to OHC damage. When the IHCs are selectively damaged, sharp tuning can remain along with nonlinearities such as two-tone inhibition. When there is selective damage to OHCs, the tuning becomes quite broad and most nonlinearities disappear [16]. If these cat data are applicable to man, one might expect there to be significant performance differences between humans with IHC vs. OHC lesions on a wide variety of auditory tasks including speech discrimination. Thus, in analyzing psychophysical studies of patients with sensorineural hearing loss, it might be fruitful to group individuals based on the shapes of psychophysical tuning curves, rather than simply based on the nature of the behavioral audiogram.

ACKNOWLEDGEMENTS

Research supported by PHS grant #NS18339.

REFERENCES

1. H. W. Ades, C. Trahiotis, A. Kokko-Cunningham and B. Averbuch, Comparison of hearing thresholds and morphological changes in the chinchilla after exposure to 4 kHz tones, Acta Otolaryngol. 78:192 (1974).
2. A. R. Cody and D. Robertson, Variability of noise-induced damage in the guinea pig cochlea: electrophysiological and morphological correlates after strictly controlled exposures, Hearing Res. 9:55 (1983).
3. B. Engstrom, A. Flock and E. Borg, Ultrastructural studies of stereocilia in noise-exposed rabbits, Hearing Res. 12:251 (1983).
4. E. F. Evans, Peripheral auditory processing in normal and abnormal ears: physiological considerations for attempts to compensate for auditory deficits by acoustic and electric prostheses, Scand. Audiol. Suppl. 6:1 (1978).
5. N. Y. S. Kiang, E. C. Moxon and R. A. Levine, Auditory nerve activity in cats exposed to ototoxic drugs, in: "Sensorineural Hearing Loss," Ciba Symposium, G.E.W. Wolstenholme and J. Knight eds., J. and A. Churchill, London (1970).
6. N. Y. S. Kiang, T. Watanabe, E. C. Thomas, and L. F. Clark, "Discharge Patterns of Single Fibers in the Cat's Auditory Nerve," MIT Press, Cambridge (1965).
7. M. C. Liberman, Auditory nerve response from cats raised in a low-noise chamber, J. Acoust. Soc. Amer. 63:442 (1978).
8. M. C. Liberman, Morphological differences among radial afferent fibers in the cat cochlea: an electron microscopic study of serial sections, Hearing Res. 3:45 (1980).
9. M. C. Liberman, Single-neuron labeling in the cat auditory nerve, Science 216:1239 (1982).
10. M. C. Liberman, The cochlear frequency map for the cat: labeling auditory nerve fibers of known characteristic frequency, J. Acoust. Soc. Amer. 72:1441 (1982).
11. M. C. Liberman, Single neuron labeling and chronic cochlear pathology, I: Threshold shift and characteristic frequency shift, Hearing Res. 16:33 (1984).
12. M. C. Liberman and D. G. Beil, Hair cell condition and auditory nerve response in normal and noise-damaged cochleas, Acta Otolaryngol. 88:161 (1979).
13. M. C. Liberman and L. W. Dodds, Single neuron labeling and chronic cochlear pathology, II: Stereocilia damage and alterations of spontaneous discharge rates, Hearing Res. 16:43 (1984).
14. M. C. Liberman and L. W. Dodds, Single-neuron labeling and chronic cochlear pathology, III: Stereocilia damage and alterations in threshold tuning curves, Hearing Res. 16:55 (1984).
15. M. C. Liberman and N. Y. S. Kiang, Acoustic trauma in cats: cochlear pathology and auditory nerve activity, Acta Otolaryngol. Suppl. #358:1 (1978).
16. M. C. Liberman and N. Y. S. Kiang, Single-neuron labeling and chronic cochlear pathology, IV: Stereocilia damage and alterations in rate and phase-level functions, Hearing Res. 16:75 (1984).

17. M. C. Liberman and M. J. Mulroy, Acute and chronic effects of acoustic trauma: cochlear pathology and auditory nerve pathophysiology, in: "New Perspectives on Noise-Induced Hearing Loss," R. P. Hamernik, D. Henderson and R. Salvi, eds., Raven Press, New York.
18. D. Lim and W. Melnick, Acoustic damage of the cochlea, Arch. Otolaryngol. 94:294 (1971).
19. J. D. Miller, C. S. Watson and W. P. Covell, Deafening effects of noise on the cat, Acta Otolaryngol. Suppl. 176:1 (1963).
20. D. Robertson, Effects of acoustic trauma on stereocilia structure and spiral ganglion cell tuning properties in the guinea pig cochlea, Hearing Res. 7:55 (1982).
21. W. F. Sewell, The effects of furosemide on the endocochlear potential and auditory nerve fiber tuning curves in cats, Hearing Res. 14:305 (1984).
22. N. Slepecky and S. C. Chamberlain, Distribution and polarity of actin in the sensory hair cells of the chinchilla cochlea, Cell Tissue Res. 224:15 (1982).
23. N. Slepecky, R. Hamernik, D. Henderson and D. Coling, Correlation of audiometric data with changes in cochlear hair cell stereocilia resulting from impulse noise trauma, Acta Otolaryngol. 93:329 (1982).
24. H. H. Spoendlin, Innervation of the organ of Corti of the cat, Acta Otolaryngol. 67:239 (1969).
25. H. H. Spoendlin, Primary structural changes in the organ of Corti after acoustic overstimulation, Acta Otolaryngol. 71:166 (1971).
26. L. G. Tilney, D. J. DeRosier and M. J. Mulroy, The organization of actin filaments in the stereocilia of cochlear hair cells, J. Cell Biol. 86:244 (1980).
27. L. G. Tilney, J. C. Saunders, E. Egelman and D. J. DeRosier, Changes in the organization of actin filaments in the stereocilia of noise-damaged lizard cochleae, Hearing Res. 7:181 (1982).

DISCUSSION

Shaddock: I would like some comments on some very preliminary results we have in a monkey that was noise exposed. We did not quantify stereocilia damage, but we did do a cytocochleogram three months after exposure; then we sectioned serially through the areas that were adjacent to the lesion. The interesting thing about the hair cells is that the cuticular plate region and the stereocilia are perfectly normal, but the subcuticular regions show all sorts of strange swellings on their lateral membranes and a number of very odd pathologies. This is an octave band exposure centered at 500 Hz. The level was 110 dB for 8 hours a day for 2 consecutive days.

Liberman: I would not have any comment other than it is certainly possible, but in material with the type of lesion we have produced, that is not the situation that we have seen.

Patuzzi: Everything you've shown seems to me to be consistent with changes in basilar membrane mechanics or Cody's suggestion that inner hair cells can be desensitized. You seem to have demonstrated that you can desensitize inner hair cells and still maintain basilar membrane mechanics if you've got outer hair cells. The only problem is the hypersensitive tails of the tuning curves that you see. My question is, are your tuning curves based on rate functions or synchrony functions?

Liberman: The tuning curves are Iso-rate functions.

Patuzzi: Have you ever looked at iso-synchrony tuning curves to see whether you may not get an elevation in firing rate and yet the neurons are responding synchronously at lower levels? That may be important because hypersensitive tails suggest that there may be two mechanisms involved. Although the mechanics changed, we have never seen any evidence that the mechanics become hypersensitive following trauma of any kind. But the W shape of the tuning suggests that there might be two stimulation mechanisms. Have you ever looked at phase locking in the hypersensitive tails or measured the phase across frequency to see if there is a change in phase as you go from the hypersensitive tail to the normal tip?

Liberman: On many units, I would take a phase measurement at the tuning curve threshold at 1 kHz, so I have a lot of data at 1 kHz as a function of CF in normal and traumatized units. In general, at that one level, the tuning curve threshold, we saw no change in the synchronization index. So at tuning curve threshold, the synchronization index is the same regardless of whether it is hyposensitive, normal or hypersensitive. With respect to what the phase is, hypersensitive tails are interesting in two regards. One is they never show a phase shift with level, i.e., what we call the 1st component and 2nd component. That nonlinearity is gone. Two-tone rates suppression also seems to be gone.

Saunders: Others have suggested that with TTS you see a proliferation of the smooth endoplasmic reticulum particles in the outer hair cells. What is your observations with regard to that?

Liberman: In this particular paradigm, I have not seen any signs of that.

Cody: When you do your VIII nerve recordings in your chronic animals, how do you know the original CF of the fiber you are recording from and how do you align that in terms of the damage in the cochleogram?

Liberman: For all of the schematics illustrated, we have single unit labeling data. Therefore, we know exactly which inner hair cell it goes to. But beyond that, the single unit labeling studies also show that in most CF regions, outside of the very highest CF regions, that CF does not shift tremendously as threshold is elevated. In the normal animal, the CF map is regular enough that based on the position of the labeled terminal you can estimate what its original CF was. Thus, in a traumatized animal, you can measure the CF of a fiber and, based on the location of its terminal, estimate what its original C.F. was. Based on those types of comparisons, it would seem that 40-60 dB of threshold shift, as is seen in these most interesting cases, is not large. It is less than 1/4 of an octave; 1/8 of an octave typically.

PSYCHOPHYSICAL AND PHYSIOLOGICAL ASPECTS OF AUDITORY TEMPORAL PROCESSING IN LISTENERS WITH NOISE-INDUCED SENSORINEURAL HEARING LOSS

R. J. Salvi, S. S. Saunders, W. A. Ahroon, B. G. Shivapuja, and S. Arehole

Callier Center for Communication Disorders
University of Texas at Dallas
Dallas, Texas 75235, USA

INTRODUCTION

One of the most serious changes in hearing that results from acoustic trauma is the deterioration in speech discrimination. However, because of the complex nature of the speech signal, it has been difficult to determine the underlying psychoacoustic and physiological mechanisms that result in poor speech perception. Consequently, many researchers have turned to simpler acoustic stimuli to investigate the performance characteristics of hearing-impaired listeners. The experiments carried out with simple acoustic stimuli have provided a wealth of information on the distortions that occur in intensity discrimination [1-3], loudness growth [4,5], frequency discrimination [6,7], frequency resolution [8,9], and temporal integration [10,11]. One area in which our knowledge has increased considerably over the past 10-15 years is in understanding the changes that occur in frequency selectivity following noise-exposure. Intense noise exposures are known to result in the loss of tuning in the basilar membrane vibration pattern (see Patuzzi this volume) and the frequency response areas of hair cell and single auditory nerve fibers (see Cody and Russell and Liberman et al. this volume). The change in physiological tuning has in turn been reflected in wider psychophysical tuning curves in noise-exposed subjects [9].

In simple resonant systems, tuning is related to damping; i.e., the broader the tuning, the greater the damping. If one assumes that the auditory system behaves like a simple resonant system, then the abnormally wide tuning curves seen in noise-exposed ears should lead to greater damping. This in turn should lead to an improvement in the ear's ability to follow rapid fluctuations in sound intensity since there should be less ringing in the system. The ability of a listener to follow these rapid fluctuations in sound intensity has generally been referred to as temporal resolution. Over the past few years, we have been looking at a number of different psychophysical and physiological measures of temporal resolution in noise-exposed ears to determine if the temporal processing characteristics of the auditory system are altered by hearing loss. Recent results, including our own, suggest that temporal resolution is, in fact, impaired in listeners with sensorineural hearing loss. The evidence for this comes from a number of different psychophysical studies involving gap detection and forward and backward masking [12-15]. One goal of this paper is to attempt to link the abnormal psychophysical measures of temporal resolution in noise-exposed subjects to the underlying physiological substrate.

METHODS

The experimental results presented below come from three different classes of experiments: psychophysical, evoked response and single unit studies. However, all of the experiments were carried out on the same species, the chinchilla, to facilitate a comparison between the different measures of temporal processing. The psychophysical experiments on gap detection were conducted with a shock-avoidance conditioning procedure which has been described previously [15,16]. The animals were restrained in a yoke-like apparatus and conditioned to respond to tone bursts (500 ms, 5 ms rise/fall time), noise bursts (500 ms, 5 ms rise/fall time, low-passed filtered at 20 kHz) and silent intervals ("gaps") embedded in a continuous noise (0.01 ms rise/fall time, low-passed filtered at 20 kHz). The animals registered a response to the stimulus by a slight upward motion of the body which closed a microswitch. Each animal's pure tone, noise burst and gap detection thresholds were determined using a modified threshold-tracing procedure. Psychophysical estimates of forward masking were also obtained using a positive reinforcement (food) conditioning technique and the method of constant stimuli [17]. The masker (100 ms, 1 ms rise/fall) and probe (10 ms, 1 ms rise/fall, 10 dB SL) were at the same frequency, and the interval between masker offset and probe onset (DT) was varied from 2-100 ms. At each DT, masker intensity was varied so that it just abolished the detection of the probe tone.

Auditory evoked potentials were obtained from another group of chinchillas using chronic bipolar electrodes implanted in the inferior colliculus [18,19]. The animals were awake during testing and restrained in the same yoke-like apparatus used for avoidance conditioning. The electrical responses were amplified (20,000 X), filtered (30-3000 Hz), and sampled (20 kHz, 600 points) by a computer for signal averaging. The evoked response was elicited by a probe tone (10 ms duration, 1 ms rise/fall time), and evoked-response threshold and forward masking recovery functions were obtained. The stimulus parameters employed in the evoked-response forward masking study were the same as those in the psychophysical experiment discussed above.

Recordings were also obtained from single auditory nerve fibers in chinchillas that were anesthetized (Dial in urethane) and tracheotomized [9,20]. A posterior fossa approach was used to expose the auditory nerve and glass microelectrodes (3M KCl, 15-40 Mohms) were used to record from single auditory nerve fibers. A ball electrode was placed on the round window to monitor the whole nerve action potential and the physiological condition of the animal. Each unit's spontaneous discharge rate was obtained and then a computer-automated threshold tracking procedure was used to estimate the tuning curve (50 ms on, 50 ms off, 1 ms rise/fall time). Single auditory nerve fiber forward masking recovery functions were obtained using a 100 ms masker and a 10 ms probe. The frequency of the masker and probe was always at the unit's CF, and the interval between masker offset and probe onset (DT) ranged from 2-200 ms. The intensity of the probe was fixed at 10 dB above the unit's threshold while masker level was varied from 10-50 dB in 10 dB steps.

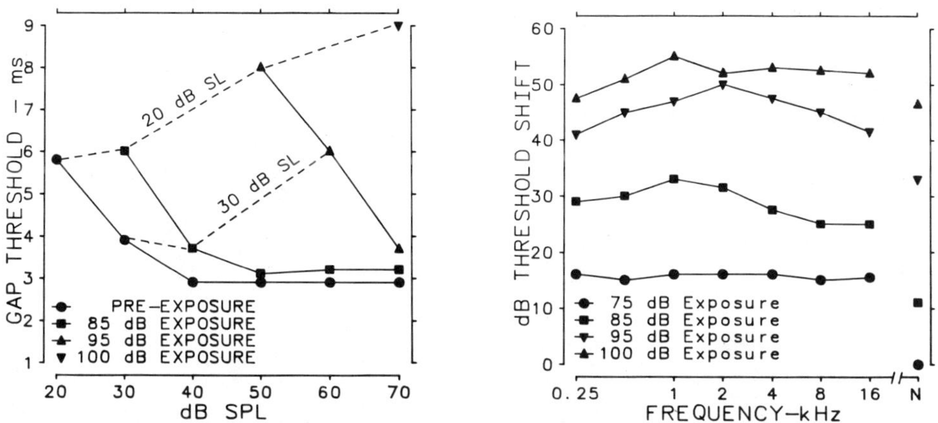

Fig. 1. Left panel shows the mean value of asymptotic threshold shift for tone and noise (N) bursts at the four noise-exposure levels. Right panel shows the mean gap detection thresholds before and during asymptotic threshold shift. Dashed lines connect gap thresholds obtained at approximately the same SL.

RESULTS

Gap Detection and Hearing Loss

There are a variety of psychophysical procedures for assessing the temporal resolving power of the auditory system, but one of the simplest and most popular techniques involves having a subject detect a brief silent interval or gap embedded in an otherwise continuous noise [21]. Gap detection thresholds presumably provide a way of estimating the minimum integration time of the auditory system. Futhermore, in hearing-impaired listeners, gap detection performance appears to be linked to poor speech perception [12]. In order to evaluate this problem, a series of experiments were carried out with chinchillas. Gap detection thresholds were first measured under normal hearing conditions and then with two patterns of noise-induced temporary hearing loss. In the first case, the animals developed a relatively flat hearing loss, while in the second case, a progressive high-frequency hearing loss was induced. The chinchillas in our first experimental group (N=5) were exposed sequentially to 4 levels (75, 85, 95 and 200 dB SPL) of octave band noise centered at 0.5 kHz. Each exposure lasted 8-11 days and resulted in a relatively stable and consistent asymptotic threshold shift (ATS). After the animals reached ATS, they were removed from the noise for audiometric testing for approximately 1 hour. Fig. 1 (left panel) shows the degree of threshold shift for tone bursts and noise bursts. There are two important points to note: first, the hearing loss was relatively flat, and second, the amount of hearing loss systematically increased with exposure level. The question of interest in this experiment is how the degree of hearing loss affects temporal resolution. Before discussing these results, it is important to consider how gap detection performance is influenced by signal level in normal listeners. As shown in the right panel of Fig. 1, the gap thresholds approach an asymptotic value of approximately 3 ms at high signal levels, but thresholds systematically increase below 40 dB SPL (approximately 40 dB SL). These results are virtually identical to those obtained from human listeners. The gap detection data from normal and impaired ears can be compared either in terms of the SL (dashed lines) or SPL (solid lines) of the signal, as illustrated in the right panel of Fig. 1 (The 75 dB

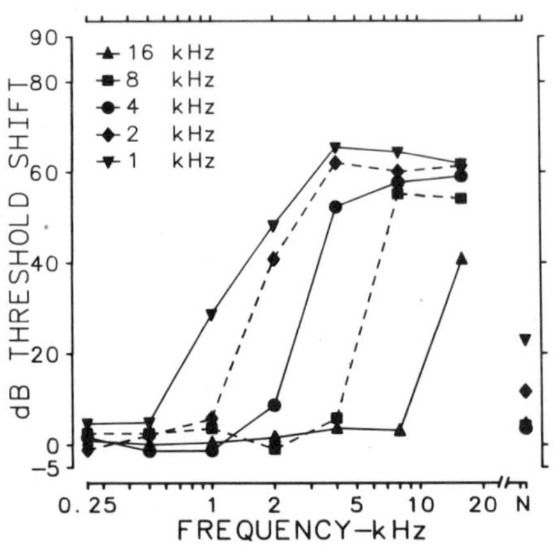

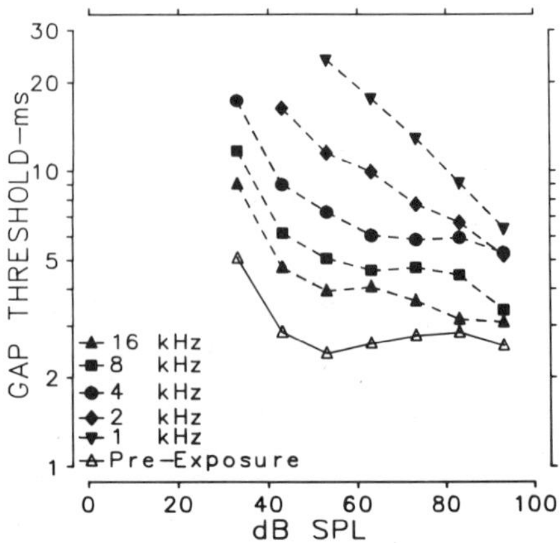

Fig. 2. Left panel shows the mean value of asymptotic threshold shift for tone and noise (N) bursts. Low-pass cutoff of the noise exposure shown in the legend. Right panel shows the gap detection thresholds as a function of signal SPL at each of the five exposure conditions.

exposure had no effect on gap detection, therefore, the results are not shown.) The simplest way of evaluating the data is simply in terms of the SPL of the test signal. As shown by the solid lines in Fig. 1, the 30 dB of hearing loss caused by the 85 dB exposure elevated the gap thresholds, but only at low intensities. The 95 and 100 dB exposures, on the other hand, produced significant elevations in the gap thresholds at all intensities. A much more conservative way of comparing the data is at a constant SL. This can be accomplished using the dashed lines in Fig. 1. When the data are analyzed at a constant SL, the gap thresholds are seen to increase only at the 95 and 100 dB exposures, i.e., after the hearing loss exceeded 30-35 dB.

Human psychophysical studies carried out with narrow bands of noise have shown that gap thresholds are shorter at the high frequencies than at the low frequencies [13,14,26]. This improvement in temporal resolution with increasing frequency was thought to be related to the increase in the width of the critical band with increasing frequency. Since noise-induced hearing loss generally involves the loss of high-frequency hearing, it seemed important to determine how gap performance was affected by the width of the high-frequency loss. This was accomplished by sequentially exposing chinchillas to 5 different bands of high-pass noise. The high-frequency cutoff of the noise remained at 20 kHz while the low-frequency cutoff was lowered from 16 to 1 kHz in octave steps. Each of the 5 exposure conditions lasted approximately 2-3 weeks so that the animals were in a state of ATS. The noise had an overall SPL of 93 dB between 1 and 20 kHz. Tone burst, noise burst, and gap thresholds were obtained from each animal before and during the exposure. Fig. 2 (left panel) shows the mean threshold shift of the 4 chinchillas. There is a progressive spread of the hearing loss towards the low frequencies as the low-pass cutoff of the noise is lowered. The first 3 exposures (16, 8 and 4 kHz) increased the high-frequency thresholds, but had little effect on either the detectability of the noise burst or the test signal used for gap detection. Nevertheless, gap detection thresholds systematically increased even when only the frequencies above 8 kHz were elevated (Fig. 2 right panel). After the 1 and 2 kHz exposures, the hearing loss migrated down to 1 kHz, and the gap thresholds increased further. However, this change in gap detection

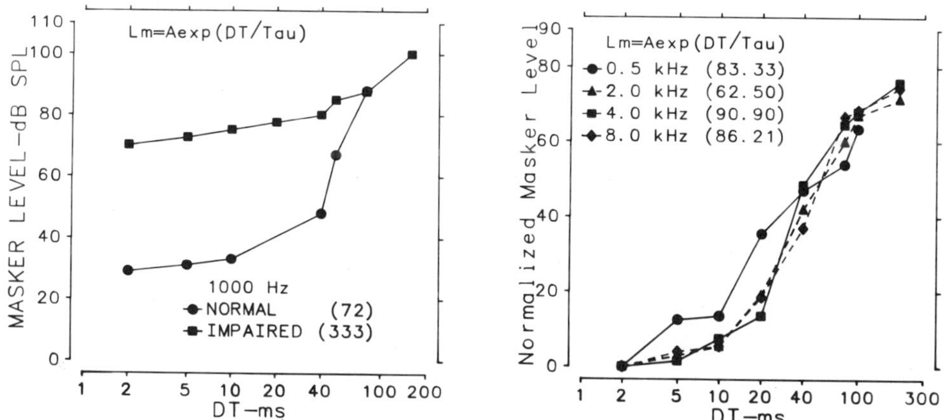

Fig. 3 Left panel redrawn from Nelson and Turner [24]. Masked threshold plotted as a function of the interval between forward masker offset and probe onset. Right panel shows the masked threshold of the auditory evoked response plotted as a function of the time interval between masker offset and probe onset. Probe and masker frequency are indicated in the figure inset.

may be partly due to a reduction in the SL of the test signal. These results, as well as other data obtained with amplitude modulated noise [22], suggest that the high frequency hearing may play a dominant role in the detection of temporal gap embedded in a broad band noise.

Forward Masking and Hearing Loss

The stimulus paradigm used in gap detection bears a close resemblance to that used in forward masking. However, in forward masking the listener is asked to detect the presence of a probe stimulus, whereas in gap detection the listener is required to detect the silent interval embedded between two test stimuli. Although the test stimuli and detection task are somewhat different, Smiarowski and Carhart [23] have shown that there is a close relationship between the results obtained with gap detection and forward masking. If the two measures are, in fact, related, then one might expect the time course of forward masking to be prolonged with sensorineural hearing loss.

One procedure for measuring forward masking is to have a listener detect a low-intensity probe tone that is preceded in time (DT) by a masking tone of variable intensity. The listener's task is to adjust the level of the masker so that it just abolishes the detection of the probe. When the procedure is carried out over a range of masker-probe intervals (DT), one obtains an estimate of the time course of masking. Since the probe is near threshold, it presumably excites a limited region of the basilar membrane and therefore provides information about the time course of forward masking from a limited frequency region. Nelson and Turner [24] reported changes in forward masking recovery functions in human listeners with sensorineural hearing loss. Fig. 3 compares the forward masking functions from a normal and an impaired listener at 1 kHz. The masked thresholds in the impaired ear are higher than those from the normal listener as a result of the hearing loss. More important, however, is the fact that the time course of forward masking is significantly different for the normal and impaired listener. A quantitative index of the time course of forward masking can be obtained from the time constant of the equation which was fit to the

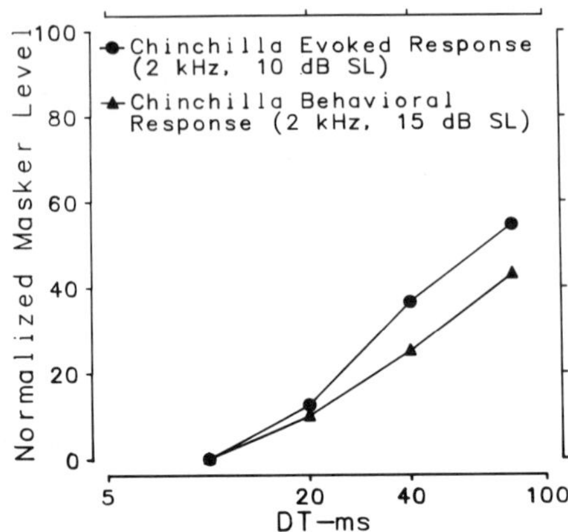

Fig. 4 Comparison of psychophysical and auditory evoked-response forward masking function from the chinchilla.

data in Fig. 3 (left panel). The time constant for the hearing-impaired listener is over 300 ms, whereas in normal listeners, it is on the order of 70 ms. This four-fold increase in the time constant provides further evidence of abnormal temporal processing in hearing impaired listeners. Unfortunately, there is relatively little anatomical and physiological evidence related to the breakdown in forward masking and temporal resolution.

Evoked-Response Forward Masking Functions and Hearing Loss

The abnormal temporal processing characteristics of impaired listeners presumably have some physiological basis. In order to gain a better understanding of the physiological mechanism(s) that might be involved, an experiment was carried out in which we measured the auditory evoked response from the inferior colliculus using a "forward masking" stimulus paradigm similar to that used in the previous psychophysical experiments. A low-level probe tone was used to elicit the evoked response. Then a forward masker was introduced and increased in level until it caused a 50% reduction in probe amplitude (i.e., the masked threshold). Fig. 3 (right panel) shows a set of evoked-response forward masking functions obtained at 4 different probe frequencies in one normal hearing chinchilla. In order to facilitate a comparison across the 4 frequencies, each function was normalized to the masked threshold at 2 ms. Several points are worth noting. First, there is very little difference across the 4 probe frequencies. Second, the evoked-response forward masking functions from the chinchilla are quite similar to those obtained psychophysically from human listeners (Fig. 3, left panel). Furthermore, the time constants for the evoked response data are comparable to those for the human psychophysical data.

Because of the inherent difficulties in making cross species comparisons, we felt that it was necessary to obtain some psychophysical data on forward masking in the chinchilla using the same stimulus paradigm that was employed in the evoked response study. Preliminary psychophysical forward masking data from one chinchilla are compared in Fig. 4 with an evoked-response forward masking function. Note the similarity between the psychophysical and evoked response data from the chinchilla as well as the similarity to the human psychophysical data shown in Fig. 3. These results suggest that it may be feasible to use the evoked response technique to study temporal processing in hearing-impaired animals.

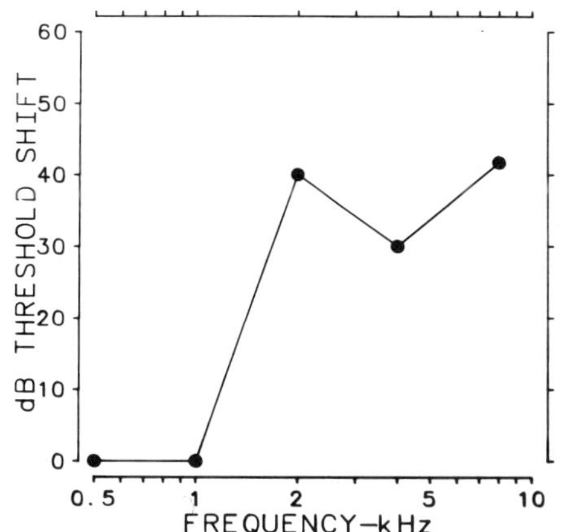

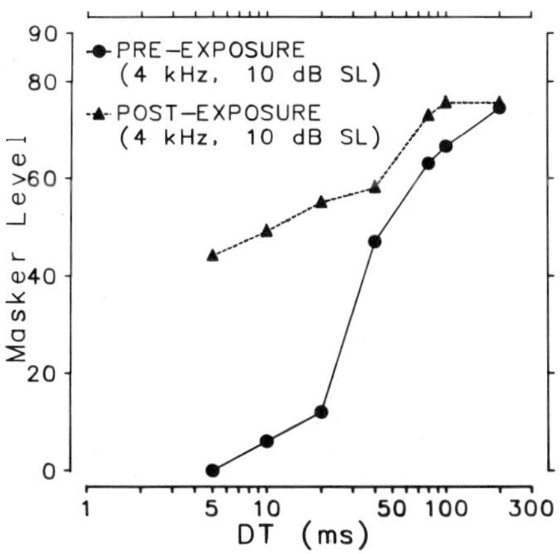

Fig. 5 Left panel shows the pattern of threshold shift resulting from the 85 dB pure tone exposure. Right panel shows the masked threshold plotted as a function of threshold shift before and after exposure.

Some preliminary experiments have been carried out in which we examined the effects of noise-induced hearing loss on the evoked-response forward masking function. The animals were exposed for approximately two weeks to a 2 kHz pure tone having an SPL of 85 dB. The typical pattern of threshold shift is shown for one animal in Fig. 5 (left panel). The exposure produced as asymptotic threshold shift at the high frequencies, but had no effect on low-frequency hearing. Fig. 5 (right panel) shows the pre- and post-exposure evoked response forward masking functions. The post-exposure function is shifted upward due to the loss in sensitivity. More importantly, the time course of recovery is slowed after exposure. The time constant that fits the data changed from 91 ms before exposure to 385 ms after the exposure. The forward masking function was also measured at 0.5 kHz where hearing was normal; this function was completely normal and thus serves as a within subject control. The results indicate that the time course of the evoked-response forward masking function can be altered by noise-induced hearing loss.

Auditory Nerve Fiber Forward Masking Functions and Hearing Loss

In order to determine if the time course of forward masking was being altered by changes in the periphery, another series of experiments were carried out on single auditory nerve fibers. The first step was to characterize the time course of recovery for single auditory nerve fibers in normal chinchillas and to determine if there were any systematic differences between fibers with different spontaneous discharge rates. The stimulus and response parameters are illustrated in Fig. 6. The unit's responsiveness was assessed with a 10 ms probe tone that was 10 dB above the threshold at the characteristic frequency (CF) of the unit. The probe tone was preceded (DT: 2-200 ms) by a 100 ms adaptor tone that varied in intensity from 10-50 dB above threshold. Neural recovery was assessed by comparing the firing rate to the probe tone when it was preceded by the adaptor tone, Rp(dt), relative to the firing rate to the probe in its unadapted state, Rp. Fig. 7 (left panel) shows the mean normalized probe rate as a function of recovery time (DT) for an adaptor level 30 dB above threshold. It appears that the high-spontaneous rate (> 18 spikes/sec) units recover faster than the low- (< 0.5 spikes/sec.) and medium-rate (0.5-18 spikes/sec) units. The results were evaluated quantitatively by fitting the equation in Fig. 7 (right panel) to the data. The time constants fit to the data are plotted as a function of adaptor level in

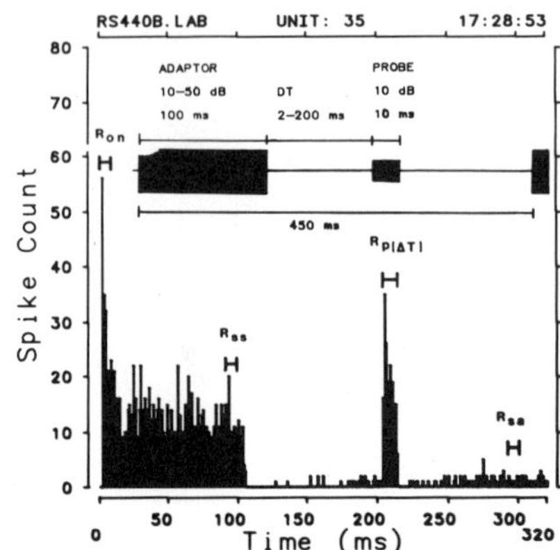

Fig. 6 Post-stimulus time histogram obtained from an auditory nerve fiber using the forward masking stimulus paradigm shown in the inset.

Fig. 7 (right panel). It is clear that the mean time constants of the high-spontaneous rate fibers are consistently shorter than the time constants for low- and medium-spontaneous rate units. This difference must be taken into account when evaluating the results from noise-exposed ears.

Auditory nerve fiber forward masking functions were also obtained from a group of chinchillas exposed at 95 dB SPL to an octave band of noise centered at 0.5 kHz. The exposure lasted 5 days and resulted in an asymptotic threshold shift of approximately 50 dB across the range of frequencies (see Fig. 1). Recordings were made over a period of approximately 12 hours after the exposure while there was a significant degree of hearing loss. The single unit thresholds were elevated approximately 50 dB, and the frequency- threshold curves of the fibers were broadly tuned as reported earlier [20]. Fig. 8 (left panel) compares the mean forward masking recovery functions from units in normal and noise-exposed animals. In order to simplify the comparison, only the results from high-spontaneous rate units are shown. The recovery functions obtained at 10 dB above threshold are essentially identical for both groups. This was generally the case at 20 dB also. However, at 30 dB, slight differences began to appear, and by 40 dB, the differences in the time course of recovery became quite noticeable. Time constants were fit to the recovery functions as discussed above and the results are shown in Fig. 8 (right panel). The time constants for the normal and noise-exposed groups are comparable at low levels. However, the time constants for the noise-exposed group diverge from those for normals at 30 dB and are significantly longer at 40 and 50 dB. The large difference between normal and noise-exposed animals at 50 dB should be interpreted cautiously, however, since few units in the noise-exposed group could be studied at this intensity level, i.e., the required intensity level exceeded the output of the sound source.

One factor that could potentially affect the time course and amount of forward masking in the noise-exposed animals would be a "recruitment-like" change in a unit's input/output function, i.e., an increase in the slope of the unit's discharge rate-intensity function. If such a change were to occur, then for a specified intensity level above threshold, the firing rate to the adaptor tone would be higher in a unit from a noise-exposed

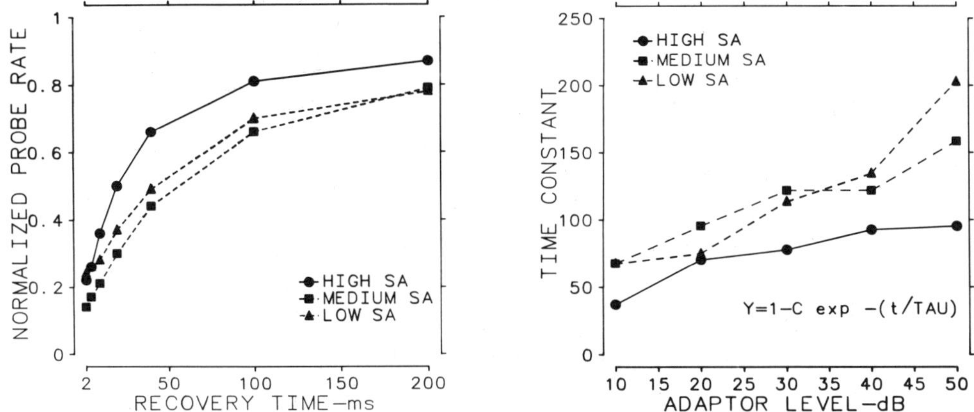

Fig. 7 Left panel shows the mean normalized probe rate plotted as a function of the interval between masker and probe. Results are shown for low-, medium-, and high-spontaneous rate units obtained at an adaptor level 30 dB above the threshold at CF. Right panel shows the mean time constants for low-, medium-, and high-spontaneous rate units as a function of adaptor level. Time constants fit to the equation in the inset using results from normal chinchillas.

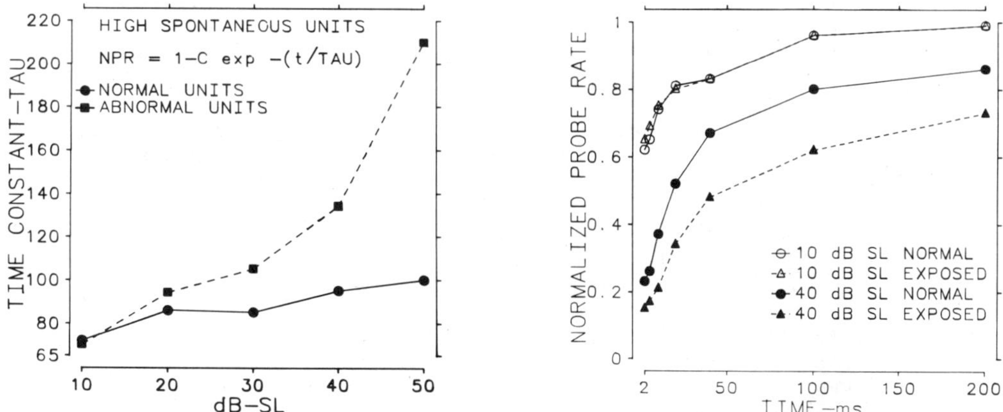

Fig. 8 Left panel shows the mean normalized probe rate plotted as a function of the interval between masker and probe. Adaptor level 10 and 40 dB above the threshold at CF. Data are from high-spontaneous rate fibers in normal and noise-exposed chinchillas. Right panel shows the time constants plotted as a function of adaptor level for high-spontaneous rate fibers in normal and noise-exposed chinchillas. Data are from high-spontaneous rate fibers.

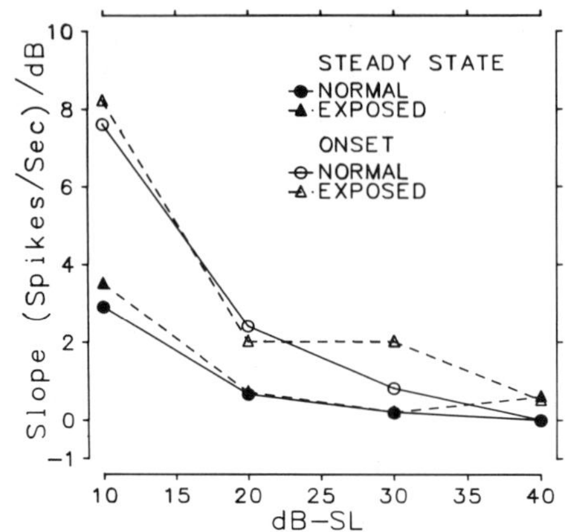

Fig. 9. Slope of the discharge rate-intensity function plotted as a function of the intensity level above the unit's threshold. Measurements were made over the onset (0-10 ms) and steady- state (90-100 ms) portions of the PST histogram to the adaptor tone.

animal than in a normal unit. The higher firing rate could in turn cause greater adaptation and prolong the time course of recovery in units from the noise-exposed animals. It is important to note, however, that this type of explanation could only account for our results at sound intensities below that needed to drive the unit to its saturation discharge rate. According to this view, all intensities that lead to saturation presumably yield the same amount of adaptation and the same amount of time to recover.

In order to examine this issue, the slope of the rate-intensity function to adaptor tone was measured over 10 dB intervals for each unit in the normal and noise-exposed animals. Measurements were made at both the onset and steady-state portions of the post-stimulus time histograms to the adaptor tone. This allowed us to measure the discharge rate-intensity function between 10 and 50 dB above a unit's threshold. The mean values of the slope measurements are shown in Fig. 9 for units in the normal and noise-exposed groups. The onset and steady-state slopes decrease with intensity as the units approach their saturation discharge rates. It is important to note, however, that the normal and noise-exposed animals have essentially the same slope and reach saturation at about the same intensity over the range of levels investigated. Thus, one cannot account for the prolonged forward masking recovery functions in noise-exposed animals on the basis of a "recruitment-like" change in a unit's discharge rate-intensity function.

DISCUSSION

Noise-induced hearing loss is a complex phenomenon that results in a broad range of psychophysical, physiological and anatomical disturbances. In recent years, there has been a growing awareness that auditory temporal resolution is disrupted in hearing-impaired ears. However, it has not been clear how the extent or pattern of noise-induced hearing loss affects temporal resolution. The two animal psychophysical studies mentioned above allowed us to systematically manipulate the degree of hearing loss as well as the band width of high-frequency hearing loss in order to determine what effect these two parameters had on temporal resolution. The degree of hearing loss was an important factor affecting temporal resolution. Prolonged gap detection thresholds were only seen when the animals sustained a noise-induced hearing loss exceeding 25-30 dB (Fig. 2). Smaller losses had no effect on gap detection performance when comparisons were made at the same SL. This fact may explain why some earlier investigators failed to report changes in temporal resolution in hearing impaired listeners [25].

It was indicated earlier that noise-induced hearing loss resulted in the broadening of psychophysical and physiological tuning curves, and it was suggested that this might lead to greater damping and better auditory temporal resolution. Our results, however, show the opposite effect, i.e., hearing loss results in poorer temporal resolution as well as abnormally broad tuning. One issue that needs to be considered is whether the breakdown in temporal resolution is closely linked to abnormal tuning. In earlier studies, we reported a systematic broadening in single unit and evoked-response tuning curves as the degree of hearing loss increased [20,26]. However, in the present study, there was an abrupt change in gap detection performance only when the hearing loss exceeded approximately 35 dB. This suggests that tuning is much more vulnerable to acoustic trauma than temporal resolution and that the underlying events giving rise to these changes may be fundamentally different.

Our results also indicate that the frequency of the hearing loss has an important effect on temporal resolution when broad band signals are used as test stimuli. Loss of high-frequency hearing, even frequencies above 8 kHz, can result in changes in gap detection performance even though the audibility of the test signal remains normal. These results suggest that the high-frequency region of the cochlea may play a dominant role in processing the rapid amplitude fluctuations contained in a broad band stimulus. When the high-frequency information is eliminated by a high-frequency hearing loss, the auditory system is forced to rely on other temporal cues relayed through the remaining low-frequency channels. The results of Fig. 2 suggest that the minimum integration time of the low-frequency channels may be longer than that of the high-frequency channels. The gap detection data obtained with high-frequency hearing loss therefore appear to be consistent with earlier human studies of temporal resolution employing narrow band signals [27] as well as studies of amplitude modulation detection in listeners with high-frequency hearing loss.

An attempt was also made to relate the changes in temporal resolution in hearing impaired subjects to alterations in the underlying pattern of neural activity in the auditory pathway. One physiological measure that appeared to be closely related to the psychophysical results on temporal processing was the evoked-response forward masking function. The evoked-response forward masking functions from normal chinchillas were nearly identical to the psychophysical temporal masking functions obtained from both humans and chinchillas. Furthermore, when the animals developed 30-40 dB of hearing loss, there was an increase in the time constants fitting the evoked-response forward masking functions; this finding is consistent with human psychophysical data on forward masking. Since we did not systematically vary the noise exposure level in our study, it is not clear what level of hearing loss is required before one sees a change in the forward masking functions.

One aspect of the forward masking paradigm that is important to consider is the use of a low-level probe tone to elicit the response. Since the probe is presented near threshold, it presumably excites a limited region of the basilar membrane. Thus, the forward masking functions should provide a metric of the time course of recovery at a relatively specific frequency region. Assuming that the auditory system behaves like a simple filter, one might expect temporal resolution to be better at the high frequencies than the lows, since internal filter bandwidths increase with frequency [28]. This expectation, however, is not supported by the evoked-response forward masking functions shown in Fig. 6. One finds that the time course of forward masking is nearly the same across a wide range of frequencies. Harris and Dallos [29] also failed to find any significant difference in the time course of forward masking in single auditory nerve fibers with different CF's. These physiological results, therefore, appear to be in conflict with gap detection results that indicate that the minimum integration time of the auditory system improves with increasing frequency [27]. Exactly why this difference exists is unclear.

The forward masking stimulus paradigm was also used to study the time course of recovery in single auditory nerve fibers. The results gathered from a large sample of normal auditory nerve fibers failed to show any significant difference in the time course of recovery as a function of the CF of the unit. Furthermore, the recovery time constants appeared to increase with adaptor level. Both of these findings corroborate earlier results obtained from the chinchilla [29]. One new result from our study is that the forward masking recovery time constants are linked to a unit's spontaneous rate. Specifically, the time constants of the high-spontaneous rate units are consistently shorter than those low- and medium- spontaneous rate units. Previous studies have shown that units with high-spontaneous rates have lower thresholds and higher saturation discharge rates than units with low-spontaneous discharge rates [30,9]. By using intracellular labeling techniques, it has been possible to relate these functional differences to the anatomical characteristics of radial afferents in the cat [31,32]. Fibers with high-spontaneous rates correspond to large diameter, mitochondrion-rich fibers while fibers with low- and medium-spontaneous rates correspond to small diameter, mitochondrion-poor fibers. It is tempting to assume that the anatomical and functional differences seen among radial afferents develop from somewhat different synaptic or pre-synaptic processes. The different forward masking time constants seen among auditory nerve fibers appear to be consistent with such a view. However, this issue will require further study.

The auditory nerve fibers in our noise-exposed animals had elevated thresholds and broad tuning curves. In addition, there was an indication that the time course of recovery from forward masking was prolonged, particularly when the adaptor tone was at least 30 dB above the unit's threshold. These results might have been predicted based on earlier anecdotal observations made by Smith [33], who noted that the time course of recovery from forward masking was prolonged in auditory nerve fibers from animals in poor physiological condition. One would assume that this prolongation in the time course of recovery in the auditory nerve would contribute substantially to any delay in the time course of recovery seen in the auditory evoked response or behaviorally. However, it is unclear if these peripheral changes can account for all of the changes that are expressed in the psychophysical data.

The pathological conditions that lead to prolonged forward masking functions at the auditory nerve are not yet understood. One mechanism that we can appear to rule out is one involving an increase in slope of a unit's discharge rate-intensity function. As mentioned earlier, the hypothesized increase in slope would have resulted in a higher masker discharge rate in pathological units compared to normal units for a given intensity above threshold. The higher rate would presumably have caused greater adaptation and prolonged the time needed for full recovery. However, we failed to detect any change in the slope of the rate-intensity function to the masking stimulus (Fig. 9). The prolonged recovery functions might also arise from some type of alteration in the mechanical properties of the hair cell cilia (see Saunders et al. this volume) or basilar membrane. Another possibility is that the prolonged forward masking recovery functions arise from some type of synaptic dysfunction. Several investigators, for example, have shown that abnormal vacuolization occurs in the neuropil beneath the inner hair cells [34,35] after acute noise exposures. These changes could potentially affect synaptic transmission and alter temporal processing at the periphery. Clearly, additional work is needed to understand the neural mechanisms that underlie the changes in temporal processing seen in noise-exposed ears.

As noted earlier, the acoustic waveform of many natural sounds such as speech is complex with considerable information being conveyed through the temporal variation in signal amplitude and signal spectrum. The deterioration in speech perception in listeners with noise-induced hearing loss undoubtedly has its roots in the altered discharge patterns which flow out the cochlea via the auditory nerve into the central nervous system. One change that has been recognized for some time is the loss of frequency selectivity. It is now becoming clear that more subtle changes in auditory temporal processing may also be linked to poor speech perception as has been suggested by recent psychophysical studies. The physiological basis for the change in auditory temporal processing needs to be clarified further, at the periphery as well as in the central auditory pathway.

REFERENCE

1. E. Luscher and J. Zwislocki, A simple method for indirect monaural determination of the recruitment phenomenon (difference limen in intensity in different types of deafness), _Acta Otolaryngol._ 78:156 (1949).
2. J. Jerger, J. L. Shedd and E. Harford, On the detection of extremely small changes in sound intensity, _Arch. Otolaryngol._ 69:200 (1959).
3. D. N. Elliott, W. Riach and H. R. Silbiger, Effects on auditory fatigue upon intensity discrimination, _J. Acoust. Soc. Am._ 34:212 (1962).
4. H. Davis, C. T. Morgan, J. E. Hawkins, R. Galambos and F. W. Smith, Temporary deafness following exposure to loud tones and noise, _Acta Otolaryngol._ S88:1 (1950).
5. D. McFadden and H. S. Plattsmier, Exposure-induced loudness shifts and threshold shifts, _in_ "New Perspectives on Noise-induced Hearing Loss," R. P. Hamernik, D. Henderson and R. J. Salvi, eds. Raven Press, New York (1982).
6. J. F. Brandt, Frequency discrimination allowing exposure to noise, _J. Acoust. Soc. Am._ 41:448 (1967).
7. R. A. Butler and J. P. Albrite, The pitch discriminative function of the pathological ear, _Arch. Otolaryngol._ 64:411 (1956).
8. B. Leshowitz and R. Lindstrom, Measurement of nonlinearities in listeners with sensorineural hearing loss, _in_ "Psychophysics and Physiology of Hearing," E. F. Evans and J. P. Wilson, eds., Academic Press, London (1977).
9. R. J. Salvi, J. Perry, R. P. Hamernik and D. Henderson, Relationships between cochlear pathologies and auditory nerve and behavioral responses following acoustic trauma, _in_: "New Perspectives on Noise-induces Hearing Loss," R. P. Hamernik, D. Henderson and R. J. Salvi, eds., Raven Press, New York (1982).
10. J. F. Jerger, Influence of stimulus duration on the pure-tone threshold during recovery from auditory fatigue, _J. Acoust. Soc. Am._ 27:121 (1955).
11. D. Henderson, Temporal summation of acoustic signals by the chinchilla, _J. Acoust. Soc. Am._ 46:474 (1969).

12. R. Tyler, Q. Summerfield, E. J. Wood and M. A. Fernandes, Psychoacoustic and phonetic temporal processing in normal and hearing-impaired listeners, J. Acoust. Soc. Am. 72:740 (1982).
13. E. Cudahy, Changes in the temporal processing of acoustic signals in hearing-impaired listeners, in "New Perspectives on Noise-induced Hearing Loss," R. P. Hamernik, D. Henderson and R. J. Salvi, eds., Raven Press, New York (1982).
14. P. Fitzgibbons and F. L. Wightman, Temporal resolution in normal and hearing-impaired listeners, J. Acoust. Soc. Am. 72:761 (1982).
15. D. M. Giraudi-Perry, R. J. Salvi and D. Henderson, Gap detection in hearing-impaired chinchillas, J. Acoust. Soc. Am. 75:1387 (1985).
16. R. J. Salvi and S. Arehole, Gap detection in chinchillas with temporary high-frequency hearing loss, J. Acoust. Soc. Am. 77:1173 (1985).
17. B. G. Shivapuja, R.J. Salvi and S. S. Saunders, Intensity discrimination in chinchillas, J. Acoust. Soc. Am. 77:S83 (1984).
18. D. Henderson, R. P. Hamernik, C. Woodford, R. Sitler and R. Salvi, Evoked-response audibility curve of the chinchilla, J. Acoust. Soc. Am. 54:1099 (1973).
19. R. J. Salvi, W. A. Ahroon, J. W. Perry, A. D. Gunnarson and D. Henderson, Comparison of psychophysical and evoked-potential tuning curves in the chinchilla. Am. J. Otolaryngol. 3:408 (1982).
20. R. J. Salvi, R. P. Hamernik and D. Henderson, Response patterns of auditory nerve fibers during temporary threshold shift, Hearing Res. 10:37 (1983).
21. R. Plomp, Rate of decay of auditory sensation, J. Acoust. Soc. Am. 36:277 (1964).
22. D. Henderson, R. Salvi, G. Pavek and R. Hamernik, Amplitude modulation thresholds in chinchillas with high-frequency hearing loss, J. Acoust. Soc. Am. 75:1177 (1984).
23. R. A. Smiarowski and R. Carhart, Relations among temporal resolution, forward masking and simultaneous masking, J. Acoust. Soc. Am. 57:1169 (1979).
24. D. A. Nelson and C. W. Turner, Decay of masking and frequency resolution in sensorineural hearing-impaired listeners, in: "Psychophysical, Physiological and Behavioral Studies in Hearing," G. Van den Brink and F. A. Bilsen, eds., Delft University Press, Delft, Netherlands (1980).
25. T. W. Tillman and L. Rosenblatt, Forward masking in normal and hearing-impaired listeners, Paper presented at the Am. Speech Hearing Assn., Washington, D. C. (1975).
26. P. Fitzgibbons, Temporal gap resolution in narrow-bank noises with center frequencies from 6000-14000 Hz., J. Acoust. Soc. Am., 75:566 (1984).
27. R. J. Salvi, W. A. Ahroon and D. Henderson, Evoked-response turing curves in normal and hearing-impaired chinchillas, Paper presented at the 19th Workshop on Inner Ear Biology, Mainz, W. Germany (1982).
28. B. Sharf, Critical banks, in: "Foundations of modern Auditory Theory," J. V. Tobias, ed., Academic Press, New York (1970).
29. D. Harris and P. Dallos, Forward masking of auditory nerve fiber responses, J. Neurophysiol. 42:1083 (1970).
30. M. C. Liberman, Auditory-nerve response from cats raised in a low-noise chamber, J. Acoust. Soc. Am. 63:442 (1978).
31. M. C. Liberman, Morphological differences among radial afferent fibers in the cat cochlea; An electron microscopic study of serial sections, Hearing Res. 3:45-63 (1980).
32. M. C. Liberman, Single-neuron labeling in the cat auditory nerve, Sci. 216:1239 (1982).

33. R. Smith, Short-term adaptation in single auditory nerve fibers: Some poststimulatory effect., J. Neurophysiol. 40:1098 (1977).
34. M. C. Liberman and M. J. Mulroy, Acute and chronic effects of acoustic trauma: Cochlear pathology and auditory nerve pathophysiology, in "New Perspectives on Noise-induced Hearing Loss," R. P. Hamernik, D. Henderson and R. J. Salvi, Eds., Raven Press, New York (1982).
35. H. H. Spoendlin, Primary ultrastructural changes in the organ of Corti after acoustic overstimulation, Acta Otolaryngol Stockh.) 71:166 (1971).

ACKNOWLEDGEMENTS

This research was supported by grants from NIH (NS16761) and NIOSH (5 R01 OH01152). The authors wish to thank K. Rockwood, L. Davis, R. Minton and G. Appleton for their generous donation of chinchillas.

DISCUSSION

Shaddock: You mentioned that the animals were exposed from 10-20 days. Were you looking for a certain threshold shift level before taking them out of the noise?

Salvi: Yes. With long duration exposures, the threshold shift stabilizes after approximately 48 hours in the noise. We wanted a long exposure so we would have enough time to obtain all the behavioral measurements. Therefore, the animals stayed in the noise until all the measurements were completed.

Cody: Your experiments reminded me of some experiments I did with Graham Yates. We used the N_1 response as the measure of the responsiveness of the cochlea. By changing the intensity or duration of the masker, we were able to plot the time between masker and probe to get an iso-voltage response from the N_1. We were able to show that as the intensity or duration of the masker increased, then you changed the recovery time constant. That would suggest to us that in those respects, we were actually mimicking TTS using a short tone.

Salvi: There is probably a continuum between your experiments, which one might call fatigue or very low-level TTS, and the experiments we are talking about here. The point which I wish to make is that when these animals have a significant hearing loss, the recovery process seems to be altered. We obviously can not say anything about the specific mechanisms right now.

Tyler: I have a question about the interpretation of your gap detection experiment with a broad band noise stimuli. Where were your progressively impaired lower and lower frequency regions? It is known that detection of a gap in broad band noise is probably dependent upon the higher frequency components. For example, with a high frequency, narrow band of noise there is a lower gap detection threshold than for a lower frequency band of noise. In your paradigm where you use a broad band noise as a stimulus, what you probably are seeing is the thresholds become more and more dependent upon the lower frequency fibers as you progressively impair the higher frequency region.

Salvi: I would agree with your interpretation of the data.

Tyler: I have a question about using sensation level as an appropriate measure as opposed to sound pressure level. I have problems with sensation level for at least two reasons, one of which is that if you take a patient with a 50 dB hearing loss and present a sound at 10 dB above the threshold, that will be fairly loud for that patient. If you take a normal hearing person and present a stimulus at 10 dB sensation level, that will be barely audible to them. So it is not exactly clear that sensation level is the appropriate measure. There are other ways of looking at it depending upon the questions you want to ask. You may want to know, for example, what the equivalent displacement would be at the stapes or, as we saw this morning, equivalent motion of the basilar membrane. Certainly using a different sensation level is going to cause a difference in the actual effect of the stimulus. I do not think it is clear cut what the appropriate level ought to be.

Salvi: This is certainly an area of concern. The reason for using sensation level to make our comparisons is that it provides the most conservative criterion for saying that there is a change in gap detection performance. We can be confident in saying there is a change in gap detection performance if the gap thresholds are compared at the same sensation level.

Patuzzi: I think Harris and Dallos showed that a single time constant was not a good fit for the forward masking data and that it was more complicated. Are the single exponentials a good fit? Second, if you are trying to factor out basilar membrane tuning from other processes, have you tried the single unit recovery data with frequencies lower than CF?

Salvi: The single exponential model gives a reasonably good fit to the data. However, other models with more parameters might give even a better fit. We used the single exponential because we wanted a relatively simple descriptor to characterize our data. The exact time constant that you get depends on a variety of parameters such as masker duration, probe duration, and probe level. The important point here is that all the conditions were held constant for both the normal and exposed animals. Under these conditions, we find an increase in the recovery curves of noise-exposed animals.

Concerning your second question, we have not looked at the recovery process above of below CF, but based on the work of Harris and Dallos in normal animals, there appears to be no difference between forward masking functions obtained below or above CF.

INCREASE IN CENTRAL AUDITORY RESPONSIVENESS DURING CONTINUOUS TONE STIMULATION OR FOLLOWING HEARING LOSS

G. M. Gerken, R. Simhadri-Sumithra and K. H. V. Bhat

Callier Center for Communication Disorders
University of Texas at Dallas
Dallas, Texas 75235, USA

Most models of hearing loss explicitly or implicitly assume that damage to the hair cells reduces the amount and distribution of input to the central auditory mechanisms according to the pattern of damage along the receptor surface. Thus, the basis for reduced psychophysical performance with hearing loss was initially sought in the pattern and distribution of cochlear damage and not in altered central mechanisms. It is now apparent that central anatomic changes follow the peripheral changes produced by acoustic trauma [1,2] or auditory deprivation in the young animal [3,4]. Central physiological differences between the normal-hearing and hearing-impaired animal have also been reported in a variety of preparations [5-9]. The argument is made herein that a contemporary model of hearing impairment not only must include impoverished transduction, but must recognize altered central processing as well.

The present paper contributes additional evidence of the central consequences of permanent threshold shift (PTS). In addition, we show that similar central effects are produced by continuous tonal stimuli of moderate intensity (65-80 dB SPL). In other words, there is a similarity in the effects of hearing loss and in the effects in the normal-hearing animal of sustained acoustic stimulation of moderate intensity. We further generalize our position by drawing parallels with the corresponding variables for vision, damage to the retina, and continuous retinal illumination. Overall, we are suggesting the need for a broader model of sensory function that links normal and impaired processing.

ELECTRICAL STIMULATION THRESHOLDS AND PTS

Relatively little work has been done with electrical stimulation of the auditory system apart from the development of auditory prostheses for humans. One important advantage of electrical stimulation, however, is that the experimental animal can behave normally and is not influenced by anesthesia, which can drastically alter auditory system performance [10].

A useful approach using electrical stimulation has been to study the interaction of an acoustic stimulus with electrical stimuli that are presented at different levels (i.e., different nuclei) within the system [11]. An even simpler procedure has proved to be very informative. This is the behavioral measurement of absolute thresholds for the detection of electrical stimulation and the contrast of these thresholds with those obtained under different experimental conditions -- one being the condition that exists in the central auditory system following a PTS. Cats trained in the operant behavioral procedures necessary for the measurement of absolute acoustic thresholds can also be used to measure absolute thresholds for electrical stimulation of auditory brainstem nuclei. The electrical stimuli are presented via permanently implanted electrodes, and the thresholds can be given in current levels (uA) which, in turn, can be specified in dB re 1.0 uA.

In terms of empirical results, it was found that electrical stimulation thresholds for auditory brainstem nuclei decreased after a PTS [11]. These threshold decreases have been termed "stimulation hypersensitivity." The threshold decreases obtained for electrodes in cochlear nucleus and inferior colliculus are illustrated in Fig. 1. The length of the bar below the abcissa shows the decrease in the electrical stimulation threshold that followed a 20 dB PTS. Electrode locations in individual animals are specified above each bar. The changes shown in Fig. 1 are the difference between mean stimulation threshold just prior to the 48 h exposure (1 kHz at 110 dB SPL) and mean stimulation threshold one month after the exposure. Stimulation hypersensitivity, however, was present at the termination of the acoustic trauma. Thus, hearing loss and the stimulation hypersensitivity both occur immediately after PTS, and both are long-term effects. Clearly, there was a functional change in the central auditory system as a result of the peripheral damage in the cochlea.

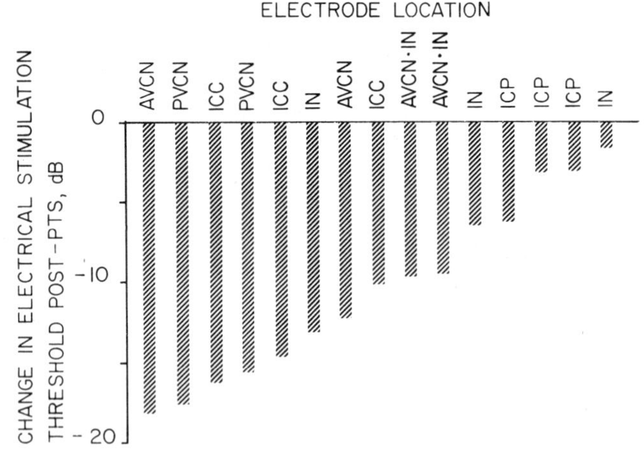

Fig. 1. Change in electrical stimulation threshold following a 20 dB PTS. Abbreviations used in Figs. 1 and 2 are: AVCN, anteroventral cochlear nucleus; DCN, dorsal cochlear nucleus; ICC, central nucleus of the inferior colliculus; ICP, pericentral nucleus of the inferior colliculus; ICX, external nucleus of the inferior colliculus; IN, interstitial nucleus; PVCN, postero-ventral cochlear nucleus.

ELECTRICAL STIMULATION THRESHOLDS AND CONTINUOUS TONE

H-T Chang's work on the evoked responses produced by lateral geniculate stimulation showed that continuous illumination of the retina produced a striking increase in responsiveness at the level of the visual cortex [12]. In contrast, the majority of studies in the field of hearing that have used continuous sound have been psychophysical works that have yielded masking effects. In electrophysiological studies employing continuous sound, or at least long duration stimuli, single units from the auditory nerve were typically recorded, and the results obtained were generally compatible with those of the masking studies. It turns out, however, that continuous tone does produce effects within the central auditory system that are not compatible with a masking interpretation. One such study is summarized below, and others will be described in later sections of this paper.

Electrical stimulation thresholds were measured in a group of three normal-hearing animals with electrodes in auditory brainstem nuclei [13]. The thresholds for electrical stimulation were measured against a background of quiet or in the presence of a continuous tone of 80 dB SPL. The tone was present throughout the five minutes or so required to behaviorally measure each electrical stimulation threshold. Frequencies of the continuous tone were 0.5, 2.0, and 4.0 kHz. Threshold measurements with the various frequencies of tone and with quiet were made in counterbalanced order.

Generally, the presence of continuous tone resulted in stimulation hypersensitivity, and the frequency producing the largest threshold decrease varied from one electrode to another. Fig. 2 shows the distribution of the largest decreases in stimulation threshold for each electrode and the corresponding electrode locations. Note that the stimulation hypersensitivity produced by this experimental procedure lasts only as long as the tone is present.

Later in the experiment, a PTS of approximately 34 dB was produced by exposure to 110 dB SPL white noise for 48 h. Following the PTS, the permanent stimulation hypersensitivity measured for each electrode correlated with the previously measured, transient stimulation hypersensitivity

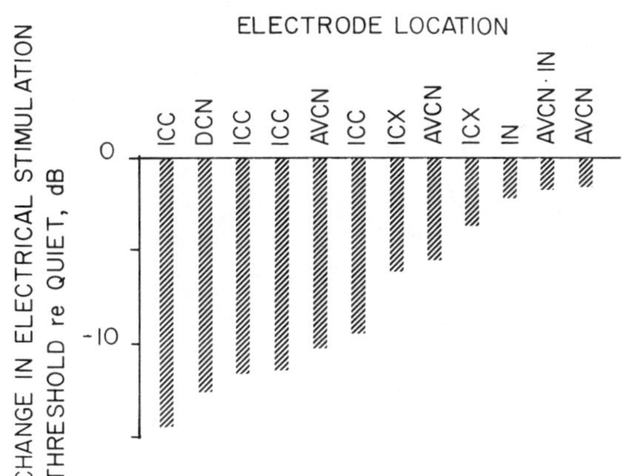

Fig. 2. Change in electrical stimulation threshold during the presentation of a continuous tone of 80 dB SPL. Abbreviations as in Fig. 1.

produced by the continuous tone with r=0.89. Thus, the hypersensitivity effects produced by continuous tone correlated highly with the hypersensitivity effects that followed PTS.

EVOKED RESPONSES IN THE HEARING-IMPAIRED CAT

Normal-appearing evoked responses can be recorded from the auditory cortex of totally deaf cats by using electrical stimulation applied to cochlear nucleus [14]. This indicates that severe, long-term hearing impairment does not render the central system nonfunctional. Hearing impairment also occurs in certain strains of mice that are used to study audiogenic seizures. To produce the seizures, the mice are briefly exposed to an intense sound during a critical age range (priming) which produces a PTS. If they are exposed to the same intense sound again at a later date, a seizure may result. It is of interest that the auditory evoked responses recorded at higher stimulus intensities from inferior colliculus in the primed animals are of considerably greater amplitude than those recorded in the unprimed animals [15,16]. In one of the studies [16], abnormally large evoked responses were also recorded from the cochlear nucleus.

In the *deafness* mutant mouse, which acquires a hearing loss through cochlear degeneration, the amplitudes of evoked responses recorded from inferior colliculus were found to be a function of age [7]. Evoked responses recorded from the inferior colliculus were larger in the *deafness* mutant at all ages in comparison with normal mice but were exceptionally large at an age of 5 to 7.5 months. Age, noise exposure, genetics and possibly species all interact with respect to evoked response amplitude.

Evoked responses that are abnormally large for higher intensity stimuli suggest a comparison with the phenomenon of recruitment. Salvi et al., [17] in seeking a physiological basis for recruitment, reviewed the findings concerning cochlea and auditory nerve after sound exposure and found no evidence that neurons in the auditory periphery have firing patterns that are altered except for reduced sensitivity.

The study described below used the same animals as the work summarized in Fig. 1. Evoked responses produced by acoustic stimuli were recorded from cochlear nucleus and inferior colliculus before and after the production of the 20 dB PTS. Acoustic stimuli were presented in 10 dB increments to determine evoked response thresholds which, in turn, were used to evaluate the hearing loss. Once threshold was exceeded in the normal-hearing animal, the evoked responses slowly increased in amplitude as the stimulus intensity was increased. In the hearing-impaired animal, however, evoked responses from some electrodes in inferior colliculus increased in amplitude very rapidly as the stimulus intensity was increased. The responses in the hearing-impaired animal were frequently of much greater amplitude than those in the normal-hearing animal. This phenomenon was not seen in any of the evoked responses recorded from cochlear nucleus.

In one animal (305), the intensity series was continued several steps above threshold. Also, the hearing loss in this animal was such that an overlapping range of intensities was used pre- and post-exposure, thus permitting comparison of the evoked responses produced by stimuli of the same intensity. Fig. 3 shows the pre- and post-exposure auditory evoked responses recorded from electrode 305-8 in left inferior colliculus. The Post-exposure evoked responses were recorded approximately one month after the acoustic trauma. The acoustic stimulus was a tone burst of 3 ms over-

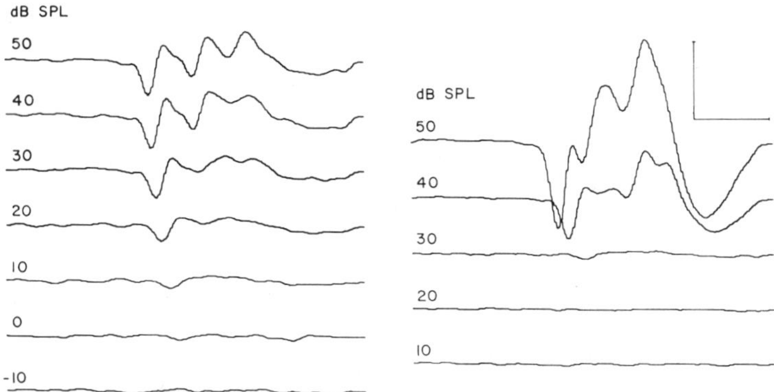

Fig. 3. Auditory evoked responses recorded from inferior colliculus before and after a 20 dB PTS. Calibration: 3 ms and 100 uV.

all duration with 1 ms rise and fall times. The intensity function for an electrode in right inferior colliculus in the same animal is shown elsewhere [11].

In these results, the developmental and genetic factors associated with the study of mutant mice are not relevant. The elevated threshold, the rapid increase in amplitude with intensity, and the abnormally large potentials would seem to relate to the phenomena of recruitment with hearing loss: namely, elevated hearing threshold, rapid increase in loudness, and uncomfortable loudness levels slightly above threshold.

ENHANCEMENT OF EVOKED RESPONSES BY CONTINUOUS TONE

The original work showing central effects from continuous stimulation was done in the visual system [12]. Later studies have suggested that the retinal dark discharge produces inhibitory effects at the upper levels of the visual system [18-21]. Interruption of the dark discharge by retinal ischemia, by enucleation, or by continuous retinal illumination produced enhancement of the visual cortical response to electrical stimulation of the lateral geniculate nucleus [19,22,23].

Chang [12] had reported that for the auditory system, continuous noise produced a small amplitude increase in the response recorded from auditory cortex to medial geniculate stimulation. Chang used anesthetized cats, but later observations on unanesthetized cats showed very strong enhancement by continuous sound of the evoked responses recorded from portions of medial geniculate nucleus and auditory cortex [24-26]. Continuous tone proved to be a much more effective stimulus for producing evoked response enhancement than continuous noise. Recently, Nomotoz [27] has shown in the pigeon that evoked responses recorded from Field L, an upper level region of the auditory system, were enhanced, unaffected, or suppressed by continuous tone.

We have begun again to study evoked response enhancement in the cat because of the constellation of effects produced by continuous tone and by hearing loss. The results presented below indicate several new aspects of evoked response enhancement and suggest that the underlying mechanisms constitute an important part of normal auditory processing.

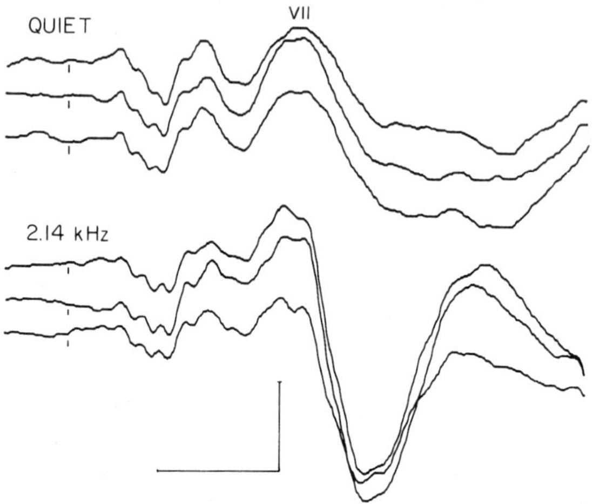

Fig. 4. Auditory evoked responses recorded from a skull electrode over right auditory cortex in cat 315. Top: background of quiet. Bottom: Same tone burst presented during a continuous tone of 2.14 kHz, 65 dB SPL. Calibration: 5 ms and 10 uV with positive up. Arrival of the tone burst at the ear is indicated by the short vertical lines.

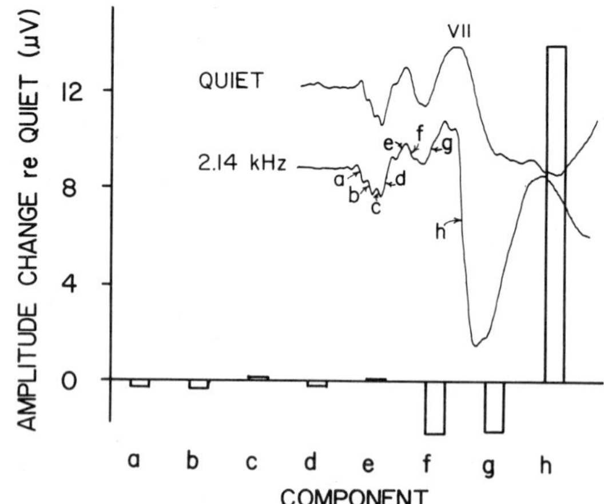

Fig. 5. Difference between the evoked responses recorded with and without a continuous tone background. Conditions were the same as in Fig. 4.

As has been indicated above for the auditory system, the presence of certain continuous acoustic stimuli can alter the central responsiveness to brief stimuli. For example, in Fig. 4 (top) three averaged evoked responses are shown that were produced by 2.83 kHz, 75 dB SPL tone bursts with 1 ms rise and fall times and 3 ms overall duration. The responses were recorded using a stainless steel screw electrode positioned in the skull over auditory cortex. The three averaged responses in the bottom half of Fig. 4 were produced by the same tone bursts but in the presence of a 2.14 kHz, 65 dB SPL continuous tone. All stimuli were presented free field to the unanesthetized, but restrained, cat.

The evoked responses in Fig. 5 show the summed responses from the two conditions in Fig. 4. The letters a through h label the peak to trough (or vice versa) measurements that were made on the two waveforms. The bar graphs in Fig. 5 show the difference in the magnitude of corresponding components such that a positive difference means the evoked response component was larger in the presence of continuous tone. It can be seen that the major change took place in the vicinity of wave VII. The latency of the peak amplitude of wave VII in quiet was 9.4 ms.

The interaction between the frequency of the tone burst and the frequency of the continuous background tone is shown in Fig. 6. Recordings were made from the same electrode as in the previous two figures. Three frequencies (2.14, 2.46, and 2.83 kHz) separated by 0.2 octave were presented in all combinations of tone burst and continuous tone with the exception that the two tones could not be of the same frequency. The amplitudes of some of the components are affected by the particular tone-burst and background frequencies used. Both component amplitudes and the waveform itself were altered. The 2.83 kHz continuous tone was particularly effective in producing a marked change in the evoked response waveform. There is clearly an interactive effect between the frequency of the tone burst and the frequency of the background tone.

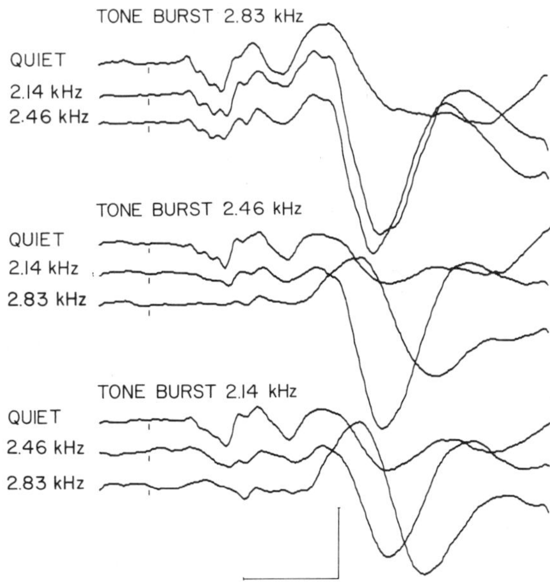

Fig. 6. Evoked responses to tone bursts in quiet and in the presence of continuous tone. Tone bursts were always 75 dB SPL while all background tones were 65 dB SPL. Calibration: 5 ms and 10 uV.

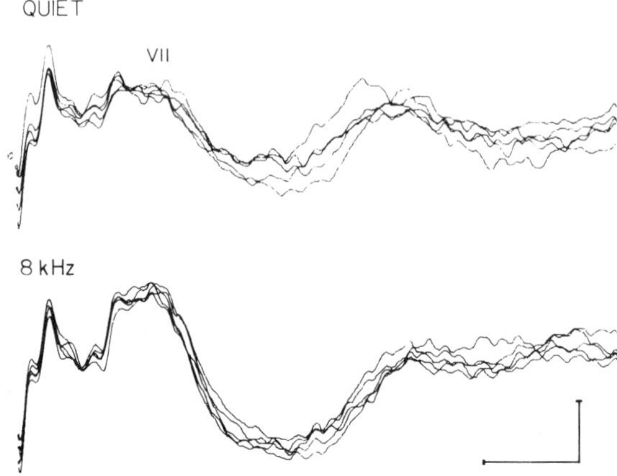

Fig. 7. Averaged evoked responses recorded from the right skull electrode (same as for Figs. 4-6) with electrical stimuli applied to left cochlear nucleus in cat 315. Top: background of quiet. Bottom: background of 8.0 kHz, 65 dB SPL continuous tone. Calibration: 5ms and 5 uV.

Given that evoked response enhancement can be produced by two acoustic stimuli, the next step was to produce evoked response enhancement using an electrical stimulus to cochlear nucleus in place of the tone burst. This procedure rules out interactions in the cochlea as a source of the enhancement. Five evoked response averages are shown in Fig. 7 (top) for electrical stimulation of 8.2 uA intensity applied to cochlear nucleus. The cathodal pulses were presented to a monopolar electrode with interpulse intervals of 200 ms and pulse duration of 0.27 ms. For each evoked response average, 100 pulses were presented. The same stimulus parameters and averaging procedures were also used for all of the remaining figures so that electrical stimuli will be specified only in terms of current level. In Fig. 7 (bottom), another five averages are shown with the same electrical stimulus but with a 8.0 kHz, 65 dB SPL continuous tone present. For the averages shown in Fig. 7 and in the following figures, the A/D converter was not enabled until 1 ms after the presentation of the electrical pulse in order to reduce the stimulation artifact.

To illustrate which components changed when the evoked response was produced by electrical pulses, the organization in Fig. 8 parallels that of Fig. 5. The top tracing in the insert is the sum of three averaged evoked responses recorded from a skull electrode on the right side and produced by an electrical stimulus of 11 uA applied to the same electrode as in Fig. 7. Note that in Fig. 8 the labeling of components is not the same as in Fig. 5 because of differences in waveform. The latency of wave VII after a 2.4 ms correction for ear, cochlear, and eighth nerve transit time was 10.12 ms. The bottom tracing in the insert shows the sum of three averages produced by the same electrical stimulus but in the presence of an 8.0 kHz, 65 dB SPL continuous tone. The bar graph indicates that there was again a change in the components in the vicinity of wave VII, but in contrast to Fig. 5, components on the leading side of wave VII also increased.

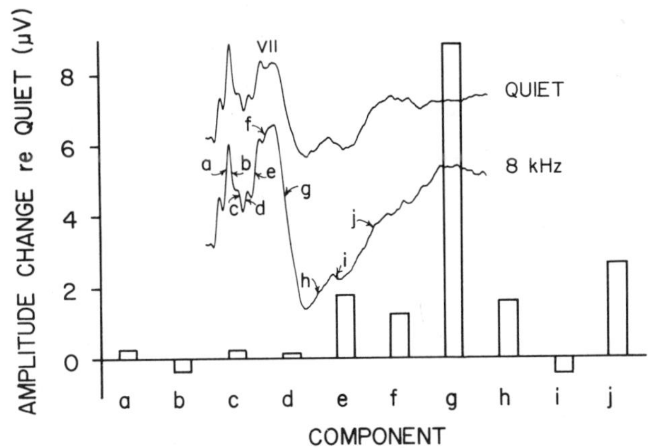

Fig. 8. Difference between the evoked responses recorded with and without a continuous tonal background. The electrical stimulus was 11 uA, but otherwise conditions were the same as for Fig. 7.

A comment is appropriate here in regard to representing the changes in the amplitudes of the components of the evoked response as absolute changes as was done in Figs. 5 and 8. Such a procedure favors large components and may underemphasize small components. Expressing the changes as percentages of the amplitudes in quiet, components a through e in Fig. 5 changed an average of 9.1% (disregarding the sign of the change) while f through h changed 61.9%. Similarly, components a through d of Fig. 8 changed 10.4% while e through i changed 77.5%. Thus, Figs. 5 and 8 do not misrepresent the changes that occurred in the evoked response wareforms. It is too early yet, however, to dismiss the smaller changes that occurred in the earlier potentials as not significant. Such small changes could prove to be a prerequisite for the large amplitude increased in the vicinity of wave VII.

Frequency of Continuous Tone

The frequency of the continuous tone proved to be an important variable. Sets of averaged evoked responses were obtained for several electrodes using backgrounds of quiet and 16 frequencies spaced at one-third octave intervals between 0.5 and 16.0 kHz. The intensity of the continuous tone, when present, was 65 dB SPL. The insert in Fig. 9 shows a series of summed responses (each response based on six averages) from an electrode in left cochlear nucleus (anteroventral division) for octave increments in the continuous tone. The electrical stimuli were 33 uA pulses. The bottom response (16.0 kHz) in this series also shows the peak to trough (or vice versa) amplitudes that are plotted in Fig. 9. The component designated by the triangle, representative of the early components in general, showed little change across the range of continuous tone frequencies.

Wave VII is indicated in Fig. 9 and its latency, corrected by the addition of 2.4 ms as in Fig. 8, was 9.84 ms. The amplitude of the leading edge of this wave (circle) showed a small but consistent increase in amplitude in the vicinity of 1.26 kHz and for 4.0 kHz and above. The later components, defined by the square and inverted triangle, increased considerably in amplitude in the presence of continuous tones of 4.0 kHz and above. The maximal effect was at 8.0 kHz. The evoked responses in the

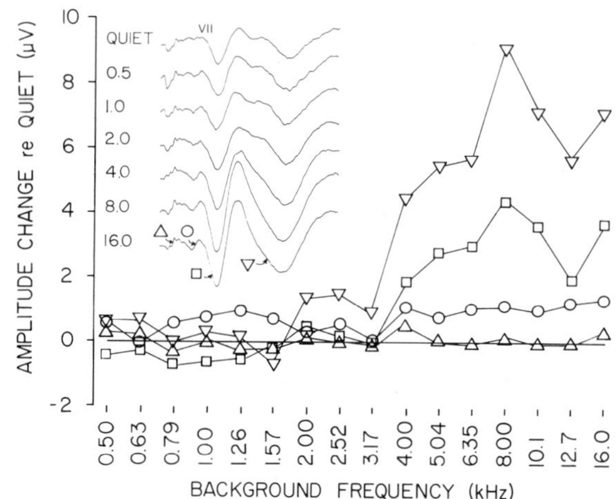

Fig. 9. Effect of the frequency of the continuous tone on the electrically evoked responses recorded from the right skull electrode in cat 312.

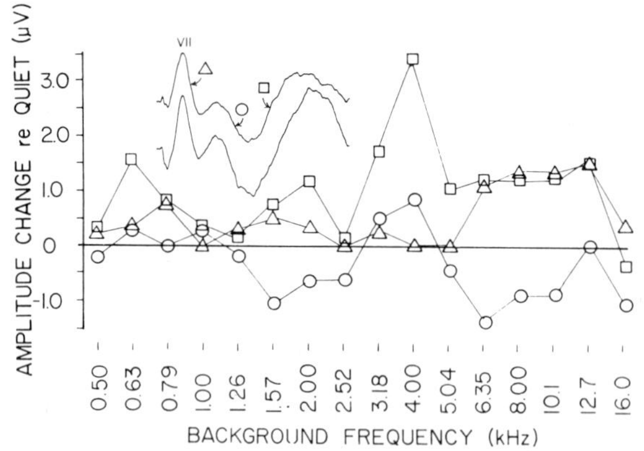

Fig. 10. Effect of the frequency of the continuous tone on the responses recorded from a skull electrode over left auditory cortex. The representative evoked responses shown were obtained in conditions of quiet (top) and a 4.0 kHz background tone (bottom).

insert also show large changes in still later waves which could not be measured because the 33.6 ms sweep time was too short.

Electrical stimuli applied to most of the electrodes positioned in cochlear nucleus produced enhancement effects in the presence of continuous tone. Typically, there was more than one major peak in the amplitude vs. frequency function. Multiple peaks might occur because the electrode was sufficiently large (75 um by 0.5 mm long) that several adjacent tonotopic areas in cochlear nucleus were stimulated. Maximal enhancement was obtained at different frequencies for different electrodes, which is probably also a consequence of the tonotopic organization of the auditory system.

Location of Stimulating Electrode

The effects of the frequency of the continuous tone were also studied with stimulating electrodes positioned in inferior colliculus. Fig. 10 shows the effect of continuous 65 dB SPL background tones spaced at one-third octave intervals. The electrical stimuli were 33 uA pulses applied to right inferior colliculus (central nucleus) in cat 314 (electrode 314-12). The evoked response waveforms in the insert are the sum of six averaged responses. The peak to trough (or vice versa) components measured

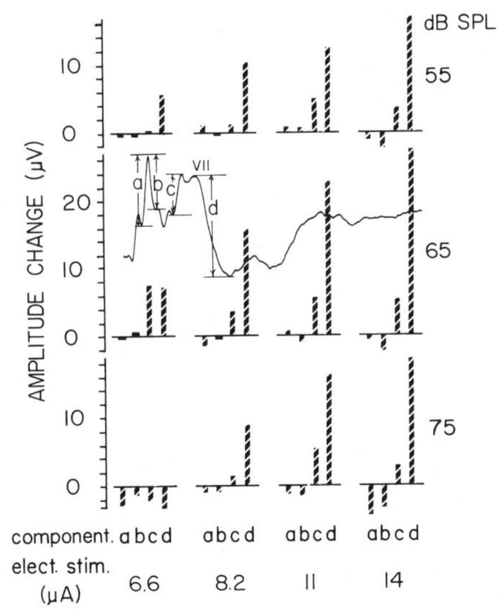

Fig. 11. Interaction of the intensity of the electrical stimulus and of the intensity of the continuous tone. Recordings were made from the same right skull electrode as in Figs. 4-8. Amplitude change is relative to the component amplitude obtained with a background of quiet. The continuous tone was 8.0 kHz, 65 dB SPL.

are indicated by the triangle, circle, and square. Latency of wave VII (or P10 in Farley and Starr) was 9.6 ms after correction by 5.0 ms to reflect the electrode position in inferior colliculus. Successive later peaks correspond to P17 (15.6 ms corrected latency) and P31 (29.7 ms corrected latency) of Farley and Starr [28].

The component on the trailing side of wave VII (triangle) showed enhancement principally for continuous tone frequencies from 6.35 to 12.7 kHz. The amount of enhancement shown by this component was not as great as for stimulation of cochlear nucleus (see square in Fig. 9 or g in Fig. 8). A later component (circle) showed a different range of frequencies that produced enhancement: namely, from 3.18 to 4.00 kHz. This range was flanked at higher and lower frequencies by regions of response reduction. A still later component (square) showed a marked enhancement for a continuous tone of 4.0 kHz although enhancement at a number of other frequencies was also obtained. It was characteristic of electrodes in inferior colliculus that enhancement effects were less pronounced, or even absent, in contrast with the more vigorous effects obtained with cochlear nucleus stimulation. Our data show differential effects in regard to the locus at which the electrical stimulus is applied, but the locus(i) of critical events underlying enhancement cannot be determined from these results.

Intensity of Electrical Stimulation and of Continuous Tone

It might be expected that the intensities of the acoustic and electric stimuli would interact with each other. This, in fact, proved to be the case. For several electrodes, four intensities of electrical stimulation were presented in conjunction with quiet and three intensities of continuous tone. Three evoked response averages were obtained for each combination of stimulus intensity and continuous tone intensity. Measurements for the results presented in Fig. 11 were based on the sum of the three averages obtained from left cochlear nucleus of cat 315 (electrode 315-17). The insert in Fig. 11 shows the response to 11 uA pulses with a background of quiet. Four peak to trough (or vice versa) components are

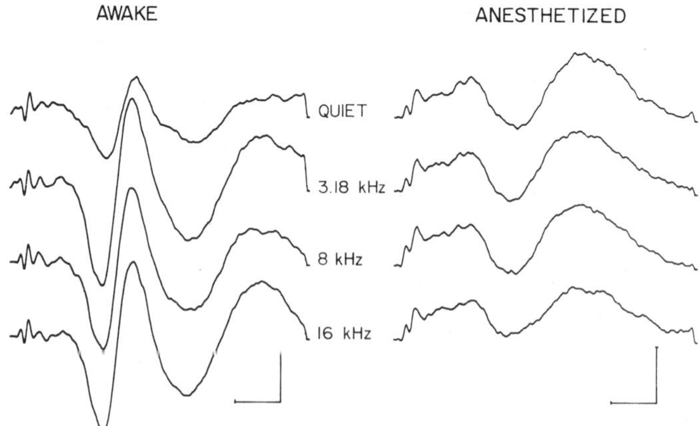

Fig. 12. Evoked responses in the awake and anesthetized animal. Intensity of continuous tone was 65 dB SPL. Calibration: 5 ms and 20 uV for the left column and 5 ms and 30 uV for the right column.

labeled a through d (again, the components are arbitrarily labeled). Fig. 11 shows the magnitude of change in each component relative to quiet for each combination of intensities.

The interaction between the intensities of the electrical and acoustic stimuli may be seen in this figure. Almost all combinations of the intensities used produced some enhancement. Typically, enhancement occurred in the components associated with wave VII. The one exception was the combination of the weakest electrical stimulus and the most intense continuous tone. The result of this combination was a reduction in the amplitude of all components; i.e., electrophysiological masking. It may also be seen in Fig. 11 that certain combinations of intensities were more effective in producing enhancement such as a 14 uA electrical stimulus and a 65 dB SPL intensity of the continuous tone.

Effect of Anesthesia

For the most part, studies involving evoked response enhancement in the auditory system have employed unanesthetized cats, so a brief study was performed to evaluate further the effect of anesthesia. It had been observed that anesthesia reduces or eliminates enhancement in the medial geniculate evoked response [29]. In general, the responsiveness of the upper portions of the auditory system is strongly affected by anesthesia. Fig. 12 shows several responses recorded from a skull electrode over left auditory cortex. Stimulus pulses of 33 uA were applied to right cochlear nucleus (junction of dorsal and anterventral divisions) in cat 312 (electrode 312-15). The responses obtained in quiet are shown at the top of the two columns which represent awake and anesthetized (Nembutal, 32 mg/kg) conditions. Enhancement may be seen in the evoked responses recorded from the awake animal with all three of the continuous tone frequencies. The anesthetized animal, however, does not show enhancement in the presence of the continuous tone and may even show response reduction (e.g., 16 kHz).

CONCLUSION

Both hearing loss and continuous tone can decrease the absolute threshold for the detection of electrical stimulation applied to auditory nuclei of the brainstem. Likewise, some of the evoked responses in the auditory system are considerably larger in the animal with hearing loss, or in the normal-hearing animal during the presentation of continuous tone.

In our experience, evoked response enhancement effects are seen at the level of midbrain or above and primarily in the unanesthetized cat. Furthermore, continuous tonal stimuli have proved to be more effective than continuous noise in producing enhancement.

The decrease in electrical stimulation threshold referred to as stimulation hypersensitivity could be an effect localizable to the vicinity of the electrode tip or it could represent a change at a higher level of the auditory system. If the latter situation is assumed with respect to the normal-hearing animal in quiet, then the electrical stimulus must still activate numerous brainstem neurons at stimulation intensities at or below detection threshold. This issue is discussed further elsewhere [11,30]. It should be noted that deafferentation results in increased responsiveness in other brain systems as well as in the auditory system [31,32].

We take the position that continuous tone and hearing loss are variables of consequence in central auditory processing. We hypothesize on the basis of the robust stimulation-hypersensitivity effect and the vigorous evoked response enhancement effect that major changes in the single unit behavior supporting these phenomena will be measureable. Psychoacoustic correlates must also be sought, but these studies may prove particularly difficult for the following reason. If the central system is, in fact, actively compensating for, or at least reacting to, the degraded input in the hearing-impaired subject, it will be very difficult to separate the sensory impairment from the altered central responsiveness with psychoacoustic methods. The use of the stimulation/recording approach in the behaving animal should continue to provide a means of studying central processing in the normal-hearing and hearing-impaired animal.

ACKNOWLEDGEMENT

This research was supported in part by NINCDS grants 16411 and 19512. We thank Sandra L. Grace for typing the camera-ready copy.

REFERENCES

1. D. K. Morest, Degeneration in the brain following exposure to noise, in: "New Perspectives on Noise-Induced Hearing Loss," R. P. Hamernik, D. Henderson, and R. Salvi, eds., Raven Press, New York, (1983).
2. D. K. Morest and B. A. Bohne, Noise-induced degeneration in the brain and representation of inner and outer hair cells, Hear. Res., 9:145 (1983).
3. D. B. Webster and M. Webster, Neonatal sound deprivation affects brain stem auditory nuclei, Arch. Otolaryngol., 103:392 (1977).
4. D. B. Webster and M. Webster, Effects of neonatal conductive hearing loss on brain stem auditory nuclei, Ann. Otol. Rhinol. Laryngol., 88:684 (1979).
5. G. Babighian, G. Moushegian and A. L. Rupert, Central auditory fatigue, Audiol., 14:72 (1972).
6. R. Salvi, D. Henderson, and R. Hamernik, Auditory fatigue: Retrocochlear components, Science, 190:486 (1975).
7. R. J. Salvi, Central components of the temporary threshold shift, in: "Effects of Noise on Hearing," D. Henderson, R. P. Hamernik, D. S. Dosanjh, and J. H. Mills, eds., Raven Press, New York, (1976).
8. K. P. Steel and G. R. Bock, Electrically-evoked responses in animals with progressive spiral ganglion degeneration, Hear. Res., 15:59 (1984).
9. J. F. Willott and S. M. Lu, Noise-induced hearing loss can alter neural coding and increase excitability in the central nervous system, Science, 216:1331 (1982).
10. W. R. Webster and L. M. Aitkin, Central auditory processing, in: "Handbook of Psychobiology," M. S. Gazzaniga and C. Blakemore, ed., Academic Press, New York, (1975).
11. G. M. Gerken, S. S. Saunders, R. E. Paul, Hypersensitivity to electrical stimulation of auditory nuclei follows hearing loss in cats, Hear. Res., 13:249 (1984).
12. H-T Chang, Cortical response to stimulation of lateral geniculate body and the potentiation thereof by continuous illumination of the retina, J. Neurophysiol., 15:5 (1952).
13. G. M. Gerken, S. S. Saunders, R. Simhadri-Sumithra, and K. H. V. Bhat, Behavioral thresholds for electrical stimulation applied to

auditory brainstem nuclei in cat are altered by injurious and noninjurious sound, Hear. Res., in press.
14. G. Rebillard, M. Rebillard, E. Carlier and R. Pujol, Histophysiological relationships in the deaf white cat auditory system, Acta Otolaryngol., 82:48 (1976).
15. K. R. Henry and M. Saleh, Recruitment deafness: Functional effect of priming-induced audiogenic seizures in mice, J. Comp. Physiol., 84:430 (1973).
16. J. C. Saunders, G. R. Bock, R. James, and C-S Chen, Effects of priming for audiogenic seizure on auditory evoked responses in the cochlear nucleus and inferior colliculus of BALB/c mice, Exp. Neurol., 37:388 (1972).
17. R. Salvi, D. Henderson and R. Hamernik, Physiological bases of sensorineural hearing loss, in: "Hearing Research and Hearing," V. 2, J. Tobias, ed., Academic Press, New York, (1983).
18. A. Arduini and M. H. Goldstein, Enhancement of cortical responses to shocks delivered to lateral geniculate body. Localization and mechanism of the effects, Arch. Ital. Biol., 99:397 (1961).
19. A. Arduini and T. Hirao, Enhancement of evoked responses in the visual system during reversible retinal inactivation, Arch. Ital. Biol., 98:182 (1960).
20. Y. Nakai and E. F. Domino, Reticular facilitation of visually-evoked responses by optic tract stimulation before and after enucleation, Exp. Neurol., 22:532 (1968).
21. J. M. Posternak, T. C. Fleming, and E. B. Evarts, Effect of interruption of the visual pathway on the response to geniculate stimulation, Science, 129:39 (1959).
22. H. Sakakura and R. W. Doty, EEG of striate cortex in blind monkeys: Effects of eye movements and sleep, Arch. Ital. Biol., 114:23 (1976).
23. H. Suzuki, Effect of reversible retinal blockage on population response of the lateral geniculate nucleus, Jap. J. Physiol., 17:335 (1967).
24. G. M. Gerken, Enhancement of the medial geniculate evoked response in conscious cat, Electroenceph. Clin. Neurophysiol., 34:509 (1973).
25. E. M. Glaser, Cortical responses of awake cat to narrowband FM noise stimuli, J. Acoust. Soc. Am., 50:490 (1971).
26. R. J. Gumnit and R. G. Grossman, Potentials evoked by sound in the auditory cortex of the cat, Am. J. Physiol., 200:1219 (1961).
27. M. Nomoto, Local auditory evoked potentials and effects of pure tones on click evoked potentials in the pigeon, Hear. Res., 17:13 (1985).
28. G. R. Farley and A. Starr, Middle and long latency evoked potentials in cat. I. Component definition and dependence on behavioral factors, Hear. Res., 10:117 (1983).
29. G. M. Gerken, Electrophysiological observations relevant to masking, Audiology, 10:97 (1971).
30. G. M. Gerken, A systems approach to the relationship between the ear and central auditory mechanisms, in: "Advances in Audiology," vol. 1, "Artificial Auditory Stimulation Theories," W. D. Keidel and P. Finkenzeller, ed., Karger, Basel, (1984).
31. J. E. Desmedt and L. Franken, Long-term physiological changes in auditory cortex following partial deafferentiation, in: "The Effect of Use and Disuse on Neuromuscular Functions," E. Gutmann and H. Pavel, ed., Elsevier, Amsterdam, (1963).
32. S. K. Sharpless, Disuse supersensitivity, in: "The Developmental Neuropsychology of Sensory Deprivation," A. H. Riesen, ed., Academic Press, New York, (1975).

DISCUSSION

Tyler: The question I have to ask actually relates to tinnitus. Most patients with tinnitus, including those with noise-induced hearing loss, seem to have a central component to tinnitus based on psychophysical studies. Related to your finding of sensitization, does the baseline spontaneneous activity in some of these more central components also increase in your subjects with hearing loss?

Gerken: Since there are several different kinds of tinnitus, I think it would be risky to categorically relate our changes to tinnitus. I am tempted to think in those terms, but there are just too many exceptions to feel comfortable with it.

Tyler: Did you see any changs in spontaneous activity?

Gerken: That is a fairly complicated story. We recorded the on going activity from the same electrodes that were used for electrical stimulation thresholds and also some that were never used for electrical stimulation. In general, the spontaneneous activity goes up when there is a hearing loss. We tried doing a correlation between the amount of increase or decrease in spontaneous activity and the change in electrical stimulation threshold. The correlations were insignificant. Consequently, we haverejected the notion that the sensitization activity is in some way causally related to spontaneous activity.

Trahiotis: Was the actual location where you got an increase in electrical activity the same place where there was sensitization?

Gerken: Our largest increases did tend to come from AVCN and PVCN or the interstial nucleus and central nucleus of inferior colliculus. Areas such as the external nucleus showed generally small changes, but the data sets are simply to small to do the kind of correlation that I think you would like to see.

Cody: When you implant these electrodes in a normal animal, do they not cause trauma? Do you find that the psychophysical detection thresholds change in the animals? Secondly, do you monitor the impedance of your electrodes over time to determine if you are polarizing the electrode? Thirdly, do you know what current you are actually passing?

Gerken: Let me try to answer these questions briefly. We use a monophasic stimulus which could produce electrode polarization, but we present them at a very slow rate, 1 every 200 millisecond. We have a paper that does examine the polarization question and concluded that it did not really produce any observable change. We monitor the currents on each presentation with an A/D converter running at a very high rate and observe the actual stimulus on the monitor screen. It is a constant current stimulus to avoid avalanche kinds of conduction. We also check the impedance of the electrode. These electrodes remain functional until we kill the cat which may be a year later. So, it is a very stable preparation. Of course, we do not start testing until the electrodes have been in for several months. We have never been able to detect a change in psychoacoustic thresholds, as a result of these electrodes.

von Gierke: How long is your continuous tone and what can you say about the time course of the response to the continuous tone?

Gerken: Well, it takes about five minutes to measure a psychophysical threshold in the cat with the methods that we use. So the continuous tone would be on for that length of time. We turn the tone on and then start the measurement procedure. After the threshold is measured, we turn the tone off. In the evoked potential studies, the tone would stay on for whatever length of time it takes to present 200 stimuli at 4 per second, a couple of minutes maybe. Based on the results of another study that I did not mention, we have a suggestion that it might take about 80 milliseconds for these effects to occur.

Patuzzi: I would like to mention the results of Desmedt and Robertson done some years ago when they saw that the attentiveness of human subjects increased the amplitude of the evoked response. Would it be possible that the background noise actually increases the attentiveness of the animals? How would you go about factoring that out?

Gerken: There are a lot of studies involving attention and the evoked potentials. Usually in humans, those are the later components like P300. This seems to be an automatic kind of response, it does not seem to make much difference what the cat is "thinking," if you will permit me to say that. Wave 7 in the cat has a latency of about 10 milliseconds.

Adams: With regard to your suggestion that you are producing disinhibition by your lesion. It would be nice to know the relationship of the best frequencies of your recording electrode and the audiogram produced by the noise trauma. Do you have any information on that?

Gerken: No. Not only that one might want to know the tuning function for the cortical screw electrode because presumably one could locate that electrode in different places.

ADJUSTMENTS IN CORONARY BLOOD FLOW WITH NOISE STIMULATION

V. Colletti,[1] F. G. Fiorino[1] and I. Sheiban[2]

ENT Department[1] and Cardiology Department[2]
University of Verona
37134 Verona, Italy

INTRODUCTION

We are all aware of the damaging action of noise on the auditory system; however, loud noises have also been thought to affect other organ systems. Among these, the cardiovascular system is considered the most involved and therefore has been given the most attention in animals and in humans. The cardiovascular system is a "stress strain" apparatus which can respond to a wide range of environmental conditions such as temperature and exercise. From a clinical point of view, it is well known that cardiovascular diseases are the major causes of death [1]. As shown in Table 1, 48.5% of the total mortality rate involves cardiovascular diseases. Among these, ischemic cardiopathies are the most prevalent cause of death, with a figure of 34.9%. Table 2 details the possible risk factors of ischemic cardiopathy. Among these hyper-cholesterolemia, smoking and arterial hypertension are statistically confirmed causes of miocardial ischemia. Other associated factors are sedentary occupations and psychological or environmental stress. In spite of the large number of risk factors, it may be noted that noise is not included. This may be due to the lack of attention given to the problem or to the negligible effects of this physical agent.

It is possible that noise, as a stress factor, may in fact increase the risk of ischemic cardiopathy. That is, noise might directly contribute to this disease by causing spasms of the main coronary arteries due to a prevalence of alpha-adrenal tone in predisposed subjects.

Table 1. CARDIOVASCULAR MORTALITY IN ITALY [1]

Deaths for all causes	554, 510	
Deaths for Cardiovascular Diseases	265,539	(47.8%)
- Ischemic cardiopathies	80,309	(30,3%)
- Cerebrovascular diseases	76,085	(28.6%)
- Hypertension	17,021	(6.4%)
- Others	92,124	(34.7%)

Table 2. Risk factors for ischemic cardiopathy [1]

- Age
- Sex
- Hereditary factors
- Hypercholesterolemia
- Diabetes mellitus
- Hypertension
- Stress
- ECG alterations
- Alcohol
- Sedentary occupation
- Cigarette smoking

A review of the literature pertaining to noise and cardiovascular problems demonstrates that noise has a specific effect on the sympathetic tone of the cardiovascular system [2-4]. Nevertheless, few specific studies on problems concerned with noise and myocardial disease have been done; although some attention has been given to the problem of noise and hypertension. Tables 3 and 4 illustrate some of the relevant studies done on animals and their respective findings. It has been demonstrated that acute exposure to a novel sound (Table 3) causes a redistribution of blood from the skin and certain inner organs to muscles [3] as a result of peripheral vasoconstriction [2]. Phasic changes in heart-rate and systolic pressure have also been detected although the size and direction of this change is still a debate. Concerning heart-rate, it may be seen from the table that an increase [2,3,5], a decrease [6,7], and a biphasic change [8] have been found.

As shown in Table 4, the most consistent effect of long-term noise exposure in animals is an increase in systolic pressure [10-13]. Table 5 shows a list of studies with the corresponding results of short-term noise exposure on several cardiovascular parameters examined in humans. Concerning acute exposures, Sokolov [4] observed that low-level sounds (below about 70 phons), especially sounds carrying information or novel stimuli, can induce vasoconstriction in the finger, vasodilation in the forehead and a decrease in heart-rate (i.e., the orienting reflex); high-level sounds

Table 3. CARDIOVASCULAR EFFECTS OF SHORT-TERM NOISE EXPOSURE IN ANIMALS.

AUTHORS	ANIMALS	HR	SBP	DBP	PF
Bolme & Novotny [9]	Dogs		>		
Caraffa & Braga [3]	Dogs	>	> <		
Hallback & Folkow [5]	Rats	>	>		
Borg [2]	Rats	>			<
Kneis [8]	Guinea Pigs	> <			
Bilsing & Schneider [6]	Guinea Pigs	<			
Turkkan & Al [7]	Baboons	<	>	>	

HR = heart-rate DBP = diastolic blood pressure
SBP = systolic blood pressure PF = peripheral blood flow
> = increase, < = decrease, > < = biphasic changes

Table 4. CARDIOVASCULAR EFFECTS OF LONG-TERM NOISE EXPOSURE IN ANIMALS.

AUTHORS	ANIMALS	HR	SBP	DBP	CO
Farris & Al [10]	Rats		>		
Medoff & Bongiovanni [11]	Rats		>		
Yeakel & Al [12]	Rats		>		
Borg [14]	Rats		=	=	
Turkkan & Al [7]	Baboons	<		<	
Peterson & Al [13]	R. Monkeys		>	>	>

HR = heart-rate DBP = diastolic blood pressure
SBP = Systolic blood pressure CO = cardiac output
> = increase, < = decrease, = = unchanged

Table 5. CARDIOVASCULAR EFFECTS OF SHORT-TERM NOISE EXPOSURE IN MAN.

AUTHORS	HR	SBP	DBP	PF
Steimann & Al [25]			>	
Lehman & Al [17]	>	> <	>	
Heinecker [16]	>	>		
Sokolov [4]	> <			> <
Eiff [19]	<			
Etholm & Egenberg [23]	=			
Jansen [26]		<		
Keefe [20]	> <			<
Klosterkotter [27]				<
Gerber & Al [15]	>			
Mosskov & Ettema [29,30]		<	>	
Ickes & Al [18]	>			
Yamamura [43,30]	=	=	=	
Fruhsthorfer & Hensel [22]	> <			<
Singh & Al [21]	> <			<
Neus & Al [31]			>	
Andren [32]			>	

HR = heart-rate DBP = diastolic blood pressure
SBP = systolic blood pressure PF = peripheral flow
> = increase, < = decrease, = = unchanged

give rise to a defense reaction characterized by a generalized vasoconstriction with an increase in heart rate. However, such reactions do not always seem to occur as may be seen in Table 5. Heart-rate, for example, has been reported to increase [15-18], decrease [19], undergo biphasic changes [20,22], or show no significant change [23,24].

Cardiac function during acute noise has also been monitored by a number of investigators. Yamamura and Aoshima [24] observed significant ischemic alteration in the ECG (a decrease in the height of the T wave and a depression of the ST segment) during eight hours of exposure to a pink noise having an SPL of 80-85 dB (A). In an epidemiological study involving prolonged noise exposure, Knipsheld [33] showed pathological heart volume and ECG altera- tions. Similar findings have been reported by Shalatov et al. [34]. Since these findings indicate an ischemic cardiopathy, it is surprising that direct studies on coronary blood flow have not been performed. The aim of this investigation therefore was to study coronary blood flow along with other cardiovascular indices by means of cardiac catheterization in subjects exposed to short-term noise. For obvious reasons, the study was performed on patients suffering from ischemic cardiopathy, namely of Variant Angina of Prinzmetal, which is a disease caused by spasm of the main coronary arteries, sometimes facilitated by exogenous stress stimuli.

The aim of the study was to ascertain whether a high-level sound inducing a defense reaction could temporarily modify coronary flow and therefore be considered as an exogenous stress stimuli such as cold or a mental task.

MATERIALS AND METHOD

Eight normal-hearing male individuals, aged 42 to 60 years (average: 53.2) participated in the present research. The subjects were in-patients admitted for cardiac catheterization, left ventricolography and selective coronarography to confirm the clinical diagnosis of Variant Angina of Prinzmetal. No subject had suffered from either myocardial infarction or any other significant (neurological or pathological) disease. Each patient was requested to sign a consent form prior to the procedure. All subjects reported negative otological histories. Pure tone audiometry was carried out in a sound-proof room using an audiometer. All patients had normal auditory function for their age [35] and passed a 20 dB HTL screening test on the experimental stimulus.

All drugs, except short-acting nitrates, were discontinued three days before the investigation. Administration of 10 mg of Diazepam was administered 30 minutes before catheterization. The subjects were studied for a period of about 25 minutes in a room maintained at 22°C. The background noise in the room was approximately 35 dB(A) SPL. During all phases of the test, the subjects remained awake. A pig-tail catheter was introduced in the femoral artery (according to the Seldinger method). Aided by X-ray, the catheter was then guided through the abdominal and thoracic aorta and then inside the left ventricle. The catheter was subsequently connected to a polygraph (Thomson Telco) which recorded the electrocardiogram and the left ventricular pressure curves.

Coronary blood flow was evaluated by means of the thermodilution method. For this purpose a venous catheterization was performed. A catheter (Edward laboratories) was introduced through the right basilic vein. The end of the catheter was guided inside the right auricle and then inserted in the coronary sinus. An opening at the extreme end of the catheter permitted the introduction of sodium chloride 0.9% into the coronary sinus. Temperature variations in the mixture of blood and normal saline were recorded by means of two thermistors situated at a distance of 20 mm from each other. The initial end of the catheter was connected to a polygraph. A 10cc solution of normal saline at 22°C was injected within 20 seconds using an automatic injector. Temperature variations were recorded simultaneously, being altered according to amount of blood flow through the sinus. The procedure used during the investigation was as follows:
(1) During the first 10 minutes after the catheterization, subjects were maintained at rest so that they could adapt to the environment. Subsequently, coronary blood flow was assessed four times in the basal condi-

tion. (2) Five acoustic stimuli lasting 30 seconds were then administered at intervals of two minutes. The stimuli consisted of 100 dB(A) broad-band noise produced by an Amplaid audiometer (Model A 200) and introduced through TDH-39 earphones and MX-42/AR cushions.

The following cardiovascular parameters were evaluated before, during and after each stimulus: (1) ECG; (2) heart-rate (evaluated by means of ECG registration); (3) left ventricular systolic pressure (LVSP); (4) left ventricular and diastolic pressure (LVEDP); and (5) dP/dT max which represents the first derivative of the pressure in a second. The last two parameters are related to the contractile efficiency of the left ventricle.

Each of the intraventricular parameters noted above were measured during the 30 seconds before noise stimulus, during the period of noise stimulation, and 30 seconds after the termination of the noise. As concerns blood flow, it was evaluated in the basal conditions, during the initial 20 seconds of noise and during the 20 seconds following its offset. The mean value was calculated for five stimulus presentations for all parameters.

RESULTS

Fig. 1 shows a tracing obtained from the polygraph. The ECG tracing is shown at the top. Shown below is the left intraventricular pressure curve from which the systolic and the end diastolic pressure may be assessed. An additional curve represents the dP/dT max. These two curves are also graphically illustrated in Fig. 2.

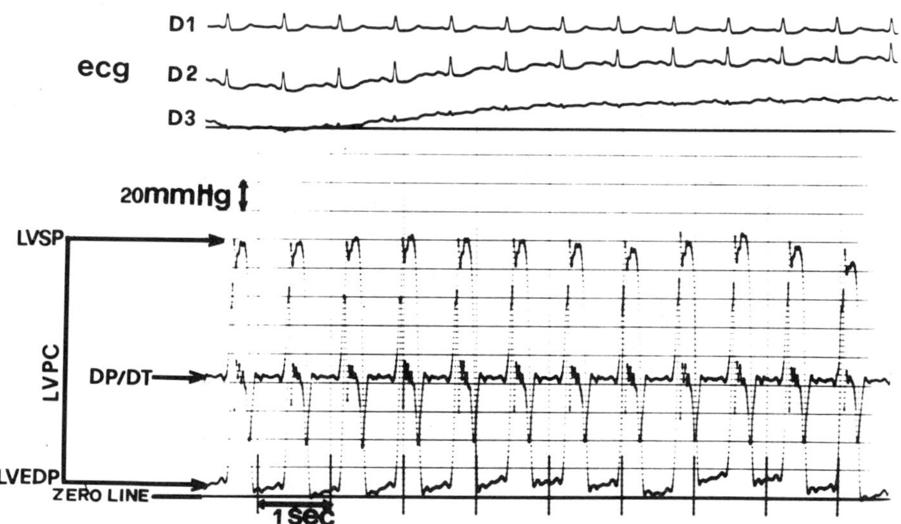

Fig. 1. Actual recordings obtained from one subject at rest. ECG tracings (D1, D2 and D3) are shown at the top. Left ventricular pressure curve (LVPC) and dP/dT are shown below. The highest value of LVPC correspond to the systolic pressure (LVSP), the lowest to the diastolic pressure (LVEDP).

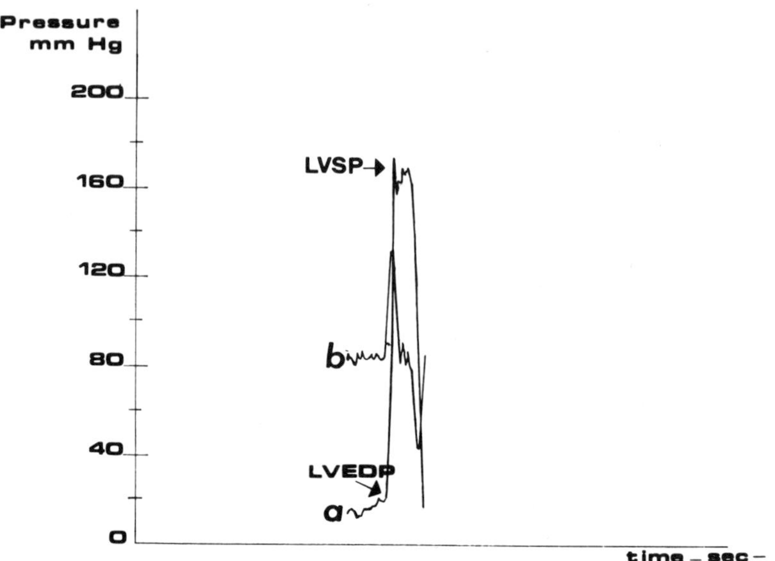

Fig. 2. Typical morphology of the two intraventricular pressure curves (left ventricular pressure curve (a) and dP/dT (b)) recorded during the present research.

No morphological variations of electrocardiogram were detected subsequent to noise. In Figs. 3 to 6, individual values for each cardiac parameter are graphically shown during the three periods. All the cardiovascular parameters were calculated at one second intervals. For each test and parameter there were originally 90 numerical values. These were converted to 15 mean values by averaging over every six values. Fig. 3 represents left ventricular systolic pressure, which shows a normal range from 120 to 170 mmHg. As may be seen, left ventricular end diastolic pressure (Fig. 4), dP/dT max (Fig. 5) and heart rate also (Fig. 6) show normal values.

The results from the periods before, during and after stimulation were statistically compared by using a Randomized Blocks Analysis of Variance (ANOVA) together with Duncan's Multiple Comparison test. A significance level of 5 percent was chosen (Table 6). This test permitted the three periods to be compared in pairs. The statistical analysis did not show any significant differences. The result were also evaluated by using data representing four arbitrarily chosen time periods in the test run. These periods are described as follows: (A) the first six seconds of noise; (B) the median value of six seconds during noise; (C) the last six seconds of the noise; (D) the first six seconds after the end of noise (Figs. 3 to 6).

The assessment of results obtained in the first phase: (A) was carried out for brief latency (approximately one second), of the vagal vegetative response; the evaluation of phase (B) is explained by the longest period of latency in the sympathetic vegetative response (approximately 15 seconds). Finally, the presence of habituation (Phase C) and the reaction on offset (Phase D) are researched.

The value of each phase was compared to the mean basal value by means of Dunnet's multiple comparison test (Table 7). As concerns heart rate, a significant difference would exist only if the value of one phase minus the basal value is greater than 1.23 beats per minute (Table 7). As may be seen from Table 7, no significant difference is present. Similarly, no

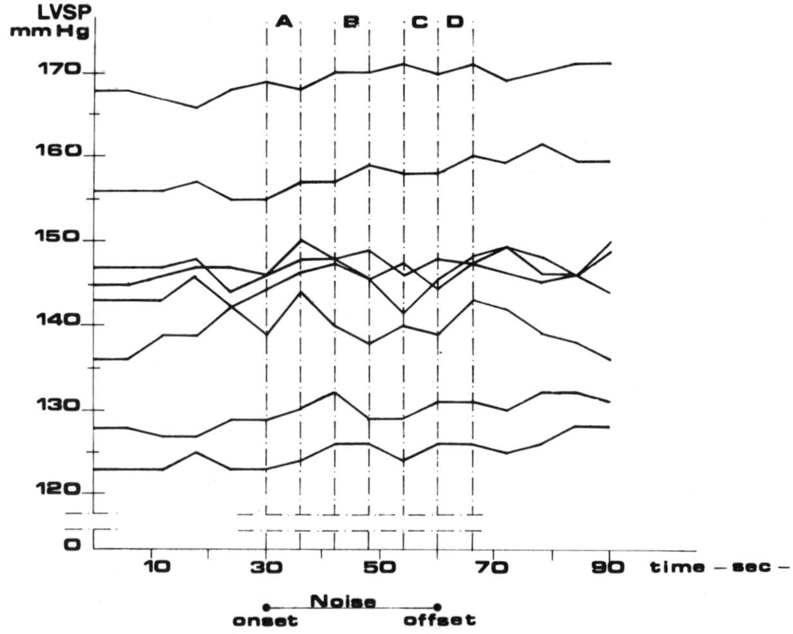

Fig. 3. Individual values for left ventricular systolic pressure (LVSP). The values are represented averaging over every six seconds. Three periods (30 seconds before noise, 30 seconds of noise administration and 30 seconds after its offset) are considered. A, B, C and D represent four time periods in the test run (see text).

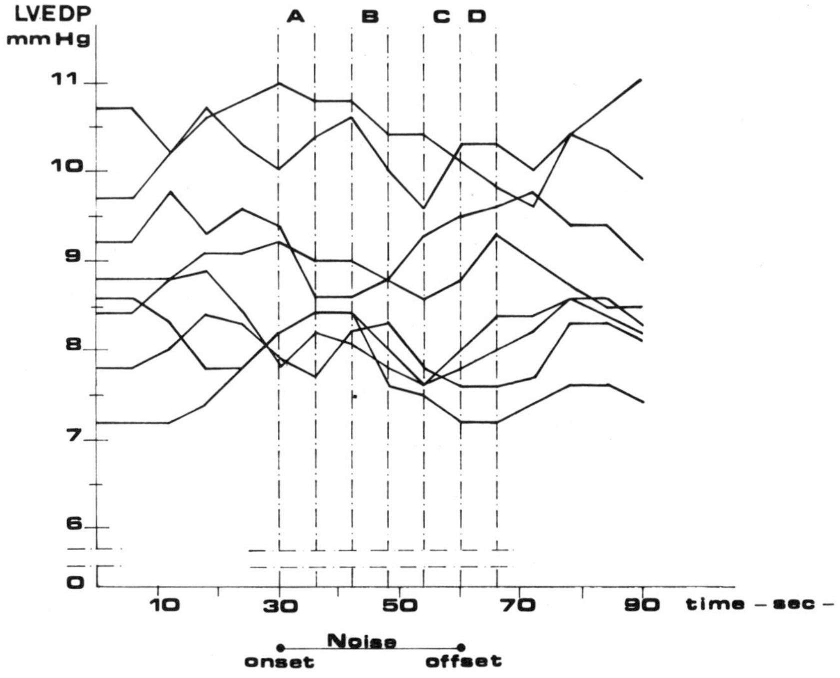

Fig. 4. Individual values for left ventricular and diastolic pressure (LVEDP); (time analysis: see legend of Fig. 3).

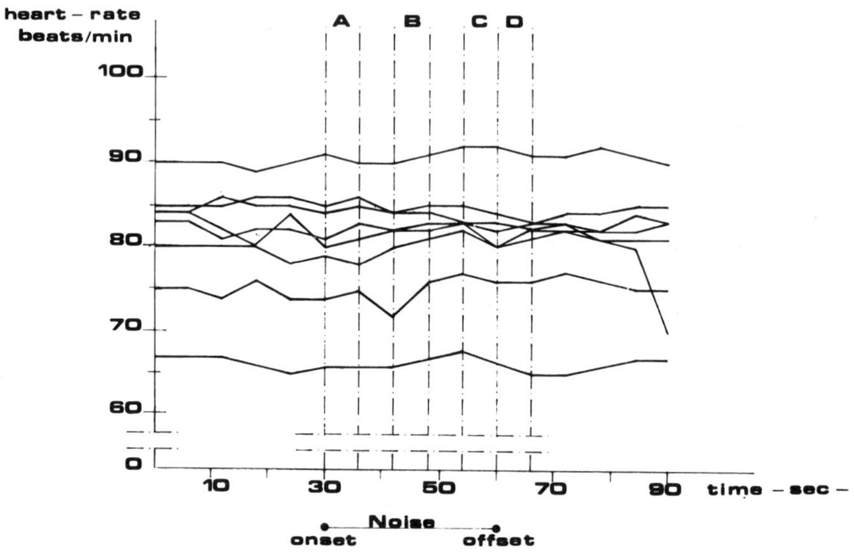

Fig. 5. Individual values for heart-rate (HR); (time analysis: see legend of Fig. 3).

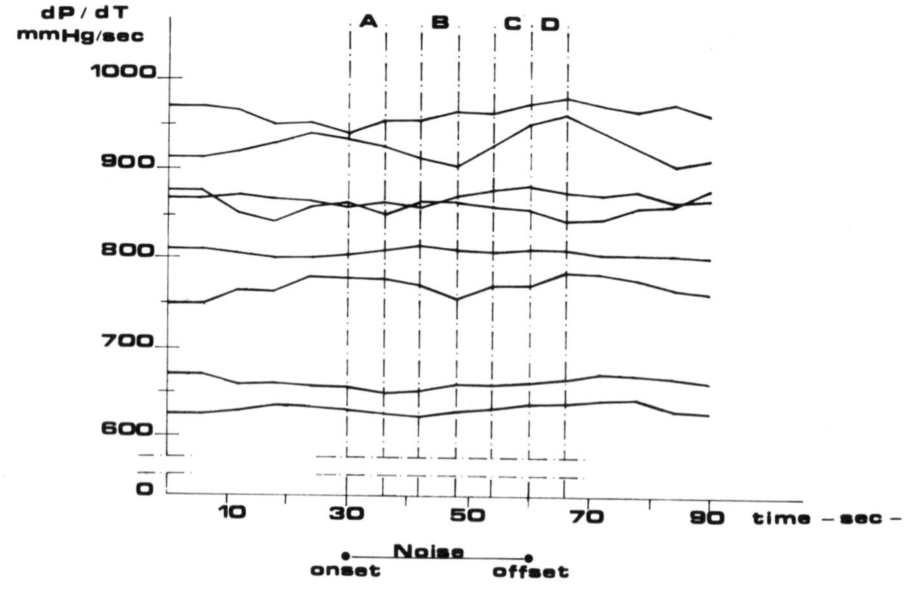

Fig. 6. Individual values for dP/dT max; (time analysis: see legend of Fig. 3).

Table 6. RANDOMIZED BLOCK ANALYSIS OF VARIANCE (ANOVA) TOGETHER WITH DUNCAN'S MULTIPLE COMPARISON TEST.

Parameters	(1)	(2)	(3)	F	ANOVA Duncan's T
Heart Rate	80.5	80.9	80.7	0.6	NS
LVSP	143.7	144.8	145.2	3.4	NS
LVEDP	8.9	8.8	8.9	2.0	NS
DP/DT Max	797	798	801	3.5	NS

Mean values (X) obtained for the periods before (1), during (2) after (3) noise exposure. NS = no-significant

Table 7. MEAN VALUES CONCERNING HEART-RATE AND INTRAVENTRICULAR PARAMETERS EVALUATED IN BASAL CONDITIONS (B.X) AND IN PHASES A, B, C AND D (SEE TEXT). THE DIFFERENCE BETWEEN EACH PHASE AND THE BASAL VALUES WOULD BE SIGNIFICANT IF HIGHER THAN 1.23 BEATS/MIN FOR HEART-RATE, 2.39 MMHG FOR LVSP, 0.46 MMHG FOR LVEDP AND 13.9 MMHG/SEC FOR DP/DT MAX (DUNNET'S MULTIPLE COMPARISON TEST; SIGNIFICANT LEVEL: 5%).

	b.X	(A)	(B)	(C)	(D)
Heart-Rate	80.5	80.5	81.0	80.4	80.4
LVSP	143.7	145.4	144.7	144.7	145.8
LVEDP	8.9	8.9	8.7	8.7	8.8
DP/DT Max	797	795	795	805	808

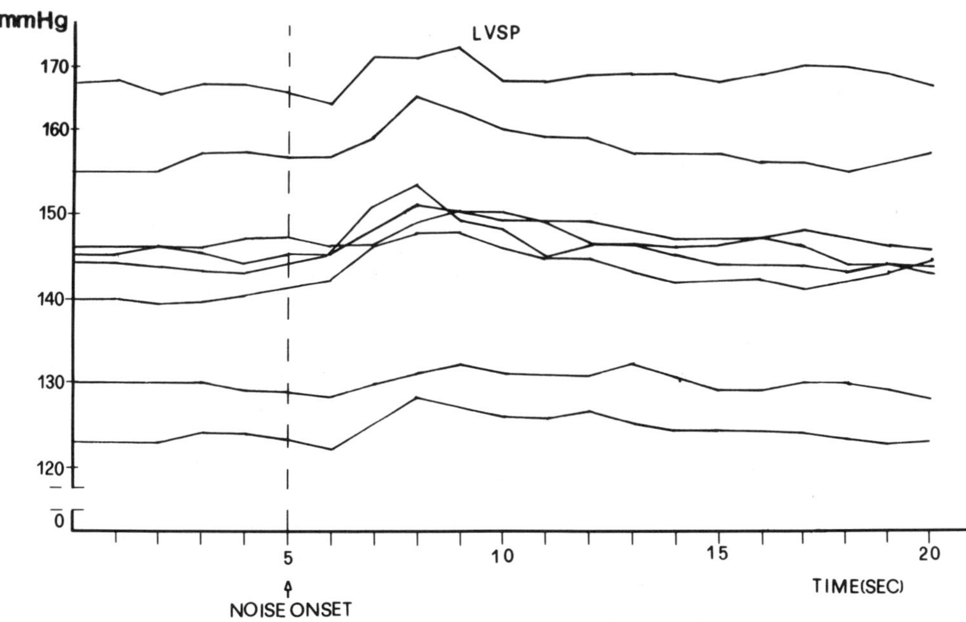

Fig. 7. Individual values for left ventricular systolic pressure plotted at one second intervals.

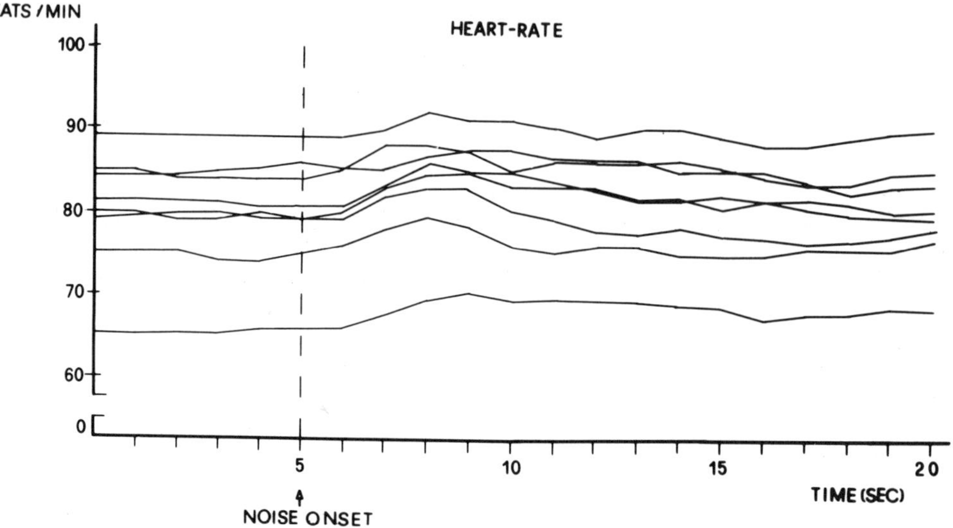

Fig. 8. Individual values for heart-rate plotted at one second intervals.

Table 8. T-TEST BETWEEN THE BASAL VALUES RECORDED FOR THE 30 SECONDS BEFORE NOISE ONSET AND THE VALUES OBTAINED 3 AND 4 SECONDS AFTER NOISE ONSET.

	X Difference	T	(P)
Heart-Rate	3.89 (+/-1.67)	6.67	(<0.01)
LVSP	4.96 (+/-2.11)	6.66	(<0.01)

differences were seen for systolic pressure, diastolic pressure and dP/dT max.

On the other hand, if the value obtained are plotted at one second intervals, a transitory and moderate increase is seen after the onset of noise. As shown in Figs. 7 and 8, increase in systolic pressure and heart rate with a latency of one to two seconds occurs, but the values return to normal limits within five to seven seconds. The maximum values are reached within three to five seconds. If we compare the values during this last period of time with those recorded in the basal interval, a significant mean difference is seen using the t-test method (Table 8).

Finally, the results of coronary blood flow are shown in Table 9. The three mean values (with the standard deviations) are shown before, during and after stimulation. The values before the noise are approximately 99.2ml/ min/100g, which is within the normal range. Note that very little modification occurs as a result of the noise exposure. A statistical comparison (Dunnet's test) of these values show no significant difference.

Table 9. MEAN VALUES (X) WITH THE STANDARD DEVIATIONS (S.D.) FOR CORONARY BLOOD FLOW.

	1	2	3
X	99.2 *	100.1 *	98.7 *
S.D.	12.0	12.8	11.2

1 = before noise   2 = during noise   3 = after noise

*The comparison in pairs of the three periods (Duncan's Test) shows no significant difference.

DISCUSSION

In the introduction of this study, we presented the most significant data in the literature related to the effects of noise exposure on the cardiovascular apparatus. Different results have been obtained both in humans and animals, but little attention has been paid to the effects of noise on coronary blood flow, in spite of its importance. In an attempt to fill this gap, we performed a study on humans recording direct and indirect parameters related to coronary blood flow. The data presented in this study show that a high-level, short-term noise exposure does not significantly alter coronary blood flow. Only transitory variations in systolic left ventricular pressure and heart rate were detected. These changes consisted of an increase of a few beats per minutes (or few mmHg) for approximately 1 to 4 seconds, but disappeared after 5 to 7 seconds. The short latency of this reaction, suggests that it is mediated by the parasympathetic system [36]. Apparently, very moderate and transitory adjustments of coronary blood flow do occur.

One aspect of the methodological procedures used in this research needs to be discussed; namely, the technique used for recording coronary blood flow. In humans, thermodilution is considered the most accurate method available. However, this technique can not be used for long term monitoring of coronary blood flow. The thermodilution technique permits the recording of the average blood flow corresponding to a duration of 20 seconds. In order to carry out long term studies of coronary blood flow, it would be necessary to permanently implant flowmeters in animals.

Another possible limitation of the present study is that we have examined pathological subjects and, in theory, the results could be different for healthy subjects. However, the group of patients investigated were suffering from a disease characterized by a hypersensitivity of coronary artery tone to some stressing factor such as those used in the diagnosis of their disease (e.g., cold, mental tasks). Therefore, the subjects selected for this study might be expected to be hypersensitive to the effects of noise. Consequently, the lack of a significant alteration in coronary blood after acute noise exposure is somewhat surprising and suggests that the same results would be obtained in healthy individuals.

The lack of significant variations in our cardiac parameters might also be due to two other factors. First, the necessary premedication with 10 mg of Diazepam may have weakened the cardiac reaction in terms of intensity and duration. Second, the surroundings and circumstances under which the investigation was carried out may have been given secondary importance by the subjects in terms of a stress factor. This could have masked out the stress effect produced by the noise.

In conclusion, the absence of significant variation in coronary blood flow with our short duration noise exposures does not imply that cardiac alterations are not possible by long-term noise exposure; however, the effect seems unlikely. If an effect does occur, it is very likely to be caused, not by direct coronary spasm, but indirectly by peripheral circulatory alteration such as arterial hypertension.

REFERENCES

1. ISTAT, Annuario di statistiche sanitarie, Roma (1981).
2. E. Borg, Tail artery response to sound in the unanesthetized rat, Acta Physiol. Scand., 100:129 (1977).
3. F. Carraffa-Braga, L. Granata, and O. Pinotti, Changes in blood-flow distribution during acute emotional stress in dogs, Pflugers Arch., 339:203 (1973).
4. E. N. Sokolov, Perception and the conditioned reflexes, Pergamon Press, New York (1962).
5. M. Hallback and B. Folklow, Cardiovascular response to acute mental stress in spontaneously hypertensive rats, Acta Physio. Scand., 90:684 (1970).
6. A. Bilsing and R. Schneider, The effect of white noise on heart-rate, open field activity and orienting response of the guinea-pig (Cavia a. porcellus), Zoo. Jahrbuch Physiol., 83:253 (1979).
7. J. S. Turkkan, R. D. Heinz, and A. H. Harris, The non-auditory effects of noise on the baboon, in: "Noise as a Public Health Problem," G. Rossi, ed. Techniche, Milano (1983).
8. P. Kneis, Influence of short acoustical stimuli on heart rate and muscular activity in the free-moving guinea-pig, Activ. Nerv. Sup., 77:58 (1969).
9. P. Bolme and J. Novontny, Conditional reflex activation of the sympathetic cholinergic vasodilator nerves in the dog, Acta Physiol. Scand., 77:58 (1969).
10. E. J. Farris, E. H. Yeakel and H. S. Medoff, Development of hypertension in emotional gray Norway rats after air blasting, Am. J. Physiol., 144-331 (1945).
11. H. S. Medoff and A. M. Bongiovanni, Blood pressure in rats subjected to audiogenic stimulation, Am. J. Physiol., 143-300 (1945).
12. E. H. Yeakel, H. A. Shenkin, A. B. Rothballer and S. M. McCann, Am. J. Physiol., 155-118 (1948).
13. F. A. Peterson, J. S. Augenstein, D. C. Tanis, R. Warner and A. Heal, Some cardiovascular and behavioral effects of noise in monkeys, in: "Noise as a Public Health Problem," G. Rossi eds, Tecniche, Milano (1983).
14. E. Borg and A. R. Moller, Noise and blood pressure: effect of lifelong exposure in the rat, Acta Physiol. Scand., 103:340 (1978).
15. S. E. Gerber, A. Mulac and M. E. Lamb, The cardiovascular response to acoustic stimuli, Audiology, 16:1 (1977).
16. R. Heinecker, Individuelle Unterschiede in der Reaktiion von Kreislauf und Gasstoffwechsel auf dosierte Belastungen: Cold Pressor Test, Flickerlicht, Larm, korperliche Arbeit, Archiv. fur Kreislaufforschung, 30:1 (1959).
17. G. Lehmann and J. Tamm, Uber Veranderungen der Kreislaufdynamik des ruhehen Menschen unter Einwirkung von Gerauschen, Int's.Z. angew. Physiol. sinschl Arbeitsphysiol. Bd 16:217 (1956).
18. W. K. Ickes, J. Espili and A. M. Glorig, Pattern A personality and noise-induced vasoconstriction, J. Speech Hear. Res. 22:334 (1979).

19. A. von Eiff, Funktionsspezifische effekte und gewohnungsphanomene bei larm von unterschiedlicher zeitstruktur, Psych. Fragen Larmfors. Colloquium Berl.-Steglitz 28 u, 29:109 (1964).
20. F. B. Keefe, Cardiovascular responses to auditory stimuli, Psychon. Sci. 19:335 (1970).
21. A. P. Singh, R. M. Rai, M. R. Bhatia and H. S. Nayar, Effect of chronic and acute exposure to noise on physiological functions in man, Int. Arch. Occup. Envir. Health, 50:169 (1982).
22. B. Fruhstorfer and H. Hensel, Extra auditory responses to long-term intermittent noise stimulation in humans, J. Appl. Physiol. 49:985 (1980).
23. B. Etholm and K. E. Egenberg, The influence of noise on some circulatory functions, Acta Otolaryngol., 58:208 (1964).
24. K. Yamamura and K. Aoshima, An investigation of biological response induced by intermittent noise, Eur. J. Appl. Physiol., 44:9 (1980).
25. B. Steinmann, U. Jaggi and J. Widmer, Uber den Einfluss von Gerauschen und Larm auf den Blutdruck des Menschen, Cardiologia, 27:223 (1955).
26. G. Jansen, Effects of noise on physiological state. ASHA report, 4:89 (1969).
27. W. Klosterkotter, Neuere Erkenntnisse uber larmwirkungen, Kampf dem Larm. Heft., 4:103-111, (1974).
28. J. L. Mosskov and J. H. Ettema, Extra auditory effects in short term exposure to aircraft and traffic noise, Int. Arch. Occup. Environ. Health, 40:165 (1977).
29. J. L. Mosskov and J. H. Ettema, Extra auditory effects in short term exposure to noise from a textile factory, Int. Arch. Occup. Environ. Health, 40:174 (1977).
30. K. Yamamura, F. Itoh and N. Maehara, Physiological responses induced by 555-min exposure to intermittent noise, Eur. J. Applied Physiol., 47:257 (1981).
31. H. Neus, A. V. von Eiff, H. Ruddel and W. Schulte, Traffic noise and hypertension. The Bonn traffic noise study, in: Noise as a Public Health Problem, G. Rossi ed., Techiche, Milano (1983).
32. L. Andren, Cardiovascular effects of aircraft noise, Acta Med. Scan. Suppl., 657:1 (1983).
33. P. Knipschild, Medical effects of aircraft noise: community cardiovascular survey, Int. Arch. Occup. Environ. Health., 40:185 (1977).
34. N. N. Shalatov, A. O. Sanitanov and K. V. Glutova, On the problem of the state of the cardiovascular system during the action of continuous noise, Labor Hygiene and Occupational Diseases, 6:10 (1962).
35. A. Spoor, Presbicusis values in relation to noise induced hearing loss, Int. Audiol., 6:48 (1967).
36. A. M. Scher and A. C. Young, Reflex control of heart-rate in the unanesthetized dog, Am. J. Physiol., 218:780 (1970).

DISCUSSION

Cody: Do you give a sedative to the patient before you insert the catheter?

Fiorimo: For this investigation, it is necessary to administer 10 mg of Diazepam. It might be that this drug could have attenuated the response to the noise both in duration and magnitude.

Manninen: What was the ambient temperature level during your experiments?

Colletti: The temperature was kept at 22°C., and the investigation was for only a short term noise exposure. It was a direct investigation of coronary blood flow. We are, of course, aware that different situations of a person working in industry might affect the results, but how much of this is from endocrinological effects? Noise, by itself, in our opinion has not changed in any significant way the parameters that we have investigated. If you are suggesting that there are changes in coronary blood flow resulting indirectly from an alteration of adrenergic and noradregenergic systems then, I would agree with you. But that is an indirect effect of noise.

Axelsson: I would like a little more information about the specific patients. Did they have coronary disease? Did they have clinical signs of arterial spasm in the coronaries? Did you have a careful history of what elicited such coronary spasm? Maybe there are emotions involved in this. Maybe this noise was not stressful enough to elicit change in coronary blood flow.

Fiorimo: All patients were suffering from variant angina of Prinzmetal which is a disease influenced by stress factor. In fact, in this disease, some stress tests such as the cold stressor test or performing mental tests gave positive results. We selected patients that were positive on cold stressor test.

Patuzzi: How much warning did the patients have that the sound was arriving?

Fiorimo: They were not aware of the arrival of the sound.

CRITICAL PERIODS OF SUSCEPTIBILITY TO NOISE-INDUCED HEARING LOSS

Marc Lenoir[1], Remy Pujol[1], and Gregory R. Bock[2]

[1]INSERM-U. 254, Lab. Neurobiologie de I'Audition, CHR St. Charles, 34059 Montpellier Cedex, France

[2]The Ciba Foundation, London, G.B.

INTRODUCTION

Deafness in children has deleterious effects on the development of speech, language and listening skills [1]. A large number of factors contribute to hearing losses in the perinatal periods. Congenital infections, such as toxoplasmosis, rubella, cytomegallo-virus and others [2] have been recognized as possible etiological factors of auditory dysfunction. Evidence for early conductive and perceptual deficits of genetic origin has been found in experimental models of hereditary hearing impairment [3]. Moreover, it has been proposed that early exposures to physical and chemical agents such as noise and ototoxic drugs, which have noxious influences on the auditory receptors in adults [4,5] may drastically increase the probability of deafness in young subjects [6-8]. This conclusion receives strong support from experimental studies, which demonstrate critical periods of susceptibility to acoustic and ototoxic trauma in young animals [9].

During these periods, exposure to noise or antibiotic treatment, which at other times would have no effect, can damage the cochlea. These periods correspond to different stages of cochlear development: the ototoxic action of the aminoglycoside antibiotics is maximum at the onset of auditory function [10] while the susceptibility to acoustic trauma appears to be greater when the cochlea has just acquired its adult functional properties [11]. Another example of a critical period in the developing cochlea is indicated by propylthiouracyl-induced thyroid hormone deprivation, which drastically alters the first stages of cochlear maturation [9].

It therefore appears that during cochlear development there are several overlapping critical periods (Fig. 1). Since the combination of different agents (for example, antibiotics and noise) exacerbates their effects in the adult cochlea [12], the risk of early auditory impairment could be dangerously increased in the developing cochlea [13,14].

This chapter essentially concentrates on periods of enhanced sensitivity to acoustic trauma. A brief review of the literature dealing with an age-dependent change in susceptibility to acoustic trauma is first presented. We then describe experiments which demonstrate a critical period for susceptibility to acoustic trauma in two animal species. Our own results are included at this point. These results are finally discussed in light of data relative to other critical periods in the developing cochlea.

AGE-DEPENDENT SENSITIVITY TO ACOUSTIC TRAUMA

The question of whether there is an age-dependent difference in susceptibility to acoustic trauma was first raised by clinicians who focused attention on the noise to which premature babies are exposed to in intensive care units [6,7]. Experimentally, they reached the conclusion that the same sound exposure could be more traumatic in young animals than in adults. Falk et al. [15] exposed three groups of guinea pigs, aged 2 days, 8 days, and 8 months, to 30 continuous hours of white noise at 119-120 dB SPL. One month later, light microscopy revealed that the cochleas of the 2-day-old and 8-day-old groups had been more affected by the white noise than the cochleas of the 8-month-old group.

Similar findings were also reported by Douek et al. [17], Dodson et al. [16] and by Coleman [17] in the guinea pig, using as traumatic sound exposures, a continuous incubator noise (80 dB SPL, 7 days), a white noise (76 dB SPL, 7 days), or a 4 kHz pure tone (119 dB SPL, 2 hours) respectively. At the same time, Price [18] demonstrated an age-dependent susceptibility to acoustic trauma in the cat using physiological techniques. Eight-week-old kittens exposed to a pure tone overstimulation (5 kHz, 50 min.) lost significantly more cochlear microphonic (CM) sensitivity than did adult cats exposed to the same tone.

These data on guinea pigs and cats clearly indicate that young animals are more susceptible to acoustic trauma than adults. However, no precise correlation between the particular sensitivity to noise and the degree of cochlear development could be established as a result of these experiments, since both neonatal guinea pigs and 8-week-old kittens have an adult-like organ of Corti [19]. The existence of a critical period in cochlear development, during which young animals are more susceptible to acoustic trauma

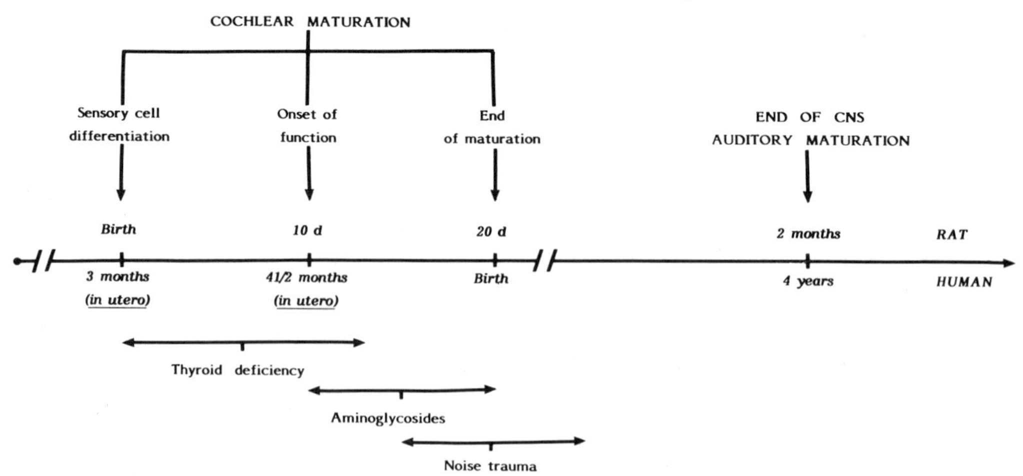

Fig. 1. Critical periods related to the main events of the rat cochlear maturation. The corresponding time course of human cochlear development is also indicated.

was first suggested by authors working on the phenomenon of priming for audiogenic seizure in mice [20,21]. Saunders and Hirsh [22] demonstrated in the C57Bl/6J strain of mice that 120 seconds of a 110 dB SPL octave-band noise (8-16 kHz) produced a 30 dB CM threshold elevation in mice exposed at the age of 18 days, whereas mice exposed before or after this date showed only minor CM changes. These results were discussed by the authors in terms of "disuse supersensitivity," a hypothesis previously proposed to account for the physiological effects of priming in mice [23]. The existence of a critical period of sensitivity to acoustic trauma in mice was recently confirmed by Henry [24] in the CBA mouse. Inbred strains of mice are, however, known to exhibit many abnormalities of hearing [25] and it was thus important to replicate these observations in a species with no genetic hearing defects [26]. Moreover, the data reviewed above did not provide any evidence concerning the locus of the developmental changes presumably underlying the observed changes in susceptibility [27].

CRITICAL PERIOD OF SENSITIVITY TO ACOUSTIC TRAUMA

The hamster was chosen by Bock and Saunders [27] as an experimental model for additional studies. This animal exhibits a more delayed cochlear development [28,29] than the mouse [30]. They subjected hamsters of various ages, ranging from 11 to 75 postnatal days to an octive band noise (5 to 10 kHz) of 125 dB re 20 uN/m^2 for 2.5 minutes. Five days after noise exposure, the CM responses were measured in the exposed animals and in control animals of the same ages. The maximum CM loss was noted in the exposed 27-day-old animals. Hamsters exposed at the ages of 11 and 75 days showed no significant changes in CM sensitivity. Identical findings were simultaneously obtained in the same animal species using a similar procedure [26]. These results demonstrated the existence of a critical period of sensitivity to acoustic trauma in the hamster. It occurs slightly before the end of cochlear maturation, but extends well after this date, according to anatomical [28,29] and electrophysiological findings [26,27] on hamster cochlear maturation. In interpreting their results, Bock and Saunders [27] considered developmental changes related to sound transmission through the middle ear: "It might be expected that a given noise exposure would not be maximally effective in producing cochlear damage before about 20 days after birth. However, given the apparent structural maturation of the ear by 20 days, there is no obvious reason to predict that the effectiveness of noise exposure in inducing threshold loss should decrease between 55 and 75 days of age." The authors made a series of measurements related to middle ear resonance and the efficiency of the acoustic reflex in 40- to 75-day-old hamsters. No developmental changes in either the middle ear cavity or ossicular chain could explain the results after the 35th postnatal day. Moreover, the CM thresholds were relatively stable after postnatal day 27 [31]. Thus, the authors reached the conclusion that the locus of the developmental process underlying the critical period of sensitivity to acoustic trauma is in the cochlea. They further confirmed this conclusion in experiments demonstrating a critical period of auditory fatigue in the hamster [31]. Since the critical period for acoustic trauma extended beyond the apparent maturation of the cochlea, the nature of the underlying developmental changes remained to be determined.

Additional experiments were clearly needed to relate hearing deficits to structural damage in the cochlea. For these reasons, Lenoir, Bock and Pujol [32] and Lenoir and Pujol [33] investigated, both physiologically and histologically, the effects of loud noise on another species, the young albino rat (Sprague-Dawley). This animal has been used for many years as an experimental model for investigating postnatal cochlear maturation [34,35]. Moreover, the authors considered that more recent studies in this species, including electron microscopic observations [36], as well as

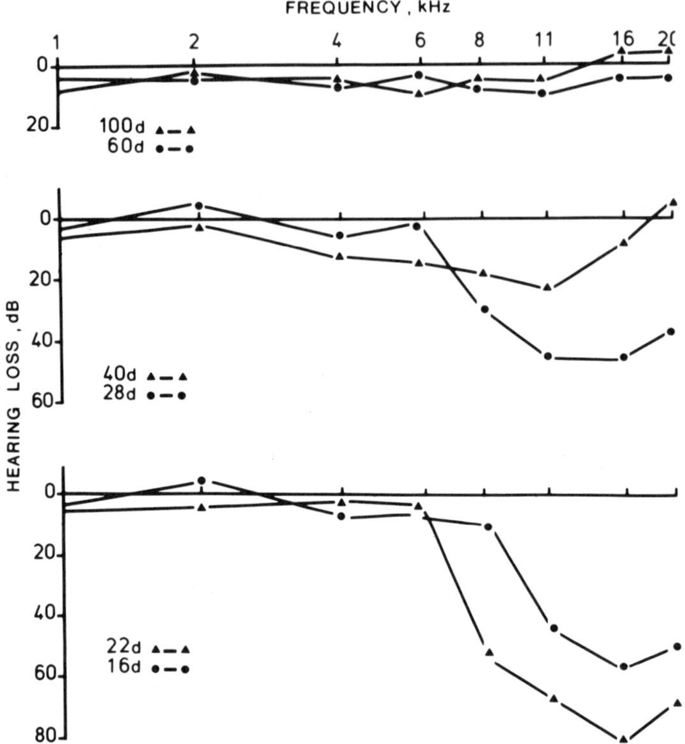

Fig. 2. Threshold elevation 7 days after white noise exposure (120 dB SPL, 30 min.) in rats exposed at 16, 22, 28, 40, 60 and 100 days of age. Each curve represents the mean values calculated for 6 animals of the same age.

measurements of the cochlear action potential (CAP) threshold [37] and frequency selectivity [38], could be useful in determining precise correlations between an enhanced susceptibility to acoustic trauma and underlying developmental events.

The experimental procedures differed from those used in the hamster, since the authors used the CAP and not the CM as the criterion for hearing function. The sound exposure was a 30-minute white noise with a total intensity of 120 dB SPL (re 2.10^{-4} ubar). Six groups of unanesthetized rats were exposed to the white noise at 16, 22, 28, 40, 60 or 100 days of age respectively. Audiograms were performed 7 and 55 days after the sound exposure. The results from each group of exposed animals were compared with recordings from control rats. One week after the white noise exposure, drastic threshold elevations (50 to 80 dB) were noted at high frequencies in the rats exposed at 16, 22 and 28 days of age. The maximum deficits appeared in the 22-day-old group. The 60- and 100-day-old rats did not exhibit any threshold shifts (Fig. 2). These results were confirmed in other groups of rats 55 days after the traumatic exposure (Fig. 3), proving that the observed hearing losses were permanent and not temporary.

In order to determine the nature of the cochlear damage responsible for the threshold elevation, the 22-day-old exposed rats were sacrificed and their cochleas were observed with light (surface preparation technique)

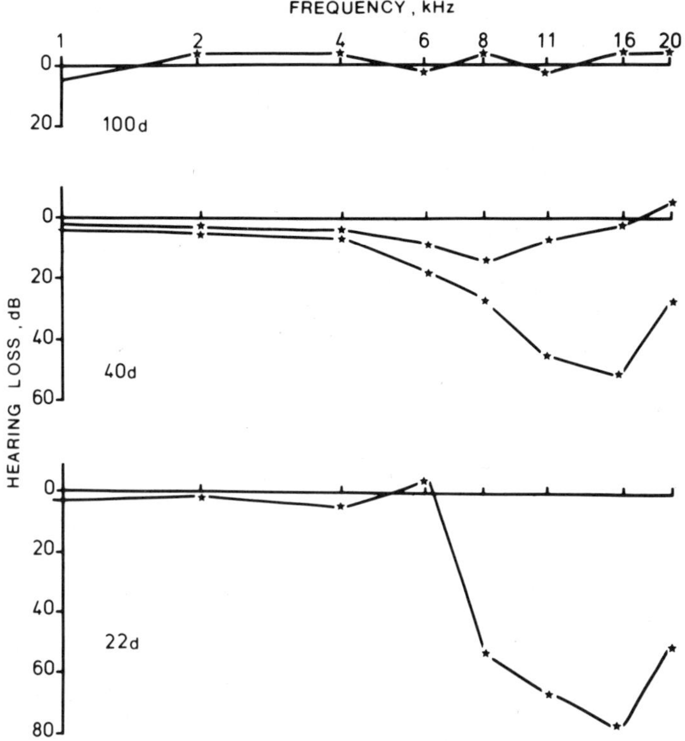

Fig. 3. Threshold elevation 55 days after white noise exposure (120 dB SPL, 30 min.) in rats exposed at 22, 40 and 100 days of age. The curves corresponding to the 22 (n = 6) and 100-day-old (n = 6) groups represent the mean values of the hearing deficit. The two curves of the 40-day-old group are taken from rats showing the greatest and smallest hearing losses.

and transmission electron microscopy [33]. In animals sacrificed 7 days after the white noise exposure, the surface preparation technique revealed only restricted areas that lacked occasional outer hair cells (OHCs) in the basal coil of the cochleas. However, with transmission electron microscopy, clear signs of cytoplasmic degeneration were found at the level of the OHCs and their afferent and efferent nerve supply (Figs. 4, 5, 6, 7) along the whole basal coil. Two months after the white noise exposure, these structures, as well as the inner hair cells and their associated afferent fibers, had completely degenerated. These results show that no immediate disruption of the organ of Corti results from 120 dB white noise exposure. On the other hand, different aspects of metabolic impairments may account for the traumatic processes [39].

Two kinds of complementary experiment were then conducted by the authors (unpublished results) to test the validity of the conclusions presented by Bock and Saunders [27] that changes in the acoustic reflex do not produce the critical period. Rats (100 days old) were subjected to 120 dB white noise for 30 minutes under deep nembutal anesthesia to abolish the acoustic reflex [40]. The results did not differ from those obtained in non-anesthetized rats exposed at the same age. The two groups of animals had no threshold shift 7 days after noise exposure. Identical findings were reported by Saunders and Bock [27] in 75-day-old animals.

In a second experiment, young (16, 20, and 28 days old) and adult (100 days old) rats were exposed to a high-frequency band of noise (6 to 16 kHz) of 110 dB SPL for 30 minutes; in this case, the acoustic reflex is less effectively activated than with a low-frequency band of noise. One month later, an evaluation of hearing function (CAP threshold) showed large threshold shifts in the young animals (60-80 dB losses), while in adults the deficits did not exceed 20 dB. These two sets of complementary experiments support the conclusion of Bock and Saunders [27] that the period of supra-sensitivity is of cochlear origin.

In summary, a critical period for acoustic trauma also exists in the rat, and this is probably a common feature of the developing mammalian cochlea. A period such as this could also exist in birds, as suggested by recent studies in chickens [41]. The critical period starts slightly before the end of cochlear maturation and extends well beyond this time. It is thus misleading to refer to an enhanced sensitivity to acoustic trauma during cochlear development. However, it must be remembered that cochlear maturation is classically determined by sensory and neural criteria. It may be that the maturational process is longer according to other criteria that take into account subtle biochemical [42] and/or micromechanical changes (e.g., coupling between OHCs and tectorial membrane).

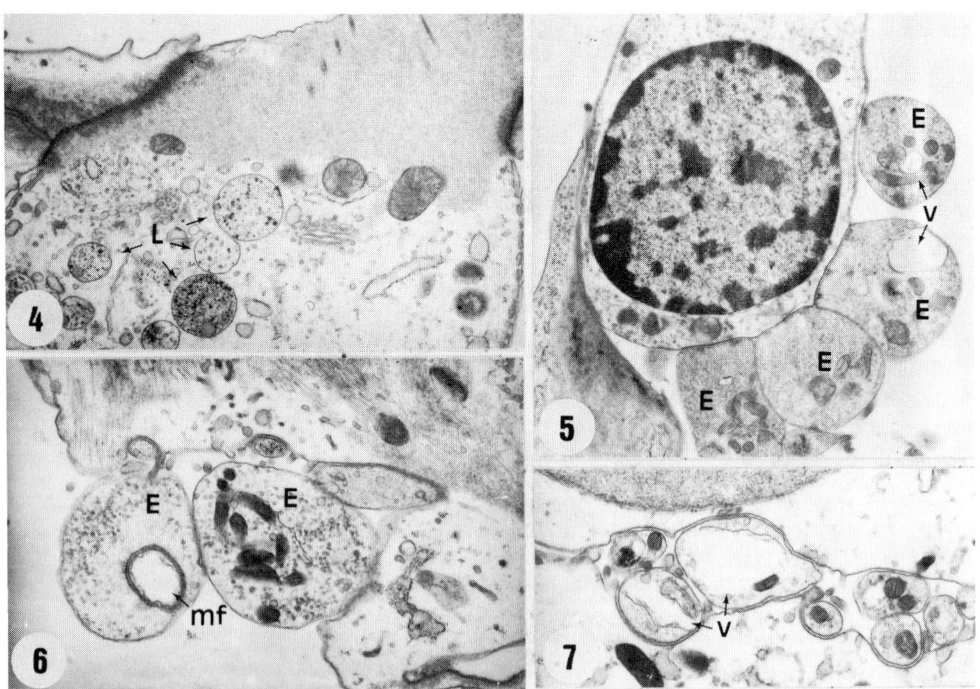

Figs. 4-7. Transmission electron microscopic aspect of cochlear structures (basal coil) in rats exposed at day 22 to the 120 dB white noise and sacrificed 7 days after. Fig. 4: Apical pole of one OHC containing numerous lysosomes (L). Figs. 4-5: Efferent endings (E) at the basal portion of one OHC. Note vacuoles (v) (Fig. 4) and myelin figures (mf) (Fig. 5). Fig. 6: Afferent spiral fibers between Deiter's cells with large vacuoles (v).

CRITICAL PERIODS DURING COCHLEAR DEVELOPMENT

The rat cochlea offers the possibility of comparing different critical periods of supra-normal sensitivity. Such a comparison could help to clarify the functional implications of these periods and improve our understanding of the basic mechanisms underlying them [43]. Considering the time course of the different critical periods (Fig. 1), we observe that a given causative agent acts preferentially during a given developmental event. However, the periods overlap, implying that two factors can simultaneously influence cochlear maturation. In the rat cochlea, for example, the period of development between 10 and 20 days after birth includes the end of the sensitive period for thyroid deficiency, the whole critical period for antibiotic ototoxicity, and the beginning of the critical period for acoustic trauma. This information, together with what is known about human cochlear development [44], indicates that there might be a period of heightened sensitivity to trauma during the second half of human pregnancy (Fig. 1), as well as during the perinatal period in premature infants. Special control of antibiotic treatment and acoustic environment is therefore advisable in premature infants.

Another issue is raised by data on the period of increased sensitivity to thyroid deficiency in the young rat [9]. It has recently been shown [45] that during this time more than one critical period is involved. With regard to the corrective effect of thyroxine injections, each cochlear structure has a slightly different critical period corresponding to the time at which the structure undergoes its main morphological changes. It can be hypothesized that multiple periods also underlie the supra-normal sensitivity to ototoxic and acoustic trauma. This notion could be of particular interest in understanding why the period of priming for audiogenic seizure overlaps the critical period for acoustic trauma [22,24,26].

Finally, we note the related findings on the supra-normal sensitivity of the cochlea to antibiotic ototoxicity with aging [46]. Anatomical and physiological studies [47-50] show that there is also a period of change within the cochlea with aging. Thus, as in the case of the developing cochlea, changes with aging could well be influenced by environmental factors that may result in an acceleration of the "normal" degenerative process.

ACKNOWLEDGEMENTS

Thanks are due to Sabine Ladrech and Pierre Sibleyras for technical support and to Anne Bara for editorial assistance.

REFERENCES

1. R. J. Ruben, Critical periods for language acquisition, Acta Oto-Laryngol., in press (1986).
2. I. Minoli and G. Moro, Constraints of intensive care units and follow up studies in prematures, Acta Otolaryngol. Suppl., 421:62 (1985).
3. K. P. Steel and G. R. Bock, Genetic factors affecting hearing development, Acta Otolaryngol., Suppl., 421:48 (1985).
4. J. H. Mills, Effects of noise on auditory sensitivity, psychophysical tuning curves, and suppression, in: "New Perspectives on Noise-Induced Hearing Losses," R. P. Hamernik, D. Henderson, and R. Salvi eds., Raven Press, New York (1982).
5. J. E. Hawkins, Drug ototoxicity, in: "Handbook of Sensory Physiology, Vol. 5: Auditory System, Part 3: Clinical and Special Topics," W. D. Keidel and W. D. Neff eds., Springer Verlag, Berlin (1976).

6. S. A. Falk and J. C. Farmer, Incubator noise and possible deafness, Arch. Otolaryngol., 97:385 (1973).
7. E. Douek, H. C. Dodson, L. H. Bannister, P. Ashcroft, and K. N. Humphries, Effects of incubator noise on the cochlea of the newborn, Lancet., 20:1110 (1976).
8. G. C. McCullagh and D. R. Watson, The noise exposure of infants in incubators, J. of Sound and Vibration, 67:231 (1979).
9. A. Uziel, Non-genetic factors affecting hearing development. Acta Otolaryngol., Suppl. 421:57 (1985).
10. R. Pujol, Period of sensitivity to antibiotic treatment, Acta Otolaryngol., Suppl., in press (1986).
11. J. C. Saunders and G. R. Bock, Influences of early auditory trauma on auditory development, in: "Studies on the Development of Behavior and the Nervous System," Vol. 4: Early Influences, G. Gottlieb ed., Academic Press, New York (1978).
12. R. P. Hamernik and D. Henderson, The potentiation of noise by other ototraumatic agents, in: "Effects of Noise on Hearing," D. Henderson, R. Hamernik, D. Dosanjh, and J. Mills eds., Raven Press, New York (1976).
13. M. Lenoir and R. Pujol, Effects combines de l'amikacine et du trauma acoustique sur la cochlee du raton pendant la periode de sensibilite critique, Acustica, 46:255 (1980).
14. H. C. Dodson, L. H. Bannister, and E. E. Douek, The effects of combined gentamicin and white noise on the spiral organ of young guinea pigs. A structural study, Acta Otolaryngol., 94:193 (1982).
15. S. A. Falk, R. O. Cook, J. K. Haseman, and G. M. Sanders, Noise-induced inner ear damage in newborns and adult guinea pigs. Laryngoscope, 84:444 (1974).
16. H. C. Dodson, L. H. Bannister, and E. E. Douek, Further studies of the effects of continuous white noise of moderate intensity (70-80 dB SPL) on the cochlea in young guinea pigs, Acta Otolaryngol., 88:195 (1978).
17. J. W. Coleman, Age-dependent changes and acoustic trauma in the spiral organ of the guinea pig, Scand. Audiol., 5:63 (1976).
18. G. R. Price, Age as a factor in susceptibility to hearing loss: young versus adult ears, J. Acoust. Soc. Am., 60:886 (1976).
19. R. Pujol and D. Hilding, Anatomy and physiology of the onset of auditory function, Acta Otolaryngol., 76:1 (1973).
20. J. C. Saunders, G. R. Bock, C. S. Chen, and G. R. Gates, The effects of priming for audiogenic seizures on cochlear and behavioral responses in BALB/c mice, Exp. Neurol., 36:426 (1972).
21. C. S. Chen, G. R. Gates, and G. R. Bock, Effect of priming and tympanic membrane destruction on development of audiogenic seizure susceptibility in BALB/c mice, Exp. Neurol., 39:277 (1973).
22. J. C. Saunders and K. A. Hirsch, Changes in cochlear microphonic sensitivity after priming C57Bl/6J mice at various ages for audiogenic seizures, J. Comp. Physiol. Psychol., 90:212 (1976).
23. K. R. Henry, Abnormal auditory development resulting from exposure to ototoxic chemicals, noise, and auditory restriction, in: "Development of Auditory and Vestibular Systems," R. Romand ed., Academic Press, New York (1983).
24. K. R. Henry, Noise and the young mouse: Genotype modifies the sensitive period for effects on cochlear physiology and audiogenic seizures, Behavioral Neuroscience, 98:1073 (1984).
25. M. S. Deol, Inherited diseases of the inner ear in man in the light of studies on the mouse, J. Med. Gen., 5:137 (1968).
26. R. Stanek, G. R. Bock, M. L. Goran, and J. C. Saunders, Age-dependent susceptibility to auditory trauma in the hamster; Behavioral and electrophysiological consequences, Transactions of the American Academy of Ophthalmology and Otolaryngology, 84:465 (1977).

27. G. R. Bock and J. C. Saunders, A critical period for acoustic trauma in the hamster and its relation to cochlear development, Science, 197:396 (1977).
28. C. B. Stephens, Development of the middle and inner ear in the golden hamster (Mesocricetus auratus), Acta Otolaryngol., Suppl. ,296 (1972).
29. R. Pujol and M. Abonnenc, Receptor maturation and synaptogenesis in the golden hamster cochlea, Arch. Oto-Rhino-Laryngol., 217:1 (1977).
30. A. Shnerson and R. Pujol, Development: Anatomy, electrophysiology and behavior, in: "The Auditory Psychobiology of the Mouse," J. F. Willot ed., C. C. Thomas, Springfield (1983).
31. G. R. Bock and E. J. Seifter, Developmental changes of susceptibility to auditory fatigue in young hamsters, Audiology, 17:193 (1978).
32. M. Lenoir, G. R. Bock, and R. Pujol, Supra-normal susceptibility to acoustic trauma in the rat pup cochlea, J. Physiol. (Paris), 75:521 (1979).
33. M. Lenoir and R. Pujol, Sensitive period to acoustic trauma in the rat pup cochlea: histological findings, Acta Otolaryngol., 89:317 (1980).
34. T. Wada, Anatomical and physiological studies on the growth of the inner ear of the albino rat, Memoirs of the Wistar Institute of Anatomy and Biology, 10 (1923).
35. D. E. Crowley and M. C. Hepp-Reymond, Development of cochlear function in the ear of the infant rat, J. Comp. Physiol. Psychol., 62:427 (1966).
36. M. Lenoir, A. Shnerson, and R. Pujol, Cochlear receptor development in the rat with emphasis on synaptogenesis, Anat. Embryol., 160:253 (1980).
37. A. Uziel, R. Romand, and M. Marot, Development of cochlear potentials in rats, Audiology, 20:89 (1980).
38. E. Carlier, M. Lenoir, and R. Pujol, Development of cochlear frequency selectivity tested by compound action potential tuning curves, Hearing Res., 1:197 (1979).
39. B. A. Bohne, Mechanisms of noise damage in the inner ear, in: "Effects of Noise on Hearing," D. Henderson, R. Hamernik, D. Dosanjh, and J. Mills, Raven Press, New York (1976).
40. R. Wersall, The tympanic muscles and their reflexes, Acta Otolaryngol., Suppl. 139 (1958).
41. H. Cousillas and G. Rebillard, Age-dependent effects of a pure tone trauma in the chick basilar papilla: Evidence for a development of the tonotopic organization, Hearing Res., in press (1985).
42. J. Dau, L. H. Bannister, D. B. Gower, R. W. Evans, and E. E. Douek, Developmental changes in the polypeptide profiles of different cochlear regions in rodents, Trans. Biochem. Soc., in press (1985).
43. J. J. Eggermont, Defining and determining sensitive periods, Acta Otolaryngol., Suppl., in press (1986).
44. R. Pujol, Morphology, synaptology and electrophysiology of the developing cochlea, Acta Otolaryngol., Suppl., 421:5 (1985).
45. A. Uziel, C. Legrand, and A. Rabie, Corrective effects of thyroxine on cochlear abnormalities induced by congenital hypothyroidism in the rat. I. Morphological study, Dev. Brain Res., 19:111 (1985).
46. K. R. Henry, R. A. Chole, M. D. McGinn, and D. P. Frush, Increased ototoxicity in both young and old mice, Arch. Otolaryngol., 107:92 (1981).
47. J. F. Corso, Auditory processes and aging: Significant problems for research, Exp. Aging Res., 10:171 (1984).
48. E. M. Keithley and M. L. Feldman, Hair cell counts in an age-graded series of rat cochleas, Hearing Res., 8:249 (1982).
49. G. Bredberg, The human cochlea during development and aging, J. Laryngol., 81:739 (1967).

50. J. F. Willott, Changes in frequency representation in the auditory system of mice with age-related hearing impairment, Brain Res., 309:159 (1984).

DISCUSSION

Borhgrevink: What if a pregnant mother was exposed to noise levels below 100 dB. Would that by any chance harm the hearing of the baby in utero?

Lenoir: I think that noise by itself is unlikely to impair the cochlea of babies in utero.

Cody: When you have an air, water interface, then something like 99.5 percent of the acoustic energy is reflected. So I would suggest for levels less than 100 dB, there is not any chance of hearing loss.

Bock: There have been a number of studies looking at hearing in babies who are born very prematurely. The main problem here is likely to arise with incubator sounds, and the evidence here is very confusing. Other studies suggest that these babies have a higher probability of having a hearing loss. Some studies show no difference. But I suspect that this is an impossible problem to resolve because a premature baby is exposed to a lot of other risk factors besides incubator noise, including toxic antibiotics and of course all the other perinatal risk factors.

Olena: I work in the audiology department at Turin University. We have performed about 10,000 audiological evaluations in babies after birth, and we have followed the babies for several years. We have never found any noise-induced hearing loss in these babies. Also, we have never found noise-induced hearing loss in babies followed up in our clinic.

Lenoir: Perhaps the hearing losses cannot be detected by the normal approach. Perhaps some subtle impairments will be reflected later in the understanding of language or frequency selectivity. These changes may not be detected with the audiogram.

von Gierke: Did you say that in animals, the period of maximum sensitivity to noise is the same as the maximum sensitivity to ototoxic drugs?

Lenoir: No. The time courses of those two factors are different. But the critical period for antibotics in rats overlaps the critical period for noise for a short period of time.

von Gierke: Is there any indication in humans that there is a period of increased sensitivity to ototoxic drugs.

Lenoir: It is very difficult to determine if there is a critical period for drugs in humans. Unfortunately, we are faced with having to extrapolate from animal studies.

THE ACOUSTIC REFLEX IN INDUSTRIAL IMPACT NOISE

Roland Nilsson

Research Department
Projekt Lindholmen
Goteborg, Sweden

SOUND ENERGY AND TRANSMISSION

The purpose of the transmission system of the ear (outer and middle ear) is to receive and transmit the sound waves to the inner ear (Fig. 1). From the viewpoint of energy, this is done by means of a number of transformations; from the acoustic energy of the air to a mechanical motion energy on the part of the eardrum and the chain of auditory bones. Then, the hydro-mechanical motion of the inner ear is converted into bioelectrical energy in the hair cells and the auditory nerve. At low and moderate sound levels, the transmission characteristic of the sound transmission system is primarily linear and the amount of energy transmitted to the cochlea is determined by the resonance of the outer ear and the amplification of the middle ear [1]. At higher sound levels, the acoustic middle ear reflex (AR) is activated causing the impedance of the system to increase and the transmission of the sound energy to decrease.

It can be assumed that relatively small individual differences in the energy transmission may significantly contribute to variations in sensitivity to noise injury. A transmission loss with the magnitude of 10 dB is regarded as being of no importance so far as actual hearing ability is concerned. At noise levels which may be injurious, e.g., 100 dB(A), a reduction by 10 dB down to 90 dB(A), however, is of considerable importance. According to ISO R 1999, the number of noise-injured persons in the 10-year-exposed population is decreased from 29% to 10% with such a reduction.

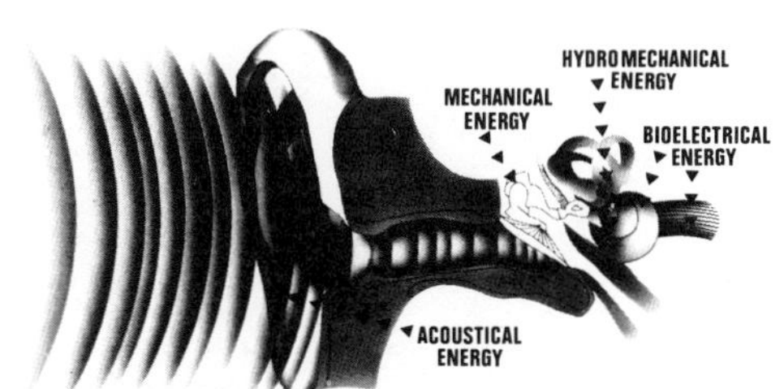

Fig. 1. Energy transformation in the auditory periphery system.

THE PROTECTIVE EFFECT OF TRANSMISSION LOSS IN THE MIDDLE EAR

Transmission losses caused by damage to the middle ear provide an example of a sound reduction which may reduce the degree of a noise injury. Observations have also shown that persons with chronic conductive loss have received a certain protective effect [2]. Results to the contrary, however, have also been reported; the sensori-neural component has been reported as greater in ears with conductive hearing loss [3]. A complicating factor is that acute and chronic infections in the middle ear, as well as otosclerosis, by themselves, can cause sensori-neural hearing loss [4]. It also seems that ears with chronic purulent otitis media or otosclerosis are more vulnerable to noise than non-infected ears.

In order to be able to draw any conclusions as to whether conductive hearing loss has a protective effect in noise which is hazardous to hearing, it is necessary to make a strict selection of the population studied and, in so doing, exclude other potential reasons for the impaired hearing than noise. With that in mind, a retrospective study of shipyard workers was carried out using individuals with one-sided transmission loss [5]. Eight persons were selected from a large population of workers who had been exposed to noise. The persons selected had one-sided conductive loss, established prior to the noise exposure period without repeated episodes of acute or chronic infection or clinically diagnosed otosclerosis. Fig. 2 gives examples of the appearance of the audiogram from one of the trial subjects. In the left ear where there is no transmission loss, there is a pronounced sensori-neural reduction, while the bone conduction of the right ear is rather insignificantly affected. All eight trial subjects showed similar results, with a pronounced sensori-neural loss at 4 kHz in ears with a normal middle ear function. Thus, the results show the value of a transmission loss as regards protection against noise injury. A direct comparison between the protective effect of chronic transmission loss and the protective effect of AR is, of course, not possible. The chronic conductive loss constitutes a static reduction in the energy transmission, without reaction time, adaptation, and dynamic adjustment as is the case with AR.

In order to evaluate the protective effect of AR in industrial impact noise, it is necessary to critically study results where the different parameters of the AR have been determined by means of clinical methods.

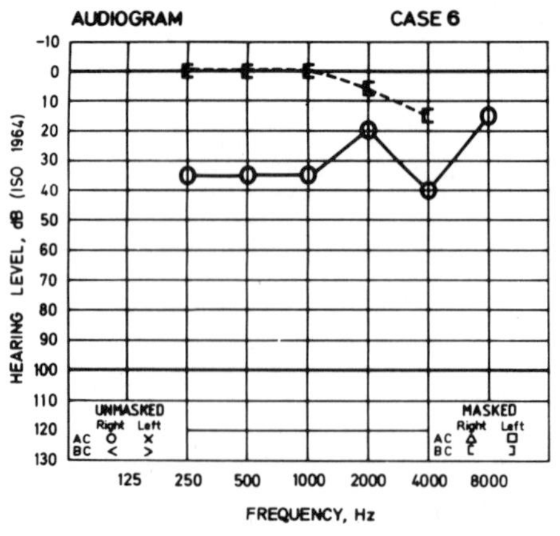

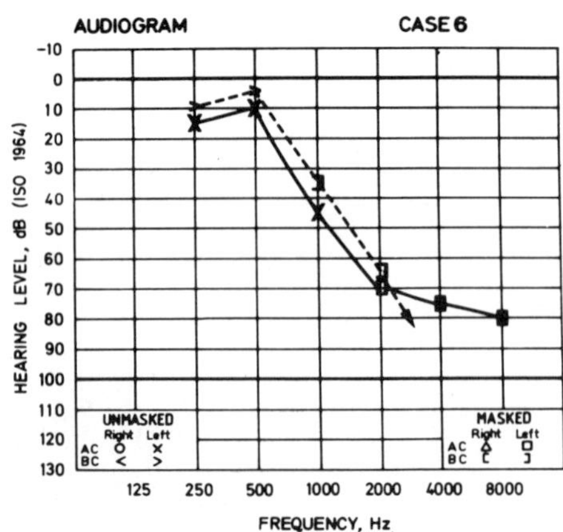

Fig. 2. Pure tone audiograms of a welder exposed to shipyard noise for 30 years. The left-hand audiogram shows air and bone thresholds of the ear with conductive hearing loss; the right-hand audiogram shows the ear without conductive hearing loss [5].

THRESHOLD VALUES IN AR

If the acoustic reflex is to give any protective effect, it must be activated at sound levels which are well below the levels hazardous to hearing. If, for instance, a person is exposed to a noise environment with levels of about 95 dB(A) and is to have a maximal contraction, the threshold value should be 70-75 dB(A). The normal values given in the literature for contralateral AR thresh (ART) are in the range 70-90 dB(A) SPL for broad-band sound stimuli [6]. It should be noticed, however, that these values refer to monaural presentation via earphones. In the case of industrial situations, lower ART values may be expected, as the activating noise most often is presented binaurally in a pseudo-free sound field. Moller [7] has shown that the ipsilateral reflex threshold may be 2 to 14 dB lower than the contralateral reflex, and that binaural stimulation may give an additional reduction in the ART by 3 dB. There are practical complications when measuring the ART under realistic noise conditions, but it can still be assumed that the ART in most persons with normal hearing is sufficiently low.

REDUCTION

In order for the AR to be an important protective factor, its reduction is of great significance. At the same time, it is probably the parameter which is most difficult to evaluate. In animals, the effect of the middle ear muscles on sound transmission in the middle ear has been studied using direct methods, e.g., cochlear microphonic (CM) determinations [8]. It has been found that frequencies up to 2-4 kHz are reduced by 20 dB in cats and rabbits [9].

In humans, however the reduction has been investigated mostly by using indirect methods. Borg [10] studied the AR in patients who had one-sided acute facial paresis, so-called Bell's palsy, with concomitant paresis of the stapedius muscle. The AR response was determined on the contralateral side before and after the recovery from the paresis. The reduction was determined by comparing the stimulus response curves, i.e., the growth function of the reflex. At 500 Hz, the reduction was about 20 dB. At higher frequencies, the reduction was lower and at 1.5 kHz, only a small reduction could be observed at maximum muscle contraction. Similar results have been reported by Rabinowitz [11] and Zakrisson [12]. Brask [13] obtained reduction on values up to 30 dB in patients with Bell's palsy. Morgan and Dirks [14], on the other hand, evaluated the reduction and found it to be only 8 dB. All reports seem to agree that AR does not give any reduction at high frequencies in the range where the noise injury is most pronounced. The development of a reliable method to determine the AR reduction in individual persons in an unselected population would be valuable.

TIME PATTERN

The long latency time in AR is a characteristic which has caused many authors to consider AR to be of no importance in the case of impulse sound exposure. Attempts to alleviate this limitation have been made, however. In humans, Fletcher and Riopelle [15] succeeded in obtaining a significant reduction in the TTS after exposure to impulse sound. They introduced a "protective tone" 200 ms prior to the impulse, sufficient to activate the AR during the course of the impulse sound. Fletchen's experiments were reproduced by Hilding [16], who worked with cats. He exposed his animals to the same type of impulse noise as Fletcher. The protective effect in the middle ear muscles was demonstrated with CM-recordings.

On the whole, latency time is regarded as a measurement of the nerve transmission time in the reflex arch. When it is determined directly by means of electro-myography, the results show the nerve transmission speed and the delays in the synapses. When the latency time is based on determinations of the impedance of the ear, other mechanisms are added, e.g., the muscle contraction time and mechanical delays in the middle ear. From the viewpoint of protection, latency time determinations based on impedance changes are the most relevant ones. This is fortunate, as most available data has been obtained by means of impedance recordings. These determinations show that latency time is of the magnitude 50-100 msec. The maximal contraction is obtained after an additional 100-200 msec. [17,18]. The rise time of an impulse (e.g., the striking sound of a sledge-hammer) is of the magnitude 50-100 microseconds. Thus, a single impulse can pass through the middle ear without any activation or with a delayed activation of the AR. With such stimulation, the AR cannot bring about any protective effect for the inner ear.

On the other hand, the impulses present in industrial noise often occur in series and often they are superimposed on a noise background. The relaxation time or the fall time in AR can in such cases be of importance. The relaxation time of the reflex is longer than the contraction time. Based on impedance determinations, the relaxation time is reported to be in the magnitude of 100-500 msec for the maximal amplitude response to decreased by 50%; in many cases, more than 1 sec. is required for total relaxation. These observations show that if the pulse frequency is sufficiently high, the stimulation can be affected by a contraction of the stapedius muscle. The importance of such mechanisms is relatively unknown so far.

FATIGABILITY

A great deal of interest has been focused on the stability and fatigability of the stapedius reflex using constant, pure tones and noise signals [19-23]. All these studies show very rapid fatigability in the AR. The obvious conclusion on the basis of these studies is that for durations that commonly occur in industrial noise exposure, (e.g., a typical 8-hour working day), the actual protective function of the AR is insignificant because of fatigability. It has also been shown, however that the AR can be reactivated after a short pause [24-26] or after a change in the intensity or frequency of the sound [27].

Industrial noise varies with respect to frequency and intensity, but has a considerably longer duration than the stimuli used by Luscher [24]. It is therefore difficult or impossible, on the basis of these data, to predict how the AR will react during a working day in an industrial environment.

In order to investigate this, two fatigability studies have been carried out [28,29]. In the first study, 18 trial subjects with normal hearing were exposed monaurally to a 30-minute-long sequence of taped shipyard noise. Fig. 3 shows the recording from one of the trial subjects. The first and the last minute of the exposure were identical, in order to make possible a comparison between the reflex activities. The results showed that the AR is conspicuously resistent to fatigability during exposure to a representative industrial noise. The inter-individual difference was considerable, however; some trial subjects showed a great deal of fatigability while others showed improvement after the exposure.

The results after exposure for about 30 minutes, however, do not provide an answer to the question of what would happen after exposure during a

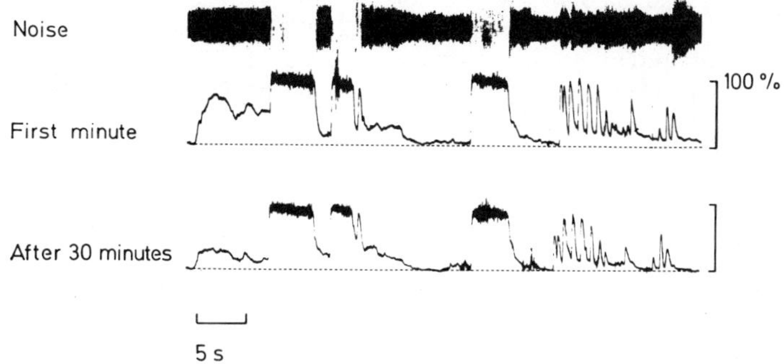

Fig. 3. Response of the contralateral stapedius reflex to shipyard noise [28].

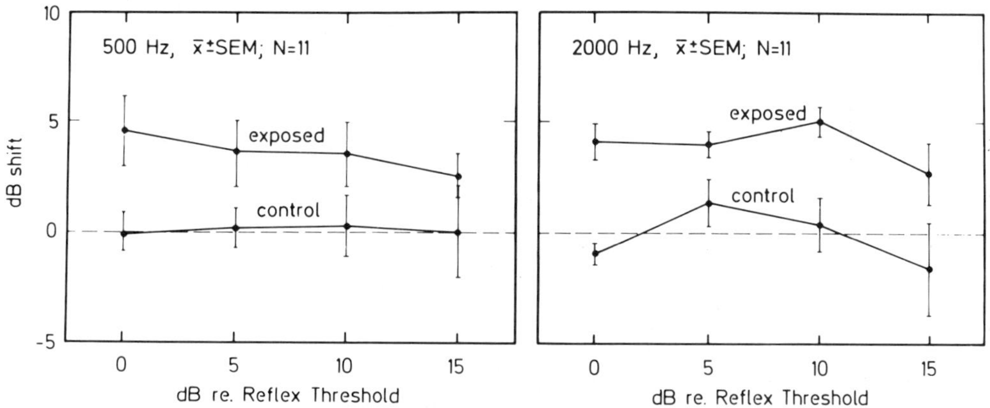

Fig. 4. Left: Average valus of AR shift at 500 Hz in the exposed ear and the control ear approximately 15 minutes after the end of the work day. Right: Average values of AR shift at 2000 Hz in the exposed ear and the non-exposed control approximately 10 minutes after the end of the work day. [29]

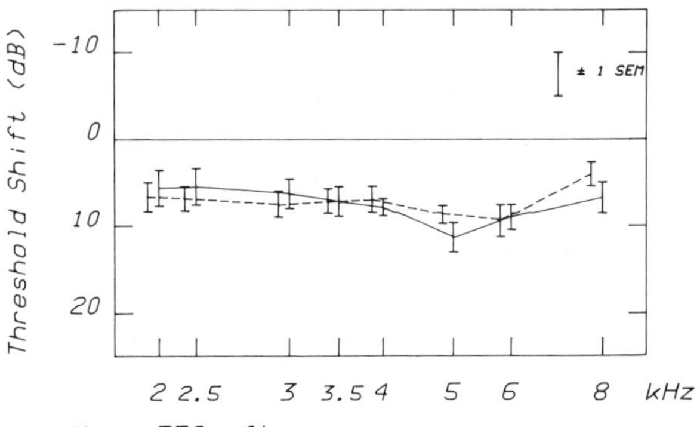

Fig. 5. TTS after exposure to continuous noise (unbroken line) and intermittent noise (broken line).

full working day. Therefore, a field study was performed. Eleven young shipyard workers with normal hearing were exposed approximately 7 hours at their regular work places. One ear was protected by means of an ear plug and served as control. Changes in the AR were evaluated using ipsilateral and contralateral reflex determinations and by comparing the stimulus response functions prior to and after the exposure. The mean values of the changes are shown in Fig. 4. The average displacement of the stimulus response curves was 3.5 dB on the exposed side while, on the whole, the protected ear was unaffected. Thus, a relatively small fatigue effect was shown. Furthermore, all the trial subjects showed reflex activity after the working day, although several of them had been exposed to noise up to 105 dB(A), (Leq = 7 h). These observations mean that the AR may provide a protective mechanism for the inner ear during noise exposure. It should be pointed out that shipyard noise exposure is extremely complex. In addition to the profuse presence of impulse noise from sledges and hammers, there is a low-frequency background noise and intermittent, intensive high-frequency noise from pneumatic hand tools. If the noise exposure consists only of continuous tones or broad-band noise, one cannot expect any endurance on the part of the AR. One way of improving such a working situation and of reaching optimal AR activity may be to introduce variations in the exposure, e.g., by taking short, silent intermissions.

In some pilot investigations, we have examined the importance of short intermissions. In the first investigation, we examined 9 trial subjects who were exposed both to a 10 minute long continuous broad-band noise (107 dB(A)) and to a 10-minute-long intermittent broad-band noise with 10-second intermissions every 50 seconds (109 dB(A)). Each trial subject participated four times. On two occasions, the reflex fatigability was determined by means of contralateral stimulus response functions. On the other two test occasions, TTS was determined by means of sweep frequency audiometry. Both exposures give, on the average, a certain AR fatigability effect, but there was no significant difference between continuous and intermittent exposures. Fig. 5 shows the TTS results. A certain displacement of the maximal TTS has occured, presumably caused by the influence of AR on the middle ear resonance. The intermittent exposure also gives a significant decrease of TTS in this range.

PROTECTIVE EFFECT

It appears that the AR under special conditions can reduce injury to the inner ear. On the other hand, it is questionable whether the hearing loss caused by industrial noise is really affected by the AR.

Arguments which have been presented against the AR as a protective function are: (1) The AR is quickly fatigued at high noise levels; (2) The AR reduces only low-frequency sound whereas the injuries appear primarily in the high-frequency region; (3) The AR reduction is too small to have a protective effect, even at low frequencies (4) The reaction time in AR is too long to affect impulse noise. If impulse noise is the main cause of impaired hearing, the AR, consequently, would have a negligible effect.

TTS experiments have been performed in man [30] and PTS experiments in rabbit [31] in order to evaluate the protective effect of the AR during exposure to industrial noise. The noise used in the exposures was similar to the noise used in the previously discussed fatigability studies. The original recordings were made using a microphone placed near the ear of a plater who worked in the welding shop of a shipyard. Noise from different hand tools, such as nut tighteners, pneumatic chisel hammers and hand sledges, contributed to the characteristic feature of the noise. The background level fluctuated between 85 and 95 dB(A) and also contained a great deal of impulse noise at very high levels. TTS was determined in 10 trail persons after exposure to taped shipyard noise. These subjects had acute one-sided facial paresis (Bell's palsy). Thus, the patients had no middle ear reflex in the affected ear. On the non-affected side, the ipsilateral reflex threshold was normal. In order to participate, the trial subjects had to have normal hearing thresholds, i.e., a threshold within 15 dB HL (ISO-389-1975) between 0.125 and 8 kHz. They were exposed for 15 minutes via earphones. On one test occasion, the affected ear was exposed; a few days later, the normal ear was exposed. The noise dose was 102 dB(A) or Leq (15 min). The hearing thresholds were determined by means of sweep frequency audiometry (type Bekesy) before and immediately after the exposure to noise.

The mean values of TTS as a function of frequency are illustrated in Fig. 6. The TTS was greatest in ears which lacked the middle ear reflex. The frequency of maximum TTS reduction shifted from about 4 kHz (3.750 kHz) to the important speech frequency range (2.075 kHz). TTS became broader with an expansion primarily toward the lower frequencies. In order to get an idea of the total reduction, the TTS surface was evaluated. This surface was significantly larger in the affected ears than in the normal ears. Summarizing the TTS test, TTS increases and expands downward in frequency after exposure to shipyard noise when there is no AR.

The PTS studies were performed in a total of seven adult rabbits. A 15-minute-long portion of the taped shipyard noise was used for exposure at three different levels: 120, 125, and 130 dB(A), Leq (15 min). Electrophysiological hearing thresholds were obtained by means of brainstem audiometry for narrow band stimuli. The AR activity prior to the exposure was determined in non-anaesthetized trial animals. Bilaterally normal reflex thresholds were considered as an indication of normal middle ears, symmetry of the inner ear function and normal hearing. In one of the trial animals, the stapedius muscle was denervated by destroying the facial nerve on one side.

Since both the stapedius muscles and the tensor tympani muscles can be triggered acoustically in rabbits, and since their common effect has a reduction which is similar to the reduction brought about by the stapedius muscle alone in man, it was desired to have a trial model with both muscles denervated. This was accomplished by means of anaesthesia (Nembutal, 40 mg/kg), as middle ear surgery should be avoided. Thus, most of the trial animals were anaesthetized on one side during the exposure. The normal and the "deactivated" ears were exposed in random order. The contralateral ear was exposed about one month after the first exposure. This was done to minimize possible interaction effects. During the noise exposure, the AR was recorded in the non-anaesthetized animals. This recording gives information about the function of the inner ear (TTS and PTS) and about the fatigability of the middle ear reflex. Finally, the inner ear specimens were examined by means of scanning electron microscopy.

In all cases, PTS was greater in ears without the AR than in those with an intact AR. At higher exposure levels, the difference was pronounced. Fig. 7 shows the threshold changes in brain stem audiometry in the protected and the non-protected ear in one of the trial animals where the stapedius muscle has been denervated on one side. A pronounced difference in PTS can be observed. PTS exceeding 25 dB at any test frequency in the protected ear could not be observed in any of the test animals. There was no clear 4 kHz dip on any side. In the unprotected ear, there was always a broad change in the brainstem audiometric thresholds. On the whole, the change corresponded to the spectrum of the noise but was about one octave higher in frequency. Logical and pronounced morphological differences between the ears were also observed. In summary, it can be said that the PTS results in trial animals were similar to the TTS in man. PTS appears in the frequency range which corresponds to the energy distribution of the noise exposure in individuals who lack a normal AR.

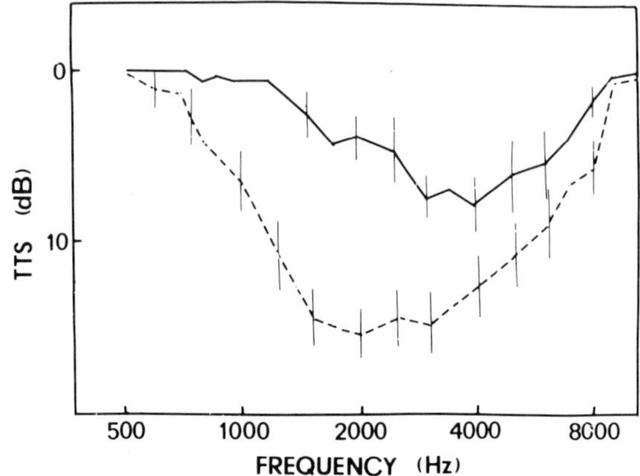

Fig. 6. Mean values and SEM of TTS in the non-affected (unbroken line) and affected ear (broken line) for 10 subjects with unilateral stapedius muscle paralysis [30].

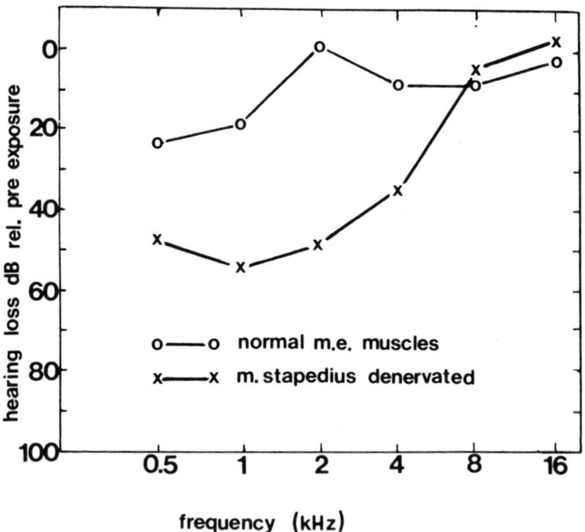

Fig. 7. Permanent threshold shift in a noise-exposed rabbit with unilaterally denervated stapedius muscle [31].

ACKNOWLEDGEMENTS

This work was supported by grant 84-1375 from the Swedish Work Environment Fund.

REFERENCES

1. J. Tonndorf, Relationship between the transmission characteristics of the conductive system and noise-induced hearing loss, in: "Effects of noise on hearing", D. Henderson, R.P. Hamernik, D.S. Dosanjh, and J.H. Mills, eds., Raven Press, New York (1976).
2. J. Temkin, Die Schadigung des Ohres durch Larm und Erschutterung, Monatsschr. Ohrenheilk Laryngol-Rhinol. 67:257 (1933).
3. D. L. Chadwik, The behavior of the pathological ear in noise, Acta Oto Rhino. Laryngol. (Belgica). 25:113 (1971).
4. M. M. Paparella, D. R. Brady, and R. Hoel, Sensori-neural hearing loss in chronic otitis media and mastoiditis, Trans. Am. Acad. Ophthalmol. Otolaryngol. 74:108 (1970).
5. R. Nilsson and E. Borg, Noise-induced hearing loss in shipyard workers with unilateral conductive hearing loss, Scand. Audiol. 12:135 (1983).
6. S. Geldfand, The contralateral acoustic-reflex threshold, in: "The acoustic reflex," S. Silman, ed., Academic Press, New York and London (1984).
7. A. R. Moller, Acoustic reflex in man, J. Acoust. Soc. Am. 34:1534 (1962).
8. F. B. Simmons, Middle ear muscle protection from the acoustic trauma of loud continuous sound. An electrophysiological study in cats, Ann. Otol. Rhinol. Laryngol. 69:1063 (1960).
9. E. Borg, Acoustic middle ear reflexes: A sensory-control system, Acta Otolaryngol. (Stockh.), Suppl. 304 (1972).
10. E. Borg, A quantitative study of the effect of the acoustic stapedius reflex on sound transmission through the middle ear of man, Acta Otolaryngol. (Stockh.), 66:461 (1968).
11. W. M. Rabinowitz, Acoustic-reflex effects on the input admittanc and transfer characteristics of the human middle ear, Thesis. Massachusetts Institute of Technology, (1977).
12. J.-E. Zakrisson, The effect of the stapedius reflex on attenuation and poststimulatory auditory fatigue at different frequencies, Acta Otolaryngol. (Stockh.), Suppl. 360:118 (1979).
13. T. Brask, Extratympanic manometry in man, Scand. Audiol. Suppl. 7:134 (1977).
14. D. E. Morgan, and D. D. Dirks, Influence of middle-ear muscle contraction on pure-tone suprathreshold loudness judgements, J. Acoust. Soc. Am. 57:411 (1975).
15. J. L. Fletcher, and A. J. Riopelle, Protective effect of the acoustic reflex for impulsive noises, J. Acoust. Soc. Am. 32:401 (1960).
16. D. A. Hilding, The protective value of the stapedius reflex: An experimental study, Trans. Am. Acad. Ophtal. Otolaryngol. 65:297 (1961).
17. B. Johansson, B. Kylin, and M. Langfy, Acoustic reflex as a test of individual susceptibility to noise, Acta Otolaryngol. (Stockh.), 64:256 (1967).
18. G. Liden, E. Nilsson, O. Laaskinen, B. E. Roos, and J. Miller, The stapedius reflex and motor reaction time: A parallel investigation of the effect of drugs, Scand. Audiol. 3:73 (1974).
19. P. Dallos, "The Auditory Periphery, Biophysics and Physiology," Academic Press, New York and London (1973).
20. T. Kato, Zur Physiologie der Binnenmuskeln des Ohres, Pflugers Arch. 150:569 (1913).
21. R. Wersall, The tympanic muscles and their reflexes, Act Otolaryngol. (Stockh.), Suppl. 139:43 (1958).
22. H. Anderson, B. Barr, and E. Wedenberg, Intra-aural reflexes in retrocochlear lesions, in: "Disorders of the skull base region," C.A. Hamberger and J. Wersall, eds., Almqvist & Wiksell, Nobel symposium 10, Stockholm (1969).

23. G. Tietze, Zum Zeitverhalten des Akustischen Reflexes bei Reizung mit Dauertonen, Arch. Ohr. Nas. Kehlkopfheilk, 193:43 (1969).
24. E. Luscher, Die Funktion des Musclulus stapedius beim Menschen, Z Hals. Nas. Ohrheilk. 25:462 (1930).
25. O. Metz, Studies on the contraction of the tympanic muscles as indicated by changes in the impedance of the ear, Acta Otolaryngol. (Stockh.), 39:397 (1951).
26. E. Borg, and B. Odman, Decay and recovery of the acoustic stapedius reflex in humans, Acta Otolaryngol. (Stockh.), 87:421 (1979).
27. K. Gjaevenes, and Th. Sohoel, Reactivating the acoustic stapedius muscle reflex by adding a second tone, Acta Otolaryngol. (Stockh.), 62:213 (1966).
28. R. Nilsson, E. Borg, and G Liden, Fatigability of the stapedius reflex in industrial noise, Acta Otolaryngol. 89:433 (1980).
29. E. Borg, R. Nilsson, and G. Liden, Fatigability of the stapedius reflex in industrial noise: A field study, Acta Otolaryngol. 94:385 (1982).
30. J.-E. Zakrisson, E. Borg, G. Liden, and R. Nilsson, Stapedius reflex in industrial impact noise: Fatigability and role for temporary threshold shift (TTS), Scand. Audiol. Suppl. 12:326 (1980).
31. E. Borg, R. Nilsson, and B. Engstrom, Effect of the acoustic reflex on inner ear damage induced by industrial noise, Acta Otolaryngol. 96:361 (1983).

DISCUSSION

Patuzzi: Studies by A. Cody and later by Rajan suggests that there may be a crossed cochlear effect which might be a confounding influence in some of your work. For example, in the Bell's palsy case, where the middle ear reflex is absent, there is still the possibility of a cochlea-to-cochlea reflex that might afford a certain degree of protection.

Nilsson: I agree, but I have no more comments about that.

Henderson: Eric Borg reported on an animal who developed a large amount of TTS and large reflex shifts. Eventually, sensitivity recovered but the acoustic reflex never recovered its normal sensitivity. Have you ever found similar results in any of your experiments or can you see any indication of permanent change of reflex sensitivity without a change in cochlear function?

Nilsson: There is a difference between man and rabbit. We can use the acoustic reflex threshold measurement as an indication of permanent noise-induced hearing loss in the rabbit, but not the case in man. Also, Barit Engstrom analyzed the cochleas and found the lesions to be almost exclusively to inner hair cells. I would like to give that question to Barit.

Engstrom: I think those animals, we later found out, had more or less pure inner hair cell damage. At the time you heard about them, they were not analyzed morphologically.

NOISE HISTORY, AUDIOMETRIC PROFILE, AND ACOUSTIC REFLEX RESPONSIVITY

V. Colletti and V. Sittoni

ENT Department
University of Verona
Policlinico, Borga Roma, 37100 Verona, Italy

INTRODUCTION

For several years there has been a debate in the literature on the effectiveness of the stapedius reflex in attenuating the acoustic input to the cochlea and its potential for reducing the amount of noise-induced hearing loss [1-10]. Several features of the acoustic reflex seemed to suggest that the attenuation provided by the stapedius contraction is irrelevant for protection of the inner ear to acoustic overstimulation: (1) the long latency and rise time of the stapedius reflex would allow single transient sounds to pass through the middle ear without being attenuated by the reflex [1]; (2) the attenuation resulting from the stapedius reflex is quantitatively too small to protect the inner ear from high sound levels and is effective outside the frequency range where noise-induced hearing loss primarily occurs [2-6]; (3) the response decays rapidly in the presence of continuous stimulation and thus the reflex is practically inactive for most of the exposure time [7-11]. Most of these conclusions had been derived from studies that had utilized simple acoustic stimuli (continuous pure tones and noise) and experimental laboratory conditions (low levels of background noise), which differ from the actual noise situation in industrial environments. Most frequently, noise encountered in industry is fluctuating with respect to both frequency and intensity. In addition, during the work period the noise may fall to levels below the stapedius reflex threshold between periods of high noise exposure. Given the profound differences between the stimuli encountered in laboratory and industrial situations, it is difficult to predict how the stapedius reflex would act in an industrial noise environment.

When studies on the acoustic reflex were performed in industrial environments or with experimental designs simulating industrial noise conditions, quite different conclusions were obtained. It was observed that the acoustic stapedius reflex was resistant to fatigue when stimulated by sounds which varied in spectrum over time [8-11]. It could be demonstrated that impulses are in fact attenuated by the acoustic reflex [12] in some experimental conditions and in many industrial noise environments where high levels of background noise result in acoustic reflex activity [13]. In addition, a series of impulses may be superimposed on the background noise and since the stapedius reflex has a slow onset-offset latency and slow rise-decay time, apart from the first impulse, all the subsequent impulses in a series will be attenuated. In fact, each of the impulses, except the first, will find the stapedius in a state of contraction. In addition, if the worker is paying attention to what he is doing and thus expecting the impulse, a preparatory or anticipatory contraction of the stapedius muscle is to be expected. Thus, even the first impulse might be attenuated.

Several studies with humans have shown that the attenuation of sound by the stapedius reflex is high (20 dB) in the low frequency range and small or absent at high frequencies [4,5,14,15]. Both animal (PTS) and human (TTS) experiments have furnished evidence that the amount of hearing loss due to noise exposure is larger and the range of frequencies affected is broader when the stapedius reflex is absent [15]. These results are in agreement with the opinion of Girolamo Fabrizi d'Acquapendente [16] who, in his work "De visione, voce et auditu," published in 1600, wrote that the middle ear muscles provide a protective function during exposure to loud sounds.

If the stapedius reflex protects the inner ear against acoustic overstimulation, the amount of the attenuation in a normal population must follow a Gaussian distribution, as many other biological phenomena. Thus, there will be some individuals in whom the stapedius reflex exhibits a low threshold, and is very active and resistant to fatigue. Conversely, others will have stapedius reflexes with high thresholds, and which are weak and adapt rapidly. If this is the case, it might be expected that in a population of workers, subjects with strong reflexes will develop less permanent noise induced hearing loss than subjects with weak reflexes.

A universal finding of all the studies in noise induced hearing loss is a significant variation in susceptibility among people exposed to noise. The fact that some individuals suffer from severe hearing impairment while others retain a fairly normal hearing function even when working in the same noise environment for an equal length of time has been known since the earliest studies on occupational hearing hazards [17,18]. The reasons for individual variability or susceptibility are still unknown, although several anatomical and functional variables from the outer to the inner ear contribute to the total variability. Certainly one such variable is represented by the sound transmission characteristics of the middle ear. It is likely that small differences in the resonant frequency (300-500 Hz) or in the sound transformation (5-15 dB), which have no practical implications at normal threshold levels, may have a significant effect and dramatically influence the noise dose reaching the inner ear over the long term. In this context, differences in the amount of attenuation provided by the reflex may also play an important role in individual susceptibility.

To investigate the possible relationship between stapedius reflex function and susceptibility to noise induced hearing loss, a systematic retrospective study of stapedius reflex parameters was performed in a population who had been exposed to a specific noise for a known number of years. Two different comparisons were made. The first comparison involved two groups of subjects, matched for age and for noise exposure time, but presenting significantly different audiometric profiles. The second comparison was made between two groups of subjects with similar audiometric profiles, but resulting from significantly different noise exposure time. This experimental design was considered necessary in order to circumvent the possible interference of hearing sensitivity on the dynamics of the stapedius reflex.

METHOD

Subjects

From a total population of 503 employees of a metallurgic and mechanic industry in Verona, we selected 85 subjects with exposure times of approximately 15 years (from 149 to 181 months). The age of this group ranged from 38 to 54 years. The hearing thresholds of each subject were analyzed and mean and standard deviations were determined (Fig. 1). On the basis of these measurements, two small subgroups were selected: Group A consisted of subjects (N=13) whose hearing thresholds were between 1 and 2 standard deviations below the mean, and Group B consisted of subjects (N=15) whose hearing thresholds were between 1 and 2 standard deviations above the mean. A third group of subjects (Group C, N=13) consisted of individuals with hearing thresholds equal to those of Group A, but with a noise exposure time limited to 5 years (58-63 months). After the first selection, all subjects available to participate in the present study were submitted to physical and otological examination and impedance testing. As a result, 18 subjects had to be excluded: 5 subjects for tympanometric abnormalities, 3 subjects for previous head injury and the remaining 6 subjects due to some minor general physical diseases. This selection reduced the 3 groups to the following figures: Group A, 7 subjects; Group B, 8 subjects; and Group C, 8 subjects. Since all of the subjects included in the present study worked in the same environment, it was reasonable to assume that all subjects within each group had received the same type of exposure to noise over the experimental period; i.e., 5 or 15 years.

Fig. 2 shows the noise conditions to which groups A, B and C were exposed during the course of a typical workday. The noise level is nearly stationary noise with levels ranging from 92 to 104 dB(A), with a peak at 125 Hz and a roll-off of approximately 6 dB per octave.

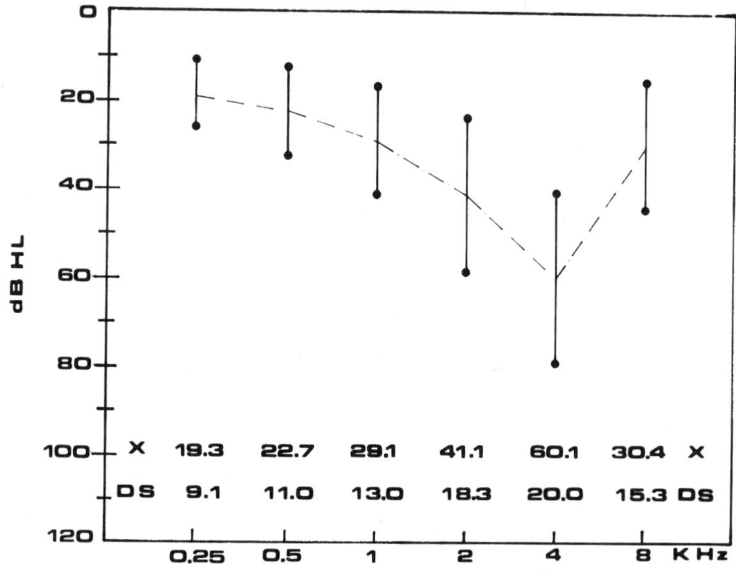

Fig. 1. Mean hearing threshold (± 1 standard deviation) of 85 subjects with exposure time of 15 years; Group A includes subjects with hearing thresholds between 1 and 2 standard deviations below the mean; Group B consists of subjects with hearing thresholds between 1 and 2 standard deviations above the mean. Group C consists of individuals with hearing threshold equal to Group A resulting from a noise exposure time of 5 years.

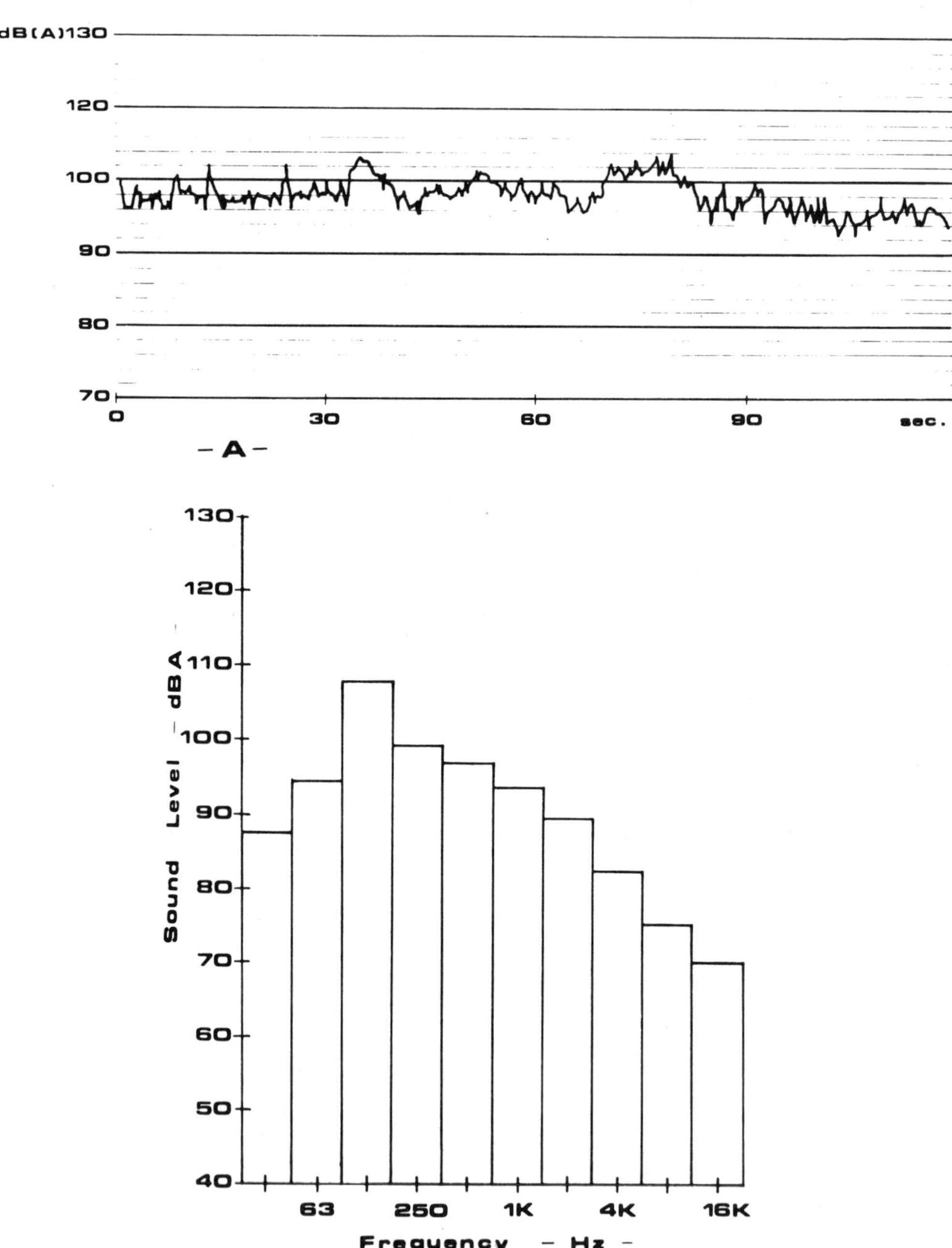

Fig. 2. Recording sequence (A) and range of octave band levels (B) for Group A, B and C during a typical workday.

Equipment

Hearing threshold determination was performed by Bekesy audiometry (Amplifon Model 270). Thresholds were obtained by using pulsed tones (250 msec with 50% duty cycle) at the frequencies of 500, 1000, 2000 and 4000 Hz. Stimuli were transmitted to the ear via TDH-39 earphones and MX-41/AR cushions.

Impedance audiometry was carried out with a modified commercial apparatus (Madsen ZO 70) equipped with a TDH-39 earphone, and MX-AR/41 cushion for elicitation of contralateral reflexes. The modifications were adopted in order to minimize temporal distortion and filtering artifacts. The time constant of the instrument was 25 msec. The acoustic stimuli for eliciting the reflex were generated by a commercial audiometer (Amplifon 300). The two outputs of the impedance bridge were connected to a two channel electronystagmograph (Galileo C 2a); one recorded the pressure values in the ear canal and the other registered the modifications of compliance. The reflex-eliciting stimuli were tone bursts at 500, 1000, 2000 and 4000 Hz. Two and five dB steps in intensity were used. Signal duration was 1000 msec (rise-fall time of 2.0 msec.) for the evaluation of the time domain parameters of the reflex and 30 sec. for the determination of peristimulatory adaptation.

Protocol

Threshold, onset latency, rise time, amplitude, offset latency, decay time and peristimulatory adaptation of the stapedius reflex were examined according to the following definitions (see Fig. 3) [19]: 1) threshold: impedance changes equal to 10% of the maximum individual amplitude; 2) onset latency: time interval between stimulus onset and 5% of the maximum amplitude of the response; 3) rise time: time required for the response to rise from 10% to 90% of its final value; 4) amplitude: height of the response at steady state (after damped oscillations) expressed in percentage of maximum individual variation of impedance; 5) offset latency: time interval for the response to fall to 95% of its value after stimulus off-set; 6) decay time: time interval between 90% and 10% of the amplitude of the response after stimulus offset; 7) peristimulatory adaptation: percentage of reduction of amplitude in relation to the steady state value during acoustic stimulation lasting 30 sec.

Onset-offset latency, rise-decay time and peristimulatory adaptation values were determined at 10 dB SL (reflex threshold). Amplitude was evaluated as a function of intensity from below threshold to maximum stimulation to determine the slope of the input-output function and to determine the satu- ration level. The static pressure in the external ear canal was continuously monitored during testing in order to check for pressure variations. Pres- sure value may in fact change during a test session and values in the ear canal have to be adjusted in order to examine the reflex at the point of maximum compliance.

Results

Individual values of the stapedius reflex threshold, along with averages, standard deviations and ranges observed in Groups A, B and C are shown in Tables I, II and III. Group A (Table I) exhibits normal values at each frequency. Table II shows reflex threshold values in Group B. The threshold is normal in each subject at 0.5 kHz; it is normal in 25% of the subjects and elevated in 75% at 1 kHz; it is elevated in 94% and absent in 6% at 2 kHz; it is elevated in 19% and absent in 81% at 4 kHz. The values for Group C are shown in Table III. Frequencies of 500, 1000 and 2000 Hz display normal threshold values. The threshold is elevated in 88% and absent in 12% of the cases at 4 kHz. The statistical analysis (student t-test) shows significant differences between group A and B at 1, 2 and 4 kHz ($p < 0.01$) and between group A and C at 2 ($p < 0.05$) and 4 ($p < 0.01$) kHz.

TABLE I - Mean, standard deviations and range of acoustic reflex threshold as a function of frequency for Group A (N=7). Noise exposure duration equals 15 years.

Hz	500	1000	2000	4000
X	81.2	82.9	85.0	87.6
SD	2.7	3.2	2.8	3.3
Range	78-89	76-91	78-92	80-93
Normal	100%	100%	100%	100%
Elevated	0%	0%	0%	0%
Absent	0%	0%	0%	0%

TABLE II - Mean, standard deviations and range of acoustic reflex threshold as a function of frequency for Group B (N=8). Noise exposure duration equals 15 years.

Hz	500	1000	2000	4000
X	84.5	100.5**	104.5**	116.0**
SD	3.7	4.1	2.8	2.9
Range	78-90	95-108	100-110	113-120
Normal	100%	25%	0%	0%
Elevated	0%	75%	94%	19%
Absent	0%	0%	6%	81%

** ($p < 0.01$)

TABLE III - Mean, standard deviations and range of acoustic reflex threshold as a function of frequency for Group C (N=8). Noise exposure duration equals 5 years).

Hz	500	1000	2000	4000
X	82.6	83.1	87.7*	101.5**
SD	2.7	2.7	2.7	3.1
Range	79-90	79-90	82-94	97-108
Normal	100%	100%	100%	0%
Elevated	0%	0%	0%	88%
Absent	0%	0%	0%	12%

** ($p < 0.01$)
* ($p < 0.05$)

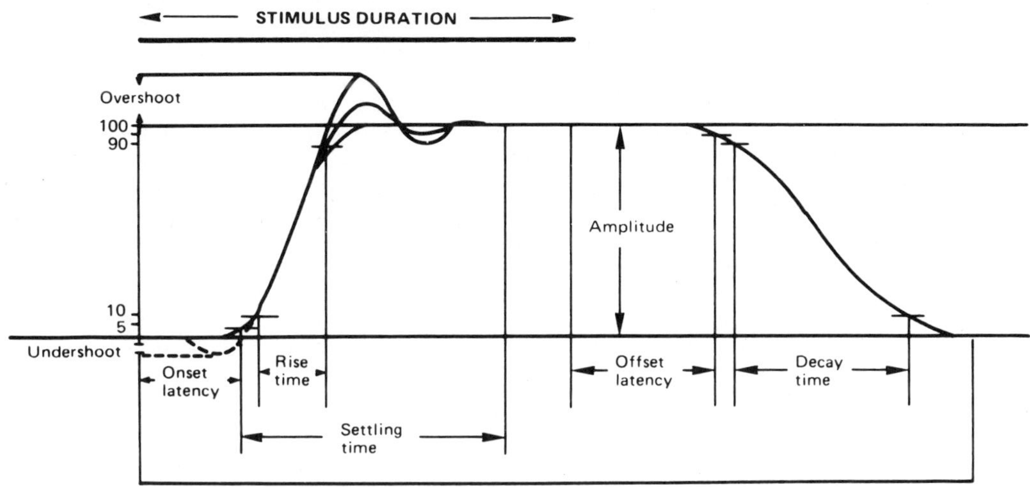

Fig. 3. Stapedius reflex parameters examined according to Colletti [19].

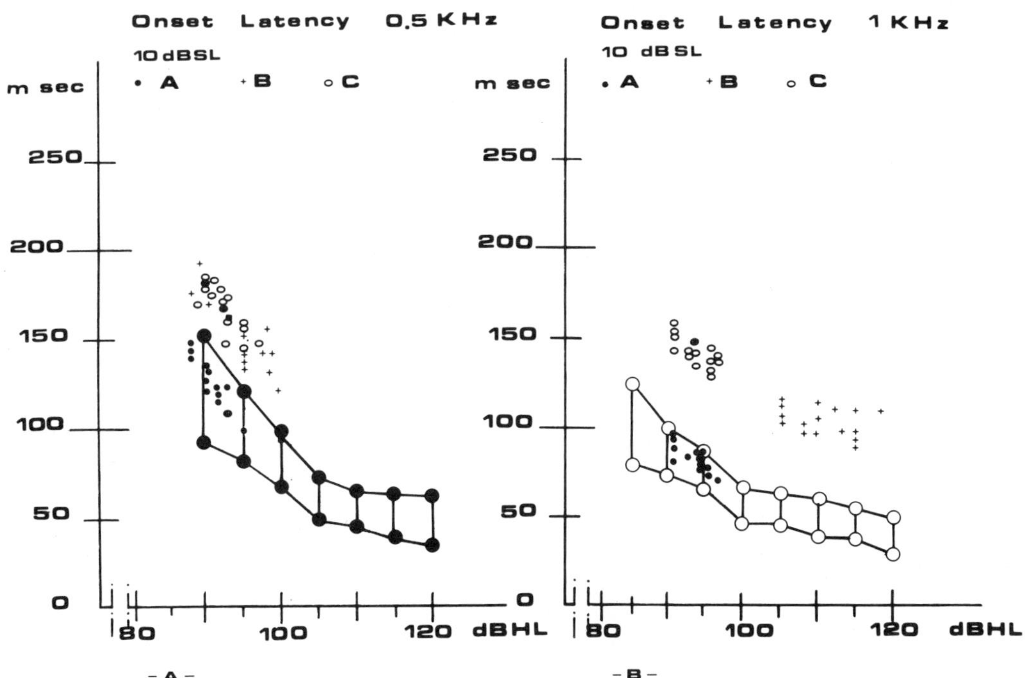

Fig. 4. Individual onset latency values at 0.5 (A) and 1 kHz (B) for Group A, B and C at 10 dB SL. Latency intensity functions (± 1 SD) previously obtained in normal hearing subjects are represented to facilitate comparison of the results among groups.

Fig. 4 shows the onset latency values at 0.5 and 1 kHz for Groups A, B and C. The mean input-output functions along with the standard deviation obtained in a previous study on normal hearing subjects [19] are represented for each parameter under investigation. Group A (Fig. 4A) shows normal onset latency values at 500 and 1000 Hz. Group B and C present significantly prolonged values at both frequencies, i.e., outside 2 standard deviations at 1 kHz and outside 3 standard deviations at 0.5 kHz. Fig. 5 shows individual onset latency values at 2 and 4 kHz in the 3 groups. The values are included in the normal range for Group A at both frequencies. Group B and C show systematically prolonged latencies with values ranging from 2 to 3 standard deviations at 2 kHz and exceeding 3 standard deviations at 4 kHz. The latency values at 4 kHz for group B are not displayed due to the abnormally elevated thresholds and the large amplitude reductions at this frequency. The statistical analysis (Fig. 6) showed significant differences between Group A and Group B and between Group A and Group C at all frequen- cies ($p < 0.01$ except for the comparison between Group A and B at 2 kHz ($p < 0.05$)).

Fig. 7 shows the rise time values of the 3 groups at 0.5 and 1 kHz. This figure also includes the input-output functions previously calculated in normal subjects [19]. The values obtained for Group A are within one standard deviation of the normal values at both frequencies. The figures for Group B and C, although definitely prolonged are still located between 2 and 3 standard deviations of normal. The rise time values for the 3 groups at 2 and 4 kHz are shown in Fig. 8. Group A presents normal values while group B and C display prolonged values which are two and three standard

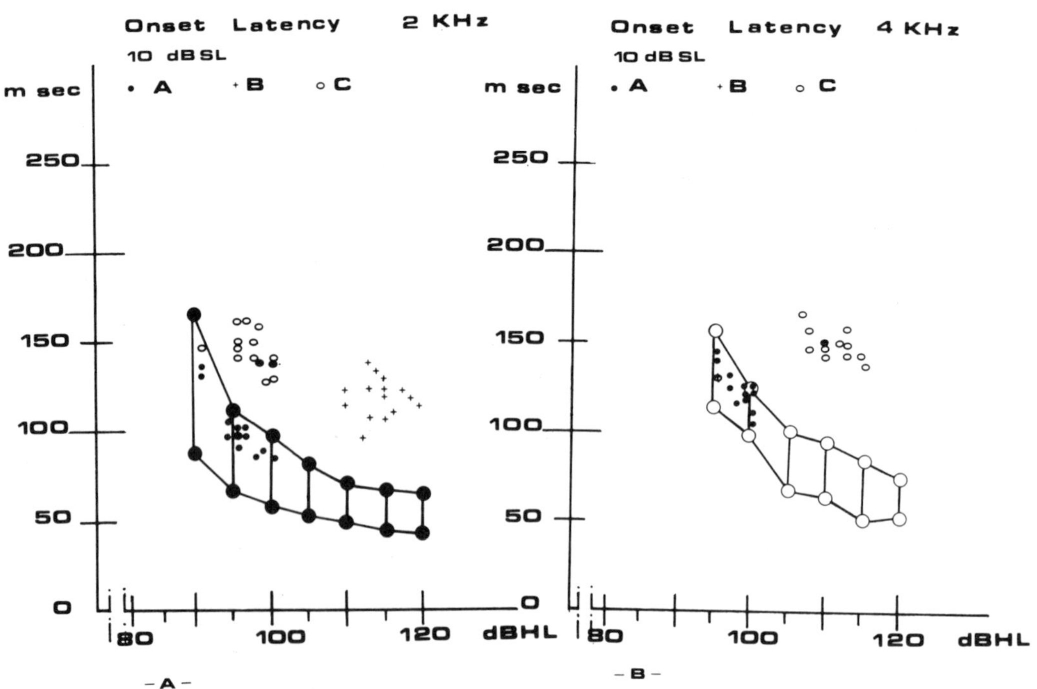

Fig. 5. Individual onset latency values at 2 (A) and 4 kHz (B) for Group A, B and C at 10 dB SL. Latency intensity functions (± 1 SD) previously obtained in normal hearing subjects are represented to facilitate comparison of the results among groups.

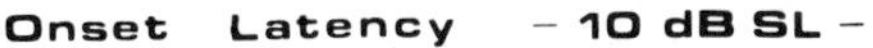

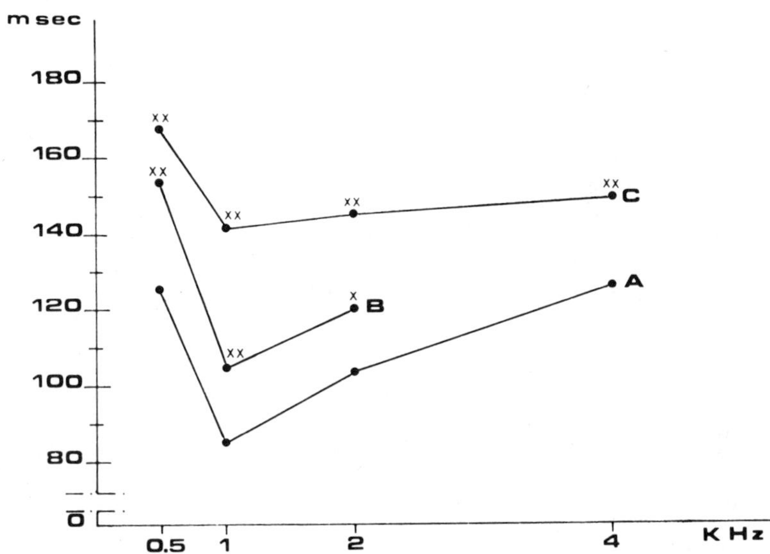

Fig. 6. Statistical analysis of onset latency examined at 10 dB SL for Group A, B and C at 0.5, 1, 2 and 4 kHz. (xx = $p < 0.01$, x = $p < 0.05$)

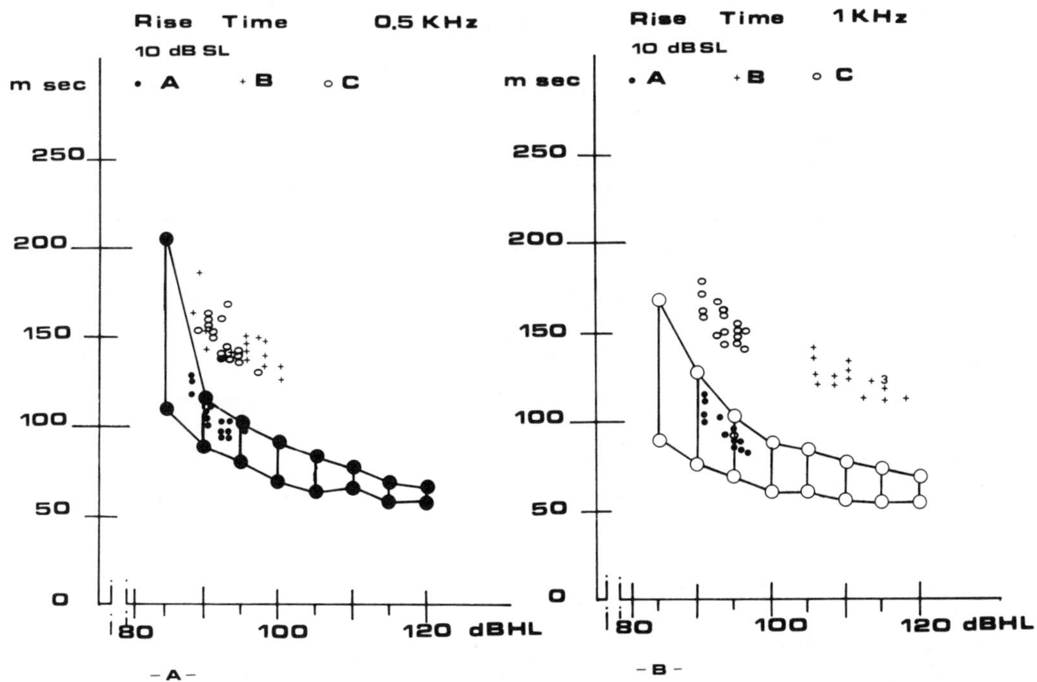

Fig. 7. Individual rise time values at 0.5 (A) and 1 kHz (B) for Group A, B and C at 10 dB SL. Rise time intensity functions (± 1 SD) previously obtained in normal hearing subjects are represented to facilitate comparison of the results among groups.

deviations from normal. The statistical analysis (Fig. 9) of rise time values shows a significant difference between Group A and B and between Group A and C at 0.5 and 1 kHz ($p < 0.01$). At 2 kHz, only Group A and Group C show a statistically significant difference ($p < 0.01$).

Figures 10 and 11 show the amplitude intensity functions (range of distribution) for the 3 groups. The amplitude is expressed as a percentage of the highest value found in each subject at 1 kHz. In addition, both figures display the range of amplitude values previously obtained in a group of normal subjects [19]. Fig. 10 (B) shows that the values for Group A are within the normal range; the functions have a linear range of 20-25 dB which is followed by saturation (around 105 dB HL). The amplitude intensity function for both Group C and B are outside the normal range (shifted to the right) and do not exhibit saturation even at the highest intensities. The value of 50% of amplitude is reached at significantly different intensities for the three groups: 85-90 dB in Group A, 105-110 dB in Group C and 115-120 dB in Group B.

Fig. 10 (A) shows the input-output function at 0.5 kHz. Group A is inside the normal distribution whereas both Group B and C are shifted significantly to the right with different slopes. At this frequency, the 50% amplitude is obtained at quite different intensities: 92-96 dB for Group A, 105-115 dB for Group B, and 112-120 dB for Group C.

Fig. 11 shows the amplitude values at 2 and 4 kHz. Again, Group A is within the normal range while Group B and C are shifted to the right. The intensity needed to reach 50% of maximum amplitude occurs at significantly different levels in the 3 groups. At 2 kHz, this value is in the range of 98-102 dB in group A and 110-120 in Group C. The amplitude function for Group B is so depressed that the 50% amplitude is never reached and is even absent at 4 kHz.

The statistical analysis (Fig. 12) performed for amplitude values at 10 dB SL shows highly significant values at 0.5 and 1 kHz for both Group A and C ($p < 0.01$). It is interesting to note that at 2 kHz the amplitude of Group B is higher than that of Group A. This discrepancy is, however, only apparent since the amplitude values were obtained at remarkably different absolute intensity values. For the same reason, the amplitude values for Group A and C appear to be equal at 4 kHz.

Fig. 13 shows the values of offset latency at 0.5 and 1 kHz. The values at 2 and 4 kHz are not shown due to abnormal amplitude depression. In addition, the mean and $\pm$ 1 standard deviation of the offset latency and the decay time previously obtained in the normal group [13] are shown. It may be observed that the individual values of offset latency at 0.5 kHz are homogeneously distributed in the normal range for all the groups. At 1 kHz (Fig. 13 B), Groups A and C are within the normal range and Group B is located between 1 and 2 standard deviations below the mean. The statistical analysis for offset latency at 10 dB SL (Fig. 14) shows significant values only between group A and C at 1 kHz ($p < 0.01$).

The decay time values at 0.5 and 1 kHz are represented in Fig. 15. Group A is distributed in the normal range, whereas the values for Groups B and C are reduced. The data for Group C fall between the mean and $\pm$ 2 standard deviations while for Group B the data are between 1 and 2 standard deviations below the mean. The statistical analysis of the decay time values at 10 dB SL displays significance at 0.5 kHz for Groups A and B and for Groups A and C ($p < 0.01$) (Fig. 16). At 1 kHz, the significance level is reached in the comparison of Groups A and C ($p < 0.01$). It should be recalled that decay time values were collected at quite different intensity levels so this representation of the data may be somewhat misleading.

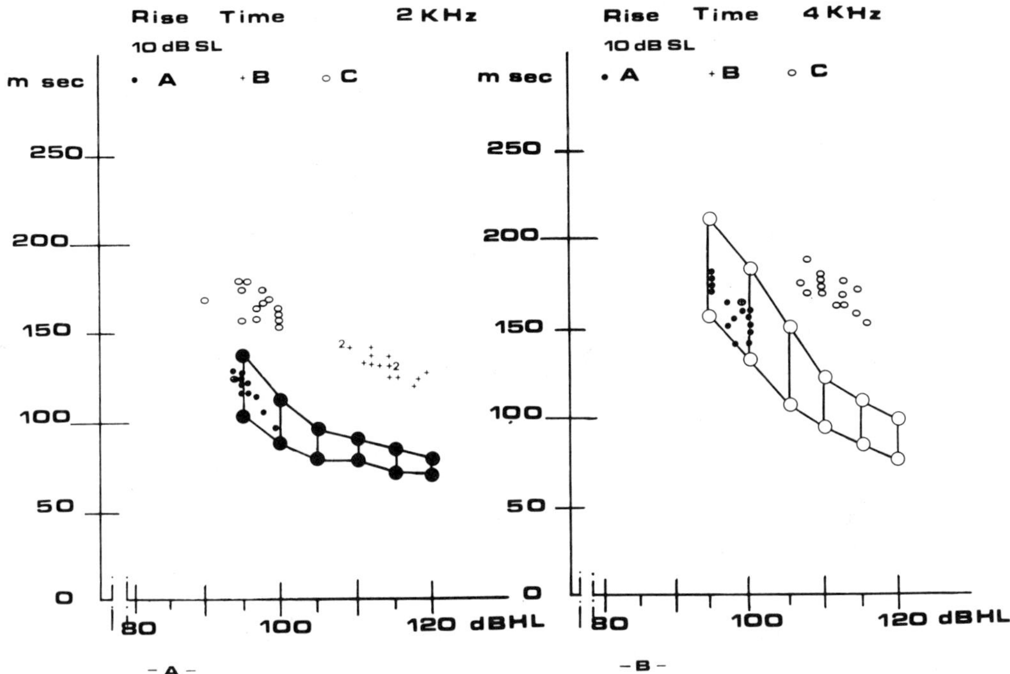

Fig. 8. Individual rise time values at 2 kHz (A) and 4 kHz (B) for Group A, B and C at 10 dB SL. Rise time intensity functions (± 1 SD) previously obtained in normal hearing subjects are represented to facilitate comparison of the results among groups.

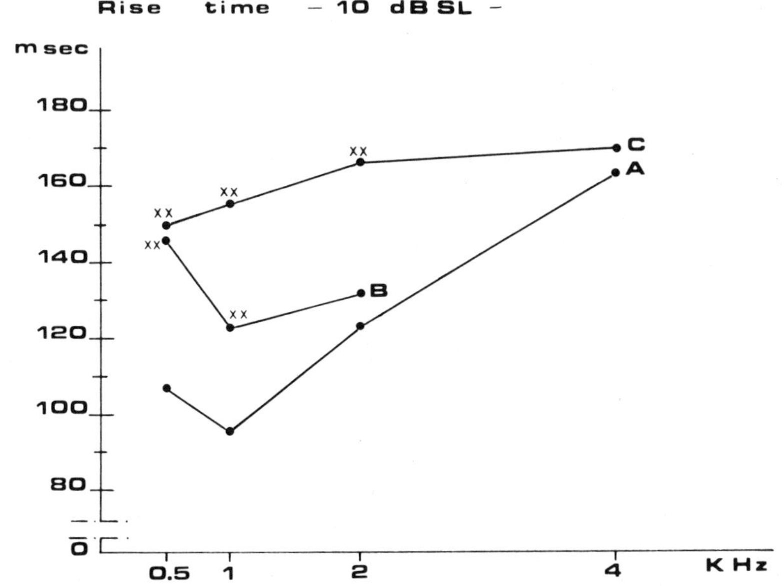

Fig. 9. Statistical analysis of rise time examined at 10 dB SL for Group A, B and C at 0.5, 1, 2 and 4 kHz. (xx = $p < 0.01$, x = $p < 0.05$)

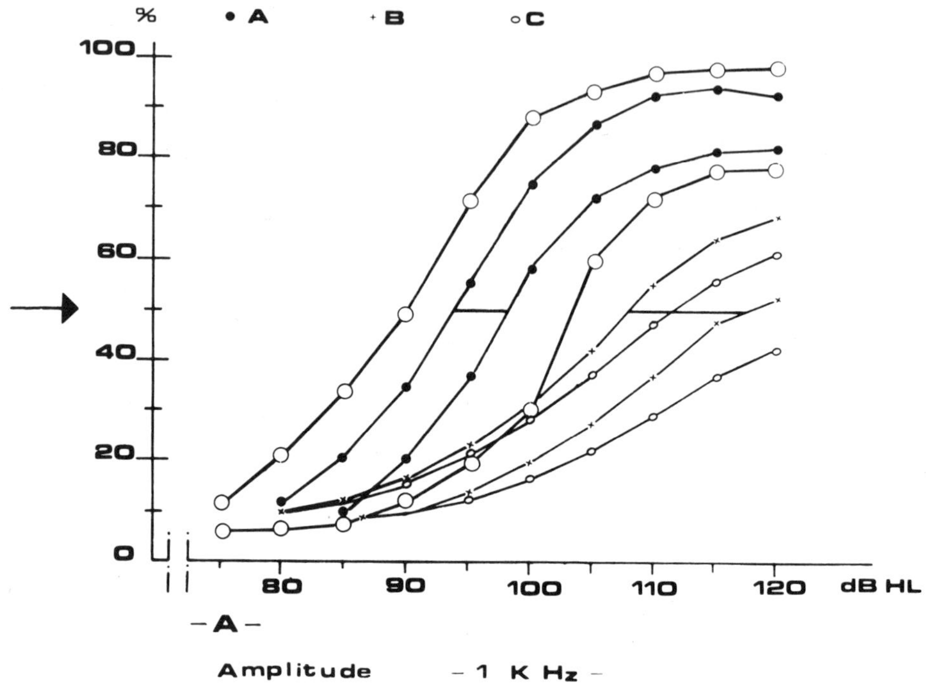

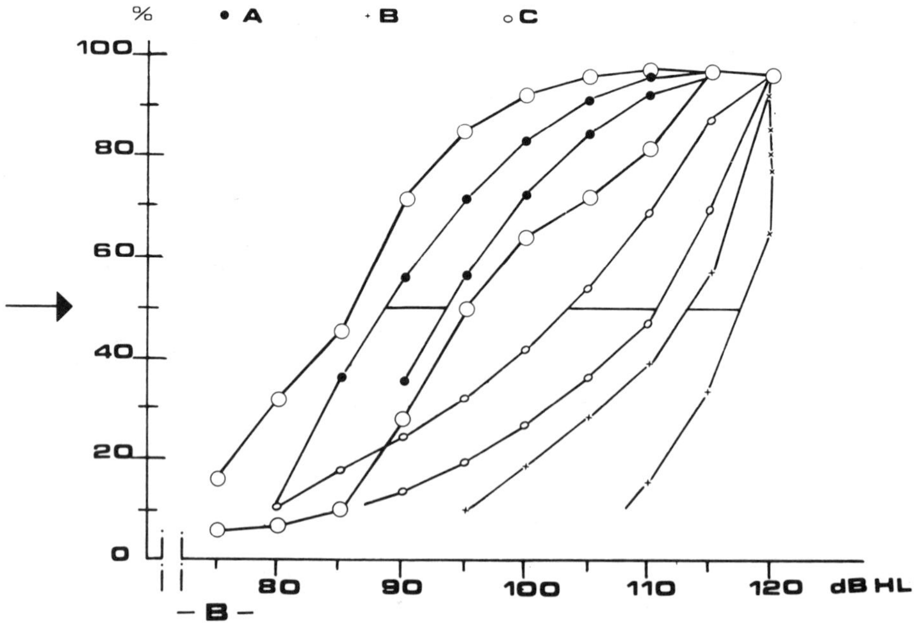

Fig. 10. Range of distribution of the amplitude-intensity functions for Group A, B and C at 0.5 kHz (A) and 1 kHz (B). The range of amplitude values previously obtained in normal hearing subjects (o-o) is included to facilitate comparison among groups.

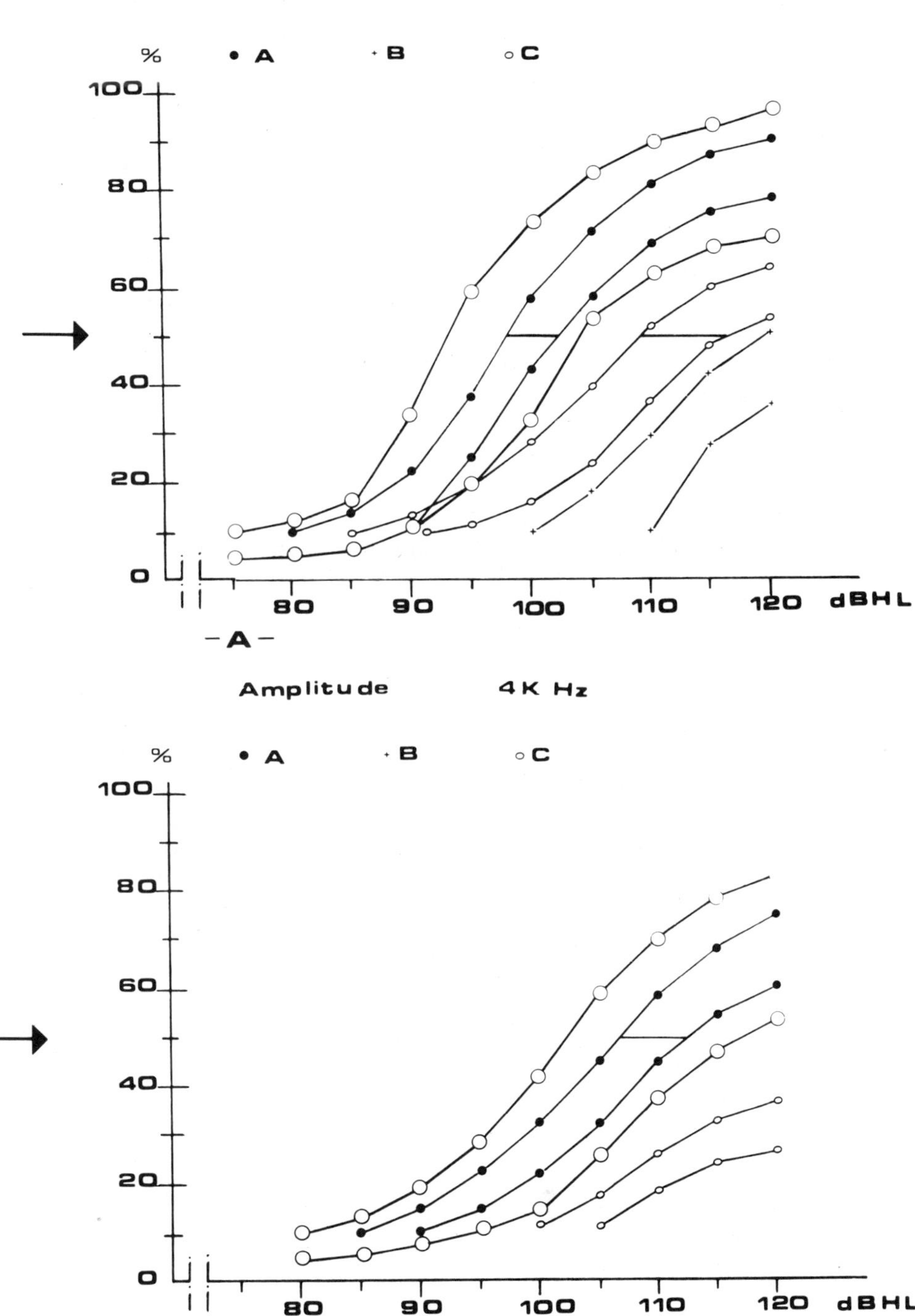

Fig. 11. Range of distribution of the amplitude-intensity function for Group A, B and C at 2 (A) and 4 kHz (B). The range of amplitude values previously obtained in normal hearing subjects (o-o) is included to facilitate comparison among groups.

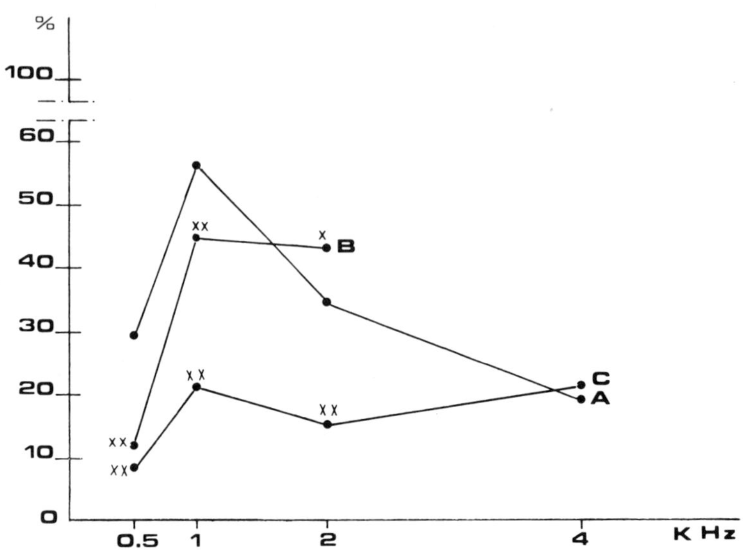

Fig. 12. Statistical analysis of amplitude examined at 10 dB SL for Group A, B and C at 0.5, 1, 2 and 4 kHz. (xx = $p < 0.01$, x = $p < 0.05$)

Fig. 17 through 19 show the peristimulatory adaptation values (mean and standard deviation) obtained at 0.5, 1 and 2 kHz in the 3 groups along with mean and standard deviations previously observed in a normal population [13]. The 3 groups (Fig. 17) display normal values at 0.5 kHz. At 1 kHz, (Fig. 18), Group A exhibits normal values and Group B and C are both located between the mean and 2 standard deviations below the mean. Fig. 19 represents peristimulatory values at 2 kHz for the 3 groups. The distribution for the 3 groups is quite similar to the one previously described at 1 kHz.

DISCUSSION

Experimental studies designed to evaluate how the middle ear muscles affect the degree of permanent noise-induced hearing loss have, for obvious ethical reasons, been primarily carried out in animals. The investigations on cats [20] and rabbits [21] demonstrated that when the stapedius muscle is inactive, permanent threshold shift is more pronounced and extends over a wider range of frequencies. Interspecies differences must, however, be taken into account when transferring the data from animals to humans. Apart from different audibility curves, it is known that in most experimental animals both the stapedius and tensor tympani muscles are activated by acoustic stimulation, whereas in man only the stapedius reflex is involved. Therefore the observations on animals cannot be easily transferred to human studies.

In order to gather detailed information on the relationship between stapedius reflex activity and noise induced hearing loss, we performed a retrospective investigation on a population that had been exposed to a specific noise for a known number of years. The rationale for the investigation is as follows. If the stapedius reflex protects the inner ear from long term noise exposure, it should be reflected in the values obtained for stapedius reflex parameters.

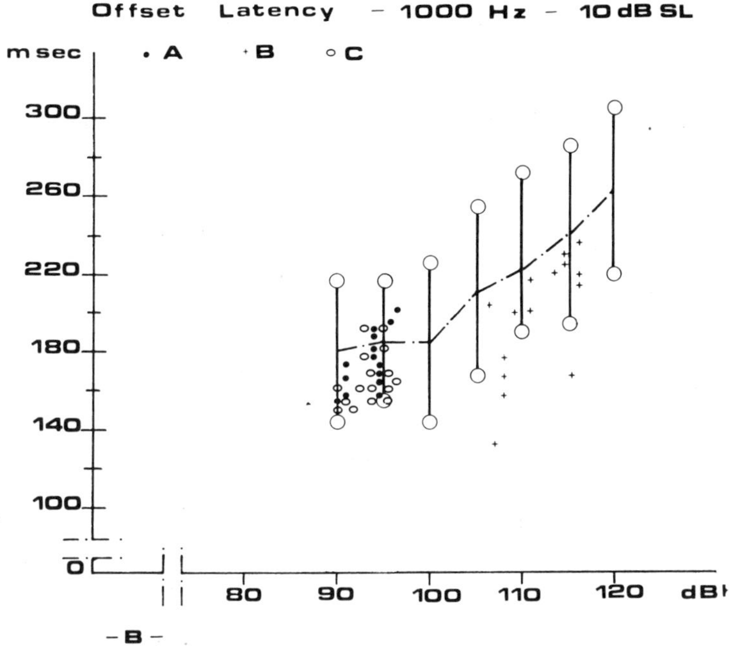

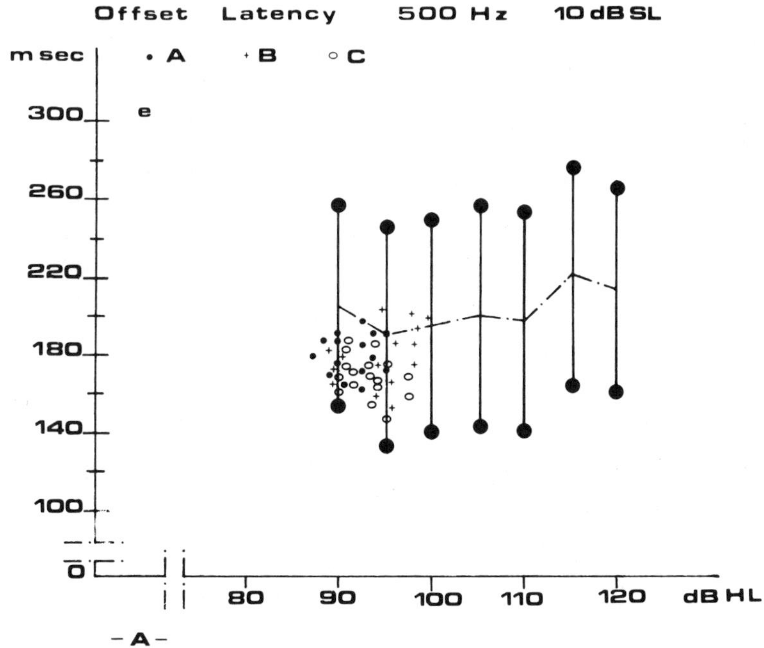

Fig. 13. Individual offset latency values at 0.5 (A) and 1 kHz (B) for Group A, B and C at 10 dB SL. Offset latency functions (mean and standard deviations) previously obtained in normal hearing subjects are superimposed to facilitate comparison among groups.

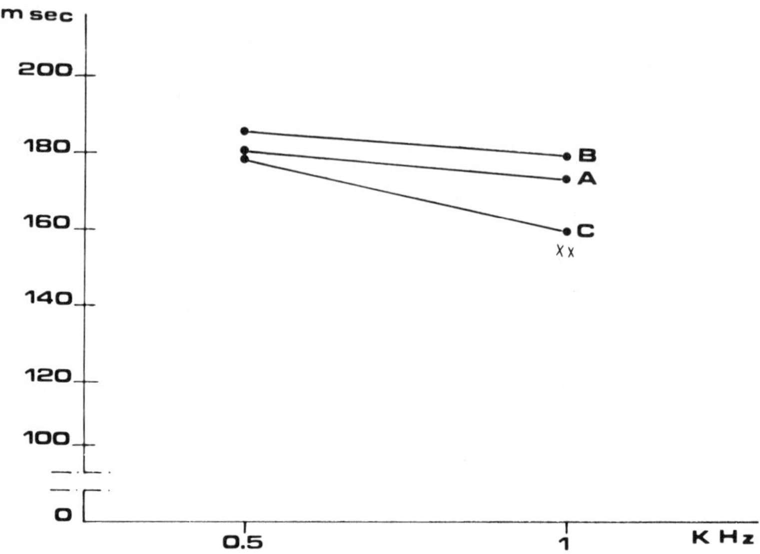

Fig. 14. Statistical analysis of offset latency examined at 10 dB SL for Group A, B and C at 0.5 and 1 kHz. (xx = $p < 0.1$)

In order to examine this issue, two groups of subjects were selected from a population of workers exposed to industrial noise for the same number of years. The two groups, matched for age, were characterized by significantly different degrees of noise induced hearing loss. Since the behavior of the stapedius reflex is dependent on the hearing sensitivity, it was necessary to control for the effects of hearing loss by comparing two groups of subjects presenting equal audiometric profiles resulting from significantly different noise exposure times (15 versus 5 years). To reduce the well known variables and biases inherent with retrospective procedures, subjects with hearing losses possibly due to causes other than noise were excluded.

The results of the present study indicate a significant difference in most of the investigated parameters between and among the three groups. Group A, characterized by a mild hearing loss resulting from 15 years of noise exposure, presented normal values of the stapedius reflex parameters at all test frequencies (0.5 - 4 kHz). Group B, with a moderate to severe hearing loss in the high frequencies resulting from 15 years of noise exposure, was characterized by important abnormalities of the stapedius reflex for both threshold and suprathreshold time domain parameters. Group C, exposed to industrial noise for only 5 years and with an audiometric profile similar to that of Group A, displayed abnormal stapedius reflex parameters mainly at suprathreshold values.

Thus, the outcomes of the present investigation indicate that the stapedius reflex may be an important factor contributing to the hearing loss in the three groups. If the different values of threshold, latency, rise time, amplitude, offset latency, decay time and peristimulatory adaptation of the stapedius reflex are taken into consideration, it can be seen that the amount of attenuation provided by the stapedius reflex differs considerably between the groups. It is not easy to specify exactly how the different parameters affect the process of attenuation. Results of this study suggests that three main factors may play an important role in this attenuation

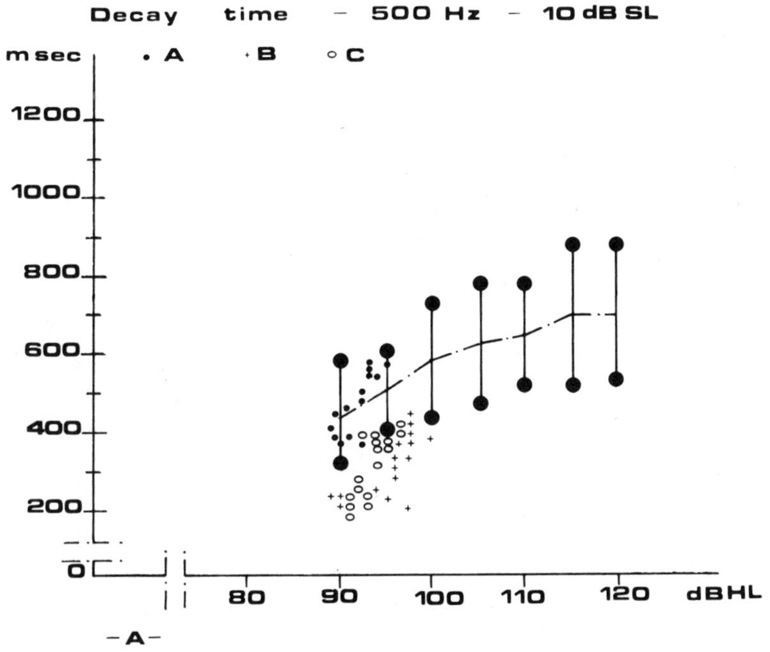

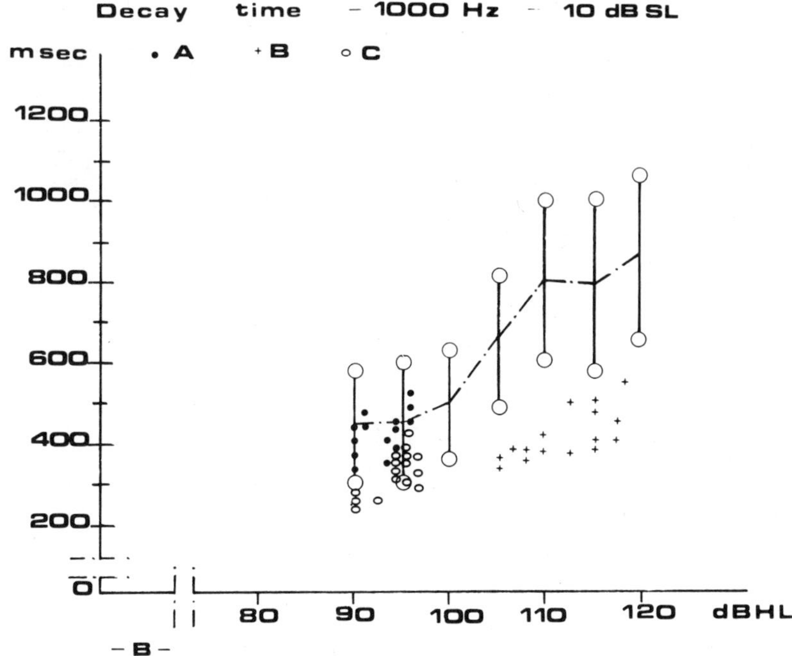

Fig. 15. Individual decay time values at 0.5 (A) and 1 kHz (B) for Group A, B and C at 10 dB SL. Decay time functions (mean and standard deviations) previously obtained in normal hearing subjects are superimposed to facilitate comparison among groups.

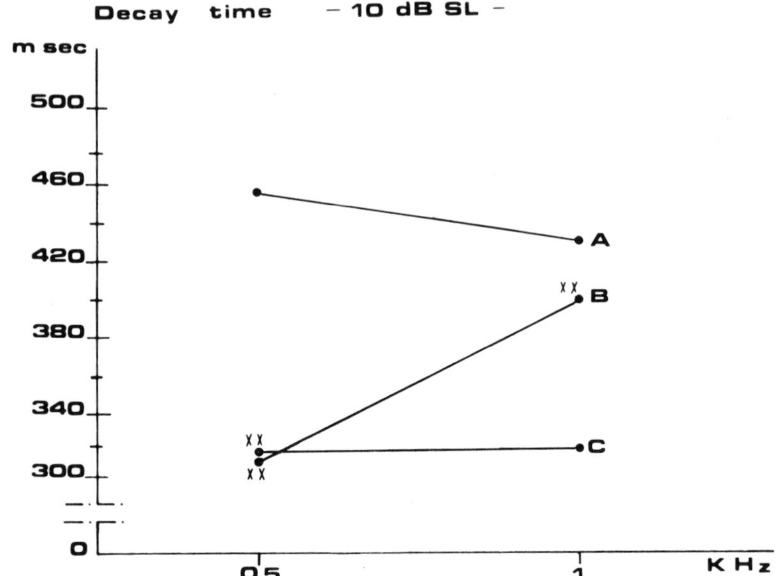

Fig. 16. Statistical analysis of decay time examined at 10 dB SL for Group A, B and C at 0.5 and 1 kHz. (xx = p < 0.01)

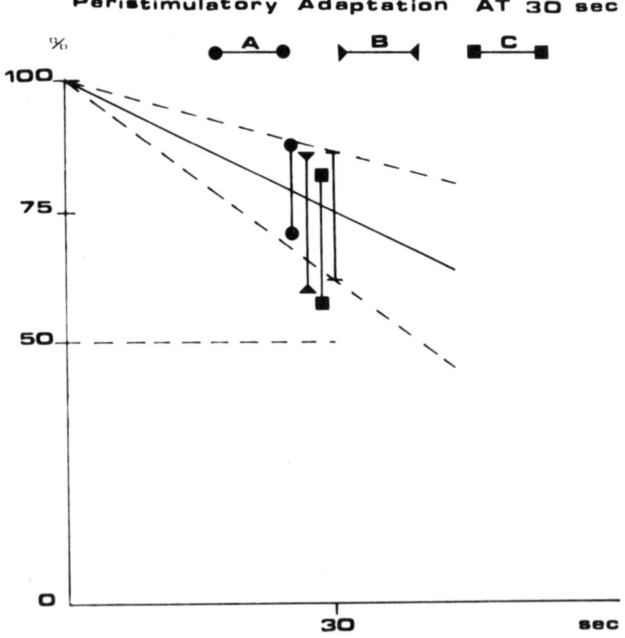

Fig. 17. Range of peristimulatory adaptation values at 30 sec for 0.5 kHz in Group A, B and C. Mean (dashed line) and standard deviation (continuous line) previously obtained in normal hearing subjects are included to facilitate comparison among groups.

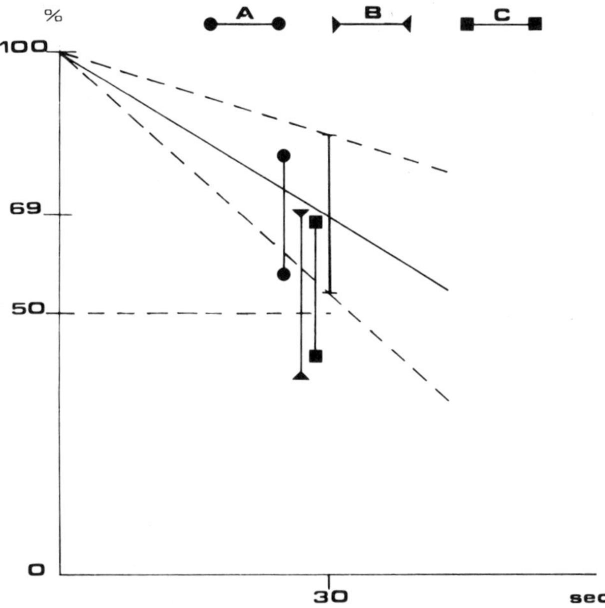

Fig. 18. Range of peristimulatory adaptation values at 30 sec for 1 kHz in Group A, B and C. Mean (continuous line) and standard deviations (dashed line) previously obtained in normal hearing subjects are included to facilitate comparison among groups.

process: threshold, amplitude and peristimulatory adaptation. It is known that the attenuation provided by the stapedius reflex starts at threshold and grows linearly at a value of 7 dB for a 10 dB increment in stimulus intensity, reaching a maximum at 20 dB [22]. Since the mean difference in stapedius reflex threshold between Group A and Group B is 18.4 dB, it is clear that Group B has a loss of attenuation at threshold equal to 12.8 dB.

The input-output functions of the reflex show a pronounced difference between groups. The amplitude functions were represented as a percentage of the maximum amplitude for each subject and not in absolute imittance values to reduce the spread of data (due to the influence of shunting impedance of the inner ear canal and the middle ear). This does not allow us to quantify in absolute terms the value of each individual amplitude function and therefore only relative calculations can be performed. Since, however, it is known that the reflex has a linear behavior of approximately 25-30 dB at supra- threshold values, the midpoints (i.e., 50%) of the amplitude function for the three groups can be used for comparison. The intensity needed to reach 50% of maximum attenuation is approximately 85-90 dB for Group A, 105-110 dB for Group C and 115-120 dB for Group B. Thus, for a given intensity level, groups B and C would show much less attenuation of the input signal than normals. Furthermore, the results of peristimulatory adaptation at 1 and 2 kHz indicates that the reduction of reflex amplitude by 50% of its original value would require only 9 sec for Group B, and 11 sec for Group C, whereas Group A would require nearly twice as long (23 sec) for the reflex to adapt. On the basis of the above mentioned considerations, we suggest that the stapedius reflex plays an important role in protecting the inner ear against

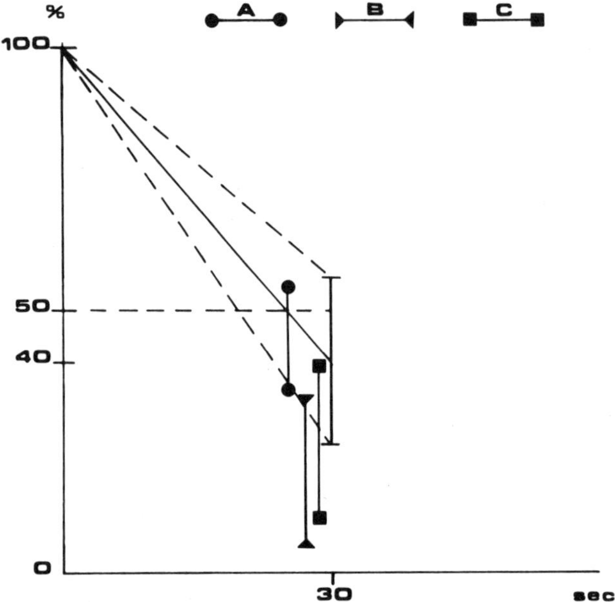

Fig. 19. Range of peristimulatory adaptation values at 30 sec for 2 kHz in Group A, B and C. Mean (continuous line) and standard deviations (dashed line) previously obtained in normal hearing subjects are included to facilitate comparison among groups.

noise and is probably also one important factor in the complex phenomenon of individual variability or susceptibility to noise induced hearing loss.

Several investigators have shown that the stapedius reflex threshold exhibits considerable intersubject variation on the order of approximately 20 dB. This amount of variability is found not only in a commonly defined normal population, but also in young subjects carefully selected for having normal hearing threshold, normal tympanometric functions and no history of otological or neurological disorders [23].

Fig. 20 reports the distribution of amplitude as a function of intensity in a normal population [24] and clearly shows the spread of threshold values calculated at 10% of maximum amplitude. It may be seen that the amplitude/intensity function of the stapedius reflex also shows a wide range of intersubject variability at 50 and at 90% of maximum ampliture, on the same order of magnitude as for threshold [17]. In a few reports, the intersubject variability for amplitude has been quantified in acoustic ohms during acoustic reflex contraction at different suprathreshold intensities [9,25-27]. The standard deviations values ranged from 1/3 to 2/3 of the mean impedance change. Furthermore, it is a common observation that subjects with low thresholds for the acoustic reflex are characterized by greater impedance changes as a function of stimulus intensity and with earlier saturation phenomena than subjects with elevated thresholds [19].

In some investigations the acoustic reflex activity following exposure to noise has been studied [28,29]. It was demonstrated that both reflex threshold and dynamic properties (temporal features) can be temporarily modified (deteriorated) with exposure to noise. Borg et al. [28] measured an

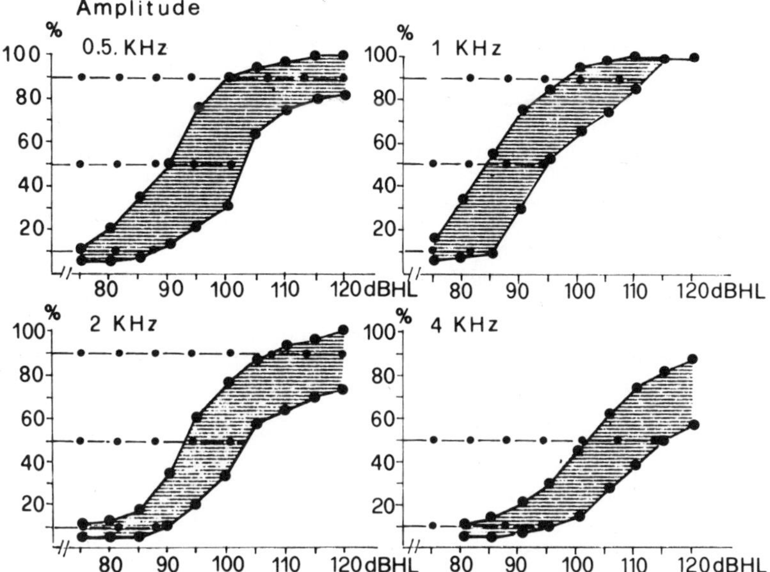

Fig. 20. Distribution of amplitude as a function of intensity at 0.5, 1, 2 and 4 kHz in a normal population. Horizontal bars indicate spread of values at 10%, 50% and 90% of maximum amplitude.

average of 4 dB of reflex threshold shift in industrial workers after a typical work-day. In addition, changes in the amplitude of the reflex were also described. More recently Gerhardt and Hepler [29] reported temporary changes in acoustic reflex threshold (5 dB) and amplitude along with behavioral temporary threshold shift (12-15 dB) in normal hearing subjects exposed to a 95 dB SPL octave band of noise centered at 1 kHz for 4 hours. Both studies reported large intersubject variability with some subjects showing a large depression and some a potentiation of the reflex after the noise exposure. Thus, it is apparent that noise exposure may depress both hearing sensitivity and stapedius reflex parameters such as threshold and amplitude. It would be interesting to know if the changes in hearing and the reflex arise from the same anatomical and physiological sites within the auditory pathway.

The observation reported by Borg et al. [28] and by Gerhardt and Helper [29] are interesting, but at the same time surprising, since we were accustomed to consider that damage to the cochlea by noise exposure does not alter the stapedius reflex threshold until the hearing loss exceeds 50-55 dB HL. However, for the present issue, it is important to realize that temporary stapedius reflex abnormalities induced by noise exposure are linked with a high degree of variability. Thus, two types of variability can be described in the stapedius reflex. (1) a general physiological variability and (2) a noise related variability. How these two are linked together and play a role in susceptibility to noise induced hearing loss can only be evaluated in prospective or longitudinal studies.

REFERENCES

1. W. D. Ward, Studies on the aural reflex. I. Controlateral remote masking as an indicator of reflex activity, J. Acoust. Soc. Am. 33:1034 (1961).
2. B. Johansson, B. Kylin and M. Langfy, Acoustic reflex as a test of individual susceptibility to nose, Acta Otolaryngol., 64:256 (1967).
3. R. R. A. Coles, Middle-ear muscle activity as a possible index of susceptibility to temporary threshold shift, Sound 3:72 (1969).
4. P. Dallos, Feedback mechanism, in: "The Auditory Periphery", Academic Press, New York (1973).
5. D. E. Morgan and D. D. Dirks, Influence of middle ear muscle contraction on pure tone suprathreshold loudness judgments, J. Acoust. Soc. Am., 57:411 (1975).
6. R. H. Wilson, J. F. Steckler, H. C. Jones and R. H. Margolis, Adaptation of the acoustic reflex, J. Acoust. Soc. Am., 64:782 (1978).
7. T. Kato, Zur physiologie der binnenmuskeln des ohres, Pflug. Arch., 150:569 (1913).
8. G. Tietze, Zum zeitverhalten des akustischen reflexes bei reizund mit dauertonen, Arch. Klin. Exp. Ohr. Nas. Kehlkopfheilk, 193:43 (1968).
9. H. Kaplan, S. Gilman and D. D. Dirks, Properties of acoustic reflex adaptation, Ann. Otol. Rhinol. Laryngol., 86:348 (1977).
10. M. E. Lutman and A. M. Martin, Adaptation of the acoustic reflex to combinations of sustained steady state and repeated pulse stimuli, J. Sound Vib., 56:137 (1978).
11. J. E. Zakrisson and E. Borg, Stapedius reflex and auditory fatigue, Audiology, 13:231 (1974).
12. J. L. Fletcher and A. J. Riopelle, Protective effect of the acoustic reflex for impulsive noises, J. Acoust. Soc. Am., 32:401 (1960).
13. V. Colletti, Meccanismi fisiologici di protezione del sensore uditivo dal rumore, in: "Recenti Acquisizioni sulla Ipoacusia da Rumore," V. Ricci and V. Colletti, eds, Piccin, Padova (1983).
14. R. Wersall, The tympanic muscles and their reflexes, Acta Otolaryngol. Suppl., 139:43 (1958).
15. E. Borg, A quantitative study of the effect of the acoustic stapedius reflex on sound transmission through the middle ear of man, Acta Otolaryngol., 66:461 (1968).
16. G. Fabrizi d'Acquapendente, De oculo, de aure et de larynge, Venezia (1600).
17. J. Haberman, Ueber die schwerhorigkeit der kesselschmiede, Arch Ohrenheilk., 30:1 (1890).
18. J. E. Zakrisson, The role of the stapedius reflex in poststimulatory auditory fatigue, Acta Otolaryngol., 79:1 (1975).
19. V. Colletti, Biometric aspects of the stapedius reflex, Acta Otorhinolaryngol., Belg., 28:545 (1974).
20. A. Sokolowski, The protective action of the stapedius muscle in noise-induced hearing loss in cats, Arch. Klin. Exp. Ohr. Nas. Kehlkopfheilkd., 203:209 (1973).
21. E. Borg, Dynamic characteristics of the intra-aural muscle reflex, in: "Acoustic Impedance and Admittance: The Measurement of Middle Ear Function," A. S. Feldman and L. A. Wilber, eds., The Williams and Wilkins, Baltimore (1976).
22. J. E. Zakrisson, The effect of the stapedius reflex on attenuation and poststimulatory auditory fatigue at different frequencies, Acta Otolaryngol. Suppl., 360:118 (1979).
23. A. R. Moller, Acoustic reflex in man, J. Acoust. Soc. Am., 34:1524 (1962).
24. V. Colletti, Impedenzometria, Ed. Tecniche, Milano (1984).
25. R. H. Wilson, The effects of aging on the magnitude of the acoustic reflex, J. Speech Hear. Res., 24:406 (1981).

26. B. H. Sprague, T. L. Wiley and M. G. Block, Dynamics of acoustic reflex growth, *Audiology*, 20:15 (1981).
27. C. G. Fowler and R. H. Wilson, Adaptation of the acoustic reflex, *Ear and Hearing*, 5:281 (1984).
28. E. Borg, R. Nilsson and G. Liden, Fatigue and recovery of the human acoustic stapedius reflex in industrial noise, *J. Acoust. Soc. Am.*, 65:846 (1979).
29. K. J. Gerhard and H. L. Hepler, Acoustic-reflex activity and behavioral thresholds following exposure to noise, *J. Acoust. Soc. Am.*, 74:109 (1983).

DISCUSSION

Tyler: How can you tell in contrasting Groups A and B whether Group A has a lower threshold because they have a stronger stapedius reflex or if Group B has a weaker stapedius reflex as a result of their noise induced hearing loss?

Colletti: That is why I analysed Group C, since I might have run into the possibility that what I observed on the reflex was exactly a function of hearing threshold.

Salvi: Were there any acute differences between Groups B and C?

Colletti: They were matched for age. That is very important, especially for subjects above 50 years old.

Nilsson: I think the relaxation time is not important for individual susceptibility because if you have a series of impulses, the first impulse can trigger the system, then you will have increased impedence during the time for the series.

Colletti: Theoretically, I agree, but as you saw in Groups B and C, both displayed shorter values or both offset latency and decay time.

SIMULATION OF THE MIDDLE EAR ACOUSTIC REFLEX APPLIED TO DAMAGE-RISK FOR HEARING PRODUCED BY BURST FIRE

Guy O. Stevin

Laboratory for Acoustics, Technical Services of the Army
SIFT/CT
Quartier Housiau - B-1801 Brussels (Peutie) - Belgium

INTRODUCTION

The middle ear muscle reflex may be described as a feedback process which reduces the sound transmission in the middle ear when the level detected in the brain is too high. The effect of this reflex is an increase of the stapedius muscle stiffness, resulting in a change of the stapes response. The contraction process of the stapedius muscle results in a reduction of the middle ear transmission, but also in an increase of resonance and of the cut-off frequency of the middle ear. Both effects, as predicted by the model, appear to be similar to those reported for animals and inferred for humans. The model is implemented in a feedback process, starting from the brain, where a threshold detector elaborates the contraction command and sends it back to the stapedius muscle through a low-pass filter.

Our aim in the present study is to establish a mathematical model of the acoustic reflex as part of the complete human auditory system, including threshold detection in the brain and feedback to the middle ear muscle. Most authors have considered that the acoustic reflex is limited to the middle ear. We are convinced that a model of the acoustic reflex should at least involve the spectral analysis of sounds carried out in the inner ear by the basilar membrane. We may indeed assume that the electrical charges transmitted to the brain along the nerve fibres are proportional to the displacements of the basilar membrane. In this case, the inner ear response is necessary to evaluate the neural phenomenon resulting in the acoustic reflex and fixing its magnitude.

MODEL OF THE MIDDLE EAR ACOUSTIC REFLEX

Experimental Description of the Muscle Reflex

The middle ear muscles (the stapedius and tensor tympani) have been the subject of interest for many years. Contraction of these muscles under high level sound stimulation leads, under certain conditions, to a reduction of the vibrations of the middle ear ossicles. This effect, known as "acoustic reflex," suggests that it may act to protect the inner ear from damage due to excessive acoustical stimulation such as high intensity industrial noise; although it is unlikely to be its primary function.

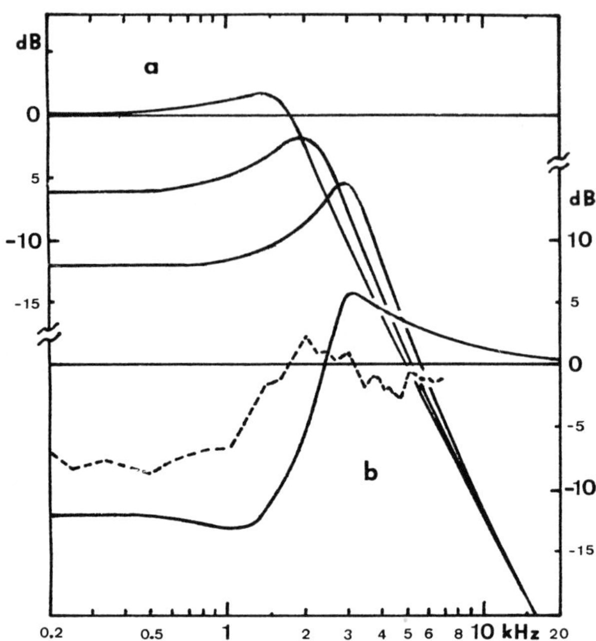

Fig. 1. Spectral response of the middle ear. (a) transfer function of the "spring-like" muscle system for increasing cut-off frequency (0 dB, 6 dB and 12 dB attenuation); (b) experimental [2] (---)curve, as observed on rabbits for a moderate reflex and computed (---) spectral response derived from (a) for a maximum reflex.

Experiments on animals [1] have shown that the main effect of reflex contraction of the middle ear muscles is the attenuation of sound transmission at frequencies below 2 kHz. Maximum attenuation values are about 20 to 30 dB. At higher frequencies there is little attenuation or slight amplification, as shown in Fig. 1. In addition, onset of the acoustic reflex is not immediate but progressive, and takes about 100 milliseconds, due to reflex latency and contraction time. It is a low-pass filter effect with cut-off frequency equal to about 5 Hz [1]. This effect corresponds approximately to an exponential decrease.

The acoustic reflex for humans, although similar to that for animals, differs by two main properties. Firstly, the maximal attenuation is lower, in order of 12 dB; secondly, the reflex only appears for high sound levels, higher than 75 dB. The maximal attenuation is obtained for stimuli of about 110 dB. The small attenuation for high frequencies and the slight amplification which were recorded for animals have also been observed [2] for humans above 1.5 kHz.

The block diagram of the acoustic reflex is shown in Fig. 2. The sound pressure p(t) at the eardrum is transmitted through the middle and the inner ear to the brain. Separation into different spectral components occurs in the cochlea according to the characteristic frequency, which appears in the transfer function of the inner ear. The

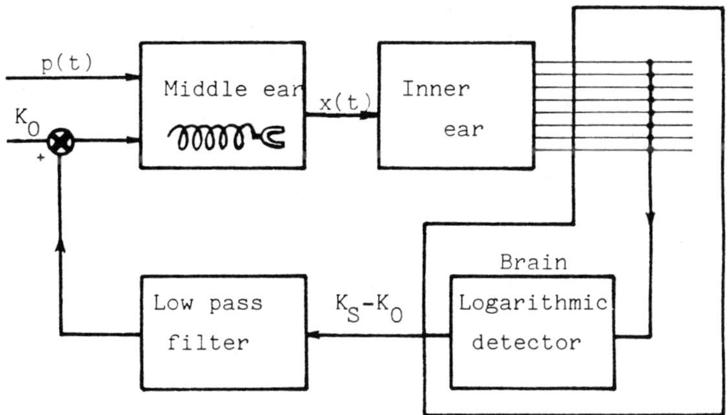

Fig. 2. Functional diagram of the ear reflex

internal process initiating the acoustic reflex is not yet known. However, it seems logical to assume that the most intense component reaching the brain is compared to an internal threshold; the magnitude of the reflex command is therefore a function of the overshoot above threshold. This command is then transmitted to the middle ear through a low-pass filter having a cut-off frequency of a few Hertz. The complete acoustic reflex thus involves three functions: two of them are located in the feedback chain - a threshold detector and a low-pass filter; the third function, being the contraction of the stapedius muscle, is located in the direct chain and is the first one to be studied hereafter.

Action of the Muscle on the Stapes

The ossicular chain of the middle ear acts as an impedance transformer between air in the ear-canal and the liquid in the inner ear. The malleus (hammer), which is shaped like a small one-sided hammer, has its handle embedded in the eardrum and its head attached in the incus (anvil). The incus, acting like a lever is connected by its long arm to the stapes (stirrup). The footplate of the stapes rest on the oval window and transmits its movement to the inner ear. The transformer ratio of the middle ear involves the ratio of the effective area of the eardrum to those of the footplate ($\sim$15) and the lever ratio ($\sim$1.3), producing [2] a value of about 20.

A mathematical model of the middle ear is found in Flanagan [3] Eq. (1) giving the transfer function of the middle ear (ratio of stapes displacement to pressure at the eardrum):

$$G(s) = \frac{C}{(1 + s/a)(s^2 + 2\,a\,s + \alpha^2)} \qquad (1)$$

In Eq. (1), s is the complex Laplace variable; the ratio of the cut-off frequencies (a/α) is equal to $(5)^{-1/2}$. This ratio is also equal to the resonance factor of the second order term. Flanagan [3] failed in determining accurately the numerical value of the cut-off frequency $F = \alpha/2\pi$; however, he found that the lower and upper limits for this frequency were 1650 and 3300 Hz respectively. The inaccuracy of this model will be discussed below.

Neglecting the first order term in Eq. (1), we may observe that the second order term is exactly the Laplace transform of the "spring" equation. We shall thus note the motion of a unit mass of the stapes by means of the equation of a damped spring whose stiffness K is due to the stapedius muscle contraction:

$$\frac{d^2x(t)}{dt^2} + F\frac{dx(t)}{dt} + K\,x(t) = C\,p(t) \qquad (2)$$

In Eq. (2), x(t) is the displacement of the stapes, F is the damping coefficient and the term C p(t) is the force applied by the eardrum to a unit mass of the ossicular chain. Comparison of Eqs. (1) and (2) shows proportionality between stiffness K and squared angular frequency α as well as between damping coefficient F and twice the angular frequency a.

According to Eq. (1), 12 dB attenuation can easily be obtained by quadrupling the stiffness, or by doubling the cut-off frequency f_α . On the other hand, it seems logical to assume that the damping coefficient F, (and thus the angular frequency a) remains constant. In this case the resonance factor is halved, resulting in a doubling (+ 6 dB) of the tuning at the frequency f_α. Fig. 1a shows the spectral responses according to Eq. (1) for different values of α , starting from 1650 Hz at rest and going to 3300 Hz when the contraction is complete. These limits are exactly the uncertainty limits stated by Flanagan [3]. This variation can thus be explained by the fact that the cut-off frequency is not constant, but varies with muscle stiffness.

It must be noted that hearing loss produced by exposure to high level noise is maximum in the vicinity of 3 kHz. This effect, mainly due to resonance of the ear canal, is also due to the higher resonance (+ 6dB) of the middle ear (with elicited reflex) at this frequency.

One should be careful when discussing the acoustic reflex in terms of the transfer function of the spring. We conclude, indeed, that attenuation is obtained in the middle ear by increasing the cut-off frequency of the filter, leading to a description of this effect by a linear differential equation with variable coefficients. Eq. (1) is therefore not appropriate, because a transfer function is only valid for a linear system with constant coefficients, which is not the case here. Spectral analysis is, however, qualitatively useful in understanding this phenomenon because the non-constant coefficients are varying at a very low rate, compared with the lowest frequency involved in the hearing process.

The differential equation completely describing the function of the middle ear is then obtained by making the stiffness $K(= \alpha^2)$ from Eq. (2) variable with time; this coefficient is given as K(t). This yields:

$$\frac{d^2x(t)}{dt^2} + 2\,a\frac{dx(t)}{dt} + K(t)x(t) = C\,p(t) \qquad (3)$$

In Eq. (3), K(t) varies with time, between K at rest and a value K depending on the magnitude of the acoustic reflex. The maximum value of K_s, noted K_M, is equal to 4 times K_o (ratio equal to 12 dB).

Threshold Detection Magnitude of the Acoustic Reflex

In the analogue model previously proposed by Lutman and Martin [7], the contraction command is an input data of the system. In order to describe the complete process, it is necessary to account for the nerve reaction in order to close the feedback loop. Although the detection mechanism is not very well known, it seems logical to suppose that the brain acts as a logarithmic detector, the detected value being an energy parameter. The brain records this value for each of the different bands. The greatest value recorded is then compared with the threshold. The ratio between this maximum value and the threshold determines the magnitude of the acoustic reflex.

Low-pass Filtering

The low-pass filter which is present in the feedback loop causes a gradual start of the ear reflex. The muscle contraction can be described by the step response of the low-pass filter to a step function with value ($K_s - K_o$). However, this input signal is a function of time, starting from zero and reaching a stable value after a certain delay. The change in muscle stiffness can be numerically expressed by a first order difference equation which corresponds to the effect of the low-pass filter:

$$K_i = \frac{K_{i-1} + K_{si-1}(T/\delta_i)}{1_i + T/\delta_i} \tag{4}$$

In Eq. (4), index i denotes the value at the time i T, T is the time interval between two numerical computations; δ is the latency of the reflex.

RESULTS OF SIMULATION

Numerical Integration

Modeling of the ear reflex requires, as stated before, the knowledge of the inner ear response. The chosen model (Eq. 4.1) in Flanagan [3] is a transfer function of the fifth order. Finally, the transfer function of the ear canal was established (see Appendix) in order to obtain a complete simulation of the entire human auditory system. The standard Runge-Kutta method of fourth order has been used in solving these differential equations. This method is known to be one of the most powerful ones in the sense of numerical stability and accuracy.

The numerical constants of the model have been chosen for a pure tone at 1000 Hz in order to fit the detection range of the acoustical reflex at sound pressure levels between 80 and 106 dB at the entrance of the ear canal. There is a good agreement between the model and experimental results. Fig. 3 shows the stapes response for some characteristic stimuli.

Effects of Impulse Noises from Weapons

The computational model has been applied to the set of impulse noises used as samples in a previous study, which statistically analyzed the hazard to hearing. For these signals, simulating weapon noises, the acoustical reflex entails a mean loudness reduction of about one decibel with regard to the previous results (without reflex). The largest variation does not exceed 3 dB for the longest impulses (20 ms). These results show that impulsive noise is not significantly attenuated by the acoustical reflex; this is due to the fact that the processed impulses contain spectral components higher than 2 kHz, and their durations are very much shorter than the latency of the muscle reaction. Consequently, it can be said that impulse noise produced by weapons results in muscle contrac-

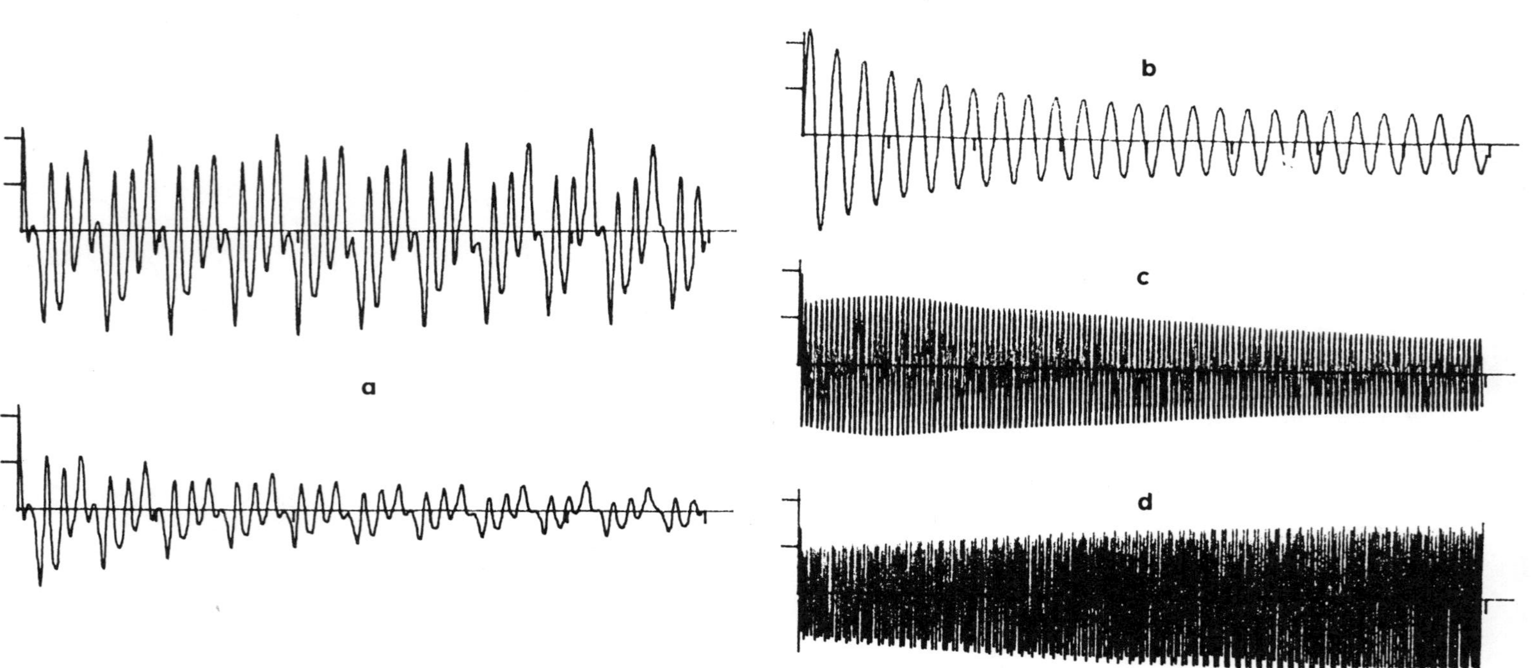

Fig. 3. Stapes response: (a) "O"-vowel without and with the ear reflex, (b) 250 Hz- sine-wave-exponential decay, (c) 2 kHz-sine-wave, increase followed by decrease, (d) 3 kHz-sine-wave-exponential increase.

tion, but this reflex is far too slow to produce an effective attenuation of the impulse noise. These conclusions fully agree with the experiments [4] on twelve small arms. For these weapons, firing single shots, the average attenuation due to the acoustic reflex is equal to 0.4 dB; the maximal attenuation remaining less than 0.8 dB.

Effects of Burst Fire

It is stated in the damage-risk criteria (DRC) for impulse noise [5] that only the first round of a burst has to be taken into account for evaluating risk to hearing. This implies that the impulses produced by the other rounds of a burst are sufficiently attenuated by the acoustic reflex; consequently, these rounds are neglected by the DRC. This rule is only applicable for short bursts (3 to 4 rounds) and provided the repetition period is greater than 100 ms (repetition rate less than 600 rounds per minute). The loudness of a burst can be computed by the usual rule for loudness addition: all rounds following more than 100 ms after the first round are identically attenuated by the middle ear. This is the case for all classical weapons whose repetition rate is less than or equal to 600 rpm. It is easily verified that one should add 16 identical rounds attenuated by a factor of 4 for having a loudness 3 dB higher than the loudness of the single shot. These figures are given for information, because they are only based on the attenuation effect, without any spectral change. In this simplified case, the loudness increase remains lower than

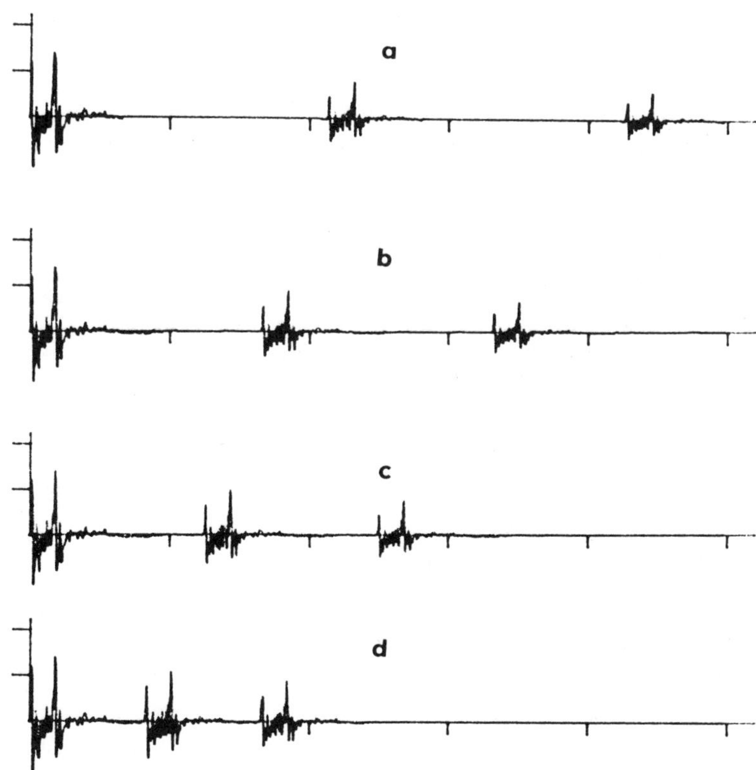

Fig. 4. Bursts of three rounds from high rate automatic weapons: (a) two-barrels AA Gun, (b) rifle G-11, (c) quad Mi.50 AA, (d) six-barrels "Vulcan".

1 dB when the burst does not exceed 4 rounds, and the approximation contained in the DRC is reasonable.

Some recent weapons, however, do have higher repetition rates. This is the case for anti-aircraft multi-barrel guns firing 600 rpm per barrel such as the Vulcan (6 barrels), quadmachine gun and two-barrel 30 or 35 mm guns. This is also the case for the novel German rifle G 11 using caseless cartridges and firing 3-round bursts at a high rate of 2000 rpm.

For each weapon, we have simulated a 3-round burst as illustrated on Fig. 4 and computed the theoretical loudness using the complete simulation. The single shot is attenuated by 0.7 dB by the ear reflex. For the classical single-barrel weapon, the loudness increase produced by the second and third rounds of the burst is equal to 0.75 dB. This value results from an overall attenuation of 10 dB for the two last rounds and confirms, on a theoretical case, the practical rules contained in the present DRC. For the high-rate weapons, however, the loudness increase is more important for the three rounds burst; the AA guns yield a loudness increase of 2.5 dB, 2 dB and 1.5 dB respectively; for the G 11 rifle, the increase is equal to 1.7 dB with regard to the single shot. These high variations, due to the two last rounds of these short bursts, may not be neglected. These values are higher than what might be predicted, due to spectral components at 2 to 3 kHz which are not attenuated, but amplified by the acoustic reflex. The number of rounds occurring within the 100 ms appears to be an important parameter for assessing the risk to hearing produced by bursts. Modern weapons with high burst-rates are more damaging to hearing than predicted by the present damage-risk criteria.

CONCLUSIONS

The middle ear model developed in the present study describes the most basic properties of the acoustic reflex. The contraction process of the stapedius muscle results in a reduction of middle ear transmission, but also in an increase of resonance and of the cut-off frequency of the middle ear. Both effects, as predicted by the model, appear to be similar to those reported for animals and inferred for humans. The computational model has been applied to forecast the loudness of impulse noise produced by bursts of gun fire. The high burst-rate for the new weapons and the presence of high frequency components in the spectrum of the impulses results in rather poor attenuation of the rounds following the first one. The present damage-risk criteria lead to an underestimate of the risk to hearing produced by this kind of impulse noise.

APPENDIX

Transfer Function of the Outer Ear

The earcanal can be represented by a uniform tube closed at one end by the eardrum. If we note u(x,t), the displacement of the air particles on the x-axis of the tube and p(x,t) the air pressure, we obtain the following system of partial differential equations (ρ is the specific mass of air and c the sound velocity):

$$\frac{\partial^2 u}{\partial t^2} = c^2 \frac{\partial^2 u}{\partial x^2} - R \frac{\partial u}{\partial t} \qquad \text{(A1)}$$

$$p(x,t) = -\rho c^2 \frac{\partial u}{\partial x}$$

The initial condition is the pressure at the entrance of the earcanal: p(0,t) equal to the acoustical stimulus. At the eardrum (x = L), there is no displacement of the air particles: the boundary condition is thus u(L,t)=0. Applying a Laplace transform to this set of equations leads to a more simple system; capitals P and U are used for the transform of functions p and u respectively; this yields;

$$(s^2 + R\, s)U = c^2 \frac{d^2U}{dx^2} \qquad \text{(A2)}$$

$$P = -\rho c^2 \frac{dU}{dx}$$

Solving this system is rather simple: the transfer function B(s) of the outer ear is obtained by computing the ratio B(s) = P(L,s)/ P(0,s). This yields:

$$B(s) = \cosh^{-1} \left[\frac{L}{c}(s^2 + R\, s)^{1/2}\right] \qquad \text{(A3)}$$

It can be easily shown that resonances are present for odd harmonics of the fundamental frequency f = c/4L = 3 kHz. A 14 dB-resonance is obtained at the fundamental frequency for value of R equal to 4800 s^{-1}.

REFERENCES

1. P. J. Dallos, Dynamics of the acoustic reflex, J. Acoust. Soc. Amer. 36:2175 (1964).
2. A. R. Moller, Function of the middle ear, The acoustic middle ear muscle reflex, in: "Handbook of Sensory Physiology - Auditory System" Vol. V/1, Springer-Verlag, Berlin, Heidelberg, New York (1974).
3. J. L. Flanagan, "Speech analysis, synthesis and perception," Springer Verlag, Berlin (1965).
4. G. O. Stevin, Spectral analysis of impulse noise for hearing conservation purposes, J. Acoust. Soc. Amer. 72:1845 (1982).
5. W. D. Ward, Proposed damage-risk criterion for impulse noise (gunfire), Report of Working Group 57, National Academy of Sciences - National Research Council, Committee on Hearing, Bioacoustics and Biomechanics (CHABA), Washington DC (1968).
6. F. Pfander, "Das Knalltrauma," Springer-Verlag, Berlin, New York (1975).
7. G. O. Stevin, A computational model of the acoustic reflex", Acustica 55:277 (1984).

DISCUSSION

Pfander: We have some field data that is revelant to your theoretical analysis. One hundred soldiers were exposed to gunfire, six shots fired quickly (presumably the reflex activated for all six shots) and a second exposure to six shots with 10 seconds between each shot (no reflex action). In the field study one group has the reflex and the other is without the stapedius. The results show that 55 persons had no TTS with the interval of 10 seconds and 54 persons had no TTS with the reflex. This field study really does not show that the reflex offers any protection.

Henderson: The data that Pfander shows does not necessarily contradict Dr. Stevins' hypothesis. An unrecognized and unappreciated variable in many noise studies is the pattern or delivery rate of acoustic energy. We have seen many times that the traumatic effects of an exposure are influenced by the rate of flow of acoustic energy. This is especially true for impulse and impact noise. It appears that a single impulse causes a state of vulnerability in the cochlea and if a second impulse (or more) "hit" the cochlea during this period of vulnerability, then the traumatic effects of that impulse will be greater. Going to Professor Pfander's data, it is possible that the slow presentation rate 1/10 sec. was an adequate amount of time for the cochlea to recover while the faster rate left the cochlea vulnerable to even the partially attenuated impulses (by the reflex). In a sense, the variable of reflex attenuation and period of vulnerability may be working in opposition.

CHANGES IN AUDITORY THRESHOLD DURING AND AFTER LONG DURATION NOISE EXPOSURE: SPECIES DIFFERENCES

Donald W. Nielsen, Mary Jane Bauman and Diane K. Brandt

Otological Research Laboratories
Henry Ford Hospital
Detroit, Michigan 48202, USA

INTRODUCTION

Because noise exposure causes physiological changes within the cochlea which cannot be investigated directly in humans, animal models must be used to study the effects of noise on human hearing. However, in choosing an animal model, one must be aware of species differences in the reaction of the cochlea to noise exposure. These differences are reflected in the behavioral temporary threshold shifts (TTS) which result from the noise exposure.

In this chapter we will discuss the growth, frequency spread, and recovery of behavioral TTS, with implications for the study of the physiological processes in the cochlea and with emphasis on species differences.

BACKGROUND

The chinchilla is the most popular animal for noise research in North America. However, all studies of noise-induced hearing loss (NIHL) using the chnichilla have shown that this animal has more hearing loss in response to a specific noise exposure than humans do. Its increased sensitivity cannot be accounted for on the basis of lower absolute thresholds for frequencies below about 8 kHz; and the chinchilla is slightly less sensitive between 500 Hz and 8 kHz [1]. Nor can the differences in NIHL sensitivity be accounted for on the basis of the acoustic properties of the chinchilla external and middle ear [2]. In fact, von Bismarck states that the "similarity between the sound pressure transfer function ...for man and chinchilla (zero middle ear pressure) is striking" [2]. Thus, the difference in response to noise exposure must occur in the inner ear or possible more centrally in the nervous system. Since NIHL is most evident in damage to the cochlea, we believe that these differences in sensitivity are due to basic differences in the way in which the inner ear of the two species reacts to noise exposure. In our efforts to find a more suitable animal model, we decided to investigate the squirrel monkey.

Squirrel Monkey Versus Human Absolute Auditory Sensitivity

The first step in evaluating the squirrel monkey as a model for the effects of noise on human hearing was a comparison of the free-field

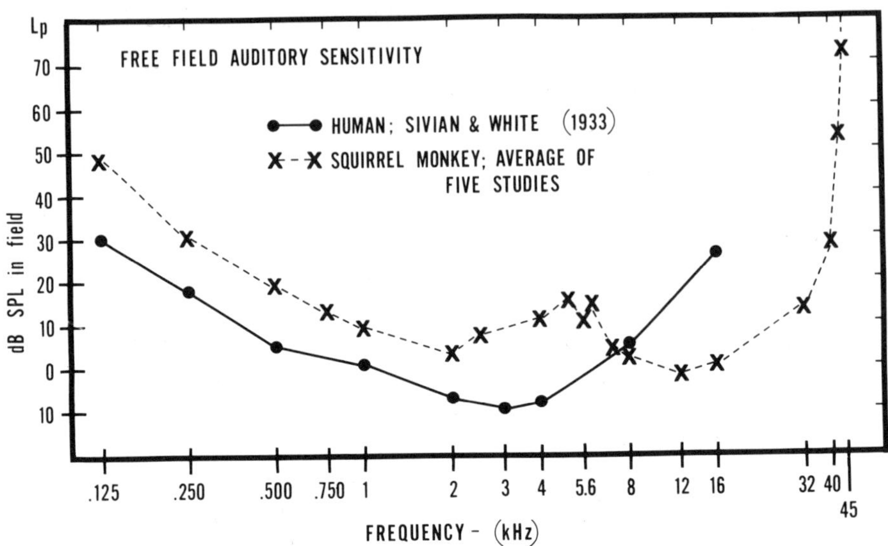

Fig. 1 A comparison of human and squirrel monkey absolute auditory sensitivity throughout the frequency range.

absolute sensitivity curves of the two species (Fig. 1). Below 6 or 8 kHz the squirrel monkey is less sensitive than the human, whereas above that point the squirrel monkey is more sensitive.

Squirrel Monkey External and Middle Ear Transfer Function

The next step was to determine the effect of the external and middle ear transfer function (EMTF) for the squirrel monkey in order to equate noise exposures for humans and squirrel monkeys in terms of the amount of sound energy reaching the inner ear. Using a probe microphone, we measured external ear resonances in squirrel monkeys. In addition, we measured the cavities of the external ear, modeled them as tubes closed at one end, and calculated the predicted resonances. These two independent sets of measures agreed. Finally, we calculated the transfer function of the middle ear from squirrel monkey Mossbauer data supplied by W. S. Rhode of the University of Wisconsin.

The combined EMTF for the squirrel monkey was compared with the behaviorally measured threshold curve (Fig. 2). While the location of the inverted transfer function is arbitrary with respect to ordinate, the agreement in the shape of the two curves below about 8 kHz is apparent. Even the fluctuation in the threshold curve between 2 and 7 kHz was predicted by the transfer function.

Thus, the differences in absolute sensitivity of the squirrel monkey and the human are most likely accounted for by acoustic characteristics resulting from the smaller size and mass of the external and middle ear of the monkey.

Since most comparisons of the auditory sensitivity of the two species involve exposure stimuli with frequencies below 8 kHz, the agreement between the two curves in that frequency range is especially important. It provides evidence that the shape of the behavioral auditory threshold curve is determined by the transfer function. That is, for stimuli below 8 kHz, the transfer function determines the complete sound pressure transformation

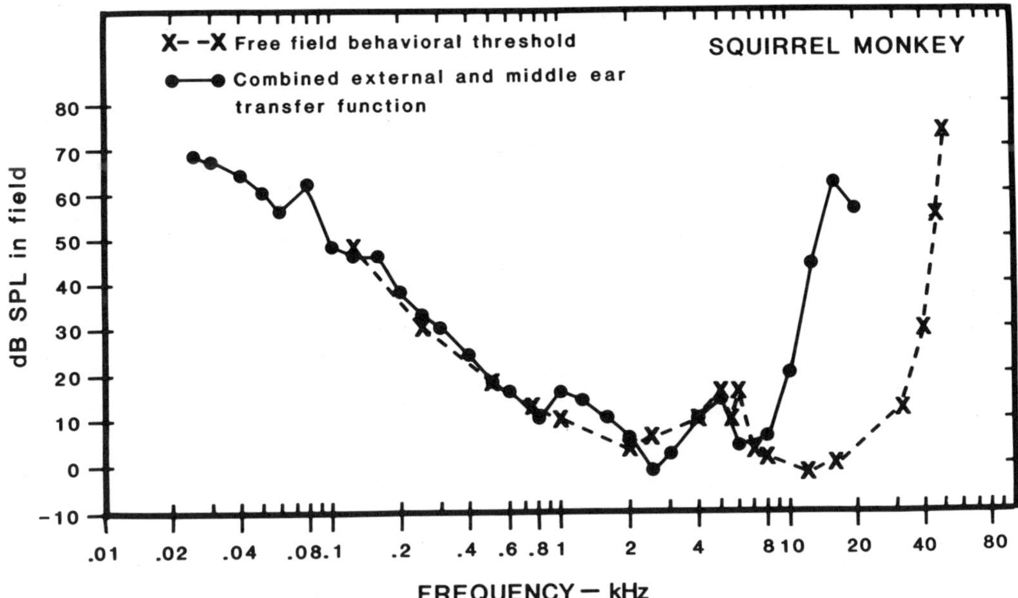

Fig. 2 The combined transfer function for the external and middle ear of the squirrel monkey is compared with the shape of the behaviorally measured absolute auditory sensitivity curve.

between the free sound field and the vestibule in the vicinity of the stapes. Numerical values for the transfer function may be interpreted as the sound pressure levels in a free field that are required to produce a constant sound pressure in the vestibule. Zwislocki [3] found similar results for humans. Thus, we can equate the sound pressure reaching the inner ear of the two species by allowing for their differences in absolute sensitivity at the frequency used.

TTS Results for Long Duration Noise Exposures

Previous research [4] with long duration noise exposures using the chinchilla as the experimental animal has shown that the TTS increases with the length of time in the noise up to about 24 hours, after which it remains constant for a long period of time. The level of TTS reached and maintained after 24 hours of exposure, which is called the asymptotic threshold shift (ATS), is thought to reflect a balance between the fatiguing and recovering processes in the cochlea.

Such chinchilla ATS studies raised the question as to whether human TTS would reach an asymptote after 24 hours of exposure. Results of experiments [5-7] in which humans were exposed for 24 hours or, in a few cases, 48 hours demonstrated that TTS growth functions did reach a plateau after about 24 hours. Since these exposures with human subjects were limited in duration, it was never established whether this plateau was a true asymptote in the mathematical sense. However, in our investigations with squirrel monkeys exposed for as long as four days, an ATS was not demonstrated [8,9]. The monkey data yielded TTS growth functions in which TTS grew at the same rate as the human TTS and which, like that of the humans, reached a plateau at about 24 hours of exposure. However, after this plateau, the TTS continued to grow. In contrast, chinchillas have a faster rate of TTS growth, reach a higher level of TTS, and their TTS reaches an asymptotic level within 24 hours. The squirrel monkeys also showed slightly less TTS than the humans, because comparatively less sound energy reached their inner ear at these low frequencies, due to the smaller size and mass of their external and middle ear.

Only one previous study has used monkeys in noise exposures longer than four days. As summarized by Moody et al. [10] in 1976, a study by Schieb et al. [11] using Old World monkeys found that "3 of 4 animals showed similar growth functions typically reaching 'asymptote' of 19 to 21 dB of loss after 8 to 12 hours of exposure." However, they go on to state that "it is readily apparent that the 'asymptote' observed after 8 hours of exposure is not a true asymptote at all, but rather a plateau in the function." Beginning at about 15 days of exposure, the threshold shift begins to be variable and eventually stabilizes at a new level about 10 dB above the original plateau. The fourth animal reached its first plateau of 56 dB TTS only after 200 hours of exposure. Therefore, their data show that Old World monkeys do not reach ATS in 24 hours, as chinchillas do, but instead reach ATS after about 15 days.

It is difficult to compare our four-day exposure TTS growth curves for squirrel monkeys to Schieb's data on Old World Monkeys, because data from only one animal were published. In that instance, ATS was reached by about 15 to 20 days of exposure. The TTS growth function for that Old World monkey is a step function consisting of an initial 11 dB step in the first hour which was maintained until about 6 hours of exposure. Between 6 and 9 hours there was a rise to 21 dB of TTS, which was maintained until about day 15 or 20 when the TTS rose to 31 dB. The other two animals also showed this step function [12]. These discrete 10 dB steps maybe due to the use of 10 dB attenuator steps in determining threshold. The growth function could actually be more gradual as we found when we used smaller attenuation steps for the squirrel monkeys.

Recent long duration exposures in the gerbil [13] have also shown that ATS is not reached in 24 hours. Those data, together with the data from the Old World monkey, raised the question of when TTS would reach asymptote for the squirrel monkey and by implication for the human. To investigate this question, we initiated some longer exposures of 60 to 90 days.

METHODS

We used six squirrel monkeys (Saimiri sciureus), 4 males and 2 females, approximately seven years of age as subjects. The behavioral testing was carried out under free field conditions using single-bar avoidance and a tracking procedure, with attenuation steps as small as 2.5 dB. Thresholds were determined by interpolation to 1.25 dB. Details of our testing procedure have been previously published [9,14].

The monkeys were exposed free field in a small reverberant room using an octave band of noise centered at either 500 Hz or 4 kHz and durations as long as 90 days. Procedural details of these studies and more detailed results will be published elsewhere.

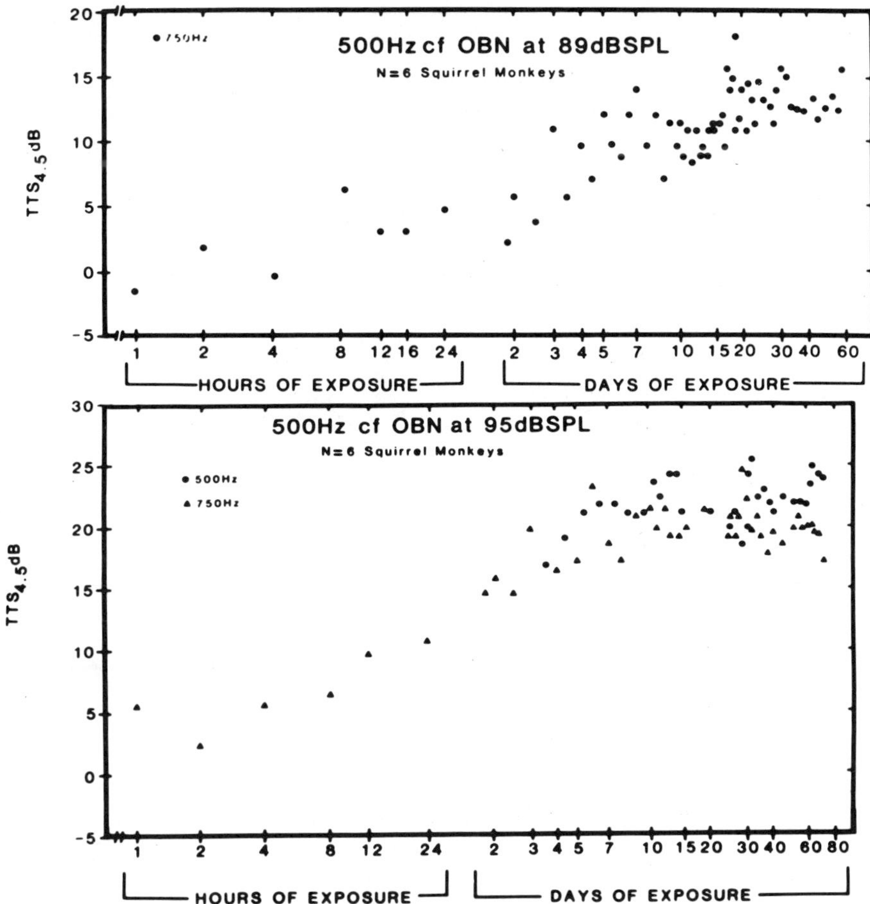

Fig. 3 Growth of TTS at either 500 or 750 Hz as a function of the length of time in the noise. The noise is an octave band of noise centered at 500 Hz and presented at 89 dB SPL (top) and 95 dB SPL (bottom).

CHANGES IN SQUIRREL MONKEY TTS TO LONG DURATION NOISE EXPOSURE

TTS Growth to an Octave Band of Noise Centered at 500 Hz

Our initial experiments used an octave band noise exposure centered at 500 Hz. In the first experiment, six squirrel monkeys were exposed to an 89 db SPL noise for 60 days; in the second experiment, the same six monkeys were exposed to a 95 dB SPL noise for 70 days.

During exposure, the thresholds were measured approximately 4.5 minutes following removal from the noise ($TTS_{4.5}$). The resulting TTS growth functions (Fig. 3) indicate that TTS grows linearly when time is plotted logarithmically. ATS was reached after about 15 to 20 days of exposure.

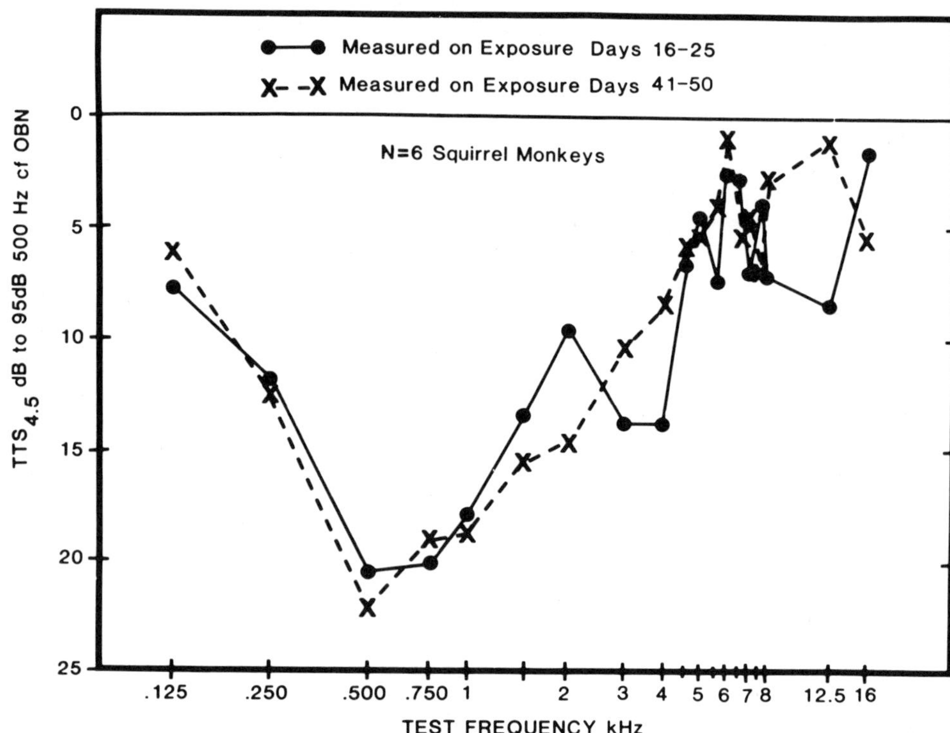

Fig. 4 TTS frequency spread to an octave band of noise centered at 500 Hz and presented at 95 dB SPL measured early in the exposure (16-25 days) and later in the exposure (41-50 days).

Thus, it appears that for this non-human primate, like the Old World monkey, the balance between fatiguing and recovering processes in the cochlea is reached in 15 to 20 days rather than in 24 hours as with the chinchilla.

TTS Frequency Spread to an Octave Band of Noise Centered at 500 Hz

During the 70-day exposure, we made two sets of threshold measurements at other frequencies to study the spread of fatigue along the cochlea and to determine whether other frequencies had reached their maximum shift by 20 days of exposure. Threshold measurements for each frequency were made 12 hours apart. Since each measurement required only five minutes out of the noise, TTS growth was not affected [10]. Test frequency selection was random, so that no two animals were tested at the same frequency during the same test period. Thus, it took nine days to make each set of measurements. In Fig. 4, TTS measurements made between exposure days 16 and 25 are compared to measurements made on days 41 to 50. No statistically significant differences between the curves were found at any frequency. Therefore, for this exposure, ATS is reached by about 15 to 20 days for all frequencies.

Recovery from an Octave Band of Noise Centered at 500 Hz

This long exposure experiment gave us a unique opportunity to study the effects of exposure duration on TTS recovery. The recovery from this 70-day exposure was compared to the recovery curve resulting from the same noise

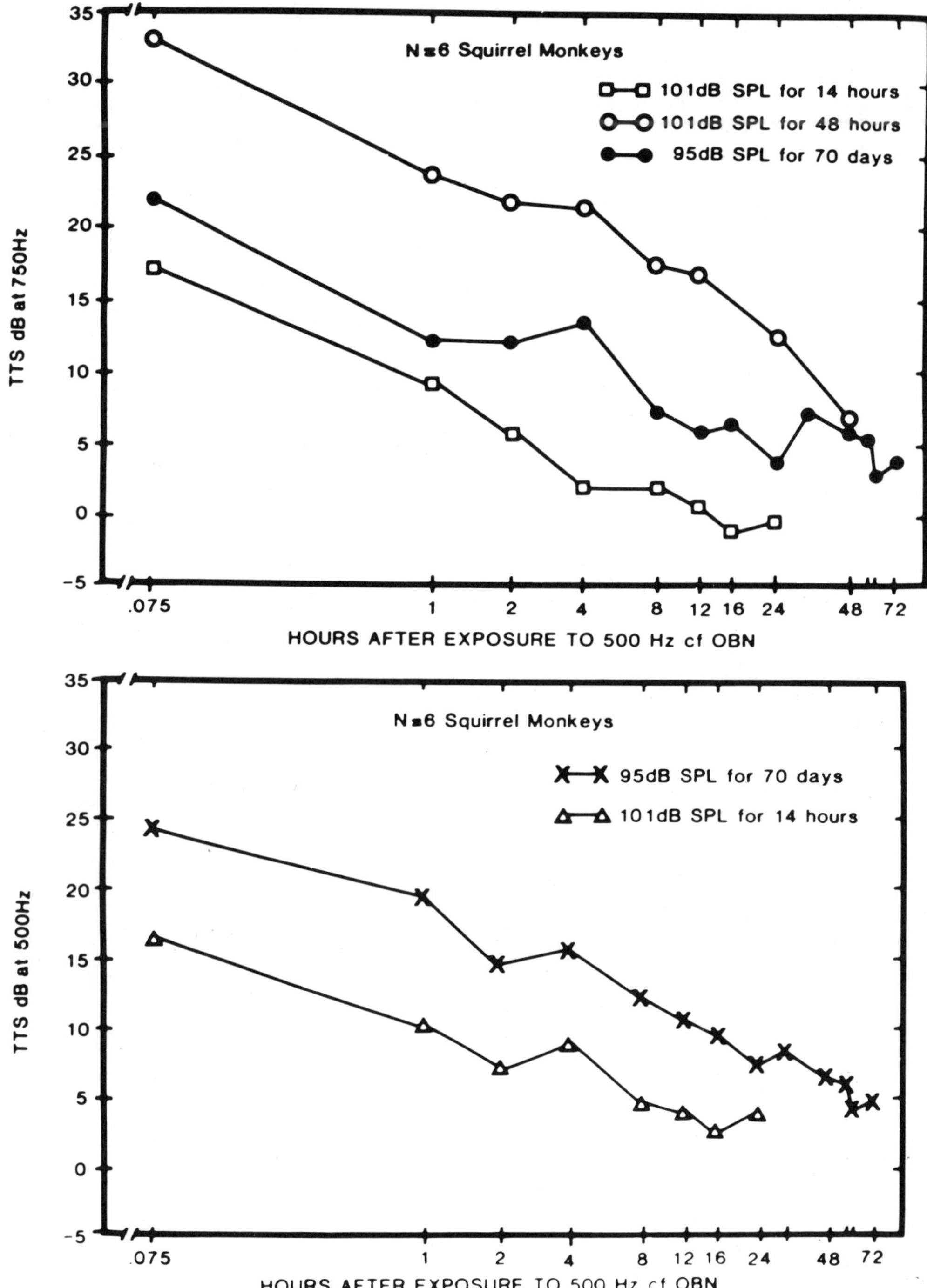

Fig. 5 Recovery of TTS from an octave band noise exposure centered at 500 Hz. Top: Recovery at 750 hZ for 95 dB SPL, 70-day exposures (solid circles); 101 dB SPL, 48-hour exposures (open circles); and 101 dB SPL, 14-hour exposures (open squares). Bottom: Recovery at 500 Hz for 95 dB SPL, 70-day exposures (x); 101 dB SPL, 14-hour exposures (open triangles).

presented at a higher level but a shorter duration; so that the shorter exposure resulted in about the same level of TTS.

After 70 days of exposure, the animals were removed from the noise and TTS recovery was measured. The recovery rate of the 750 Hz threshold from the 70-day exposure was compared with the recovery of 750 Hz from two other higher exposures (101 dB SPL), but shorter durations of 48 and 14 hours (Fig. 5). From these data, all collected on the same group of animals, it is obvious that whether the exposure is 14 hours or 70 days, the rate of recovery is the same and is linear when recovery time is plotted on a logarithmic scale. We had similar results from the 70-day and the 14-hour exposures for recovery at 500 Hz (Fig. 5). These data demonstrate that, for the squirrel monkey, the rate of recovery is not related to the length of

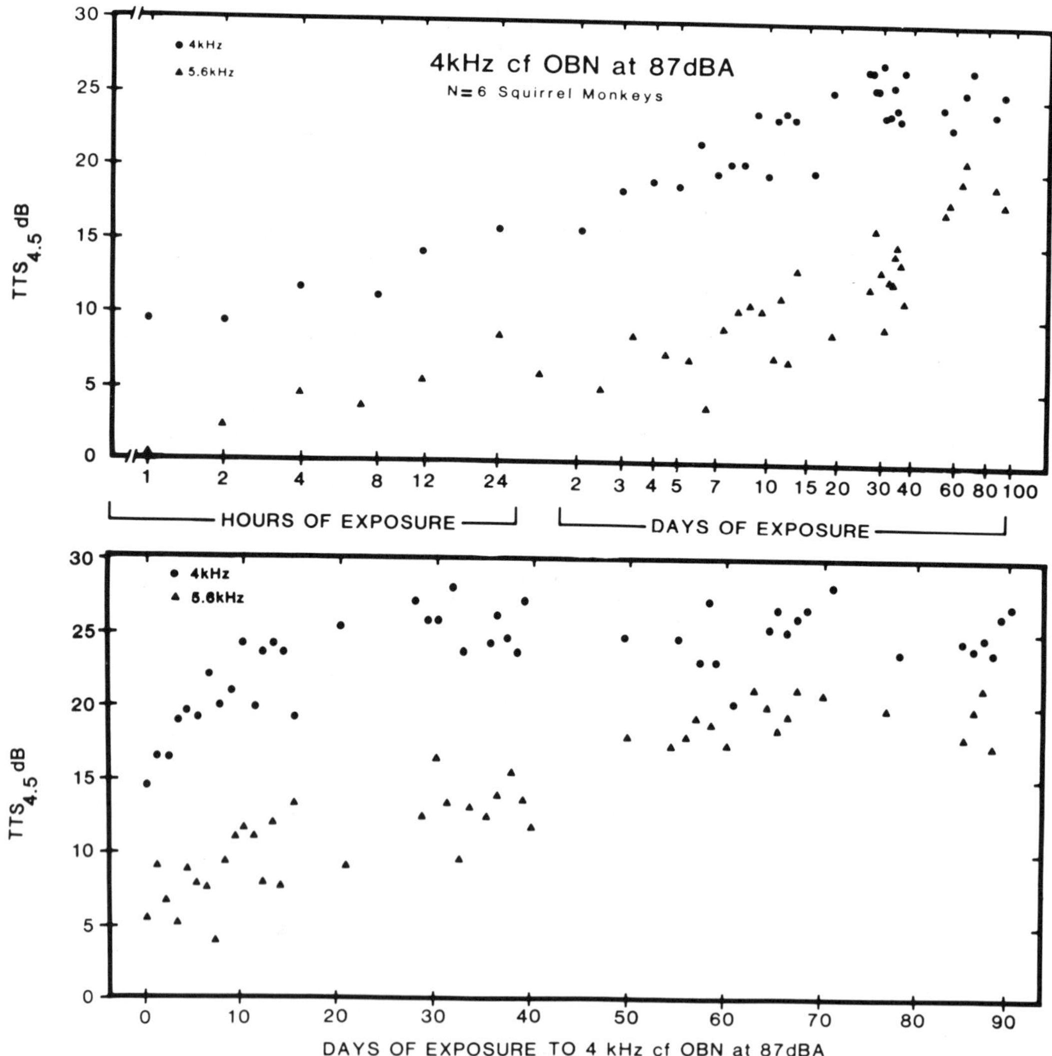

Fig. 6 Growth of TTS at 4 kHz (circles) and 5.6 kHz (triangles) to an octave band of noise centered at 4 kHz and presented at an SPL of 87 dBA for 90 days. Top: Length of time in the noise plotted logarithmically. Bottom: Length of time in the noise plotted linerarly.

time the ear is exposed to noise. For low frequency exposures of 14 hours or longer, the rate of recovery is independent of the length of the exposure. This conclusion is also consistent with the human data of Mills et al. [6] who concluded that "the magnitude of the TTS determines the time required for complete recovery" and that the "duration of the exposure was apparently not significant."

Furthermore, the linear recovery rate demonstrated for the squirrel monkey differs from the delayed recovery seen when chinchillas are used as the experimental animal. When chinchillas are removed from noise exposure, they tend to maintain a constant threshold shift for a period of time before recovery begins. Thus, TTS recovery as well as growth rates can differ significantly between species. In investigations of NIHL where one wishes to generalize to humans, and where the length of exposure and recovery time are consequential variables, it is important to choose an animal model with growth and recovery rates similar to those of humans.

TTS Growth to an Octave Band of Noise Centered at 4 kHz

After these studies using low frequency exposures were completed, we investigated the same effects with a high frequency exposure to determine if the fatiguing and recovering processes in the cochlea were similar across frequency. The exposure used in these experiments was an octave band of noise centered at 4 kHz and presented at an SPL of 87 dBA for 90 days.

The resulting growth of TTS at 4 kHz and at 5.6 kHz is shown in Fig. 6. At 4 kHz, TTS reaches an asymptote after about 20 days in a manner comparable to the 500 Hz exposure data in Fig. 3. That is, the growth of TTS at 4 kHz is linear (Fig. 6, top) where the time scale is logarithmic. By contrast, the 5.6 kHz TTS continues to grow up to about 65 days, where it appears to reach an asymptote close to the 4 kHz TTS. At 5.6 kHz, the growth of TTS is better described as linear in linear time (Fig. 6, bottom). Thus, the fatiguing processes in the high frequency region of the cochlea have different rates of growth for these two different test frequencies.

TTS Frequency Spread to an Octave Band of Noise Centered at 4 kHz

To study these differential frequency effects in more detail, we measured TTS at 17 additional frequencies at several times during the 87 dBA, 90 day exposure. When earlier measures made at 16 to 27 days of exposure were compared to later measures at 72 to 83 days, TTS at 5.6 kHz and at 6 kHz continued to grow after TTS growth at all other frequencies had reached its maximum (Fig. 7). The growth of TTS at 5.6 and 6 kHz between these two sets of data was statistically significant, whereas the differences at other frequencies were not.

Thus, for high frequency exposures, TTS must be measured at several frequencies in order to have an accurate estimate of the growth of hearing loss across frequency.

TTS Recovery from an Octave Band of Noise Centered at 4 kHz

We also measured recovery at 4 kHz and 5.6 kHz from the 90-day, 87 dBA exposure (Fig. 8). Both frequencies demonstrated a linear recovery in logarithmic time, as was seen with recovery from the low frequency exposure (Fig. 5). Surprisingly, the rate of recovery was identical for these two test frequencies, although they had different growth functions.

Since we had earlier established that the duration of the exposure did not affect the TTS recovery, it was reasonable to compare the squirrel monkey recovery data to human recovery data from an octave band noise exposure

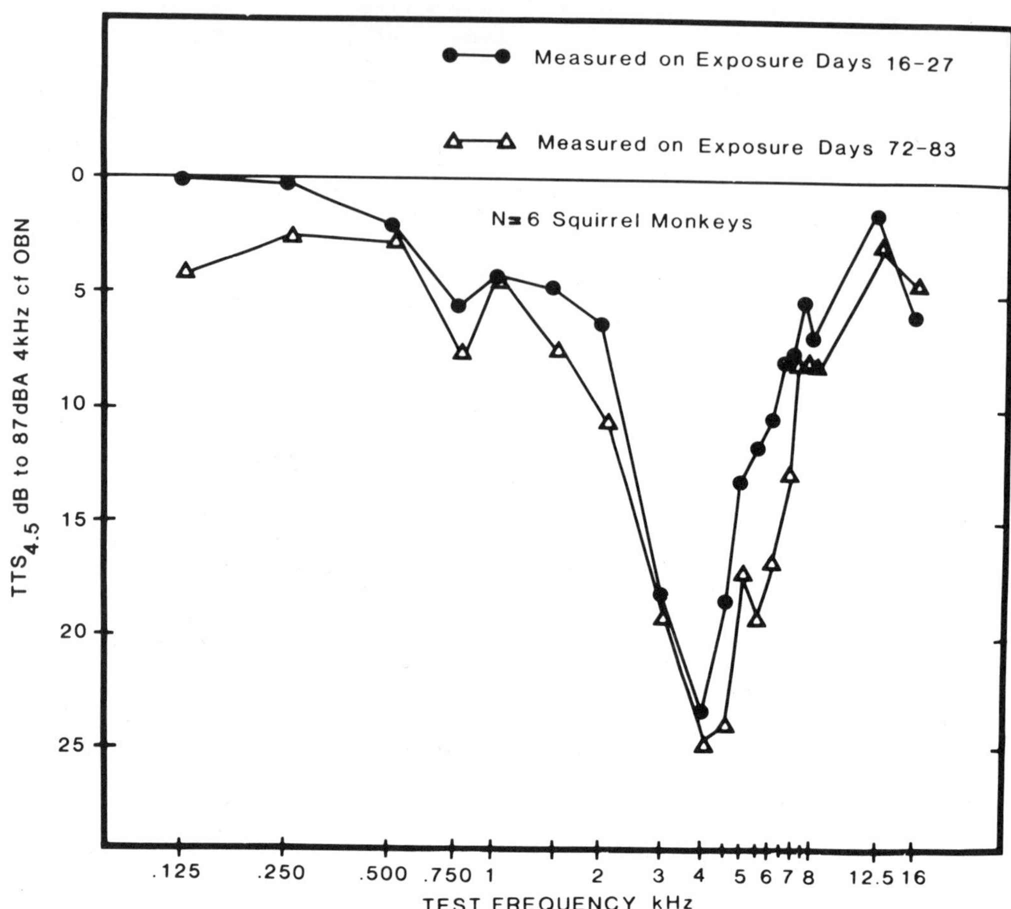

Fig. 7 TTS measured between 16 and 27 days and between 72 and 83 days after exposure to an octave band of noise centered at 4 kHz and presented at an SPL of 87 dBA.

monkey recovery data to human recovery data from an octave band noise exposure presented at 88 dB for 24 hours (Fig. 8). It is obvious from these data that when the humans and the squirrel monkeys have the same amount of TTS, the recovery rate is amazingly similar, both being linear when time is plotted logarithmically. Again such linear recovery differs from the delayed recovery seen in the chinchilla.

Experiments are underway in our laboratories comparing the recovery curves from this long duration, high-frequency exposure to recovery curves from short duration, high-intensity exposures of the same frequency. Future investigations will study permanant noise-induced hearing loss in the squirrel monkey and the resulting histopathology, in the manner described in the chapter by Liberman and with emphasis on the stereocilia abnormalities.

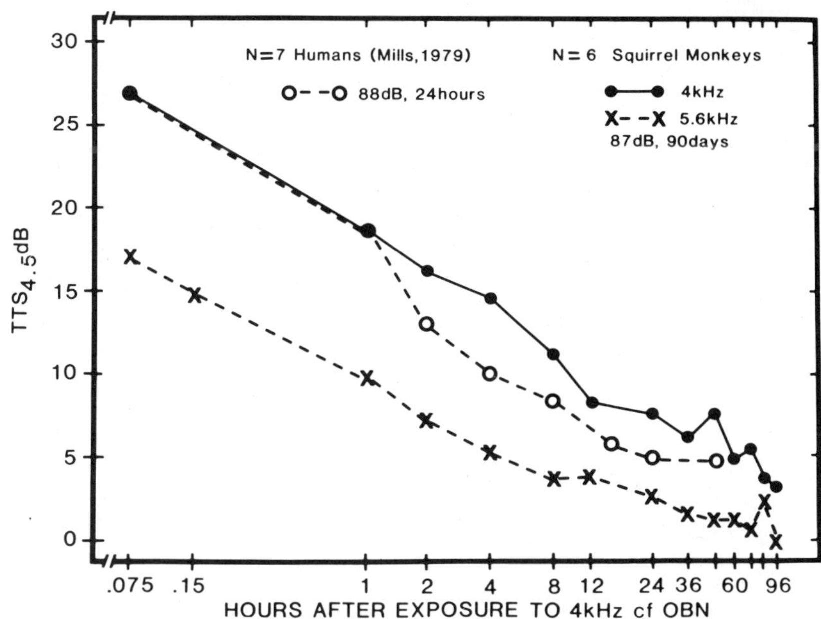

Fig. 8 Recovery of TTS at 4 kHz (solid circles) and 5.6 kHz (x) for an octave band noise exposure centered at 4 kHz and presented at an SPL of 87 dBA for 90 days. Human TTS recovery data from an octave band noise exposure centered at 4 kHz and presented at an SPL of 88 dB for 24 hours are also shown for comparison (open circles).

CONCLUSIONS

Our experiments have shown that:

1. For squirrel monkeys, as for humans, the rate of the recovery processes in the cochlea is independent of the length of time the cochlea is exposed to noise, at least for low frequency exposures of 14 hours or longer.

2. For the squirrel monkey, fatiguing processes in the high frequency region of the cochlea have different rates of growth for different frequencies, but similar rates of recovery.

3. Both Old World and New World monkeys, reach ATS at the maximally affected frequency after 15 to 20 days of noise exposure.

4. There are differences between primate and non-primate species, not only in the amount of hearing loss resulting from a given exposure, but also in the rate of growth and recovery of TTS.

Furthermore, we suggest that in investigations of noise-induced hearing loss where one wishes to generalize to humans and where the length of exposure and of time to recovery are consequential variable, it is important to choose an animal model with growth and recovery rates similar to those of humans. Finally, we also suggest that in studying physiological processes underlying noise-induced hearing loss, one must be cautious about generalizing from one species to another, especially between primates and non-primates.

ACKNOWLEDGMENTS

The authors would like to thank William S. Rhode for providing the middle ear measurements, Mike Davis for collecting the external ear measurements, and Robert G. Turner, Jr. for assistance in calculating the EMTF. Also, we wish to express our gratitude to Patricia Cornett for her editorial assistance, Barbara Williams and Susan Pierson-DiTomasso for collection of the TTS data: Thomas Boismier, Steve Dantzer, Cathy Thompson, Nancy Allar, John Wilson, and Zhi-Ping Gu. Finally, we would like to thank David B. Moody, William C. Stebbins, Constantine Trahiotis, and W. Dixon Ward for their comments on an earlier version of this manuscript. The work described above was supported in part by National Institute of Health contract NO1 RR82140, Division of Research, and in part by a grant from the Fund for Henry Ford Hospital.

REFERENCES

1. J. D. Miller, Audibility curve of the chinchilla, J. Acoust. Soc. Am., 48:513 (1970).
2. G. Von Bismarck, "The sound pressure transformation from free-field to the eardrum of chinchilla," Master Thesis, Massachusetts Institute of Technology (1967).
3. J. J. Zwislocki, The role of the external and middle ear in sound transmission, in: "The Nervous System, Vol, 3: Human Communication and its Disorders," D. B. Tower, ed., Raven Press, New York (1975).
4. H. M. Carder and J. D. Miller, Temporary threshold shifts from prolonged exposure to noise, J. Speech Hear. Res., 15:603 (1972).
5. H. M. Melnick and M. Maves, Asmptotic threshold shift (ATS) in man from 24-hour exposure to continuous noise, Ann. Oto. Rhinol. Laryngol., 83:824 (1974).
6. J. H. Mills, R. M. Gilbert and W. Y. Adkins, Temporary threshold shifts in humans exposed to octave levels of noise for 16 to 24 hours, J. Acoust. Soc. Am., 65:1238 (1979).
7. M. R. Stephensen, C. W. Nixon and D. L. Johnson, Growth and recovery of temporary threshold shift from 24 hour continuous, 48 hour continuous, and 48 hour intermittent noise exposure, J. Acoust. Soc. Am. Supple., 65:1238 (1979).
8. D. W. Nielsen, Asymptotic threshold shift in the squirrel monkey, in: "New Perspectives on Noise-Induced Hearing Loss," R. P. Hamernik, D. Henderson, and R. J. Salvi, eds., Raven Press, New York (1982).
9. D. W. Nielsen, J. Burnham and C. Talley, Squirrel monkey temporary threshold shift from 48 hour exposures to low frequency noise, J. Acoust. Soc. Am., 64(2):478 (1978).
10. D. B. Moody, W. C. Stebbins, L. G. Johnsson and J. E. Hawkins, Jr., Noise-induced hearing loss in the monkey, in: "Effects of Noise on Hearing," D. Henderson, R. P. Hamernik, D. S. Dosanjh, and J. H. Mills, eds., Raven Press, New York (1976).
11. B. T. Schieb, W. C. Stebbins and D. B. Moody, Temporary threshold shifts in non-human primates resulting from chronic exposure to a 2-kHz octave band of noise, J. Acoust. Soc. Am. Suppl., 57:S41 (1975).
12. D. B. Moody and W. C. Stebbins, Personal communication.
13. J. H. Mills and E. F. Elkins, Noise-induced hearing loss: State-of-the-art., Am. Speech-Hear-Lang. Assoc., 26(10):60 (1984).
14. D. W. Nielsen, L. Franseen and D. Fowler, The effects of interruption on squirrel monkey temporary threshold shifts to a 96 hour noise exposure, Audiology 23:297 (1984).

DISCUSSION

Henderson: Will you comment on the relationship between the rate of growth to ATS and the exposure level? In the chinchilla, the the rate of growth to ATS increased with stimulus level.

Neilson: I would suspect just looking at the data at 500 Hz (Fig. 3) that the same thing is true for the squirrel monkey. But we do not have enough data to answer that question more precisely.

Salvi: The work of Carder and Miller in the chinchilla showed that for many ATS exposures, there was a 10 or 15 hours period where there was little or no recovery. Thus, recovery is not linear in log time. Could you comment on the differences between the chinchilla and monkey in terms of recovery?

Neilson: We do not see the delayed recovery period in the monkey, and can not explain the differences between primates and chinchillas.

Henderson: PTS seems to depend on the amount of time in the noise. Thus, even though chinchillas may reach a stable level of ATS, those that remain in the noise for a longer period of time develop larger cochlear lesions. Also you mentioned, the rate of recovery stays essentially the same in your exposures; however, this seems unusual given that the longer exposures may lead to PTS. Could you comment on this in relationship to your results?

Neilson: We do not have data on PTS, but it is striking how fast these squirrel monkeys recover when they are taken out of the noise.

von Gierke: I think the main difference between your data and other human data is that in human data the recovery depended on the length of exposure.

Neilson: As far as I am aware, I do not believe we have recovery data from humans exposed to these long duration exposures. The longest ones I know of for humans are 48 hours.

von Gierke: Chuck Nixon exposed people for 48 hours and 24 hours and there were definite differences in recovery times even though both groups had the same TTS. From a practical point of view, this is extremely important.

THE CURIOUS HALF-OCTAVE SHIFT: EVIDENCE FOR A BASALWARD MIGRATION OF THE TRAVELING-WAVE ENVELOPE WITH INCREASING INTENSITY

Dennis McFadden

Department of Psychology
University of Texas
Austin, Texas, USA 78712

INTRODUCTION

Following exposure to an intense tonal stimulus, there may be no temporary threshold shift (TTS) at the exposure frequency, even though there is considerable hearing loss at a higher test frequency. This effect--commonly known as the half-octave shift in TTS--is among the oldest, best known, and most widely cited facts of psychoacoustics, yet it stands without a generally accepted explanation. This paper has three primary purposes: (1) to review the physiological findings apparently relevant to this upward shift of maximum effect; (2) to demonstrate that half octave-like shifts are not unique to TTS experiments, but rather, they can be found in data obtained in a wide array of psychophysical tasks not involving auditory fatigue; and (3) to present a possible explanation of the upward shift which accounts for many of the existing facts, and thus appears worthy of serious consideration by both theorists and experimentalists.

By way of historical perspective, the first reports of the maximum temporary hearing loss being shifted upward in frequency from the exposure stimulus were apparently made by Rawdon-Smith [1] and Ewing and Littler [2] (see Perlman [3] for a review and additional data). The fact was then well-documented and popularized by Davis et al. [4] in their classic monograph on auditory fatigue. Specifically, the effect is this: when narrow-band or tonal waveforms of high intensity are used as exposure stimuli, the test frequencies showing the greatest TTS are typically 0.5-1.0 octave above the exposure [4-6]. Indeed, Davis et al. [4]--and many others since--sometimes measured essentially no hearing loss at the exposure frequency, even though sensitivity at higher frequencies was reduced 15-20 dB or more. Upward shifts of maximum hearing loss are evident in measures of permanent threshold shift (PTS) as well as in TTS. Looking across studies and paradigms, there are some indications that the mechanisms producing the upward shift of effect may differ somewhat in the frequency regions above and below about 1000 Hz. Below about 1000 Hz, shifts are sometimes absent, small, or in the opposite direction [4, 7-10], or they appear to behave in accord with rules different from those above 1000 Hz [11]. If confirmed, this difference may prove to be a reflection of the apparent change in the characteristics of the cochlear partition in that region (at least in humans) that also produces linear rather than logarithmic frequency spacing below about 1000 Hz [12].

Over the years, this upward displacement of maximum hearing loss has universally come to be called the half-octave shift in TTS; however, it must be emphasized that the term is merely descriptive, not explicit--the maximum TTS can occur at the half-octave frequency, at the octave frequency, or above or below either of these. But while there may be nothing particularly magical about the half-octave frequency itself, the effect the term denotes is truly curious, and it is surprising that the half-octave shift has received so little experimental and theoretical attention during the 50 years it has been known.

The student seeking an explanation of the upward shift in maximum hearing loss following exposure is naturally drawn to look for possible structural bases for the effect. In this regard, the auditory periphery appears to offer a wealth of possibilities. For example, there are two, mutually dependent populations of transducers--inner and outer hair cells--which (1) have different gross and ultrastructural morphologies and different patterns of distribution along the cochlear partition; (2) synapse with different populations of primary afferents; (3) have different patterns of innervation, both afferent and efferent; (4) are thought by some to be stimulated by different modes of shearing; (5) are known to be differentially sensitive to such insults as anoxia, reduction in blood supply, and drug toxicity; etc. In addition to differences between the two populations of hair cells, the shift of maximal effect to adjacent frequency regions might be attributed to factors such as possible changes in the mechanics or micromechanics of the cochlear partition [13,14], and surely there are various metabolic, biochemical, or other nonstructural features that might also be suggested as relevant to the half-octave shift.

But even though the cochlear partition offers numerous possible candidates for the basis of the upward shift in hearing loss following exposure, to my knowledge none of these has ever been proposed or investigated. Indeed, as far as I can determine, only one explanation of the half-octave shift has received repeated mention over the years, and even these mentions have often been somewhat off-handed; certainly no one has attempted to systematically examine the various implications of this explanation, or to test it directly. The essence of this recurring idea is that the peak of displacement of the traveling-wave (TW) envelope may not occur at the same point along the cochlear partition for all stimulus intensities, but rather the peak may gradually move basally as intensity is increased. If the peak of displacement of the TW envelope does move basally along the cochlear partition as intensity is increased, that is tantamount to having a multiplicity of intensity-dependent tonotopic maps of the cochlear partition--the map for each successively higher intensity being displaced slightly toward the base. Thus, the cochlear location maximally "fatigued" by a high-intensity exposure would be basal to the point at which the exposure tone produced its maximal displacement when presented at a <u>low intensity</u>. That is, at threshold intensities, the frequencies activating the maximally fatigued portion of the partition would be ones <u>higher</u> than the exposure frequency--which would itself maximally activate a slightly more apical region. This point is illustrated in the left panel of Fig. 1.

Place theorists of pitch perception long ago suggested such changes in position as an explanation of the claim that high tones get higher in pitch and low tones get lower in pitch with increasing intensity [15]. In recent times, the basic idea has been mentioned in various contexts [8, 16-26].

Davis [27] recently advanced a "conceptual model" of cochlear mechanics that suggests a possible mechanism for the basalward migration of the peak of the displacement envelope with increasing stimulus intensity. Davis argued that the <u>total</u> envelope of membrane displacement produced by a tonal stimulus is always the point-for-point sum of two components. First,

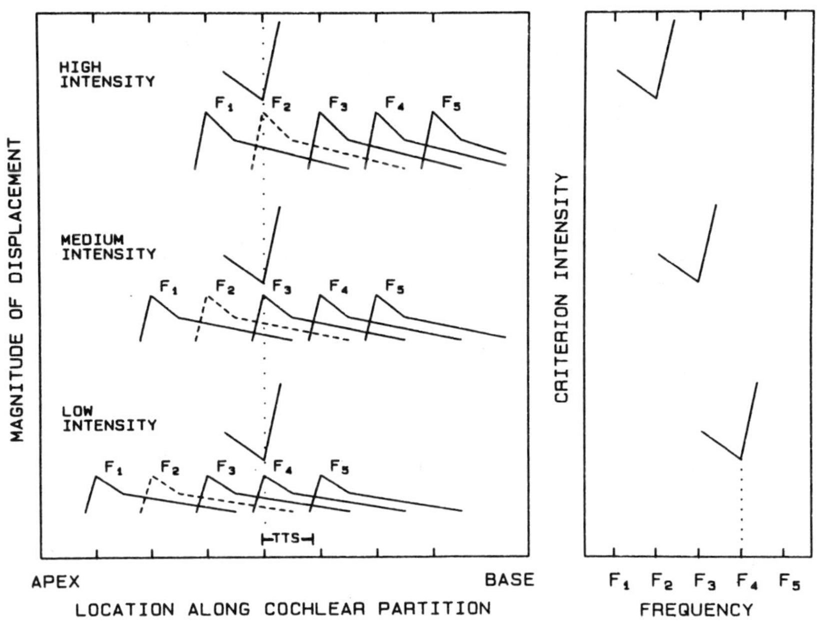

Fig. 1. Schematic representation of migration of the traveling-wave envelope with increasing intensity. Shown at the left, on the dimension of cochlear position, are the top halves of the displacement envelopes for five tones at each of three intensities. For each intensity, a neural tuning curve is shown above the TW envelopes, and then is shown again in the right panel, now correctly located on the frequency dimension. The bar marked TTS at the bottom left is meant to indicate the region of "fatigue" produced by tone F2 at the highest intensity shown; at "threshold" intensities, F2 itself would show little or no aftereffect of the exposure, but frequencies above the exposure frequency would.

there is the mechanical TW of displacement that is the result of the physical properties of the cochlear partition, and which has a relatively broad peak of displacement; this is the classical TW envelope described by von Bekesy and which Davis regards to be basically a passive response to the input signal. Second, there is a steeply rising, horn-shaped pattern of displacement located at the apical foot of the classical TW that is the product of active elements residing in the cochlea which Davis refers to collectively as the cochlear amplifier (CA). In Davis' model, the CA is subject to a saturating non-linearity, so its relative contribution to the total envelope of membrane displacement is greatest at low intensities; thus, at low intensities the peak of the total envelope of displacement lies 2-3 mm apical to the peak of the classical, mechanical TW envelope. As intensity increases, the contribution of the apically located CA to the total envelope of displacement continuously diminishes, and the relative contribution of the basal, mechanical TW grows, with the result that the peak of the total envelope of displacement gradually migrates basally. In exposure situations, then, the "elements" maximally "fatigued" or "injured" are those located near the peak of the mechanical envelope of displacement-elements tuned to frequencies higher than the exposure tone when measured at low stimulus intensities.

While appealing in many ways, Davis' conceptual model does appear to contain a limiting condition that seems not to exist in the data. Namely, once the stimulus intensity reaches the point that the total displacement envelope coincides with the mechanical envelope, there can apparently be no further upward shift. Yet, there are numerous physiological and psychophysical demonstrations of the maximum effect being upward in frequency by an octave or more and apparently growing without bound [4,6,28].

As we shall see, there is considerable evidence in support of the idea of a basalward migration of the point of peak displacement with increasing intensity, but there are also some gaps and contradictions in the story. One point to remember during the following summary of the evidence is that even when some physiological or psychophysical measure does migrate in the correct direction for our purposes, the magnitude is seldom adequate to account for a half-octave shift--which corresponds to approximately 2 mm along a human cochlear partition [29]. (On the other hand, it is also rare for these measures to cover the 90-100 dB range typically covered in TTS paradigms.) In addition, it is important to remember that there is no intent here to suggest that migration is the sole explanation for any fact considered; surely most of these effects are at least partially the result of other aspects of cochlear behavior. Thus, in the following we will be emphasizing qualitative, not quantitative, agreements.

PHYSIOLOGICAL AND ELECTROPHYSIOLOGICAL EVIDENCE

By now, most auditory scientists are sufficiently familiar with the twin concepts of the spatial pattern of the TW envelope and the tuning characteristic of a single point along the cochlear partition that they can easily alternate their thinking between them. However, when one adds the factor of basalward migration of the TW envelope, the potential for confusion grows. One fact for the reader to remember is that if the maximum of the TW envelope does migrate basally with increasing intensity, then any measurements obtained from a fixed position along the membrane (e.g., tuning curves obtained from the basilar membrane, a hair cell, or a primary fiber) should appear displaced <u>downward</u> in frequency as intensity is raised--reference to Fig. 1 should make this point clear. (Note that the same downward shift is also expected in these various measurements following any manipulation that reduces or eliminates the cochlear amplifier segment of the TW envelope, but that type of shift is different from an intensity-dependent one.) It is sometimes helpful to think about this downward shift in tuning in terms of the input/output functions underlying it. If the input/output functions are parallel for all individual frequencies within the passband of a fixed point on the partition, then the tuning curves associated with that point would have both the same nominal characteristic frequency (CF) and essentially the same shape at all intensities. But if, for any reason, the input/output functions are not parallel, the nominal CF will be different at different intensities. Now, migration of the peak of the TW envelope <u>ought</u> to produce non-parallel input/output functions for frequencies located in different regions within the passband of the cochlear position being studied. The reason is that input/output functions for frequencies on the high side of the "actual" CF (the CF measured at near-threshold intensities) should be relatively shallow because the peaks of membrane displacement for those frequencies are gradually sliding basalward, "out from under" the membrane location being measured; in contrast, the input/output functions for frequencies on the low side of the actual CF ought to be steeper since their points of maximal displacement will remain apical to the membrane location being studied. (Again, this is not to argue that factors other than migration might not also contribute to these different input/output functions.)

Early data on basilar membrane mechanics did show some of the expected characteristics described above [30,31], but since early data have become suspect in light of findings about the effects of inadvertent damage to the delicate structures in the cochlea [32], we shall concentrate upon data obtained under procedures designed to minimize cochlear damage. Using Mossbauer techniques, Sellick et al. [33] obtained non-parallel input/output functions of the sort suggested above. For data they felt were among their best (their Fig. 5a), the CF for the location of their Mossbauer source was 19 kHz at low displacement amplitudes (actually velocities); it dropped to 18 kHz at higher amplitudes and to 16 kHz at the highest displacement amplitudes. Rough estimates indicate that the rate of migration was about 0.07 octave/10 dB in this 16-19 kHz region. The basilar membrane data of LePage and Johnstone [34] also indicated shallow input/output functions at frequencies above CF. Thus, an expectation that follows directly from the idea of basalward migration of the peak of the TW envelope is confirmed--the apparent CF for a fixed basilar membrane location decreases with increasing stimulus intensity.

Similar effects on input/output functions and tuning curves were observed by Russell and Sellick [35] in their studies of high-frequency inner hair cells, but while the magnitudes of the effects appear large, estimates of migration rate are not possible from their published figures. The inner hair cell data of Dallos [10] do not show these effects as strongly as the above data do, but interestingly, he was studying hair cells located in the 800-Hz region of the cochlear partition, where half-octave effects are sometimes problematic.

While cochlear microphonic (CM) data do provide weak support for a basalward migration of the displacement peak with increasing intensity [36], Dallos [18] has clearly shown that the non-linear input/output functions of CM can produce the appearance of a basalward migration without there actually being a translation of the displacement peak along the cochlear partition. Thus, we shall ignore CM data.

Not surprisingly perhaps, the primary fibers show the same downward shift in tuning that Russell and Sellick [35] observed in the inner hair cells. At high intensities, the peak firing rate often moves to a lower frequency [7], as does the CF of the tuning curve [37-39]. Again, the 1000-Hz region appears to be a dividing line; Evans [37], Liberman and Mulroy [38], and Liberman and Kiang [39] all reported downward shifts for cells with CFs above 1000 Hz and upward shifts for cells with CFs below 1000 Hz. Sachs and Abbas [40] showed that the slopes of the functions relating primary-fiber discharge rate to stimulus intensity are increasingly less steep as the test frequency is raised above CF, and Abbas and Sachs [41] showed that two-tone suppression is less at high levels of excitor and suppressor than at low levels when the frequency of the suppressor is above CF. Both of these outcomes are in accord with a basalward migration of the TW envelope with increasing intensity.

Kim and Molnar [42] attempted to gain insight into the pattern of excitation along the cochlear partition for different intensities by stimulating about 1400 primary fibers with identical sets of tonal stimuli and then plotting the population response to each stimulus. Unfortunately, this interesting procedure is hindered by the problem of saturation in neural firing rates, so that as the intensity of the tone was increased, the peak of activity in the population response first broadened and then simply flattened, and while Kim and Molnar [42] did report hints of a basalward shift, the evidence is not unequivocal. Also relevant, perhaps, is that the stimulating tone used by Kim and Molnar was 1000 Hz.

Physiological Aftereffects of Intense Stimulation

Of the various physiological measurements that have been made during and following exposure to intense sounds, only a few are relevant to the idea of a basalward migration of peak displacement with increasing stimulus intensity. Lonsbury-Martin and Meikle [8] obtained post-exposure measures in primary fibers after exposures of one minute to moderately intense tones of different frequencies--at CF, one-half octave below CF, and one-half octave above CF; they monitored both driven and non-driven firing rates. For our purposes, the principal result was that exposure to a tone one-half octave below CF produced the greatest, and the longest lasting, post-exposure depression in firing rate (measured at CF). The second most effective exposure was the CF stimulus itself, and the least effective was the stimulus one-half octave above CF. Cody and Johnstone [43] repeated the Lonsbury-Martin and Meikle [8] experiment using more exposure frequencies at more intensities, with the same general outcome. Cody and Johnstone alluded to mechanical explanations of the effect, without specifying or embracing a particular one. Since the exposure duration was only one minute in both the Lonsbury-Martin and Meikle and the Cody and Johnstone experiments, both can be thought of as analogous to TTS experiments. These results clearly square with the explanation being considered here; exposures with frequencies at and above the CF of the fiber produced maximal displacement of the cochlear partition, and thus maximal "fatigue," at points basal to the one served by the fiber being monitored, whereas the point being served by that fiber was maximally displaced, and fatigued, by exposures to frequencies somewhat below CF.

Results parallel to those of Lonsbury-Martin and Meikle and to Cody and Johnstone have been obtained with the whole-nerve action potential (AP). The AP shows greater aftereffects above the exposure frequency than at it [44-46], and there is a tendency for the maximum effect to shift to higher frequencies with increasing exposure intensity [45-48]. In a related paradigm, Abbas [49] used the AP to obtain tuning curves before, and soon after, presentation of adapter tones of varying intensity and duration. In accord with the idea of a migrating peak of displacement in the TW envelope, he found greater post-adaptation decrements in the AP at frequencies above the adapter than at it, and this effect was greater for the more intense adapters.

Other physiological findings obtained following exposure to intense sounds will be mentioned for the sake of completeness, even though they reveal little about the possibility of a basalward migration with increasing intensity. To my knowledge, no experiment on basilar membrane mechanics has ever systematically manipulated the exposure variable, but as noted above, it is now believed that many early experimenters--including von Bekesy himself--inadvertently studied noise-damaged cochleas [32]. The effects of noise damage, and of numerous other sorts of damage, are less-sharp tuning and a downward shift in the measured CF [28, 32, 33, 50]. It is comforting to those seeking parsimony that essentially identical changes are believed to occur in hair cells and primary fibers following damage and/or exposure [26, 51-53]. Cody and Johnstone [47] monitored single primary fibers during prolonged exposures to intense tones one-half octave below CF. Beginning about one minute after the onset of the exposure, there was a downward shift in the nominal CF that continued and progressed for about the first hour of exposure. In that time, sensitivity had declined by about 60 dB on the average, and nominal CF was approximately half an octave below original CF. As the exposure continued, the tuning curves became increasingly flatter and less sensitive, and somewhere between 2-3 hours of continuous exposure, all cells failed to respond to test tones of 110 dB. This experiment clearly involved both TTS and PTS, but there is no information as to the dividing line between them. Liberman

[26] worked with a PTS-like paradigm and also found a downward shift in apparent CF (of as much as 0.66 octave) in primary fibers following noise exposures that induced varying degrees of localized damage to cochlear structures. Averaged across neurons of differing sorts (his Fig. 2), the downward shift in CF was at a rate of about 0.08 octave/10 dB of PTS, but the variability was high. Finally, Van Heusden [54] has obtained downward shifts in nominal CF of nearly two octaves in the tuning curves of cells in the anteroventral cochlear nucleus following exposure to intense noise.

COMMENT

The preceding section revealed that there are considerable physiological data in qualitative agreement with the idea of a migration of the peak of displacement of the TW envelope with increasing stimulus intensity. In the following section, a comparable array of psychophysical evidence is presented in support of the idea. However, most of the psychophysical demonstrations we will examine differ in an important way from most of the physiological demonstrations just considered, and the difference points up an important feature of the migration effect not yet mentioned.

The physiological experiments discussed above typically involved measurements made using single tones as stimuli. In contrast--with the exception of TTS paradigms--psychophysical manipulations capable of establishing whether or not a slightly different segment of cochlear partition is being stimulated by different intensities always require the presence of a second tone, or set of tones; logically, one cannot hope to measure a tuning curve or filter characteristic psychophysically with single-tone stimuli. This necessity raises an interesting and potentially difficult problem. Clearly, if <u>both</u> the signal and the auxiliary tones were subject to migration, and their rates of migration were the same, no psychophysical experiment could possibly reveal evidence of that migration, even if it were substantial. As the following sections will show, a number of psychophysical tasks <u>do</u> provide evidence for migration of the TW envelope with increasing intensity, implying that--under some conditions at least--the signal and auxiliary tones are either not both migrating, or not both migrating at the same rate. Let us consider two general possibilities for the form of the migration. First, below some "critical intensity" there may be no migration of the displacement peak with increasing stimulus intensity, and above that critical intensity, migration may proceed in the same linear manner for all frequencies (illustrated at the top in Fig. 2). For the sake of the example, let us consider the implications of this alternative for a tone-on-tone masking situation. Increases in the intensity of a relatively weak signal--necessitated by increases in the intensity of the masker--cannot erase the evidence for a migration in the masker tone as long as the signal stays below some critical value of intensity. Once the intensity of the signal also exceeds the critical value, however, migration will appear to cease, and the masker will appear to have migrated less than it actually has.

Alternatively, it might be that migration occurs over the entire range of intensity, but that the rate of migration is greater at high intensities than at low (illustrated at the bottom in Fig. 2). According to this version, a relatively weak signal is itself subject to some migration, but as long as there is a reasonable difference in the intensities of the signal and the masker(s), migration will be revealed. Note that in this case the magnitude of migration will be underestimated by psychophysical measures, but that, unlike the first version, the apparent magnitude will (correctly) increase continuously over the entire range of intensities studied. From this consideration of these two possibilities, it should be clear that--unlike physiological measures--psychophysical procedures can, at best,

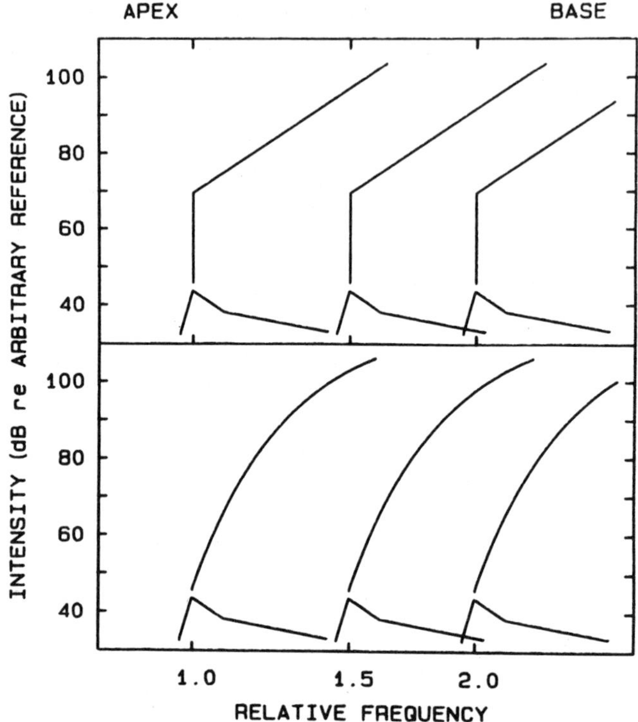

Fig. 2. Schematic representations of two simple versions of the process of migration of the traveling-wave envelope. The curves shown describe the loci of the peaks of the displacement envelopes for each of three tonal stimuli. In the top panel, the peak of displacement does not migrate along the partition until the intensity reaches some "critical" value; above that value, the peak migrates basally at a fixed rate. In the bottom panel, the peak of displacement migrates over the entire range of intensity, but, for a unit change in intensity, the magnitude of the basalward shift is greater at high intensities than at low. Psychophysical measures necessarily reveal only differences in rate of migration.

measure *differential* rates of migration of stimuli, and thus, it would be remarkable indeed to find good quantitative agreement between physiological and psychophysical results.

PSYCHOPHYSICAL EVIDENCE

Masking

If different intensities of the same frequency do maximally activate different portions of the cochlear partition, one might expect this fact to be revealed in tone-on-tone masking experiments in which maskers of different intensity and test tones of varying frequency are used. The expectation would be that at low and moderate masker intensities, the masking pattern would peak at the masker frequency, whereas at high masker intensities, the peak of masking would be displaced toward higher frequencies. The classical data of Wegel and Lane [55] and of Egan and Hake [56] naturally come to mind in this context, and while there are no marked shifts of the masking peak in those data--just a general broadening of the extent of masking with increasing masker intensity--Fig. 3 of Egan and Hake does show more masking at 1000 and 1400 Hz than near the 400-Hz masker at high masker intensity [57]. While this evidence is obviously not compelling, simultaneous masking procedures using two tones are known to be plagued by the problem of beats. When this problem is circumvented, more satisfying evidence for migration is obtained.

Zwislocki developed a simultaneous contralateral masking procedure for use in his studies of central masking. Zwislocki et al. [58] used a fixed signal frequency in one ear and a slowly varying masker frequency of fixed intensity in the other; the subject adjusted signal intensity for threshold. If there were migration, this fixed-signal procedure should yield a downward shift in the maximally effective masking frequencies, and the peaks of the masking functions obtained by Zwislocki et al. (their Figs. 9-11) do show a displacement downward in frequency with increasing masker intensity. The rate was about 0.04 octave/10 dB.

Vogten [22] minimized the problem of beats in simultaneous presentations of tonal signal and masker through the use of a phase-locking technique that obviates uncontrolled intensity fluctuations. He has reported experiments conducted in two ways: with the signal level held constant and the masker level adjusted at a number of masker frequencies (yielding what is commonly known as a psychophysical tuning curve or PTC; see his Fig. 6) and--like Zwislocki et al. above--with the masker level held constant and the signal level adjusted at a number of masker frequencies (see his Fig. 7). Both methods reveal a monotonic decrease in the "peak" frequency of the masking function with increasing intensity. In a second article, Vogten [59] argued that the shift in the peak seen at low intensities is due to a contribution from a suppression mechanism, but he accepted the possibility that the shifts at higher intensities may be related to a migration in the peak of displacement along the cochlear partition. He estimated the migration to be about 0.04-0.07 octave/10 dB in the 1000-Hz region. In related research, a rate of migration similar to that reported by Vogten [59] was obtained by Florentine and Houtsma [60] in a single impaired ear; the simultaneous PTCs of Carney and Nelson [61] also showed a downward shift of the "peak" at higher signal intensities; and while the simultaneous masking data of Zwicker and Jaroszewski [62] contain no obvious shifts, perhaps this is owing to the use of weak maskers only.

Temporal masking is the most commonly used procedure for avoiding the unwanted interactions between signal and masker that occur in tone-on-tone experiments. If the frequency of a forward masker were fixed, the migration idea would lead us to expect that at moderate and high masker intensities, the signals most masked would be slightly <u>higher</u> in frequency than the masker. The classical data of Munson and Gardner [63] confirm this expectation (their Figs. 8 and 18)--the peaks of the forward-masking patterns they obtained migrate from their 1000-Hz masker frequency toward 1500 Hz as masker intensity is increased. The results of a forward-masking experiment by Zwislocki and Pirodda [64] were similar; for two of their three subjects, the maximum of the masking function moved upward in frequency by about 1000 Hz as the intensity of their 3150-Hz masker was increased from 60 to 100 dB SPL (about 0.11 octave/10 dB). In the intervening years, numerous investigators have published temporal masking patterns or PTCs that contain shifts which are in accord with the idea of a basalward migration of the peak of the TW envelope with increasing intensity, and which are often substantial [65-71]. Abstracting across studies, it does appear that shifts of reasonable magnitude are most reliably obtained in the frequency regions above 1000 Hz. McFadden and Yama [9] obtained shifts of about 0.10-0.15 octave/10 dB, and they suggested that shifts are more likely to be seen when the signal duration and masker-to-signal interval are longer than typically used nowadays (at least 50 msec).

We saw, in our earlier consideration of tuning curves for fixed basilar membrane locations, that there is a necessary relation between tuning curves and the input/output functions measured for individual frequencies within the passband of the point of interest, and this is no less true for PTCs than for basilar membrane tuning curves. The migration idea predicts relatively steeper growth-of-masking functions for masker frequencies below CF, and relatively flatter ones at and above CF, because in the latter case the maskers are "moving away" from the signal as masker intensity is increased, necessitating greater increases in level to achieve a fixed increment in masking. Results of this sort have been reported by Widen and Viemeister [69], among others. In related, unpublished measurements, Pasanen used forward masking to determine the psychometric function for a 20-msec, 6500-Hz tone of 12 dB SL masked by preceding 200-msec tones of higher or lower frequency and variable intensity. In accord with the idea at hand, the psychometric function obtained with the higher frequency masker was less steep than that with the lower frequency masker--approximately 9 dB of change in the masker was required to cover the range from 60% to 90% correct with the high-frequency masker, and only about 3 dB with the low-frequency masker.

Lateral Suppression

Were the migration idea under examination here correct, one might expect to see manifestations of it in lateral suppression data. Specific predictions are made difficult by the complex of possible interactions between suppression, masking, and migration, but there are indications that effects compatible with the migration idea do occur [22]: suppressors on the high-frequency side of the signal become decreasingly effective with increasing level [21]; the asymmetry of lateral suppression toward the high-frequency side of the signal which is seen at relatively low suppressor intensities appears to reverse at high suppressor intensities [72]; and, as noted previously, the effects on two-tone suppression in primary fibers are different when suppressor level is varied for frequencies above, versus below, cell CF [41].

Pitch Shifts

The initial reaction of nearly everyone meeting the migration idea for the first time is, "But if that were right, pitch ought to shift upward with increasing intensity, and it doesn't." In fact, there now appears to be general agreement that the pitch of high-frequency tones does get higher (and the pitch of low-frequency tones gets lower) with increasing intensity [73-75], but it is necessary to qualify this fact as it pertains to the migration idea. First, the pitch shifts observed typically amount to only a small percentage change in frequency (although Kim reported data for several subjects who showed upward shifts of 10-15%, about 0.04-0.06 octave/10 dB, at 5000 Hz [19]). Second, the middle frequencies (about 1000-4000 Hz) typically show little or no pitch shift with intensity; the effect is restricted to more extreme frequencies. These qualifications are generally unnecessary for the various other psychophysical and physiological effects described above that are in accord with the proposition at hand. Thus, the relative constancy of pitch unquestionably stands as the most troublesome fact to rationalize with the other evidence pertaining to migration. To paraphrase an old saw, "pitch is a witch." (Perhaps the relative invariance of pitch across wide ranges of intensity is evidence that pitch constancy has had great evolutionary value and--since the "problem" of migration has presumably existed for a long time--that the nervous system has developed ways to achieve constancy despite migration.)

Aftereffects of Intense Stimulation

Given that the half-octave shift was first noticed in TTS research, it is natural to expect to find considerable detailing of the effect in the TTS literature. Surprisingly, and unfortunately, this is not the case; the half-octave shift has itself not been the object of much research. In the vast majority of TTS experiments, hearing loss and/or recovery are measured at only one or a few test frequencies, and these are chosen with the presumption that there will be a half-octave shift rather than to test for its presence. But while the TTS literature is not packed with crucial information relevant to the possibility of migration of the peak of the TW envelope with increasing intensity, some facts are worth mentioning.

As already noted, the data of Davis et al. [4], Ward [5], Cohen and Baumann [6], and others, do show more TTS above the exposure frequency than at it. Also, the finding by Reger and Lierle [76], Hirsh and Bilger [77], Selters [78], and Young and Sachs [79] that a _low_-intensity exposure tone produces more TTS at the exposure frequency than does a high-intensity exposure comes into accord with the migration idea once it is appreciated that this decline _is_ accompanied by increasing TTS at higher test frequencies as exposure intensity increases [19,20,77,80]. Note that at very high exposure levels--above about 115-120 dB--there is evidence of a different sort of decline in TTS with increasing exposure intensity [5]; this decline can exist across a wide array of test frequencies, and thus it appears to be due to mechanisms quite different from migration of the TW envelope. For the sake of completeness, we note that there is at least one report of the peak of TTS moving _toward_ the exposure band with increasing exposure intensity [81].

Following exposure to an intense tone, McFadden and Plattsmier [25] measured changes in both detection threshold and in suprathreshold loudness at both the exposure and the half-octave frequencies. In accord with past research, there was little or no TTS at the exposure frequency, even though there was as much as 15-20 dB of TTS one-half octave higher. But interestingly, there was as much as 15 dB of loudness change at the exposure frequency, even though its threshold was unchanged. An outcome of this sort is expected if the peak of basilar membrane displacement migrates basalward with increases in intensity, because absolute sensitivity for the exposure frequency would be mediated via a relatively apical and unaffected segment of the partition, whereas the loudness measures--involving as they do a match to a stimulus of suprathreshold intensity--would be mediated over a slightly more basal segment of the cochlear partition, one including the (more basal) region of maximal "fatigue" (Fig. 1).

If there were a gradual basalward migration of the peak of displacement along the cochlear partition with increasing intensity, the TTS induced by a relatively weak exposure stimulus should all be at, or close to, the exposure frequency, whereas the TTS induced by more intense stimuli should gradually move toward increasingly higher frequencies as exposure intensity increases. As noted previously, the TTS data of Hirsh and Bilger [77] support this idea, but they only monitored post-exposure performance at two frequencies-- the exposure and the half-octave frequencies. Hood [80] and Kim [19,20] did test at several frequencies other than the exposure frequency, and both did find evidence for a gradual upward shift of the peak TTS frequency, but both used exposures of only 30 sec, and as a consequence, obtained only small amounts of TTS (less than 4 dB in most cases). Since both experimenters used tracking procedures to estimate post-exposure sensitivity, such small values of TTS are problematic. Ward [5] reported TTS for a series of exposure intensities, but the weakest was sufficiently intense (115 dB) that migration was already well-established. McFadden and Plattsmier [24] described experiments in which frequency patterns of TTS were obtained for a number of intensities of the exposure tone; the intensities were less extreme than Ward's, and longer and more intense than Hood's and Kim's, and data were collected for more test frequencies than is typical. The expectation was that the peak in the TTS pattern would gradually migrate from the exposure frequency at low intensities toward higher frequencies with increasing exposure intensity, but the results were not this simple. These detailed TTS patterns did not have single, well-localized peaks that just shifted upward in frequency with increasing exposure intensity. Instead, the patterns had at least two, apparently reliable, local maxima whose relative sizes changed with exposure intensity (calculated "centers of balance" for these TTS patterns shifted upward at a rate of about 0.03-0.12 octave/10 dB). Indications of a two-peaked pattern of effect can also be seen in the data of Hood [80], Munson and Gardner [63], Zwislocki and Pirodda [64], Zwislocki et al. [58], Kim [19,20], and Pirodda and Ceroni [67]. Perhaps these complex patterns are reflections of the transition envisioned by Davis [27] from an overall TW envelope dominated by the cochlear amplifier component to one dominated by the mechanical TW component. If so, detailed TTS patterns may be providing us with more information about cochlear mechanics than has previously been appreciated.

It is well-known that there can be substantial shifts in pitch induced by exposure to intense sound [82]. Davis et al. [4] did not even begin their pitch measurements until 60 minutes following the exposure, yet they often measured shifts of 40-80%. For our purposes here, perhaps the most important fact about these pitch shifts is that they were minimal or nonexistent for test frequencies below and at the exposure frequency, and they were maximal for frequencies a half to a full octave above the exposure frequency. This locus of maximum effect is exactly what the migration idea predicts, of course, especially when it is recalled that Davis et al. used quite intense exposures. Also of interest is that the direction of the pitch shifts was <u>always upward</u> in the Davis et al. experiment, which is in accord with what is now known about the neural aftereffects of exposure. Following exposure, a primary fiber loses its sensitive tip and is thereby "re-tuned" to a lower frequency. Thus, presenting a test tone in the region of maximal post-exposure "fatigue" will lead to greatest activity in fibers whose actual CF is higher than the test tone, and since those fibers are presumably still "labeled" by the higher neural centers as being higher in pitch than the test tone, a higher frequency is needed contralaterally to achieve a pitch match [46]. The pitch of the tonal tinnitus that is often induced by narrow-band exposures is also located well above the exposure frequency [83].

Form of the Migration Process

Now that the psychophysical data have been presented, we can return to the questions raised previously about the form of the migration process--specifically, whether there exists a "critical intensity" at which migration begins, and whether migration proceeds at the same rate for all intensities once it has begun.

In the data of Hirsh and Bilger [77], the upward shift in TTS appears to begin somewhere between 60 and 80 dB SL. In the Kim [19,20] data, there are hints of an upward shift of TTS beginning at 45 dB SL for some subjects. (In the McFadden and Plattsmier data [25], there appears to be an upward displacement of the TTS pattern even for the lowest exposure intensity used--82 dB SPL--so they are uninformative on the issue of a critical intensity.) In the forward-masking data of Zwislocki and Pirodda [64], the earliest evidence of an upward shift in the masking pattern is for maskers of about 80 dB SPL; the same is true for Pirodda and Ceroni [67]. For Munson and Gardner [63], a shift first appears between 70 and 90 phons. The observations of Selters [78] further muddy the waters; Selters monitored the growth of TTS at 1000 Hz as a function of the intensity of a 1000-Hz exposure tone (of 10-sec duration, so adaptation may be a better term than TTS--but no matter). After growing continuously for exposures of 5-30 dB SL, TTS plateaued from 30-60 dB SL, and from 60-80 dB SL, TTS declined from its value at lower exposure intensities before rising again at exposure intensities of 90-100 dB SL. The plateau and the decline are to be expected if there is a "critical intensity" for migration, but the final rise is not. A similar plateau is also present in the forward-masking data of Munson and Gardner [63]. In contrast, at the physiological level, the basilar membrane input/output functions for frequencies above CF are shallow, with no obvious inversion point, from the lowest intensities tested [33]. It is obviously difficult to generalize across these disparate studies, but--recalling the earlier observation that psychophysical measures have the potential to obscure the details of the migration process --it may be prudent to side with the still-sparce physiological data, and tentatively conclude that migration exists over the entire range of audible intensities.

The psychophysical data also provide a blurred picture of how migration proceeds once it does begin. Recall that, were the parallel version at the top of Fig. 2 correct, migration should appear to cease once the weaker of the two test tones begins to migrate, but if the non-parallel version were correct, migration should (correctly) appear to grow continuously with increasing intensity. There is precious little experimental evidence available on this point, and what little does exist unfortunately goes in both directions. There are some indications that maximum TTS moves continuously upward in frequency with increasing exposure intensity [4,25], but in other cases, maximum TTS appears to remain in the vicinity of the half-octave frequency in the face of large increases in exposure intensity [5]. At this time, the available physiological data are of little assistance with this question.

SUMMARY

Over the years, numerous investigators have suggested that the displacement peak of the TW envelope may migrate basalward with increasing intensity and that this migration is the basis of the so-called half-octave shift in TTS, as well as of other effects. Recently, the physiological evidence relevant to this issue has become less contradictory, and it now stands in qualitative agreement with the migration idea. Considerable psychophysical data have been in qualitative accord with it for years, so the migration idea carries the strong attraction of being a parsimonious and unifying concept covering a broad spectrum of effects. To be sure, no single piece of evidence examined can yet be viewed as conclusive, and the magnitudes of the various effects are not in perfect agreement, but taken together, the evidence is impressive. Not to be ignored is the fact that there is presently no alternative explanation with anything like the breadth of coverage possessed by the migration explanation. Perhaps an implication of this argument requires emphasis--half octave-like shifts appear to be normal consequences of the basilar membrane's response to increasing intensity; they are not just the result of over-driving and fatiguing the system as in TTS paradigms. At the very least, the migration explanation deserves to finally be put under the microscope of experimental investigation, so that its future acceptance or rejection can be based on more than hints and trends extracted by looking across experiments, paradigms, and decades.

ACKNOWLEDGMENTS

Versions of this paper have existed since 1981. In this time I have been supported in part by grants from the National Institute of Neurological and Communicative Disorders and Stroke (NS 08754 and NS 15895) and the National Institute for Environmental Health Sciences (ES 03539). Special thanks are due Wilson S. Geisler and Craig C. Wier for their numerous valuable comments on a preliminary draft, and to E. G. Pasanen and H. S. Plattsmier for assistance of various sorts.

REFERENCES

1. A. F. Rawdon-Smith, Auditory fatigue, Brit. J. Psychol., 25:77 (1934).
2. A. W. Ewing and T. S. Littler, Auditory fatigue and adaptation, Brit. J. Psychol., 25:284 (1935).
3. H. B. Perlman, Acoustic trauma in man: clinical and experimental studies, Arch. Otolaryngol., 34:429 (1941).
4. H. Davis, C. T. Morgan, J. E. Hawkins, Jr., R. Galambos, and F. W. Smith, Temporary deafness following exposure to loud tones and noise, Acta Oto-Laryngol., 88:4 (1950).
5. W. D. Ward, Damage-risk criteria for line spectra, J. Acoust. Soc. Am., 34:1610 (1962).
6. A. Cohen and K. C. Baumann, Temporary hearing losses following exposure to pronounced single-frequency components in broad-band noise, J. Acoust. Soc. Am., 36:1167 (1964).
7. C. D. Geisler, W. S. Rhode, and D. T. Kennedy, Responses to tonal stimuli of single auditory nerve fibers and their relationship to basilar membrane motion in the squirrel monkey, J. Neurophysiology, 37:1156 (1974).
8. B. L. Lonsbury-Martin, and M. B. Meikle, Neural correlates of auditory fatigue: frequency-dependent changes in activity of single cochlear nerve fibers, J. Neurophysiology, 41:987 (1978).
9. D. McFadden and M. F. Yama, Upward shifts in the masking pattern with increasing masker intensity, J. Acoust. Soc. Am., 74:119 (1983).
10. P. Dallos, Response characteristics of mammalian cochlear hair cells, J. Neuroscience, 5:1591 (1985).
11. J. H. Mills, J. D. Osguthorpe, C. K. Burdick, J. H. Patterson, and B. Mozo, Temporary threshold shifts produced by exposure to low-frequency noises, J. Acoust. Soc. Am., 73:918 (1983).
12. A. Wright, Dimensions of the cochlear stereocilia in man and in the guinea pig, Hearing Research, 13:89 (1984).
13. D. McFadden, Intense sounds may alter the mechanical properties of the cochlear partition, J. Acoust. Soc. Am., 74:447 (1983).
14. W. E. Brownell, C. R. Bader, D. Bertrand, and Y. De Ribaupierre, Y., Evoked mechanical responses of isolated cochlear outer hair cells, Science, 227:194 (1985).
15. S. S. Stevens, The relation of pitch to intensity, J. Acoust. Soc. Am., 6,150 (1935).
16. R. F. Galambos, C. D. Geisler, H. Davis, and J. L. Zwislocki, Discussion, in: "The Physiology of the Auditory System," M. B. Sachs ed., National Educational Consultants, Baltimore (1971).
17. A. E. Hubbard and C. D. Geisler, A hybrid-computer model of the cochlear partition, J. Acoust. Soc. Am., 51:1895 (1972).
18. P. Dallos, The auditory periphery, Academic Press, New York (1973).

19. D. O. Kim, Role of place cue in simple-tone pitch perception assessed with temporary threshold shift, J. Acoust. Soc. Am., 56, S44, (1974) and unpublished manuscript.
20. D. O. Kim, Discussion, in: "New Perspectives on Noise-Induced Hearing Loss," R. P. Hamernik, D. Henderson, and R. Salvi eds., Raven Press, New York (1982).
21. H. Duifhuis, Cochlear nonlinearity and second filter--a psychophysical evaluation, in: "Psychophysics and Physiology of Hearing," E. F. Evans and J. P. Wilson eds., Academic Press, New York (1977).
22. L. L. M. Vogten, Simultaneous pure-tone masking: the dependence of masking asymmetries on intensity, J. Acoust. Soc. Am., 63:1509 (1978a).
23. S. D. Anderson, Some ECMR properties in relation to other signals from the auditory periphery, Hearing Research, 2:273 (1980).
24. D. McFadden and H. S. Plattsmier, Exposure-induced loudness shifts and threshold shifts, in: "New Perspectives on Noise-Induced Hearing Loss," R. P. Hamernik, D. Henderson, and R. Salvi eds., Raven Press, New York (1982).
25. D. McFadden and H. S. Plattsmier, Frequency patterns of TTS for different exposure intensities, J. Acoust. Soc. Am., 74:1178 (1983).
26. M. C. Liberman, Single-neuron labeling and chronic cochlear pathology, I. Threshold shift and characteristic-frequency shift, Hearing Research, 16:33 (1984).
27. H. Davis, An active process in cochlear mechanics, Hearing Research, 9:79 (1983).
28. D. Robertson, A. R. Cody, G. Bredberg, and B. M. Johnstone, Response properties of spiral ganglion neurons in cochleas damaged by direct mechanical trauma, J. Acoust. Soc. Am., 67: 1295 (1980b).
29. G. Ehret, Comparative psychoacoustics: perspectives of peripheral sound analysis in mammals, Naturwissenschaften, 64:461 (1977).
30. W. S. Rhode, Observations of the vibration of the basilar membrane in squirrel monkeys using the Mossbauer technique, J. Acoust. Soc. Am., 49:1218 (1971).
31. W. S. Rhode, Some observations on cochlear mechanics, J. Acoust. Soc. Am., 64:158 (1978).
32. D. G. B. Leonard and S. M. Khanna, Histological evaluation of damage in cat cochleas used for measurement of basilar membrane mechanics, J. Acoust. Soc. Am., 75:515 (1984).
33. P. M. Sellick, R. Patuzzi, and B. M. Johnstone, Measurement of basilar membrane motion in the guinea pig using the Mossbauer technique, J. Acoust. Soc. Am., 72:131 (1982).
34. E. L. LePage and B. M. Johnstone, Nonlinear mechanical behaviour of the basilar membrane in the basal turn of the guinea pig cochlea, Hearing Research, 2:183 (1980).
35. I. J. Russell and P. M. Sellick, Intracellular studies of hair cells in the mammalian cochlea, J. Physiol. (London) 284:261 (1978).
36. V. Honrubia and P. H. Ward, Longitudinal distribution of the cochlear microphonics inside the cochlear duct (guinea pig), J. Acoust. Soc. Am., 44:951 (1968).
37. E. F. Evans, Frequency selectivity at high signal levels of single units in cochlear nerve and nucleus, in: "Psychophysics and Physiology of Hearing," E. F. Evans and J. P. Wilson eds., Academic Press, New York (1977).
38. M. C. Liberman and M. J. Mulroy, Acute and chronic effects of acoustic trauma: Cochlear pathology and auditory nerve pathophysiology, in: "New Perspectives on Noise-Induced Hearing Loss," R. P. Hamernik, D. Henderson, and R. Salvi, eds., Raven Press, New York (1982).
39. M. C. Liberman and N. Y.-S. Kiang, Single-neuron labeling and chronic cochlear pathology. IV. Stereocilia damage and alterations in rate- and phase-level functions, Hearing Research 16: 75 (1984).

40. M. B. Sachs and P. J. Abbas, Rate versus level functions for auditory-nerve fibers in cats: tone-burst stimuli, J. Acoust. Soc. Am., 56:1835 (1974).
41. P. J. Abbas and M. B. Sachs, Two-tone suppression in auditory-nerve fibers: extension of a stimulus-response relationship, J. Acoust. Soc. Am., 59:112 (1976).
42. D. O. Kim and C. E. Molnar, A population study of cochlear nerve fibers: comparison of spatial distributions of average-rate and phase-locking measures of responses to single tones, J. Neurophysiology, 42:16 (1979).
43. A. R. Cody and B. M. Johnstone, Acoustic trauma: Single neuron basis for the 'half-octave shift,' J. Acoust. Soc. Am., 70:707 (1981).
44. C. Mitchell, R. Brummett, and J. Vernon, Frequency effects of temporary N1 depression following acoustic overload, Arch. Otolaryngol., 103:117 (1977).
45. D. Robertson, B. M. Johnstone, and T. J. McGill, Effects of loud tones on the inner ear: a combined electrophysiological and ultrastructural study, Hearing Research, 2:39 (1980).
46. D. P. Gans, Computing auditory fatigue of the whole nerve action potential, J. Acoust. Soc. Am., 70:711 (1981).
47. A. R. Cody and B. M. Johnstone, Single auditory neuron response during acute acoustic trauma, Hearing Research, 3:3 (1980).
48. D. Robertson and B. M. Johnstone, Acoustic trauma in the guinea pig cochlea: early changes in ultrastructure and neural threshold, Hearing Research 3:167 (1980).
49. P. J. Abbas, Recovering from long-term and short-term adaptation of the whole nerve action potential, J. Acoust. Soc. Am., 75:1541 (1984).
50. D. Robertson and G. A. Manley, Manipulation of frequency analysis in the cochlear ganglion of the guinea pig, J. Comp. Physiol., 91:363 (1974).
51. E. F. Evans, Auditory frequency selectivity and the cochlear nerve, in: Facts and Models in Hearing, E. Zwicker and E. Terhardt eds., Springer-Verlag, New York (1974).
52. D. Robertson, Effects of acoustic trauma on stereocilia structure and spiral ganglion cell tuning properties in the guinea pig cochlea, Hearing Research, 7:55-74 (1982).
53. D. Robertson and B. M. Johnstone, Aberrant tonotopic organization in the inner ear damaged by kanamycin, J. Acoust. Soc. Am., 66:466 (1979).
54. E. Van Heusden, Effects of acute noise trauma on cochlear response times in cats, in: "Psychophysical, Physiological and Behavioral Studies in Hearing," G. van den Brink and F. A. Bilsen eds., Delft University Press, The Netherlands (1980).
55. R. L. Wegel and C. E. Lane, The auditory masking of one pure tone by another and its probable relation to the dynamics of the inner ear, Phys. Rev. 23:266 (1924).
56. J. P. Egan and H. W. Hake, On the masking pattern of a simple auditory stimulus, J. Acoust. Soc. Am., 22:622 (1950).
57. J. V. Tobias, Low-frequency masking patterns, J. Acoust. Soc. Am. 61:571 (1977).
58. J. J. Zwislocki, E. Buining, and J. Glantz, Frequency distribution of central masking, J. Acoust. Soc. Am., 43:1267 (1968).
59. L. L. M. Vogten, Low-level pure-tone masking: a comparison of 'tuning curves' obtained with simultaneous and forward masking, J. Acoust. Soc. Am., 63:1520 (1978b).
60. M. Florentine and A. J. M. Houtsma, Tuning curves and pitch matches in a listener with a unilateral,low-frequency hearing loss, J. Acoust. Soc. Am., 73:961 (1983).

61. A. E. Carney and D. A. Nelson, An analysis of psychophysical tuning curves in normal and pathological ears, J. Acoust. Soc. Am., 73:268 (1983).
62. E. Zwicker and A. Jaroszewski, Inverse frequency dependence of simultaneous tone-on-tone masking patterns at low levels, J. Acoust. Soc. Am., 71:1508 (1982).
63. W. A. Munson and M. B. Gardner, Loudness patterns--a new approach, J. Acoust. Soc. Am., 22:177 (1950).
64. J. J. Zwislocki and E. Pirodda, On the adaptation, fatigue and acoustic trauma of the ear, Experientia, 8:279 (1952).
65. R. H. Ehmer and B. J. Ehmer, Frequency pattern of residual masking by pure tones measured on the Bekesy audiometer, J. Acoust. Soc. Am., 46:1445 (1969).
66. H. Fastl, Transient masking pattern of narrow band maskers, in: "Facts and MOdels in Hearing," E. Zwicker and E. Terhardt, eds., Springer-Verlag, New York (1974).
67. E. Pirodda and A. R. Ceroni, Some experiments on temporary threshold shifts produced by short tones, Acta Otol. 85:191 (1978).
68. B. C. J. Moore, Psychophysical tuning curves measured in simultaneous and forward masking, J. Acoust. Soc. Am., 63:524 (1978).
69. G. P. Widin and N. F. Viemeister, Intensive and temporal effects in pure-tone forward masking, J. Acoust. Soc. Am., 66, S9 (1979).
70. G. Kidd, Jr. and L. L. Feth, Patterns of residual masking, Hearing Research, 5:49 (1981).
71. E. M. Burns, Pure-tone pitch anomalies. I. Pitch-intensity effects and diplacusis, J. Acoust. Soc. Am., 72:1394 (1982).
72. R. Shannon, Two-tone unmasking and suppression in a forward-masking situation, J. Acoust. Soc. Am., 59:1460 (1976).
73. E. Terhardt, Pitch of pure tones: its relation to intensity, in: "Facts and Models in Hearing," E. Zwicker and E. Terhardt eds., Springer-Verlag, New York (1974).
74. J. Verschuure and A. A. van Meeteren, The effect of intensity on pitch, Acustica, 32:33 (1975).
75. W. Jesteadt and D. L. Neff, A signal-detection-theory measure of pitch shifts in sinusoids as a function of intensity, J. Acoust. Soc. Am., 72:1812 (1982).
76. S. N. Reger and D. M. Lierle, Changes in auditory acuity produced by low and medium intensity level exposures, Trans. Amer. Acad. Ophthal. Otolaryngol., 58:433 (1954).
77. I. J. Hirsh and R. C. Bilger, Auditory-threshold recovery after exposure to pure tones, J. Acoust. Soc. Am., 27:1186 (1955).
78. W. Selters, Adaptation and fatigue, J. Acoust. Soc. Am., 36:2202 (1964).
79. E. Young and M. B. Sachs, Recovery of detection probability following sound exposure: comparison of physiology and psychophysics, J. Acoust. Soc. Am., 54, 1544 (1973).
80. J. D. Hood, Studies in auditory fatigue and adaptation, Acta Oto-Laryngol., 62:5 (1950).
81. J. H. Mills, R. M. Gilbert, and W. Y. Adkins, Temporary threshold shifts in humans exposed to octave bands of noise for 16 to 24 hours, J. Acoust. Soc. Am., 65:1238 (1979).
82. D. McFadden and H. S. Plattsmier, Suprathreshold aftereffects of exposure to intense sound, in: "New Perspectives on Noise-Induced Hearing Loss," R. P. Hamernik, D. Henderson and R. J. Salvi eds., Raven Press, New York (1982).
83. D. McFadden, Tinnitus: Facts, Theories and Treatments. National Academy Press, Washington, D.C. (1982).

NOTE ADDED TO WORKSHOP

In the above paper, much of the physiological evidence cited in support of a migrating TW envelope was necessarily indirect. In the absence of direct measurements of basilar membrane motion made over a wide range of intensity, and made with the required fine grain in frequency. I was forced to make inferences about the behavior of the cochlear partition from tuning curves and input/output functions taken from hair cells and primary fibers. While I hope this evidence was adequate to convince most readers, new direct evidence was presented at this Workshop that should help to convince skeptics as well. In his Fig. 3, Dr. Patuzzi shows measurements supporting Davis' suggestion that the broad, and more basally located, mechanical component of the TW envelope should come to dominate the more apical cochlear-amplifier component at high stimulus intensities, with the result that peak displacement will migrate basally with increases in intensity. Now that this missing link in the argument has finally been supplied, I hope that both physiological and psychophysical investigators will be motivated to study more fully the numerous interesting concomitants of this migration.

DISCUSSION

Salvi: Some of your psychophysical data suggests that at high levels there was a dramatic jump in the data, whereas some of the explanations you have given sounds like the shifts are very gradual. Is it a shift or is it a jump?

McFadden: There are two options to explain the migration data. The critical intensity idea, or there is the continuously varying idea. On the basis of the available data, it is difficult to decide. The psychophysical data looked like there is very little or no migration at first over a reasonable range of intensity and until some break occurs. But the electrophysiological shows that the differences begin at the lowest intensities. So it appears that the migration physiologically starts right at the very beginning.

HUMAN NOISE EXPERIMENTS USING A TEMPORARY THRESHOLD SHIFT MODEL

Fredrik Lindgren and Alf Axelsson

Department of Audiology, Sahlgrens Hospital
S-413 45, Gothenburg, Sweden

INTRODUCTION

Measurement of temporary threshold shift (TTS) may serve as an experimental method to study possible interactive effects of factors that increase or decrease TTS. Interaction studies should preferably be conducted as controlled studies (i.e., each subject is exposed both to noise only and to noise in combination with the factor of interest) rather than exposing two different groups of subject and drawing conclusions from group differences. The amount of TTS acceptable from ethical standards is limited. Consequently, "the dosage" of both noise exposure and the interactive factor also have to be limited. Therefore, it is important to reduce the intra-individual variance in order to distinguish even small shifts between test conditions.

Early parametric investigations of TTS showed a considerable variability among subjects, as well as for the same subject on different test occasions, when they were exposed to equal noise doses under similar test conditions. Davis et al [1] obtained reliable pre-exposure hearing thresholds (HTL), but in test-retest sessions (i.e., when the subject was exposed twice to an equal stimulus) only 30% exhibited equal TTS's within 5 dB, and only 50% within 10 dB. In some cases the difference in TTS was as large as 52 dB. Later investigations showed less variability. Lightfoot [2] studied the TTS recovery at time intervals from 20 seconds to 9 minutes after cessation of exposure for test-retest sessions in 24 subjects. His results showed an inter-individual standard deviation (SD) of 4.3 to 9.5 dB. Comparisons of test- and retest-data showed a positive but low correlation between TTS's in the same subject. Ward [3] found test-retest SD of 3.5 dB for 95% of the subjects, when the average TTS was 20 dB. In the frequency region of 2000 to 5600 Hz, Ward [4] obtained values for SD between 3.9 and 4.6 dB for test-retest experiments. Mustain and Shoeny [5] found a correlation coefficient of 0.66 between test and retest TTS_2-values at 4 kHz when 10 subjects were exposed to a 3 min 110 dB SPL 2 kHz pure tone. A corresponding value of 0.95 was found for TTS_2 at 1 kHz when subjects were exposed to a 3 min 115 dB SPL 500 Hz pure tone. Chermak et al [6] exposed 20 subjects on three occasions to a 3-min 110 dB SPL white noise. The two first exposures were presented to the subject on the same day, while the third exposure was presented with an interval of one week between the two first and the last exposures. They found a strong correlation between TTSs the same day (0.54 at 4 kHz and 0.65 at 8 kHz). However, correlations were poor between TTS-values obtained at the first or second session and TTS at the third session (0.23 and 0.33 respectively).

These investigations have one thing in common: the subjects were exposed and tested at only two sessions, and in most cases, the TTS was monitored only at one or two frequencies. Also, technical and biological factors, which might have influenced the test situation, were seldom clearly defined. In clinical noise studies using TTS as a measure of individual noise susceptibility, accuracy and reliability of the pure tone threshold determinations, prior to and following noise exposure, are essential. Variation in pure tone thresholds at different test sessions can be due to many variables. The variation may depend on biological causes, e.g., differences in motivation, alertness, reaction time and central auditory masking as well as related to the subjects' middle ear sound transmission. But, Ward [4] reported the diurnal variability in threshold sensitivity and found no evidence that susceptibility to TTS varied cyclically. Further, technical factors may influence the test situation, e.g., differences in background sound level in the test room; in test equipment and earphones; in placement of earphones from test to test. It is probable that these technical difficulties influence intra-individual variability more than the above mentioned biological factors.

In order to determine TTS-variations within and between individuals accurately, it is obvious that we must control the test situation as rigorously as possible, both from the technical and biological points of view. Thus, the aim of the present investigation was to study the reliability in TTS when variations in test- and retest-procedures as well as in noise exposures were kept at a minimum.

MATERIAL AND METHOD

The experimental subjects were 16 male volunteers, with a mean age of 27.4 years. Each individual showed normal hearing (<20 dB HL at all test frequencies) on manual pure-tone audiometry (Interacoustics AC-4 with TDH-39 headphones in MX42/AR cushions) in the frequency range 0.25 to 8 kHz. Middle ear pressures were within 0 +/- 0.25 kPa for all subjects at all sessions, confirmed by tympanometry using a Madsen ZO-72 impedance audiometer with a 220 Hz probe tone.

The noise exposure consisted of 1/3 octave band filtered noise with 2 kHz center frequency presented at 105 dB SPL for 10 minutes. Each subject was exposed to the noise on ten successive occasions. All exposures were presented to each subject within a minimum interval of 24 hours. At each session, each subject's HTLs before and after noise exposure were established for the left ear with a computerized sweep-frequency audiometer (type Bekesy) in the frequency range 2 to 8 kHz [7]. In order to minimize variations caused by earphone placement, the test tone as well as the noise exposure was delivered to the subject via a test fixture consisting of a TDH-39 earphone attached to an ear speculum [8]. Pre- and post-exposure audiograms were calculated by a computer from the sweep recordings at test frequencies 1, 2.5, 3, 3.5, 4, 5, 6, 7 and 8 kHz. The threshold was calculated as the mean value of the excursions encompassing these frequencies.

The post-exposure pure tone threshold determination started at 800 Hz 1 min after cessation of the exposure. The computerized audiometer is tailored to use a linear frequency sweep-rate of 20 Hz/sec. Consequently, the post-exposure delay for the test-frequencies were: 2.0 min for 2 kHz (TTS_2), 2.4 min for 2.5 kHz, 2.8 min for 3 kHz, 3.2 min for 3.5 kHz, 3.7 min for 4kHz, 4.5 min for 5 kHz, 5.3 min for 6 kHz and 7.0 min for 8 kHz. The computerized evaluation of the sweep recordings made it possible to calculate a mean hearing level over an arbitrary range of frequencies. This was accomplished by taking all excursions into consideration and by calculating the threshold in steps of 1 Hz. The calculated mean values of all excursions were connected with a fitted line. The threshold at individual frequencies in 1 Hz steps were determined as the difference in dB between the fitted line and the 0 dB level. The thresholds in 1 Hz steps were then summed over the actual frequency region and finally divided by the number of steps in the range. This measurement then corresponds to a mean HL in the specified frequency ranges: 2 - 2.5, 2.5 - 3, 3 - 3.5, 4 - 5 and 2 - 8 kHz. The TTS was calculated as the difference in dB between pre- and post-exposure HTLs at above given specific frequencies as well as between the thresholds at above given areas. All hearing tests were carried out in a sound-proof booth, with background sound pressure levels below those recommended by ISO/DIS 6189 DRAFT. The audiometers were regularly calibrated in accordance with ISO-389 1975. All hearing tests and noise exposures were conducted by the same audiometric technician at all sessions.

RESULTS

Usage of the test-fixture resulted in an increased HTL at frequencies below 3.5 kHz and a decreased threshold above 3.5 kHz, when compared to thresholds obtained with standard earphones in cushions. However, since this study dealt with TTS, the absolute threshold is of less interest than the relative differences in pre- and post-exposure HTLs.

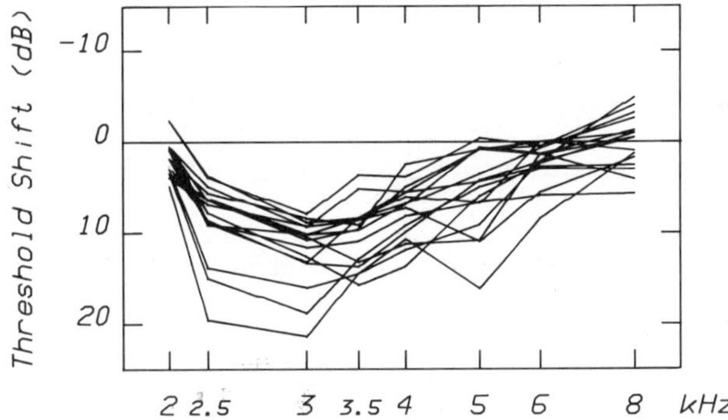

Fig. 1. Mean individual TTS in 16 subjects.

Table 1. Mean and standard deviation of hearing thresholds and TTS-values in 16 subjects.

	Frequency (kHz)									Frequency area (kHz)					
	2	2.5	3	3.5	4	5	6	7	8	2-2.5	2.5-3	3-3.5	3.5-4	4-5	2-8
mean HTL	3.5	3.9	0.2	-1.5	-0.1	-3.5	3.4	-5.4	-3.2	3.8	1.6	-1.5	-0.6	-0.6	-0.8
SD*	6.7	7.9	5.5	6.0	5.7	6.3	4.5	3.8	5.3	7.3	6.3	5.8	5.7	6.1	4.5
mean TTS	1.6	8.5	12.1	10.4	7.7	5.4	2.4	1.1	0.0	4.9	10.5	11.7	9.2	6.1	5.2
SD*	2.2	4.3	3.8	3.4	3.1	4.6	2.4	2.1	3.0	3.2	3.4	3.1	2.8	3.8	2.3

*SD of 16 individual means.

The HTLs varied considerably between subjects and resulted in a standard deviation between subject means (i.e., inter-individual variation) in the range 3.8 - 7.9 dB (Table 1).

Table 2. Standard deviations of difference, pooled SD and reliability coefficient of HTL's and TTS's in 16 subjects tested 10 times.

	Frequency (kHz)									Frequency area (kHz)					
	2	2.5	3	3.5	4	5	6	7	8	2-2.5	2.5-3	3-3.5	3.5-4	4-5	2-8
HTL															
$\frac{\text{SD diff}^{a}}{\sqrt{2}}$	3.9	3.1	3.1	2.5	2.0	2.5	3.4	2.5	4.3	2.8	2.5	2.6	2.4	1.4	1.5
SD pooled[b]	3.4	2.9	2.9	3.0	2.6	2.8	3.7	3.0	4.4	2.8	2.7	2.4	2.6	2.1	1.8
1-p 10[c]	.02	.01	.02	.02	.02	.02	.07	.06	.07	.01	.01	.01	.02	.01	.01
TTS															
$\frac{\text{SD diff}^{a}}{\sqrt{2}}$	5.3	3.7	4.0	3.7	3.5	4.7	3.9	4.1	4.3	3.5	3.2	4.2	3.5	2.8	1.7
SD pooled[b]	4.1	3.5	3.5	3.7	3.7	4.0	4.0	3.6	5.6	3.1	3.1	3.3	3.3	3.2	2.0
1-p 10[c]	.37	.06	.09	.11	.14	.08	.29	.29	.37	.10	.08	.10	.14	.07	.07

[a] SD of the difference between test no. 1 and test no. 2.

[b] Square root of the mean individual session variances.

[c] 1 - reliability coefficient for 10 repeated measures, index of inconsistency.

The amount of TTS from all 160 exposures showed a large inter-individual variation. Fig. 1 shows individual mean TTS-values for the 16 subjects. The most TTS-sensitive frequencies for this 2000 Hz stimulus were 3 - 3.5 kHz, where inter-individual differences also were greatest, with a SD in the range 2.1 - 4.6 dB (Table 1).

The TTS-distributions showed uniform shapes at all test frequencies, but with a wide inter-individual range, e.g., at 3500 Hz one individual on one occasion showed -6 dB TTS compared to +26 dB TTS for another subject. The assessment of reliability was established in four different ways for both HTLs and TTS-levels. One calculation simulated a test-retest situation; data from the first and second tests only were taken into consideration. The intra-individual variability was assessed by calculating the individual differences between the tests and computing the mean and SD of these differences. The SD divided by the square root of 2 then corresponds to the population's estimated intra-individual SD in the range 1.4 - 4.3 dB for HTLs and 1.7 - 5.3 dB for TTSs over frequencies (Table 2). Further, we used data from all 10 repeated sessions and computed each individual's variance over sessions and then calculated the square root of the subject's mean variances (pooled SD). The reliability expressed as the pooled individual SD was found in the range 1.8 - 4.4 for HTL's at specific frequencies and for frequency areas. Corresponding figures for TTS-levels were 2.0 - 5.6 dB. The lowest SD-values were, in most cases, found for frequency area thresholds (Table 2). The reliability was also analyzed by calculating the reliability coefficient [9]. The reliability coefficient expresses the amount of measurement error in repeated measures. This analysis indicated a limited amount of measurement error in HTL determinations (i.e., at 4 kHz, only 2% of the total variation could be explained by measurement errors). It was found that the reliability coefficients were better when HTL's were expressed in areas than at specific test frequencies (Table 2). Reliability coefficients for TTS-values were generally poorer than corresponding figures for HTL's, and showed a considerable variation in TTS-levels at specific frequencies. However, TTS-values monitored in frequency areas showed an improved reliability (Table 2). A further attempt to calculate the reliability was made by computing Pearson product-movement correlation coefficients (r). All subsets of correlations reveal a substantial set of figures, and, therefore, we choose to compute the mean

Table 3. Correlation coefficients between sessions in HTL's and TTS's.

	Frequency (kHz)									Frequency area (kHz)					
	2	2.5	3	3.5	4	5	6	7	8	2-2.5	2.5-3	3-3.5	3.5-4	4-5	2-8
HTL															
r mean[a]	0.80	0.89	0.82	0.82	0.83	0.84	0.61	0.64	0.63	0.92	0.90	0.89	0.85	0.93	0.92
r min[b]	0.71	0.84	0.76	0.74	0.75	0.66	0.20	0.44	0.49	0.83	0.83	0.84	0.80	0.87	0.82
r max[c]	0.90	0.94	0.94	0.96	0.86	0.92	0.83	0.84	0.79	0.96	0.95	0.94	0.90	0.97	0.98
TTS															
r mean[a]	0.25	0.68	0.56	0.51	0.44	0.54	0.27	0.16	0.22	0.59	0.58	0.46	0.42	0.60	0.59
r min[b]	-0.20	0.47	0.34	0.36	0.11	0.43	0.00	-0.04	-0.02	0.42	0.42	0.20	0.18	0.39	0.39
r max[c]	0.73	0.80	0.75	0.73	0.76	0.67	0.56	0.52	0.65	0.75	0.70	0.76	0.75	0.75	0.73

[a]Mean value of Pearson correlation coefficients. Test 1 vs test 2, test 1 vs test 3 etc. Mean of 9 r values.
[b]Minimum r value found when computing above described mean.
[c]Maximum r value found when computing above described mean.

of the correlation coefficients for values obtained at the first session, compared to values obtained at the second session, the third session, etc. The presented mean value then consists of a mean value of 9 correlation coefficients (Table 3). In addition, the minimum and maximum correlations are also presented. The correlation between the first and subsequent tests were high in HTL measurements (r 0.63 - 0.89), and area-thresholds showed the highest correlations (r 0.85 - 0.93). Correlations between TTS-levels at the first and subsequent sessions were weaker, but significant at frequencies where most TTS was exhibited (r 0.51 - 0.68).

The present material showed a substantial inter-individual variation for initial HTL's, admitting possibilities to calculate the influence of the HTL's upon the resulting TTS. It was found that the amount of TTS was dependent upon the subject's initial HTL. This relationship was most marked at 3.5 kHz, i.e., the frequency where the largest TTS occurred, indicating that the better HTL-values at 2, 2.5 and 3 kHz, the more pronounced TTS at 3.5 kHz (r -0.69 - -0.70) (Table 4). Somewhat surprisingly, TTS at 3 kHz (i.e., the second frequency in order of TTS magnitude) showed a relatively poor correlation coefficient against HTL's (Table 4). The table shows that HTL at 2 kHz best predicted TTS at 2.5 kHz, that KTL's at 2.5 kHz best predicted TTS's at 3.5 kHz. At 4 kHz TTS's were best predicted by HTL's at 6, 2, 7 and 2.5 kHz in rank order. The correlations between TTS's at different frequencies revealed a strong relationship between TTS at adjacent frequencies, but a reduced correlation between TTS at frequencies far apart (i.e., a marked TTS at 2.5 kHz would predict a large TTS at 3 kHz (r=0,9), while TTS's at or about 5 kHz could not be predicted with accuracy.

Pearson correlation coefficients were also calculated between HTL's in frequency areas and TTS's in frequency areas (Table 5). It was found, that in spite of a strong correlation between HTL's, TTS's were best predicted by the HTL area 2-8 kHz rather than from any other HTL area or HTL at any specific test frequency.

DISCUSSION

As discussed in the introduction, previous authors investigating the reliability of one test-retest session report a SD of TTS in the same individual of approximately 4 - 10 dB. However, one test-retest session provides only limited information about TTS reliability and might disguise

Table 4. Pearson correlation coefficients between HTL and TTS at specific test frequencies.

	HTL								TTS								
	2.5	3	3.5	4	5	6	7	8	2	2.5	3	3.5	4	5	6	7	8
HTL 2	0.86	0.82	0.67	0.66	0.60	0.69	0.36	0.49	-0.67	-0.53*	-0.42	-0.69	-0.58*	-0.46	-0.51*	-0.42	-0.29
2.5		0.95	0.83	0.79	0.66	0.73	0.47	0.35	-0.59*	-0.46	-0.40	-0.76	-0.53*	-0.39	-0.30	-0.43	-0.29
3			0.91	0.83	0.56*	0.62	0.39	0.23	-0.43	-0.33	-0.25	-0.70	-0.46	-0.18	-0.26	-0.36	-0.19
3.5				0.85	0.53*	0.50*	0.36	0.06	-0.21	-0.04	-0.05	-0.57*	-0.43	-0.15	-0.22	-0.48	-0.19
4					0.49	0.65	0.29	0.11	-0.15	-0.20	-0.09	-0.55*	-0.51*	-0.13	-0.22	-0.38	-0.27
5						0.83	0.57*	0.40	-0.38	-0.29	-0.28	-0.51*	-0.40	-0.52*	-0.36	-0.53*	-0.42
6							0.64	0.54*	-0.40	-0.45	-0.48	-0.63	-0.63	-0.43	-0.32	-0.31	-0.37
7								0.62	-0.17	-0.36	-0.44	-0.62	-0.58*	-0.36	-0.24	-0.39	-0.13
8									-0.48	-0.49	-0.48	-0.49	-0.43	-0.30	-0.42	-0.26	-0.22
TTS 2										0.56*	0.43	0.44	0.25	0.48	0.36	0.35	0.28
2.5											0.90	0.64	0.53*	0.42	0.41	0.16	0.18
3												0.66	0.56*	0.44	0.28	-0.06	0.16
3.5													0.85	0.46	0.38	0.21	0.08
4														0.49	0.45	0.17	0.25
5															0.64	0.50*	0.50*
6																0.62	0.46
7																	0.50*

* p<0.05 ______ p<0.01

Table 4. Pearson correlation coefficients between HTL and TTS at specific test frequencies.

Table 5. Pearson correlation coefficients between HTL and TTS in frequency area.

	HTL					TTS					
	2.5-3	3-3.5	3.5-4	4-5	2-8	2-2.5	2.5-3	3-3.5	3.5-4	4-5	2-8
HTL 2-2.5	0.92	0.84	0.77	0.87	0.91	-0.53*	-0.51*	-0.56*	-0.67	-0.57*	-0.68
2.5-3		0.92	0.82	0.83	0.88	-0.44	-0.54*	-0.58*	-0.59*	-0.40	-0.55*
3-3.5			0.92	0.77	0.83	-0.17	-0.23	-0.39	-0.49	-0.28	-0.39
3.5-4				0.77	0.80	-0.12	-0.12	-0.31	-0.48	-0.29	-0.37
4-5					0.91	-0.35	-0.42	-0.57*	-0.57*	-0.46	-0.59*
2-8						-0.39	-0.47	-0.64	-0.71	-0.57*	-0.67
TTS 2-2.5							0.82	0.65	0.59*	0.56*	0.72
2.5-3								0.77	0.58*	0.51*	0.68
3-3.5									0.84	0.69	0.16
3.5-4										0.82	0.77
4-5											0.92

* p<.05 ______ p<.01

a trend effect in repeated measures. Thus, an average of many TTS seasurements may increase reliability. In the present study, based upon 160 TTS observations in 16 individuals, the calculated pooled intra-individual TTS SD for all frequencies was < 4.2 dB (8 kHz excluded). These results are comparablt to those given in TTS investigagions by Ward [4], who showed a test-retest TTS SD between 3.9 - 4.6 dB in the frequency region 2 - 5.6 kHz. Interestingly, in our study the specific frequency that showed most TTS (3000 Hz) showed a calculated mean TTS SD of only 3.5 dB over 10 sessions, which is less than the value obtained when only two exposures (i.e., test-retest values) were taken into consideration.

The technique of calculating the HTL's and TTS's in frequency areas, rather than at specific test frequencies, resulted in a considerable improvement in reliability. Expressing TTS in area values makes it possible to distinguish between small TTS-values in controlled studies. For example, in a study comprising 10 subjects, it is possible to statistically verify a TTS-difference of 1.3 dB in the frequency area 2-8 kHz as significant, while a corresponding value at specific frequencies must exceed 2.5 dB. This finding is useful in designing interactive TTS-experiments.

If a study includes several repeated sessions, it is important to analyze if the TTS's are influenced by "trend-effects" (i.e., increasing or decreasing over sessions). In this study, we computed the mean correlation coefficients over the ten sessions. We choose to build the mean by using the correlation between the first and all subsequent tests rather than the correlation between the first and the second, the second and the third, etc. If a trend was present, the mean correlation would decrease when the number of sessions included in computations of the mean value increased. However, this was not the case, and no apparent trend-effect was obvious.

The major advantage with use of the test-fixture was the reduced TTS-variation compared to the variation using standard earphones. This reduction in variation is probably explained by the improvement in accuracy in threshold determinations as well as improved accuracy in the repeated noise exposures.

CONCLUSION

In order to diminish variations of TTS due to technical causes, the following measures are recommended:

- sweep frequency audiometry rather than standard manual audiometry.
- thresholds expressed in frequency areas.
- regular calibration of the test equipment.
- fixed consistent earphone placement.
- noise exposure levels regularly monitored before each session.
- participating subjects familiar with the test situation.
- the entire experiment conducted and performed by one operator.

If these conditions are met, it seems possible to obtain TTS-measurements on an individual basis highly reliable and with less variability than commonly reported.

ACKNOWLEDGEMENTS

This work was supported by Grant 81-0236 from The Swedish Work Environment Fund.

REFERENCES

1. H. Davis, C. T. Morgan, J. E. Hawkins, R. Galambos and F. W. Smith, Temporary deafness following exposure to loud tones and noise, _Acta. Otolaryngol. (Stockh)_, suppl. 88:1 (1954).
2. C. Lightfoot, Contribution to the study of auditory fatigue, _J. Acoust. Soc. Am._, 27:356 (1955).
3. D. W. Ward, The concept of susceptibility to hearing loss, _J. of Occupational Medicine_, 7:595 (1965).
4. D. W. Ward, Susceptibility to auditory fatigue, _in_: "Advances in sensory physiology," Vol. 3, W. D. Neff, ed., Academic Press, New York (1967).
5. W. D. Mustain and Z. G. Shoeny, Psychoacoustic correlates of susceptibility to auditory fatigue, _Ear Hear_, 10:91 (1980).

6. G. D. Chermak, J. E. Dengerink and H. A. Dengerink, Test-retest reliability of auditory threshold and temporary threshold shift, Scand. Audiol., 12:237 (1983).
7. A. Ivarsson, B. Erlandsson, H. Hakansson and P. Nilsson, Advantages with a new Bekesy audiometer in the measurement of noise-induced hearing loss, Scand. Audiol., suppl. 12:265 (1981).
8. B. Erlandsson, H. Hakansson, A. Ivarsson and P. Nilsson, The reliability of Bekesy sweep audiometry recording and effects of the earphone position, Acta. Otolaryngol. (Stockh.), suppl. 336:99 (1980).
9. B. J. Winer, Statistical principles in experimental design, 283-296, McGraw-Hill, New York (1971).

DISCUSSION

Pfander: I find it quite astonishing that your subjects have so much TTS. We made quite similar experiments with hundreds of people. After exposure to 90 dB white noise for several minutes, approximately 80 percent of the persons have no TTS. Increasing it to 110 dB, another 5 percent developed TTS, and when we tested people after exposure to gunfire, the percent increased to about 30 percent. I think if you test people, you will see very different results.

Lindgren: We have succeeded in inducing TTS in all our subjects. We also see a relationship between the initial hearing threshold and the amount of TTS. If you have a poor hearing threshold, then you will not experience much TTS.

Question: There is at least one paper showing that carbon monoxide will accelerate TTS under noise exposure. Therefore, I would like to know what is the most important chemical component with smoking, is it nicotine or carbon monoxide? The second questions is, what are the cutoff frequencies in your noise? We know that cutoff frequencies have a very important role on the development of TTS values.

Lindgren: The first question about the smoking, I wish I could answer you, but I can't. Animal studies using laser doppler shows that carbon monoxide acts like an asphyxia with a very high tendency to bind hemoglobin. The effects of nicotine are not only on the vascular system but can also influence enzymes in the cilia. So, we can not give a good explanation for which agent dominated the interaction effects of smoking and noise.

Patuzzi: I think one of the statements you made earlier is that TTS may be a protective mechanism, but I would just like to point out that if TTS does involve mechanical changes in the basilar membrane, those changes only occur for the mechanical response at very low intensities. If you look at some of the results I presented the other day, the point is that at high exposure intensities, the vibration pattern is virtually normal. So, if TTS does turn out to be protective mechanism of some sort for PTS or further TTS, the point is it is not because there is a change in mechanics at high intensities.

Phillips: As smoking and performance is becoming a very important concern in the U. S. Army, do you have any data on smoking and intra subject variability of TTS? Smoking can be a complicated variable to control, i.e., if you withhold smoking from a smoker, wake him up in the morning, make him do a task he doesn't do very well until he has the first cigarette, how to you categorize this subject? The effects of a single cigarette on carbon monoxide level is really relatively modest. It is at the end of the day, when the cigar, pipe and cigarette smokers have relatively elevated levels of carbon monoxide.

Answer: We are studying the effect by exposing subjects and letting them smoke prior to noise exposure, during noise exposure and during the recovery time. So far, we have not seen any major effects.

Phillips: Have you taken the same subject, measured their hearing level and then retested after they have had a cigarette without noise exposure?

Answer: No.

Phillips: I would do that to make sure they do not do better after they have had their first cigarette. That may be a possible explanation for some of your data.

Pujol: Smoking a cigarette is known to release some enkephalins, and we now know that these are in some of the efferent synapses in the cochlea. So, maybe, there is a relationship there.

McFadden: Is it fair to presume that the resting thresholds of the smokers and the non-smokers are the same?

Lindgren: Yes. We have the came criteria when choosing subjects. There would be no difference there.

Alberti: In a Canadian study, I examined PTS and smoking in several thousand industrial workers. Those smoking at least 20 cigarettes a day showed much higher noise induced hearing loss.

THE RELATIONSHIP BETWEEN SPEECH PERCEPTION AND PSYCHOACOUSTICAL MEASUREMENTS IN NOISE-INDUCED HEARING LOSS SUBJECTS

Richard S. Tyler and Nancy Tye-Murray

Department of Otolaryngology--Head & Neck Surgery
Department of Speech Pathology and Audiology
The University of Iowa
Iowa City, IA 52242, USA

INTRODUCTION

One of the most devastating effects of noise exposure is the potential loss in speech recognition abilities. While individuals with noise-induced hearing losses can detect speech, they often cannot discriminate its message (particularly when there is competing background noise). This often leads to frustration and communication breakdown.

Relating noise-induced hearing loss (NIHL) to the concommitant loss of speech understanding is difficult. The speech signal is multidimensional, changing rapidly in intensity and frequency characteristics as a function of time, and it is fairly robust (at least for normal listeners) to distortions and noise. Several basic auditory processing skills contribute to speech perception; certainly no single psychoacoustical ability can account for the multifaceted perception of speech.

DOES NIHL RESULT IN UNIQUE PSYCHOACOUSTICAL MANIFESTATIONS?

One characteristic feature of NIHL is its audiometric configuration (the loss in sensitivity is initially restricted to the 3000-6000 Hz region, with a peak loss around 4000 Hz). With further noise exposure, decreased sensitivity may be noted in the adjacent frequency regions as well. While decreased sensitivity to pure tones greater than 8000 Hz may also signal early NIHL, this can also be attributed to other causes, such as ototoxicity or presbycusis.

There are surprisingly few studies that examine other psychoacoustical differences between NIHL listeners and individuals with other types of cochlear impairments. Hood [1] measured loudness growth as a function of intensity in 13 patients with NIHL, 26 patients with deafness following head injury, and 200 patients with Menieres disease. He noted that the 'recruitment angle' (a measure of the rate of loudness increase for a given increase in level) was similar in the NIHL and Menieres group. The loudness increased at a slower rate in the head trauma group, which was attributed to a combination of sensory and retrocochlear abnormalities in this group.

Owens [2] compared tone decay (a measure of adaptation to a continuous tone) in 13 NIHL patients and 53 patients with Menieres disease. He reported that "tone decay occurred only at frequencies showing noticeable hearing loss," and that his findings did not differentiate the two groups. In the largest study of tone decay, Palva, Karja and Palva [3] tested 305 patients, 58 with NIHL. No differences were apparent across patient groups. Eight patients with NIHL had a threshold shift greater than 30 dB. Other work on NIHL patients suggest that loudness adaptation is limited to levels slightly above threshold [4,5], and that the amount of tone decay is related to the amount of threshold loss [6].

It has also been noted that the NIHL patients show reduced temporal integration abilities [7,8] and increased ability to detect intensity increments [9], but these findings cannot be differentiated from those obtained from other types of cochlear hearing loss. Others [10-13] have noted that the reduced frequency resolution in NIHL patients is similar to that found in other types of cochlear impairment.

NIHL patients generally process low-frequency sounds normally and typically demonstrate normal masking level differences [14]. However, some NIHL subjects with normal low-frequency thresholds demonstrate abnormal results in the low-frequency region on tasks of frequency resolution [12,15], frequency discrimination [16], threshold adaptation [17], and temporal integration [18].

We must conclude that, at present, there is no measure distinguishing the psychoacoustical abilities of NIHL subjects from those with other types of cochlear hearing loss. Since ample physiological evidence suggests different anatomical abnormalities, we suggest that basic psychoacoustic differences exist, but either we have not yet found the appropriate measures, and/or we have not made the measurements with sufficient precision. We need some direction from the physiologists and theorists regarding what type of perceptual consequences should follow specific anatomical lesions.

WHAT IS THE INFLUENCE OF THE THRESHOLD LOSS ON SPEECH PERCEPTION?

The loss of threshold sensitivity will result in some speech sounds not being heard and others being misidentified. Fig. 1 shows the significant relationship (r = -0.76) between threshold loss at 2000 Hz and percent correct word recognition (after Lindeman [19]) tested on 679 NIHL patients. The speech tests are an averaged score obtained at four signal-to-noise ratios (from -5 dB to 10 dB). At other frequencies between 1600 Hz and 6300 Hz, correlations with word recognition were also high (see Table 1), but the correlation at 2000 Hz was the highest. In another study, Plath [20] tested word recognition in quiet in 130 NIHL patients. It is noteworthy that the highest correlation with any of the frequencies tested was at 2000 Hz (r = -0.59), in agreement with Lindeman's [19] study. Correlations between speech perception and the threshold loss at any single frequency are greater at high than at low frequencies. Tyler et al. [12], for example, found a correlation of r = -0.39 at 500 Hz and r = -0.71 at 4000 Hz in a speech-in-noise task.

Perhaps the threshold at 2000 Hz shows the highest correlation because it is the best indicator of the encroachment of the damage from the high-frequency region into the lower frequencies. In addition, important speech information, including formants 2 or 3 of many vowels and consonants, is centered around 2000 Hz, and may be lost with decreased sensitivity.

Note in Fig. 1 the substantial individual variability. Some patients have mild threshold losses and poor word recognition, while others have

Table 1. Correlations among threshold and word recognition in NIHL patients.

Study	Subjects	Background Noise	Frequency (Hz) 500	1000	2000	4000
Lindeman[19]	679 NIHL	yes		-.75[a]	-.77	-.67[b]
Plath[20]	130 NIHL	no	-.48	-.54	-.59	-.53
Tyler et al.[12]	12 NIHL 10 normals	yes	-.39			-.71

a. 1600 Hz; b. 6300 Hz

severe threshold losses but good word recognition (c.f. Niemeyer [21]). Both Plath [20] and Tyler et al. [12] also observed negative correlations between word recognition and age, so the combination of aging and noise exposure cannot be overlooked.

It may also be that correlations are higher with speech in noise compared to speech in quiet. Fig. 2 shows the results of a study by Suter [22]. Word recognition for the 16 normals and 16 NIHL subjects were similar in quiet, but when noise was added, the decrease in performance by the NIHL subjects was much worse.

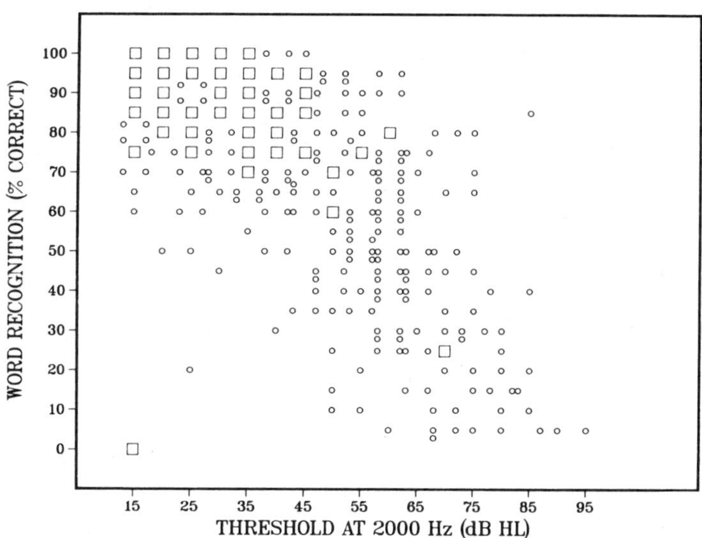

Fig. 1. The relationship between hearing threshold at 2000 Hz and word recognition in noise (data from Lindeman [19]). Circles represent individual data points, squares represent five or more data points of the same value. The correlation coefficient for the data shown is r = -0.76.

It is of interest to examine the kinds of perceptual speech errors that occur when thresholds are elevated in the 3000 - 6000 Hz region. Vowel perception is thought to rely heavily on the frequencies of the lower three formants. For male talkers, only the vowel /i/ has a typical third formant (F_3) above 3000 Hz, so one would predict few vowel confusions. For women, the /i, I, ɛ/ typically have F_3 in the region of 3000 Hz, but again few confusions would be expected. For children, all F_3 values for the vowels except (3^r) are typically above 3000 Hz, and so is the second formant for /i/. In this instance we might expect more errors, for example, between /i/ and /u/, both having similar F_1s.

In general agreement with these comments, several researchers have observed that vowel confusions are infrequent in the cochlear-impaired among all but those with severe threshold losses across the frequency range. However, these tests have almost uniformly utilized adult male speakers. Future research may revise these conclusions for female and child speakers.

Consonant perception depends on a variety of cues. A NIHL loss might eliminate important energy that can be used to distinguish sounds within the group /f, θ, s, ʃ/ or within /v, ð, z, ʒ/. In addition, the stops /p, t, k/ and /b, d, g/ might be confused, depending on the degree of threshold loss and the vowel context. But are consonant confusions different for NIHL compared to other cochlear-impaired subjects? Oyer and Doudna [23], and Schultz [24] (33 NIHL subjects) both failed to find different types of phonetic errors in different types of hearing losses.

We have completed a pilot study evaluating the effects of a '4000-Hz notch' on consonant recognition. Three subjects with normal hearing listened to 13 consonants embedded in an /iCi/ context (a male speaker with general American dialect). In the simulated NIHL condition, information from 3000-5000 Hz was eliminated by filtering (115 dB/octave). In the second condition, which simulated some other types of cochlear impairment, all information above 3000 Hz was eliminated. The only errors committed by eliminating the information between 3000-5000 Hz were the confusion of /m/ and /n/. From an examination of the spectrograms, it appeared that the frequency location of F , about 4600 Hz for /n/ and about 4200 Hz for /m/, was a key difference. The elimination of all information above 3000 Hz also resulted in /m/ and /n/ confusions, but also /f/ and /s/ errors. Fig. 3 shows the spectrograms of /f/ and /s/. The /s/ has more intense

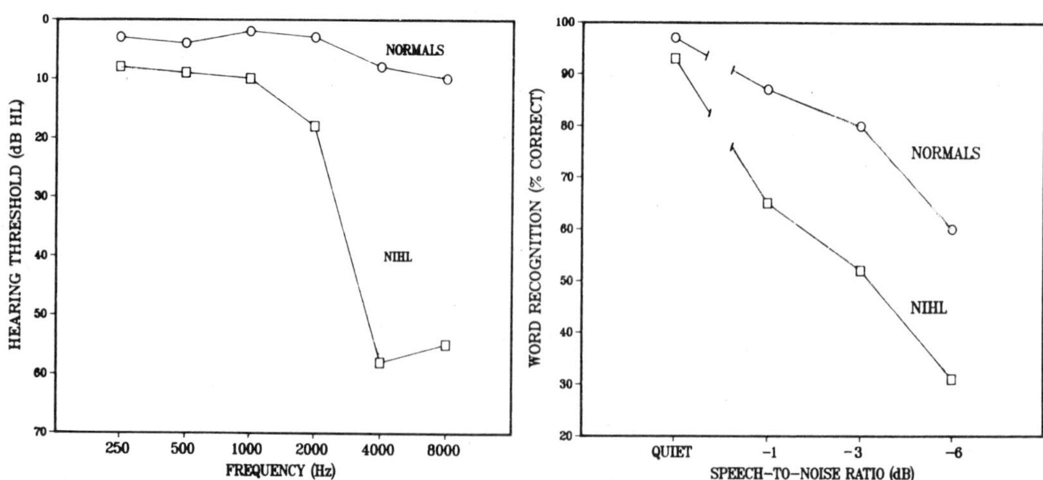

Fig. 2. Audiograms (left) and word recognition (right) in a group of 11 normal and 16 NIHL patients (after Suter [22]).

high-frequency frication. Eliminating the information between 3000 Hz and 5000 Hz does not eliminate the distinction, but eliminating all information above 3000 Hz does. While this is not a good simulation of NIHL, it does attest to the importance of receiving speech information above 5000 Hz. At later stages of NIHL this will be lost, and performance will deteriorate.

WHAT IS THE RELATIONSHIP BETWEEN PSYCHOACOUSTICAL PERFORMANCE AND SPEECH PERCEPTION?

One step in examining the relationship among word recognition and psychoacoustical tasks is to determine if correlations exist among them. There are few studies that examine this question strictly for a NIHL population. Plath [20] measured word recognition, the ability to detect changes in amplitude modulation, and the ability to detect increments in a continuous tone in 'more than 500' patients with NIHL and 63 patients with other types of hearing loss. Significant correlations (see Table 2) existed for both groups between word recognition and the intensity increment detection at 4 kHz (r = -.25) and with amplitude-modulation detection at 10 dB SL at 4 kHz (r = -0.19), although the correlations were small.

Tyler et al. [12,13] computed correlations between word recognition and several psychoacoustical measurements (see Table 2). These findings suggested moderate correlations between word recognition and detecting a 4000 Hz tone in noise background (critical ratio) (r = -0.63), the low (r = -0.50) and high (r = 0.64) frequency slope of a 4000 Hz psychoacoustical tuning curve, and temporal integration for a 4000 Hz tone.

From our previous discussion, we noted that psychoacoustical measures have not clearly differentiated between NIHL patients and other types of cochlear hearing loss. Therefore, it may be fruitful to examine studies of hetereogeneous groups of cochlear hearing loss.

Table 3 shows several correlations from a few such studies. While it is difficult to compare across studies because of differences in subjects and procedures, a few generalizations can be made. First, there are several tasks that show high correlations, particularly for measurement of frequency and temporal resolution. Tyler et al. [25] for example, noted a

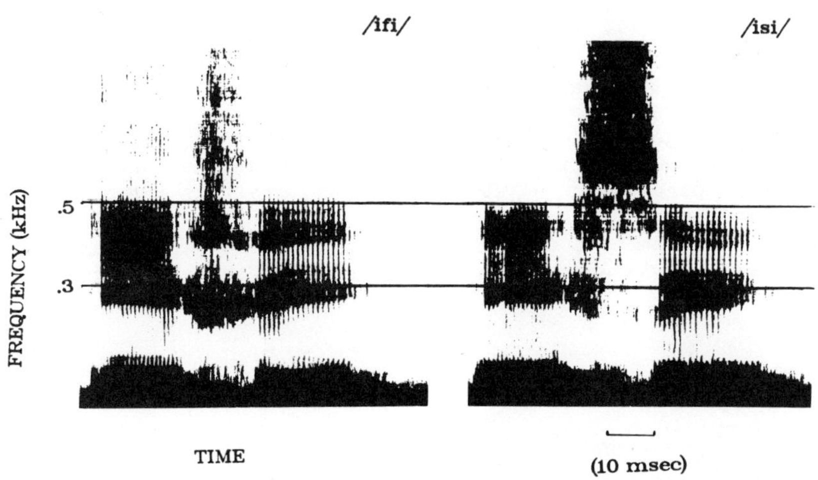

Fig. 3. Spectrograms of the sounds /ifi/ and /isi/.

Table 2. Correlations among speech perception and psychoacoustical tasks for normals and NIHL subjects (*statistical significance).

	Plath[20]	Tyler et al.[12]
age	-.51*	-.69*
intensity increments 4000 Hz	-.25*	
amplitude modulation	-.19*	
500-Hz threshold	-.48*	-.39
4000-Hz threshold	-.48*	-.71*
4000-Hz critical ratio		-.63*
4000 Hz PTC low-frequency slope		-.50*
4000-Hz PTC high-frequency slope		.64*
4000-Hz temporal integration		-.45*

PTC = psychoacoustical tuning curve

significant correlation between word recognition and gap detection and between word recognition and temporal difference limens, even after the effects of threshold were partialled out (see Fig. 4). Frequency resolution measurements have typically shown moderately high correlations, with the exception of the high-frequency slope. The correlations with the two measures of intensity resolution mentioned in Table 2 are notably lower. However, we should keep in mind that speech recognition likely depends on several basic abilities, and correlations obtained from any single ability would be predictably moderate at best.

The next stage in such an analysis could be a multiple regression analysis, where the results of several psychoacoustical tasks are used to predict speech perception. Tyler et al. [25] did this for a number of temporal and frequency resolution measures (see Table 4). They were able to account for 85 percent of the variance on a word recognition test with seven measures. This again emphasizes the multifaceted nature of speech recognition.

DISCUSSION

Although it may not always be evident when tested in quiet situations with adult male speakers, NIHL patients have difficulty recognizing speech.

Table 3. Correlations among speech perception in noise and psychoacoustical tasks at 4000 Hz for normal and cochlear-impaired listeners. Numbers in brackets represent correlation partialling out the effect of threshold (*statistical significance).

	Dreschler and Plomp[26]	Tyler et al.[25]	Tyler et al.[27]	Festen and Plomp[28]	Stelmachowicz et al.[29]
Subjects	10 coch	16 norm 16 coch	12 norm 12 coch	22 coch	11 norm 13 coch
4 kHz threshold	-.90*a	-.73*	-.71*	-.38*a	
temporal integration		-.67* (-.35)		-.24b	
gap detection		-.73* (-.48)*			
gap difference limen (30-msec standard)		-.50* (-.15)			
temp difference limen (30-msec standard)		-.74* (-.42)*			
peak-trough temporal masking				..34b	
forward masking				-.24b	
backward masking				.22b	
PTC Q_{10} dB				-.63*b	-.69*c (.60)*
low-frequency slope of PTC		-.64* (-.28)		-.60*b	-.62*c
high-frequency slope of PTC		.25 (-.06)	.50* (-.24)	-.08b	.62*c
PTC tip-to-tail		.69* (.27)	-.49* (.17)		-.53*
critical ratio	.90*b			.63*b	
comb-filter noise	.79*b				
frequency difference limen*			-.63* (.49)		
frequency transition difference limen			-.55* (.26)		

a average of .5, 1., and 2 kHz
b at 1 kHz; c at 2 kHz

PTC = psychoacoustical tuning curve

These difficulties cannot be predicted reliably from the audiogram for an individual. Psychoacoustical abnormalities, not related to threshold, are sometimes present, and the results suggest that these contribute to the difficulty in speech perception. It is critical that more sensitive tests be developed. We should be able to measure psychoacoustical differences between NIHL and other types of cochlear hearing loss. Large scale, multivariate studies (for example, using Path Analysis [30]) are required to clarify the relationship between basic measurements of frequency, intensity temporal processing and speech perception. Furthermore, measurements utilizing speech-like stimuli should be helpful to more clearly define the relationship between psychoacoustics and speech perception in NIHL patients.

Table 4. Multiple regression of psychoscoustical measures on word recognition correct scores for 16 normal and 16 hearing-impaired listeners. Multiple regression analysis evaluates the overall dependence of one variable on a set of independent variables (adapted from Tyler et al. [25]).

Variable	kHz	Simple R	Multiple R^2
Temporal difference limen	4.0	-0.74	0.55
Temporal Integration	4.0	0.67	0.68
Gap detection	4.0	-0.73	0.75
PTC Tail-tip difference	0.5	0.02	0.79
PTC high-frequency slope	4.0	0.25	0.82
Temporal integration	0.5	0.03	0.83
PTC low-frequency slope	4.0	-0.64	0.85

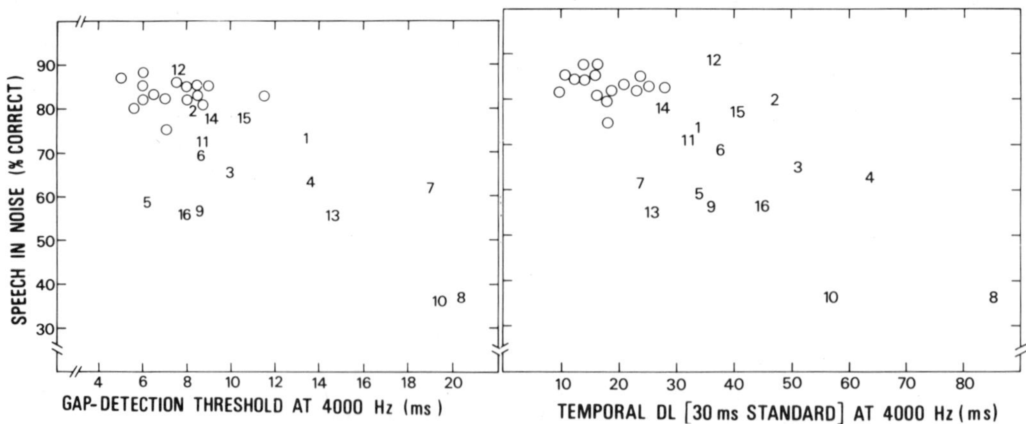

Fig. 4. Correlations between word recognition and gap detection (left) and with temporal difference limen (30 msec standard) obtained from 16 normals (circles) and 16 cochlear-impaired listeners (adapted from Tyler et al. [25]).

REFERENCES

1. J. D. Hood, A comparative study of loudness recruitment in cases of deafness due to Menieres disease, head injury and acoustic trauma, Acta Oto-Rhino-Laryngol. Belg. 14:224 (1960).
2. E. Owens, Tone decay in VIIIth nerve and cochlear lesions, J. Speech Hear. Dis. 29:14 (1964).
3. T. Palva, A. Karja, and A. Palva, Auditory adaptation at threshold intensities, Acta Otolaryngol. Suppl. 224:195 (1967).
4. D. D. Dirks, D. E. Morgan, and D. A. Bray, Perstimulatory loudness adaptation in selected cochlear impaired and masked normal listeners, J. Acoust. Soc. Am. 56:554 (1974).
5. T. L. Wiley, D. J. Lilly, and A. M. Small, Loudness adaptation in listeners with noise-induced hearing loss, J. Acoust. Soc. Am. 59:225 (1976).
6. W. D. Ward, R. E. Fleer, and A. Glorig, Characteristics of hearing losses produced by gunfire and by steady noise, J. Aud. Res. 1:325 (1961).
7. W. O. Olsen, D. E. Rose, and D. Noffsinger, Brief-tone audiometry with normal, cochlear, and eighth nerve tumor patients, Arch. Otolaryngol. 99:185 (1974).
8. C. B. Pedersen, Brief-tone audiometry, Scand. Audiol. 5:27 (1976).
9. H. Fastl, and K. Schorn, Discrimination of level differences by hearing-impaired patients, Audiology 20:488 (1981).
10. E. Zwicker, and K. Schorn, Psychoacoustical tuning curves in audiology, Audiology 17:120 (1978).
11. M. Florentine, S. Buus, B. Scharf, and E. Zwicker, Frequency selectivity in normal-hearing and hearing-impaired observers, J. Speech Hear. Res. 23:646 (1980).
12. R. S. Tyler, M. Fernandes, and E. J. Wood, Masking, temporal integration and speech intelligibility in individuals with noise-induced hearing loss, in: "Disorders of Auditory Function III," I. Taylor and A. Markides, eds., Academic Press, New York (1980).
13. R. S. Tyler, E. J. Wood, and M. Fernandes, Frequency resolution and hearing loss, British J. Audiol. 16:45 (1982b).
14. W. O. Olsen, D. Noffsinger, and R. Carhart, Masking level differences encountered in clinical populations, Audiology 15:287 (1976).
15. L. E. Humes, D. M. Schwartz, and F. H. Bess, Two experiments on subtle midfrequency hearing loss and its influence on word discrimination in noise-exposed listeners, Audiology 18:307 (1979).
16. C. A. Turner, and D. A. Nelson, Frequency discrimination in regions of normal and impaired sensitivity, J. Speech Hear. Res. 25:34 (1982).
17. R. C. Findlay, Auditory dysfunction accompanying noise-induced hearing loss, J. Speech Hear. Dis. 41:374 (1976).
18. J. Komovic, Auditory temporal integration in subjects with cochlear pathology due to noise exposure, unpublished master's thesis, University of Pittsburgh.
19. H. E. Lindeman, Relation between audiological findings and complaints by persons suffering from noise-induced hearing loss, Amer. Ind. Hyg. Assoc. 32:447 (1971).
20. P. Plath, Signal perception in noise induced hearing loss, Acustica 29:47 (1973).
21. W. Niemeyer, Speech discrimination in noise-induced deafness, Int. Audiol. 6:42 (1967).
22. A. H. Suter, The ability of mildly hearing-impaired individuals to discriminate speech in noise, EPA Report NO. 550/9-78-100, AMRL Report No. TR-78-4, Washington, D.C.: U. S. Environmental Protection Agency; Ohio: Aerospace Medical Research Laboratory (1978).
23. H. J. Oyer, and M. Doudna, Structural analysis of word responses made by hard of hearing subjects on a discrimination test, AMA Arch. Otolaryngol. 70:357 (1959).

24. M. C. Schultz, Suggested improvements in speech discrimination testing, J. Aud. Res. 4:1 (1964).
25. R. S. Tyler, A. Q. Summerfield, E. J. Wood, and M. A. Fernandes, Psychoacoustic and phonetic temporal processing in normal and hearing-impaired listeners, J. Acoust. Soc. Am. 72:740 (1982a).
26. W. A. Dreschler, and R. Plomp, Relation between psychophysical data and speech perception for hearing-impaired subjects I., J. Acoust. Soc. Am. 68:1608 (1980).
27. R. S. Tyler, E. J. Wood, and M. Fernandes, Frequency resolution and discrimination of constant and dynamic tones in normal and hearing-impaired listeners, J. Acoust. Soc. Am. 74:1190 (1983).
28. J. M. Festen, and R. Plomp, Relations between auditory functions in impaired hearing, J. Acoust. Soc. Am. 73:652 (1983).
29. P. G. Stelmachowicz, W. Jesteadt, M. P. Gorga, and J. Mott, Speech perception ability and psychophysical tuning curves in hearing-impaired listeners, J. Acoust. Soc. Am. 77:620 (1985).
30. J. R. Duffy, J. Watt, and R. J. Duffy, Tutorial Path analysis: A strategy for investigating multivariate causal relationships in communication disorders, J. Speech Hear. Res. 24:474 (1981).

COMMENTS

Flottorp: We talk about noise induced hearing loss as if it was a single entity with a characteristic audiogram, when in fact it is many audiograms with a number of complicating factors. In our studies, we tend to factor noise induced hearing loss into old vs. young, predominantly high frequency losses vs. flat losses. These are potentially central components. So I am not sure that one can draw conclusions right across the spectrum.

Tyler: We have found a significant correlation between age and speech recognition. Using partial correlation techniques, we have tried to factor the effects of age, temporal DL's and gap detection. We found that age was not a confounding factor. Although it certainly is true, that it would not be surprising if these patients do have some central processing difficiencies based on age, which would be an additional handicap to which noise exposure would add.

Salvi: In one of the papers you showed that there was not very much correlation between AM processing and speech perception. Yet, another test of temporal resolution, gap detection, seemed like it was fairly well correlated with speech perception. Are AM detection and gap detection sampling the phenomena, because both are supposed to be tests of temporal resolution.

Tyler: Certainly there are different factors that go into different psychoacoustical tests. For example, gap detection and forward masking might be considered more direct measures of decay of excitation and recovery again. These correlational studies are done on fairly small numbers of subjects. But I do think there are some fine differences in the actual procedures to make them non-compatible.

Salvi: Do you see changes in temporal difference limen as a function of hearing level, i.e., do you need a certain amount of hearing loss to see a change in the temporal difference limen?

Tyler: I am not certain what that would be off hand. I would have to look back at some of our data.

von Gierke: Have you or anyone else looked at those psychoacoustic tests in noise induced hearing loss patients compared to the same or similar tests in people with temporary threshold shift?

Tyler: I certainly have not.

Question: In your conclusion, you pointed out the urgent need to carry out more multi-variate study in this field. I just wanted to point out a potential problem. When we are carrying out multi-variate studies and adding predictors and if those predictors are correlated with each other. Do you have any idea how to develope this kind of multi-variate methods, how to understand these potential interactions?

Tyler: The strategy that I began using was to look at initially a number of measures of frequency resolution and correlate those with speech intelligibility. Given one or two best predictors based on the preliminary data, select the most powerful prediction and then undertake a larger scale study. In fact, a study like that has been undertaken with a large number of patients at the Institute of Human Research in Nottingham where they have a very large data base available.

SPEECH PERCEPTION IN INDIVIDUALS WITH NOISE-INDUCED HEARING LOSS AND ITS IMPLICATION FOR HEARING LOSS CRITERIA

Guido F. Smoorenburg

Institute for Perception TNO
Postbox 23, 3769 ZG Soesterberg
The Netherlands

HEARING HANDICAP INDICES

Assessment of hearing handicap is one of the objectives of audiometry. Regrettably, this objective has received much attention because of the growing incidence of financial claims that should compensate hearing loss due to occupational noise exposure; whereas quantification of the hearing handicap also pertains to evaluation of ear surgery and hearing-aid fitting, to examination of hearing in relation to job requirements, and to adequate provisions for groups with a certain hearing handicap (such as the aged). In this paper, however, we shall address ourselves to the main issue of current interest, the handicap due to noise-induced hearing loss.

A number of indices have been proposed to quantify hearing handicap. Most are based upon the (pure) tone audiogram. Tone audiometry provides objective measures, is relatively easy to obtain, and is insensitive to abuse. Financial claims led to the concept of 'onset of handicap', the so-called 'fence', and to the definition of percentage of impairment of hearing. This percentage increased in a monotonic fashion with the hearing loss in excess of the fence. The indices are usually based on the average value of the audiometric threshold at some selected frequencies. The most familiar indices and fences are listed in Table I.

Table I. Hearing handicap indices and fences. The reference fence is the corresponding fence for 1, 2 and 3 kHz; r gives the correlation between the listed index and the index based on 1, 2 and 3 kHz.

Source	Year (kHz)	Frequencies	Fence (dB)	Reference Fence	r
AAOO [1]	'59	0.5,1,2	25 (26)	42	.86
AAO [2]	'79	0.5,1,2,3	25	29	.99
NIOSH [3]	'72	1,2,3	25	25	1.00
DHSS [4]	'73	1,2,3	50	50	1.00
BADL/BSA [5]	'83	1,2,4	20	18	.96
OSHA-STS [6]	'83	2,3,4	10	6.5	.96
LAFON [7]	'81	2,4	20-30	13-20	.94

To facilitate a comparison of the fences based on different sets of audiometric frequencies, a reference fence has been included in Table I. This reference fence presents the corresponding average hearing loss at 1, 2 and 3 kHz. The frequencies 1, 2 and 3 kHz take a central position among the quoted indices. The reference fence was calculated from the losses expressed in the listed index plotted against those at 1, 2 and 3 kHz by way of a linear fit minimizing the variance perpendicular to the fitting line. The data base consisted of 400 ears with different degrees of noise-induced hearing loss. These ears are included in the speech-perception study to be summarized below. The coefficient of correlation between the indices is given in the right column of Table I.

Table I shows a wide range of fence values. The oldest sources put forward the highest fences. The fence of 25 dB (in some versions 26 dB), which is the average loss across 0.5, 1 and 2 kHz proposed by the American Academy of Ophthalmology and Otolaryngology (AAOO) [1] has received the widest acceptance. It was based on "the ability to hear everyday speech under everyday conditions." Similar considerations underlie the other high fence in Table I of the British Department of Health and Social Security (DHSS) [4]. By including 3 kHz instead of 0.5 kHz, the British index was tuned more closely to the noise dip. This inplies a more accurate measure, but also a more restricted validity (see Tempest [8]).

The early fences were criticized because the "ability to hear everyday speech under everyday conditions" was interpreted as correct repetition of sentences presented at 60-70 dB SPL in a quiet environment. Interference of ambient noise was excluded because the question of what ambient noise is representative of everyday conditions was not solved [9]. Kryter [10] argued that the fence should be lowered to a 15 dB average across 0.5, 1 and 1 kHz, or preferably a 25 dB average across 1, 2 and 3 kHz (c.f. NIOSH '72 in Table I), because even in quiet conditions, a person with a hearing loss corresponding to the AAOO-fence would be unable to correctly perceive individual speech sounds, and even some sentences, whenever the speech level would be lower than the normal level of 60-70 dB at 1 m from the talker. After discussing the DHSS-fence, Tempest [8] introduced a grouping scheme for assessment of hearing handicap in which he distinguished a significant loss of hearing at high frequencies, the criterion being a loss of 25 dB or more at 4 and/or 6 kHz. A loss of this nature is considered to reduce the quality of hearing, such as not fully hearing music and natural sounds, impairment of phoneme discrimination (e.g., between 's', 't' and 'th', and a limited ability to follow speech in noisy situations.

Arguments like those presented above led to reconsideration of the fences first proposed. The AAOO (meanwhile AAO [1]) adjusted the fence by including the hearing loss at 3 kHz, while leaving the average value of the thresholds at 25 dB and thus effectively lowering the fence. In 1983, the British Association of Otolaryngologists (BAOL) and the British Society of Audiology (BSA) [5] proposed a fence of 20 dB average hearing level across 1, 2 and 4 kHz. They included into their criterion, noisy backgrounds and the perception of everyday sounds, not just everyday speech.

Amongst other studies, they took into consideration the results of the pilot study [11,12] preceding the study to be summarized below. Quite independently, Lafon [7] proposed an index based on the frequencies 2 and 4 kHz. He derived his percentage-disability measure from phonemic confusions. At the lowest level of 30 dB included in his study, he found a disability of 3 percent. The remaining fence in Table I is the Standard Threshold Shift of the USA Occupational Safety and Health Administration [6]. This fence is of a different nature. It is the shift in an individual's hearing level at or above which action must be taken for better hearing protection. For this fence, the reference fence in Table I also represents a shift in threshold rather than a threshold level.

OBJECTIVE OF THIS STUDY

At the end of the '70s, we felt that the hearing handicap indices and fences in use at the time were not properly justified. In particular, we felt that speech perception in noisy situations, although recognized as an important factor, was insufficently represented in the measures of handicap. When one sets out to define an onset of handicap (a fence), attention should be focused on those situations in which people with hearing loss first experience a handicap. It is generally reported that this occurs with speech perception in noisy situations. Therefore, we started this study on speech perception in quiet and noisy conditions for individuals with noise-induced hearing loss.

The concept of 'onset of handicap' is closely linked with the question of what hearing loss is acceptable. This is an ethical problem. The only proper answer is none whatsoever. However, many people are subject to involuntary noise exposures. While it is not presently feasible, from an economical and a technical point of view, to reduce all noise exposures below the risk level, it is important to show what hearing handicap is associated with the tone-audiometric losses known to arise from the noise exposure. In our opinion, an involuntary noise exposure should not cause a noticeable hearing handicap. Therefore, in this study the fence is defined as that hearing loss for which an individual begins to notice a handicap in everyday (noisy) situations. A higher loss is definitely not acceptable. A smaller loss is also not acceptable. From the point of view of preventive medicine, we should strive to reduce the noise exposures to levels at which the exposed population does not show any noise-induced hearing impairment.

METHODS

The present study is based on 400 ears, using the left and right ears of 200 subjects. These subjects were divided into 5 groups of 40 subjects each. Each group of subjects worked in a different noisy environment. The five noisy environments included three types of construction workplaces, locomotive engines and shooting ranges. The ears were virtually free of conductive hearing loss. All subjects were younger than 55 years, to minimize the effects of presbyacusis. The medical history was used to exclude subjects with hearing loss of an origin other than noise exposure. The subjects were selected with respect to their degree of tone-audiometric hearing loss, in order to evenly cover the full range of hearing loss (i.e., no hearing loss at all to the highest measurable loss).

Tone-audiometric thresholds were determined with an automatic audiometer (the Audiomat) for use in occupational audiometry [13]. The Audiomat automatically runs an audiometric program using a microprocessor. The measurement procedure is an optimized up-and-down threshold tracking procedure with fixed frequencies. The tones are presented in bursts of 200 ms duration. The accuracy of the measurement is 3 to 4 dB. Fig. 1 shows the distribution of the audiometric thresholds for all 400 ears. The losses in the left and right ear are quite symmetric. The correlation between the average values of the thresholds at 2 and 4 kHz in the left and right ear is $r = 0.82$. Therefore, one might argue that only one ear per subject should be considered. There is, however, no essential difference between the results for one ear per subject and those for two ears per subject.

In spite of the selection of subjects according to their degree of tone-autiometric hearing loss, the intersubject variance in hearing loss, as apparent from Fig. 1, was smaller than we had hoped to find. An

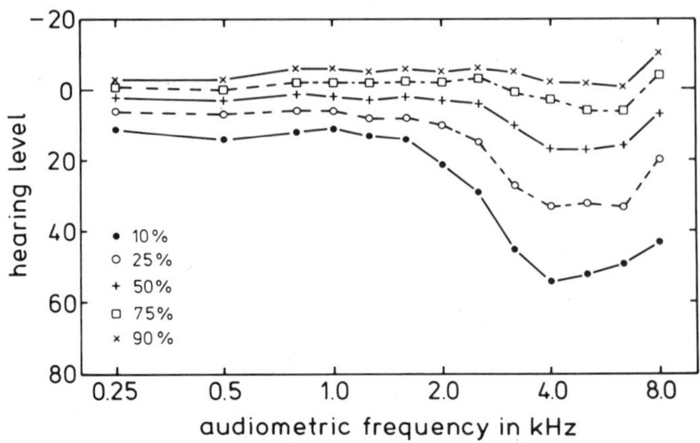

Fig. 1. Median value, quartiles and upper and lower decile of the thresholds for the 400 ears included in this study.

increase of intersubject variance could be obtained by excluding all subjects younger than 45 years of age. An additional interesting aspect of such a subgroup is that 'age' becomes a less important variable. Statistical analysis of the results for this subgroup shows higher correlation coefficients when the tone-audiometric data are compared with the speech perception data. The increase in correlation stems from variability in the speech reception thresholds becoming less important with a higher intersubject variance. There is, however, no essential difference between speech perception in relation to the tone audiogram for this subgroup and for all 400 ears. Therefore, we will continue with the data for all 400 ears.

Since we were interested in hearing handicap, speech perception was measured using sentences. We followed the method introduced by Plomp and Mimpen [14,15]. Simple sentences, consisting of eight or nine syllables, were recorded on tape using a male voice. The set of sentences was homogenized by excluding sentences that required more than 1 dB level correction in order to arrive at the average score. After a run-up phase using three sentences, the speech reception threshold (SRT) was measured with a sequence of ten sentences. The level of the sentence was increased by 2 dB when a sentence was not completely correctly repeated by the subject, and it was decreased by 2 dB when it was repeated completely correctly. The SRT (50% sentence intelligibility) was determined by averaging the sound pressure level during this up-and-down sequence. The sentences were presented without interfering noise and with noise at 35, 50, 65 and 80 dBA. The spectrum of the noise matched the spectrum of the male voice. In our opinion, the social handicap is mainly determined by speech-born noise interfering with speech perception. In spite of this, there are, of course, many occupational situations in which machine noise interferes with communication on the job.

SPEECH PERCEPTION IN RELATION TO HEARING LOSS AT 1, 2 AND 3 kHz

Here we shall only summarize the results of our study. Elsewhere, the results will be reported in full detail. Fig. 2 shows the coefficients of the correlation between the SRTs and the tone-audiometric losses. For speech in quiet situations, the highest correlations are found at low audiometric frequencies, whereas high-frequency hearing loss appears to be important for speech perception in noisy situations. There is little

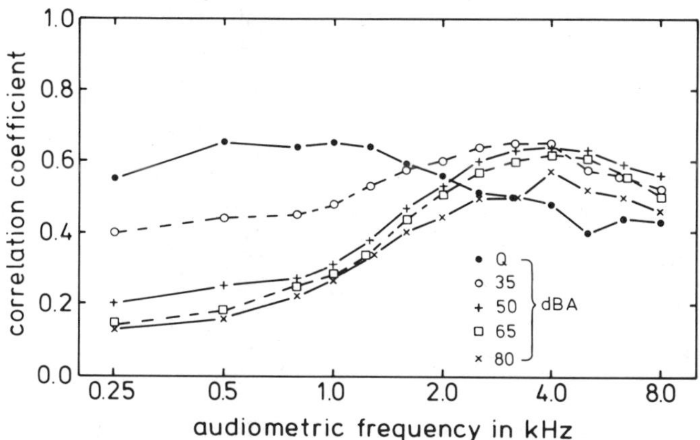

Fig. 2. Correlation coefficients for the relation between the speech reception threshold and the tone-audiometric threshold. Q: quiet situation; 35, 50, 65 and 80 dBA: noisy situations.

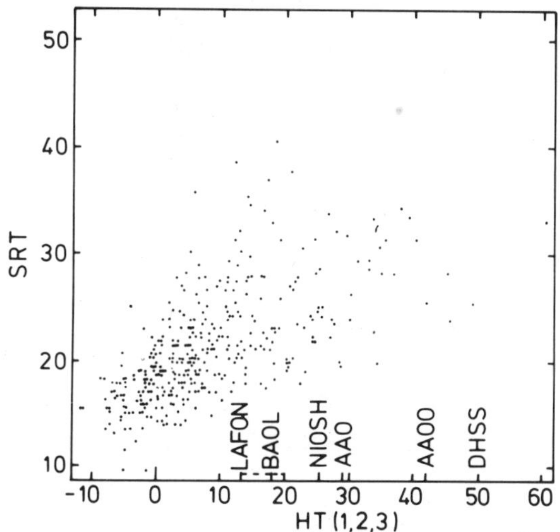

Fig. 3. Speech reception threshold for quiet situations (in dBA) in relation to the hearing thresholds averaged across 1, 2 and 3 kHz. Several fences are indicated along the abscissa. The correlation coefficient is 0.63. It is based on 400 data points.

difference between the correlation coefficients for noise at 50, 65 and 80 dBA. Therefore, we will distinguish only two situations: speech perception in quiet and speech perception in noise at 50-80 dBA. The intermediate condition of 35 dBA will be discarded. For noise at 50-80 dBA, the SRTs expressed relative to the noise level (i.e., the signal-to-noise ratios, S/N), are very close to one another. Hence, the SRTs for the combined noise conditions will be expressed in average S/N values.

The SRTs in the quiet condition are plotted as a function of the reference index based on 1, 2 and 3 kHz, HT (1,2,3), in Fig. 3. The correlation coefficient for these data equals 0.63. The fences of Table I are indicated along the abscissa. Fig. 3 shows that, except for one SRT at about 52 dBA, the SRTs in quiet conditions range up to about 40 dBA. Thus, even for the AAOO or DHSS fence, there is no handicap in understanding sentences at normal speech levels of 60-70 dB in quiet environments. However, Kryter's [10] argument should also be considered. A near perfect perception of the weakest phonemes like 'f' requires sound levels at least 35 dB higher than the SRT for sentences. Thus, a SRT above about 30 dBA for sentences presented in quiet situations implies imperfect perception of individual speech sounds at normal speech levels of 60-70 dB. According to Fig. 3, the SRT of 30 dB corresponds to about HT(1,2,3) = 34 dB; a value lower than either the AAOO or the DHSS fence. Fig. 3 shows, however, considerable scatter of the data points. Therefore, a reliable fence cannot be derived from those data. Earlier, we stated that speech perception in noisy environments is the important condition for determining the onset of handicap. We shall therefore continue with the SRTs for noisy situations.

Fig. 4 shows the relation between the SRTs in noisy conditions (expressed S/N) and HT (1,2,3). The correlation coefficient equals 0.66. Above 15 dB, the average loss across 1, 2 and 3 kHz shows a clear increase of the SRT. An increase of the SRT by 1 dB corresponds to a decrease in sentence intelligibility of 15 to 20% when S/N is kept constant. Above the NIOSH, AAO, AAOO and DHSS fences, the increase in SRT approaches 3 dB or more which implies a decrease in sentence intelligibility of 50% or more. This means an unacceptable hearing loss.

In this section, the SRTs were presented with respect to the reference index based on 1, 2 and 3 kHz. However, this index is not the best measure to predict the SRT for noisy conditions. In the next section, we shall indicate fences based on the best predicting tone-audiometric index.

FENCES BASED ON HEARING LOSS AT 2 AND 4 kHz

Statistical analysis of the tone audiograms and of the speech reception thresholds (principal components, canonical correlation and multiple regression) shows that the SRT in noisy situations can adequately be predicted from the tone audiometric thresholds at 2 and 4 kHz. The predictor based simply on the average value of these two thresholds [HT(2,4)] suffices. This result is based, of course, on our noise-induced hearing loss data only. The SRT as a function of HT(2,4) is presented in Fig. 5. The correlation coefficient equals 0.72. Increasing the intersubject variance in hearing loss by restricting the data base to the worse ear and to all subjects at or above 45 years of age raises this coefficient to 0.80.

Splitting up the data according to HT(2,4)-intervals of 10 dB, and even of 5 dB, shows that there is no change in SRT up to HT(2,4)=10 dB. Above 10 dB, the SRT starts to rise. Thus, from the point of view of preventive medicine, the target fence that we should strive for is HT(2,4) = 10 dB.

For the ears satisfying HT(2,4)<10 dB, the mean SRT equals -4.6 dB, while the standard deviation is 1.1 dB. This means that an individual shows a significantly increased SRT at the 5% level when SRT = -2.8 dB and at the 1% level when SRT = -2.0 dB. These SRT values correspond to about HT(2,4) = 24 dB and HT(2,4) = 32 dB, respectively. The lower value of 24 dB corresponds in turn to about HT(1,2,3) = 15 dB; a hearing loss that we previously suggested as a fence on the basis of the pilot study [11,12].

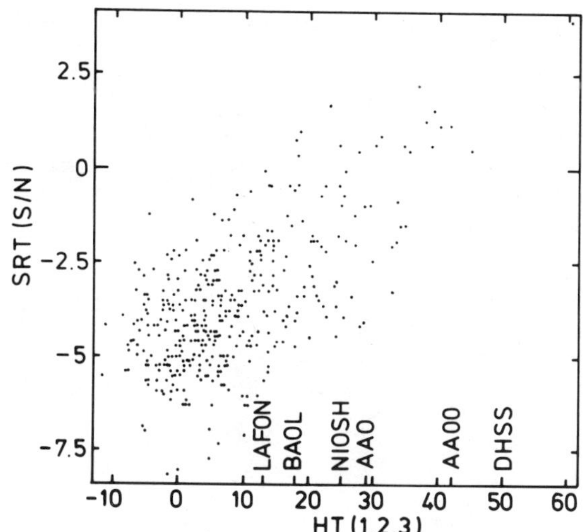

Fig. 4. Speech reception threshold for noisy situations (in dB signal-to-noise ratio) in relation to the hearing threshold averaged across 1, 2 and 3 kHz. Several fences are indicated along the abscissa. The correlation coefficient is 0.66. It is based on 400 data points.

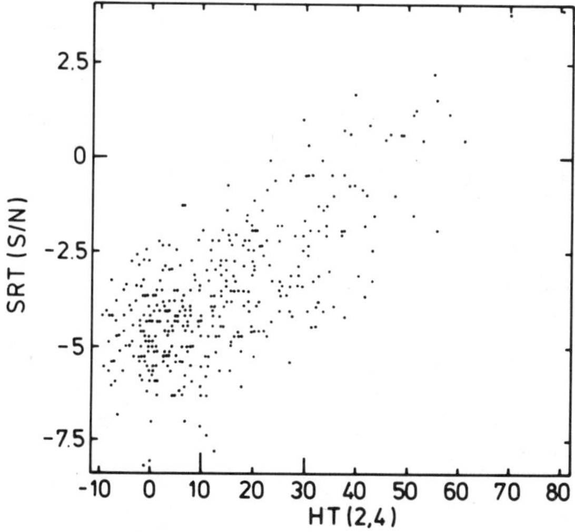

Fig. 5. Speech reception threshold for noisy situations (in dB signal-to-noise ratio) is relation to the hearing threshold averaged across 2 and 4 kHz. The correlation coefficient is 0.72. It is based on 400 data points.

The present study shows somewhat less impairment of speech perception given the tone-audiometric hearing loss than the pilot study. The higher value of HT(2,4) = 32 dB corresponds to about HT(1,2,3) = 22 dB. This higher value, associated with an increase of the SRT by 2.6 dB, implies an unacceptable hearing handicap. Plomp and Mimpen [14] found a median increase of the SRT by 2.5 dB for people about 65 years of age with presbyacusis only. The median handicap of these people will be familiar to the readers. In addition, an increase of the SRT by 2.6 dB means a critical distance (50% sentence intelligibility) of 74 cm between speaker and talker compared to 100 cm for normal-hearing people in the same situation. Thus, people with this increase of SRT have to bend forward noticeably when listening.

In conclusion, the results for speech perception in noisy situations show that a hearing loss, averaged across 2 and 4 kHz, of 30 dB or more is definitely not acceptable. From the point of view of preventive medicine, we should strive for noise exposures that do not induce hearing loss exceeding a 10 dB average across 2 and 4 kHz.

ACKNOWLEDGMENT

The author is much indebted to A. M. Mimpen for developing the sentence-intelligibility test and to W. G. van Golstein Brouwers for collecting and processing the data.

REFERENCES

1. AAOO, see Glorig and Baughn.
2. AAO, Guide for the evaluation of hearing handicap, JAMA 241:2055 (1979).
3. NIOSH, see Kryter [10].
4. DHSS, See Tempest [8].
5. BADL/BSA method for assessment of hearing disability, Brit. J. Audiol., 17:203 (1983).
6. OSHA, Occupational Noise Exposure; Hearing Conservation Amendment, Final Rule, Part II:9738 (1983).
7. J.-C. Lafon, Measurement of hearing level in occupational noise-induced hearing loss, Audiology, 20:79 (1981).
8. W. Tempest, The assessment of hearing handicap, J. Soc. Occup. Med., 27:134 (1977).
9. A. Glorig and W. L. Baughn, Basis for percent risk table, in: "Proceedings of the International Congress on noise as a Public Health Problem," Superintendent of Documents, U. S. Government Printing Office, Washington, DC (1973).
10. K. D. Kryter, A critique of some procedures for evaluating damage risk from exposure to noise, "Proceedings of the International Congress on Noise as a Public Health Problem," Superintendent of Documents, U. S. Government Printing Office, Washington, DC (1973).
11. G. F. Smoorenburg, J. A. P. M. de Laat and R. Plomp, The effect of noise-induced hearing loss on the intelligibility of speech in noise, "Proceeding of the AGARD Specialists' Meeting on Aural Communication in Aviation, AGARD CP-311," National Information Services (NTIS), Springfield, VA (1981).
12. G. F. Smoorenburg, J. A. P. M. de Laat and R. Plomp, The effect of noise-induced hearing loss on the intelligibility of speech in noise, Scand. Audiol. Suppl., 16:123 (1982).
13. G. F. Smoorenburg, J. L. van Raay and A. M. Mimpen, "The Audiomat: an Automatic Audiometer for use in Occupational Audiometry," Defense Research Information Centre, DRIC-T-7318, Station Square House, Orpington, Kent, UK (1984), translated from: G. F. Smoorenburg,

J. L. van Raay and A. M. Mimpen, De audiomaat; "Een Automatische Audiometer voor de Bedrijfs-Audiometrie, "Institute for Perception TNO, Report 1983-17.
14. R. Plomp and A. M. Mimpen, Improving the reliability of testing speech reception threshold for sentences, Audiology, 18:43 (1979).
15. R. Plomp and A. M. Mimpen, Speech-reception threshold for sentences as a function of age and noise level, J. Acoust. Soc. Amer., 66:1333 (1979).

DISCUSSION

Question: I appreciate the use of principle component analysis. However, one problem I have is that you broke down the hearing losses into three principle components and then ignore principle component 3, which was the low-frequency conductive hearing loss. What evidence is there that showed it was a conductive loss? Is it valid to throw away the low frequency component in hearing loss and then refer to the correlation between low frequency hearing losses and perception in quiet and noise?

Smoorenberg: In the multiple correlation analysis, the low-frequency loss was still there, and that analysis shows that there is quite a good correlation between the speech perception threshold in quiet and the low-frequency loss. There is no straightforward evidence that the low-frequency losses are of a conductive type. However, it correlates very highly with the attenuation component in the speech intelligibility data, which I think it's fair to say is due to a conductive loss.

Alberti: We went into the question of hearing aids with our compensation patients, of whom we have seen about 10,500. They are often told by their own audiologist that a hearing aid will not help them. Surprise, they do help, and over the past five or six years we have completely changed our view. We are trying to work out why these aids work; whether it is the newer hearing aid or whether it is the new methods of fitting with perhaps an open mold or high frequency emphasis. Also, a comment about your handicap scales. Initially we had 1/2, 1, 2 and 3 kHz in Canada in 1974, five years before the AAO. But the truth is, if you go back to the old AMA standards, they were much better than the original AAO, but I gather just too complicated to put into place.

Smoorenberg: With respect to the high frequency hearing loss and the effects of hearing aids, I would like to stress again sometimes we too find that patients profit from hearing aids. But, we should not have too high expectations.

Tyler: You have a large number of patients and you have focused on the strong correlation between quiet thresholds and speech intelligibility. However, one should keep in mind that there are other important factors. I would like to make that point in three ways: (1) from your own data, there is indeed quite a bit of scatter between an individual's hearing loss configuration and the performance on the speech and noise task. Of course, we all know that patients with similar audiograms may have differing performances on a speech recognition task, particularly in noise. (2) In correlating frequency resolution measurements with speech intelligibility, when the effects of thresholds are partialled out, the correlation between frequency resolution and speech intellibibility dropped considerbally. (3) In your particular task of speech recognition, it is more likely to be speech reception threshold in noise.

Forrest: The different "fences" corresponded to very different definitions of ability or disability; some far more lax than others. I wonder about the relation between either speech reception threshold or audiometric threshold or any other measurement and disability in terms of difficulty at work or at home. The question really is how can we define disability? Can we use a more realistic measure than speech reception threshold in noise? At what point in other words do people feel they are to some extent disabled?

Smoorenberg: I do not think I have an answer to that. I do not think that it is up to me as a scientist to set a level.

Forrest: My point is that ultimately we have to define handicap in terms of quality of life or what people can do. Speech perception thresholds in noise is a good way to find the answer. I think ultimately we have to look at various measures of quality of life. It is obviously a very difficult thing to do.

Alberti: A practical point on fences. It would be delightful to move the fence down. The effect of moving the fence of 1/2, 1, 2 and 3 kHz from 35 to 30 dB would have major economic implications. We now compensate in our province of 8 million people, approximately 1,500 new claimants a year, for noise-induced hearing loss with the 35 dB fence and we give them hearing aids with a 25 dB fence. We would have added about 52% to the cost of the annual cost of the pensions by moving the fence down 5 dB. I hope we will, but I am skeptical the government will accept it. Those are the practical aspects of the work we are doing here.

Smoorenberg: I think, in a way, you are illustrating my point. It is not up to the scientist to decide on the tradeoff between the amount of money in compensation and the hearing handicap.

THE PERCEPTION OF SYNTHETIC SPEECH IN NOISE

Charles W. Nixon, Timothy R. Anderson, and Thomas J. Moore

Harry G. Armstrong Aerospace Medical Research Laboratory
Wright-Patterson AFB, Ohio 45433, USA

INTRODUCTION

Although much information about synthetic speech has been acquired over past decades, we have been unable to find in the literature a systematic examination of the perception of synthetic speech in noise. Simpson [1] has reported that synthetic speech altitude callouts to airline pilots in widebody jet cockpit noise at a S/N of -10 dB for the first time were 99.7% intelligible and that synthetic speech voice warnings to helicopter pilots in simulated helicopter noise at a S/N ratio of -22 dB were 99.2% intelligible [2]. Nusbaum [3] has reported that perceptual confusions for synthetic CV and VC syllables were quite different than confusions observed for natural speech degraded by noise. Pisoni (personal communication) indicates that one of two synthetic speech systems with very high levels of segmental intelligibility in quiet, showed greater decrements in the intelligibility of CV syllables in noise than did the other system. Clark [4] reported little difference in the intelligibility of vowels in noise for synthetic and natural speech, whereas natural CV syllables were clearly superior to synthetic CV syllables under all noise conditions.

Research in our laboratory has examined the performance of various speech coding systems (analysis-synthesis) in a wide range of ambient noise conditions and found differing amounts of degradation of intelligibility among these systems due to the noise [5-7]. Most of these studies were accomplished for a specific communication or operational situation, and results cannot be readily generalized to synthetic speech. Beyond these studies, little information was found on the effects of noise on synthetic speech perception.

Digital representations of speech can be produced by a variety of coders, processors and systems. The most straightforward form is simply to digitize natural speech in the format in which it will be utilized. Other forms range from complex coding and processing schemes to the storing of various segments of speech in memory and the subsequent use of these segments to construct new, synthetic speech according to various rules. This study examined three commercially available text-to-speech synthesizers and three digital speech coders. The intelligibility of the synthetic and coded speech produced by these systems was evaluated relative to natural speech in the presence of a pink noise. The term synthetic speech is used in this paper to refer to the speech generated by synthesizer systems and coded speech refers to that produced by the coders-decoders.

DIGITAL SPEECH SYSTEMS

A brief description is provided below of the six digital speech systems of interest in this study.

Text-to-Speech

In general, synthetic speech systems operate using segments of speech which are stored in memory and used to construct synthetic speech according to the rules of the system. The three text-to-speech systems in this study were a low, a medium and a high quality system selected on the basis of ratings of their natural sounding quality and relative intelligibility in non-noisy environments. Synthetic speech has a mechanical or unnatural sounding quality.

Low Quality Speech Synthesizer. The low quality synthesizer utilizes procedures that convert ASCII text into phoneme strings which are then synthesized to generate synthetic speech. Pitch of the output can be varied, however, the system uses no phonological or prosody rules.

Medium Quality Speech Synthesizer. The medium quality system operates in a similar mode as the high quality system, however, the phonological and prosody rules are less sophisticated.

High Quality Speech Synthesizer. The high quality system utilizes a three level processing scheme. At the first level, ASCII text is converted into a pronunciation code using a unique combination of dictionary and letter-to-sound rules. The second level of processing deals with the effect of surrounding words on individual pronunciations. Rules of intonation, duration, and word stress are also applied. The third step generates the speech from the above assumptions.

Digital Coding Systems

Digital coding systems, also called analysis-synthesis systems, operate using a natural speech input signal which is segmented, coded, processed and later decoded to provide the coded speech output. Coded speech has a natural speech quality that appears to be transmitted over a noisy communication channel.

Continuously Variable Slope Delta Modulation (CVSD). CVSD is a coding technique that uses Delta Modulation, which has an inherently poor dynamic range. CVSD overcomes this limitation by companding or compressing the voice input and output. This process decreases the amplitude of the high signal levels and increases the amplitude of the low level signals. The compressed signal is then encoded by the conventional Delta Modulation without the constraint of the poor dynamic range.

Time Domain Harmonic Scaling/Sub Band Coding (TDHS/SBC). TDHS and SBC can be combined to produce a medium to high complexity voice encoder at a bit rate of 9600 bps. The TDHS algorithm compresses the input voice signal bandwidth and sampling rate by a factor of two. The compression is performed over a localized pitch period of the input signal. Pitch extraction is needed. The SBC is a waveform coding technique which segments the bandwidth of the input waveform into several frequency bands. Each band is then encoded and the output multiplexed to produce the SBC data stream. Decoding the data stream is just the reverse procedure.

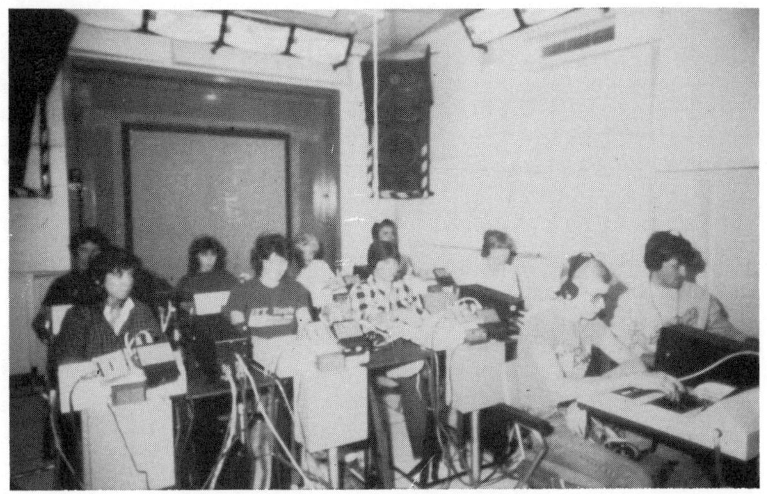

Fig. 1. Volunteer subjects seated at the ten listening stations in the audio communications laboratory facility

Linear Predictive Coding (LPC). LPC predicts a present speech sample from a linear combination of past speech samples. The prediction is based on three characteristics of speech, the excitation parameters (pitch period and voicing), reflection coefficients (which are the vocal tract filter parameters), and the speech RMS amplitude. The analyzer normalizes the amplitude and low-pass filters in the input speech. The excitation parameters are then found. Next, ten reflection coefficients are calculated. Then the speech RMS amplitude is found. This information is processed into a standard LPC data format. The LPC algorithm used in this study was the government standard LPC 10, which operates at 2.4 kbps.

APPROACH

Facility

These experiments were accomplished in an audio communications research laboratory. This facility duplicates the total audio communications link from talker to listener and includes the system, operator and environmental variables that may influence voice communications effectiveness. A master experimenter station controls ten individual communications stations inside a large reverberation chamber that houses a programmable high intensity sound system. Each station is integrated with a Computer Display-Response System in which the central processor is a Hewlett-Packard 9845T. Each station contains an LED display, which is used to present data and information to the listener, and various subject response buttons. In this study, each listening station was configured as a wide band frequency response intercommunication system (100-6000 Hz bandwidth) terminating in wideband frequency response headsets (Yamaha YH-1, 20 to 20,000 Hz bandwidth). Prerecorded speech signals were input to the audio communications test facility directly from tape recorders. Presentation of the speech materials to the subjects and their responses were automatically controlled by the Computer Display-Response System.

Subjects

Eighteen volunteer subjects participated in the experiment, with a mix of half male and half female. All were recruited from the general population and were paid an hourly rate for their participation with a cash bonus when all sessions of an experiment were completed. The hearing of all subjects was considered to be normal, with no hearing levels greater than 15 dB at any standard audiometric test frequency from 100 to 6000 Hz. Although the subjects were well trained and were experienced in listening to digital coded speech, additional training in listening to synthetic speech was given over several days.

Criterion Measure

The Modified Rhyme Test (MRT), a standardized measure of intelligibility, was used as the speech recognition task. The MRT was developed [8] from the Rhyme Test of Fairbanks [9] as an instrument for measuring audio communications effectiveness. Materials consist of lists of 50 one-syllable words that are essentially equivalent (lists) in intelligibility. The response format consists of a six foil, multiple-choice answer set for each of the 50 test words. The subject selects from the set of six words the stimulus word that was recognized. The MRT is automated on the audio communications research facility, so that the multiple-choice response foils are presented on LED displays at the individual listening stations where subjects respond by pushing appropriate buttons.

The criterion measure for this instrument is percent correct response. During data analyses, a correction factor was applied to compensate for correct answers obtained by guessing [#correct - #incorrect/(possible choices - 1)]. The MRT is easy to administer and score and it does not require extensive training of subjects.

Communication System Calibration

The basic communication test system consisted of the tape recorder, pink noise generator, wideband intercommunications systems and the high fidelity earphones. The ten listening stations have a common input and a gain control that equally affects all stations. In addition, each station is equipped with an individual gain control. A calibration signal at 75 dB(A) was presented through the communication test system to all headsets. One headset was then placed on the artificial ear and its gain control adjusted to provide an output at the earphones of 75 dB(A). The gain control of that headset was "set" and was not moved from that position for the duration of the study. This procedure was repeated for the headsets at the other nine listening stations providing an output of 75 dB(A) at all headsets for the 75 dB(A) input. The calibration procedure for each presentation was accomplished with the common gain control and with only one of the headsets positioned on the artificial ear.

Signal-to-Noise Ratio

The MRT word lists were utilized in this study without a common carrier phrase. Calibration signals were recorded at the beginning of all tape presentations to allow the programmed signal-to-noise ratios to be presented to the subjects. The calibration signals were used to adjust the speech materials to a presentation level of 75 dB(A). A precision attenuator at the output of the pink noise generator was then adjusted to provide S/N ratios of -8, -4, 0, +4, +8, and +12 dB at the earphones.

The average speech levels of the word lists were determined by taking the arithmetic average of the peak reading on the A-weighted scale of a sound level meter, slow meter response, for each of the fifty words in a list. To accomplish these measurements, the subject earphone was placed on a Bruel and Kjaer (B&K) artificial ear and the output fed into the sound level meter. The word list was played through the instrumentation and the 50 peak readings were averaged.

Natural Speech

The natural speech word lists were recorded inside a large anechoic chamber by a male talker with average mid-western American speech that exhibited no accent or regional dialect. A B&K 4145, one-inch, free field microphone that fed a TEAC four-channel, professional tape recorder was positioned twelve inches in front of the lips of the talkers. The talker maintained the desired level of his speech output by monitoring a VU meter. The average speech levels of the word lists were determined in the manner described in the section on Signal-to-Noise Ratios. A 1000 Hz calibration tone was recorded at the beginning of each list at an A-weighted sound level equivalent to the average speech level of the word list. The 1000 Hz tone was used to calibrate all presentations of natural, coded and synthetic speech to the listening panels.

Coded Speech

Natural speech word lists were presented to the three "coders" which digitized, stored, and synthesized the words, which were then recorded on high quality magnetic tape. The tapes of the coder processed natural speech were used for calibration of the speech signals and for presentation to the listening panels. The average speech levels of the recorded materials processed by the three coder-decoder speech systems were determined as described earlier. A 1000 Hz calibration tone equivalent in level to the average speech level of the list was recorded at the beginning of that tape.

Synthetic Speech

The synthetic speech tapes used in this study were provided by Dr. David Pisoni, Director, Speech Research Laboratory, Indiana University. The word lists were generated by three text-to-speech synthesizers rated as generating low, medium and high quality synthetic speech. The average speech levels for the synthetic word lists were derived in the same manner as for the natural and coder processed speech. A 1000 Hz tone equivalent to the average speech level was recorded for calibration at the beginning of the tape.

PROCEDURE

During the listening sessions, the experimenter adjusted the 1000 Hz calibration tone for each word list to a level of 75 dB(A). The average speech level remained at 75 dB(A) for all conditions. The experimenter then set the attenuator dial to correspond to the S/N ratio called for by the experimental design.

Subjects occupied the same listening station and wore the same headset for all test sessions. When subjects were ready and headsets were properly worn, the experimenter began the tape presentation. The subjects heard the first word and immediately the six word multiple-choice response foil corresponding to the test word appeared on the LED display. The subject depressed the response button that corresponded to the word that was recognized. This procedure was repeated for the 50 words in each list. Typically, six 50-word lists were accomplished in one listening session. Subjects were given fifteen minute breaks in a lounge area between test sessions.

The sequence of evaluating the seven different types of speech and the order of presentation of the six S/N ratios for each type of speech were random. Measurements were taken consecutively for one system until all S/N

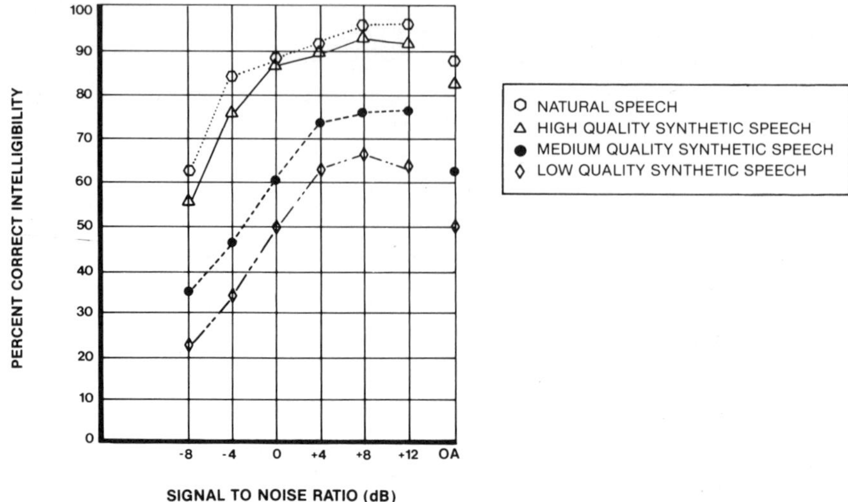

Fig. 2. MRT word intelligibility in noise of three text-to-speech synthesizers

conditions were completed, then evaluation of the next system was initiated.

Primary interest in this effort was the relative speech intelligibility in noise of the types of speech studied and to better understand why differences were observed. To further this understanding, spectrograms were produced of samples of the various speech types in quiet, again measured at the headset, to observe the distribution of energy in terms of the sounds of speech.

RESULTS

Speech Recognition

Word intelligibility scores for a particular condition were obtained as the average number of right answers, corrected for guessing, and converted to percent correct.

Test-To-Speech Systems. The average word intelligibility values in noise for the three text-to-speech systems are shown in comparison to natural speech in Fig. 2. Natural speech is clearly most intelligible for all measured conditions. The high quality synthetic speech intelligibility values are surprisingly close to those of natural speech. The high quality synthetic speech is slightly more susceptible to the masking noise at the two worse signal to noise ratios, but overall the performance is very good. Even though recognition values for these two types of speech are relatively close, the quality of the synthetic speech is clearly unnatural and subjectively might be expected to be less intelligible in the noise than was indicated by the measured values.

The relative performance of the three synthetic speech systems was similar to the qualitative ratings given to them. The intelligibility of the high quality system exceeded that of the medium quality system by as much as 20 to 30 percent and that of the low quality system by an additional 15 percent. The most significant reductions in performance due to

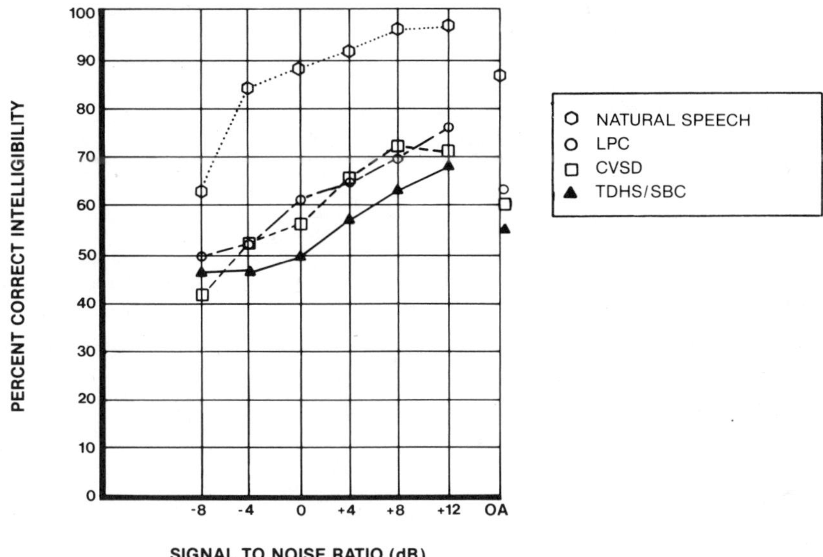

Fig. 3. MRT word intelligibility in noise of three digital speech coders

the noise occurred at 0 S/N ratio for the two lower quality systems, at -4 S/N for the high quality system and at -8 S/N for natural speech. The overall average of the intelligibility of all conditions for each type of speech is shown on the right portion of the figure.

Digital Speech Coders-Decoders. The intelligibility scores for the natural speech exceeded those for the three speech coders at all S/N conditions (Fig. 3). The differences were quite large and ranged from about 15 percent at the -8 S/N condition to about 30 percent at the -4 S/N condition. The relative intelligibility among the three systems is close with an envelope or range of approximately 10 percent. The TDHS/SBC speech was clearly the worst of this group even though the magnitude of the difference was only about 10 percent. The performance of the LPC and CVSD were very similar, however, on the basis of intelligibility in noise alone, the LPC might have a very slight edge. The LPC and TDHS/SBC appear to be slightly more resistant to the highest noise condition than the CVSD.

Synthesizers and Coders. The word intelligibility scores for natural speech and the coded and synthesized speech are compared in Fig. 4. As noted earlier, the high quality text-to-speech synthesizer exhibited word intelligibility that ranged from about equal to 10 percent less than the natural speech, depending on the S/N condition. Performance was significantly better than for the other synthesizers and the coders-decoders at all the noise conditions.

The word intelligibility of the coder-decoder systems was generally equivalent to that of the low quality synthesizer and less than the medium and high quality systems under the higher speech to noise ratios. However, the performance of all the synthesizers dropped off sharply in the low signal to noise conditions, whereas the coders showed some resistance to the noise and better performance than both of the lower quality synthesizer systems.

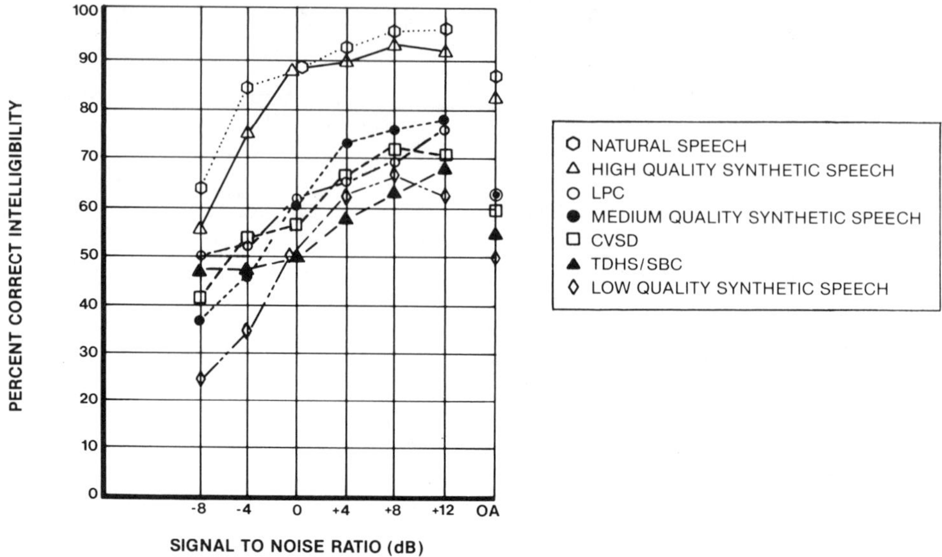

Fig. 4. MRT word intelligibility in noise of three text-to-speech synthesizers and three digital speech coders

Speech Spectrograms

The phrase "Welcome to the speech research laboratory" was produced by the natural talker and by the six digital representations of speech in the absence of masking noise. Speech spectrograms of these phrases were generated by a List Processing Language (LISP) on a Symbolics 3670 artificial intelligence computer. The spectrograms display a 2-second sample of the speech along the abscissa, a frequency response of 0 to 7225 Hz along the ordinate and relative level is represented by a "darkness scale" of the signature. The denser or darker the signature, the higher is the level of the speech signal, and the absence of any signature indicates the absence of acoustic energy in that region.

The quality and intelligibility of the natural speech sample were better than those of the digital speech samples examined in this study. Assuming that there is some relationship between these qualities and the spectrogram, natural speech was used as a basis for comparison with the others.

The spectrograms of the three synthetic speech phrases (Fig. 5) vary in richness, with the high quality system showing the greatest detail. There appears to be less energy at the highest frequencies in the low and medium quality spectrograms than in natural speech. The medium quality synthetic speech shows similarities to the high quality speech, however, the formant regions are less clearly defined, the transitions are not as smooth as for the high quality speech, and it appears to contain less acoustic information.

The spectrograms of the speech from the three coders appear much less like natural speech than do the synthetic speech displays (Fig. 6). The acoustic information is concentrated in the frequency region of 0 to 4000 Hz. There is clearly less vowel, consonant and transition information, except for LPC. LPC is most similar to the natural speech spectrogram in the lower frequency bands. CVSD contains poorly defined speech information and a reasonable amount of noise corresponding to the speech sounds across

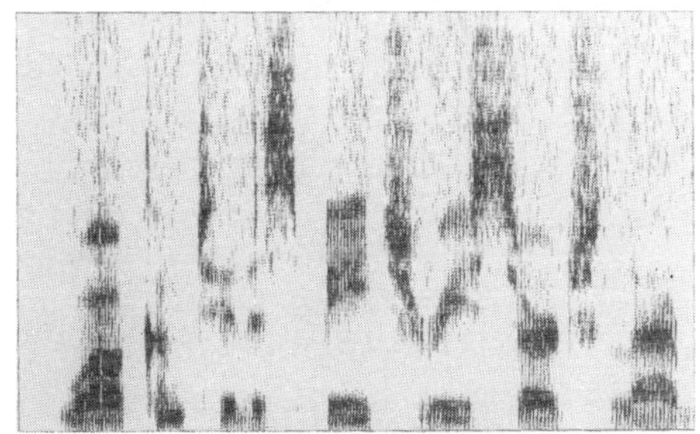

NATURAL SPEECH

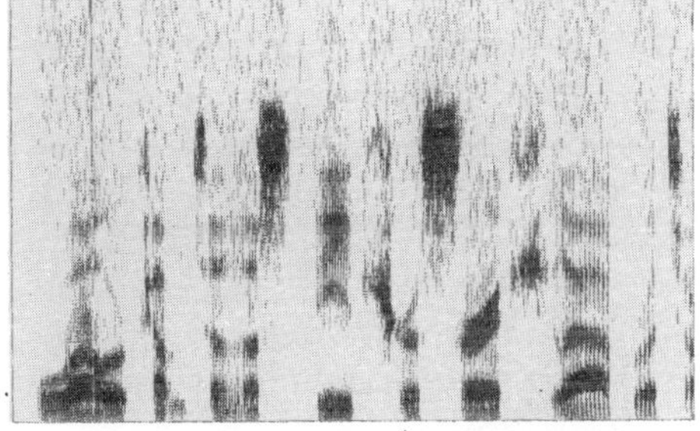

MEDIUM QUALITY SYNTHETIC SPEECH

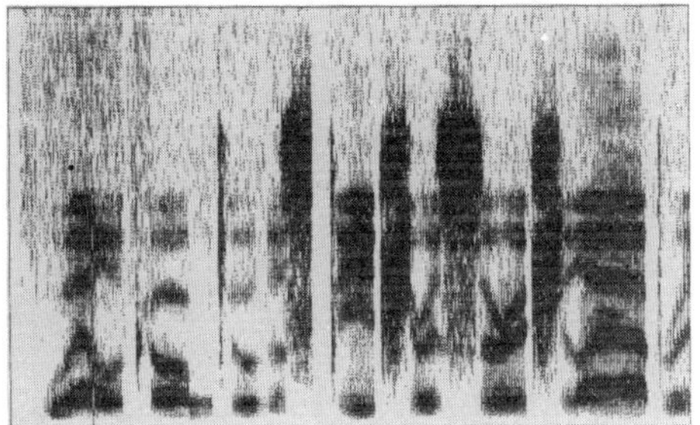

HIGH QUALITY SYNTHETIC SPEECH

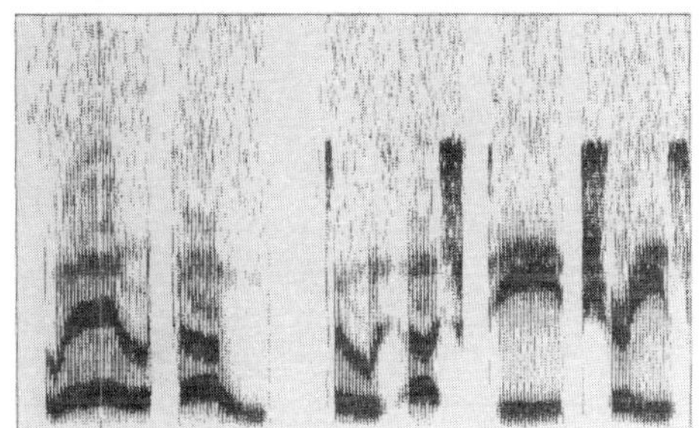

LOW QUALITY SYNTHETIC SPEECH

Fig. 5. Speech spectrograms

the full frequency range. TDHS/SBC appears to contain the least amount of information, with little definition of the speech sounds.

Samples of the seven types of speech were subjectively rated on the basis of their "general quality" or "what sounds best." LPC seemed to have features that were closest to natural speech, except at the higher frequencies, and it was chosen third following the high quality synthetic speech. The medium and low quality synthetic speech followed in that order with CVSD, followed by TDHS/SBC. Some relationship is seen among the patterns of the spectrograms and the subjective rating of the speech samples.

The LPC spectrogram through about 5000 Hz is most similar to that of natural speech. The others appear to follow an order that very generally relates to the subjective ratings. The highest quality synthetic spectrogram contains the most detailed speech information, and the progression of lesser information proceeds through the other synthetic speech to the two coders.

DISCUSSION AND CONCLUSIONS

This study demonstrated a differential effect of noise on selected digital representations of speech. The performance of the natural speech in noise was better than that of all six samples of the digital speech. The perception of the high quality speech should appear to be very similar to that of natural speech and superior to all others evaluated in this study.

The measured intelligibility of the synthetic speech corresponded to the subjective ratings with the high quality system providing the highest intelligibility and the others following in rank order. Also, the poorer quality synthetic speech showed adverse effects of the noise at lower S/N ratios than did the high quality speech. This may suggest that the per-

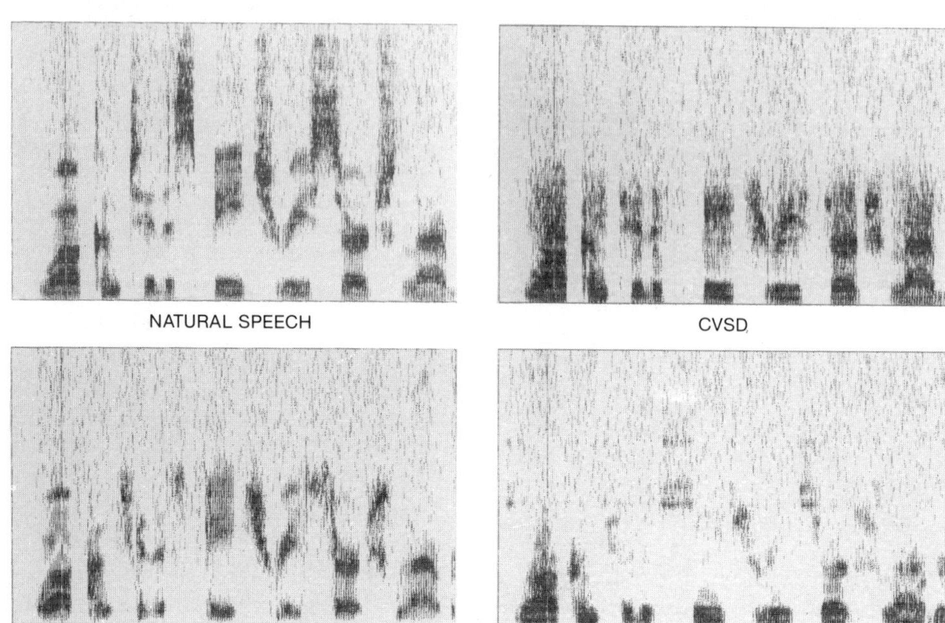

Fig. 6. Speech spectrograms

ceived quality of a synthetic speech is a good indicator of its intelligibility in relative quiet. The data are considered inadequate to extend this observation to noisy environments.

The word intelligibility of the digitally coded speech in noise was very similar among the three systems. On the basis of our experience with the speech produced by these systems, LPC was expected to be the best performer of the three. The differences between the performance of LPC and the other two coders was rather small. Also, the performance of CVSD and TDHS/SBC was expected to be equal to or lower than the two lower quality synthetic speech samples. The performance of the coders was expected to be better than the two lower quality synthetic speech samples. Intuitively, the coders or analysis-synthesis systems process a natural speech input, whereas synthesizers utilize segments of speech assembled according to various rules. Also, the coded speech sounds like natural speech, with some distortion, on a noisy communication channel instead of the unnatural quality of synthetic speech. The higher performance expected with natural speech input and natural sounding output was not reflected in the results.

The spectrogram data did demonstrate some very general correspondence between the rated "general quality" of the speech and word intelligibility. The synthetic speech spectrograms contained well defined speech energy regions that rather clearly reflected the various speech sounds and transitions. The substantially greater detail displayed for the high quality speech over natural speech indicates that much of that information is not being used in the determination of word intelligibility. A final observation is that even the poor systems were relatively intelligible in quiet, in spite of spectrograms which displayed very little speech information.

All of the synthetic speech sounded unnatural. The feature of naturalness of synthetic speech is considered to be highly important for most applications, however, it does not appear to be visible in the standard speech spectrogram. Whenever this characteristic is sufficiently understood to be readily identified in such analyses of speech as the spectrogram, synthetic speech will be developed that cannot be readily discriminated from that produced by the natural voice.

A systematic research program focusing on the perception of synthetic speech in noise must encompass a rather broad scope. It must include not only the science and technology of digital representations of speech, projected applications, and operating environments, but it also must concentrate on the operator well beyond the recognition level. Work in this area must include the full range of cognitive functions represented by comprehension, storage, retrieval and operator actions. Recent results from Pisoni's laboratory have demonstrated that the perception of synthetic speech generated by text-to-speech systems requires more effort and time to process than natural speech, even in quiet. These differences were found when the task involved lexical decisions, naming, and sentence verification [10,11]. It has also been reported that text-to-speech generated stimuli place greater capacity demands on short term memory than natural speech [12]. Much remains to be accomplished in the perception of digital speech in quiet and in noise.

This effort confirms that the perception of digital speech, including synthesis and analysis-synthesis, is a rather complex process and that perception in noise, even at the recognition level, is not well understood nor easily explained at this time.

REFERENCES

1. C. Simpson, "Synthesized Voice Control Callouts for Air Transport Operations," NASA CR-3300, NASA Ames Research Center (1980).
2. C. Simpson and Marchionda, "Synthesized Speech Rate and Pitch Effects on Intelligibility of Warning Messages for Pilots," Proc. of the Second Symp. on Aviation Psychology, Department of Aviation, Ohio State University, Columbus, Ohio, USA (1983).
3. H. C. Nusbaum, M. J. Dedina, and D. B. Pisoni, "Perceptual Confusions of Consonants in Natural and Synthetic CV Syllables," Speech Research Laboratory Technical Note 84-02, Bloomington, Indiana, USA (1984).
4. J. E. Clark, Intelligibility Comparisons for two synthetic and one natural speech source, _J. Phonetics_ 11:37 (1983).
5. R. L. McKinley, T. R. Anderson, and T. J. Moore, "Evaluation of Speech Synthesis for Use in Military Noise Environments," Proceedings of National Bureau of Standards Workshop on Standardization of I/O Technology, Gaithersburg, Maryland, USA (1982).
6. J. Freedman and W. A. Rumbaugh, "Accuracy and Speed of Response to Different Voice Types in A Cockpit Voice Warning System," Air Force Institute of Technology Report LSSR 89-83, WPAFB, Ohio, USA.
7. R. L. McKinley and T. J. Moore, "The Effect of Audio Bandwidth on Selected Digital Speech Coding Algorithms," MILCOM '85 Conference Record, IEEE, 345 East 47th Street, New York, New York, USA (1985).
8. A. S. House, C. E. Williams, M. L. H. Hecker, K. D. and Kryter, Articulation testing methods: consonantal differentiation with a closed-response set, _J. Acoust. Soc. Am._ 37:158 (1965).
9. G. Fairbanks, Test of phonemic differentiation: the Rhyme test, _J. Acoust. Soc. Am._ 30:596 (1958).
10. D. B. Pisoni, Speeded classification of natural and synthetic speech in a lexical decision task, _J. Acoust. Soc. Am._ 70:598 (1981).
11. L. M. Manous, M. J. Dedina, H. C. Nusbaum, and D. B. Pisoni, "Speeded Sentence Verification of Natural and Synthetic Speech," Research on Speech Perception, Progress Report No. 11. Indiana University, Bloomington, Indiana, USA (1985).

12. P. A. Luce, T. C. Feustel, and D. B. Pisoni, Capacity demands in short-term memory for synthetic and natural word lists, Human Factors, 25:17 (1983).

DISCUSSION

Smoorenberg: The word reception thresholds are rather low (50% score) for a 9 dB S/N ratio. What is the spectrum of the noise and how do you measure the level of the speech words?

Nixon: The spectrum of noise was white noise. The speech signal was calibrated according to the ISO draft and the new ANSI draft which recommends A-weighting and a slow meter average the peak or the a weighting on a slow meter (the recommended 150 and ANSI).

Manninen: We have found that speech production itself deteriorates in noise, especially spectral characters of the speech. It implies that there is a type of vicious cycle i.e., not only is it harder to perceive speech in noise, but the actual signal generator is degraded in the noise, thereby further compounding the difficulty.

Nixon: The algorithm designers recognize that the acoustic phonetic features are very important, and when we speak in noise there are subtle changes in speech that are different from speech in quiet. If we are dealing with an automatic speech recognition system that we want to employ in noise environment, then we can not train it in quiet because the subtle features of the speech signal will be different and its recognition accuracy not as good.

Tyler: I am surprised with the observation that putting the words in a carrier pharse resulted in poorer performance. I believe there is some evidence from normal hearing listeners with distorted speech that typically improves performance. It seems like as long as they knew where the word was going to be, i.e., say the word _______.

Nixon: Our presentation was: "You will mark the word same please, you will mark the word gun please," etc. Yes, we found that using this system there is no significant differences in the perception of isolated words versus words in a carrier phrase. Once the subjects are trained using the MRT. So yes, we were also quite surprised.

CONCEPT - REFERENCE COHERENCE IN SPEECH PERCEPTION: CONSEQUENCES FOR NATIVE AND SECOND LANGUAGE SPEECH COMPREHENSION IN NOISE

H. M. Borchgrevink

Joint Medical Service of the Norwegian Armed Forces
FSAN, Oslo mil/Huseby, Oslo 1

SUMMARY

Simple Norwegian [10] and English [10] every-day sentences were read by a bilingual adult, tape recorded and presented individually to adults with English (n=13) or Norwegian (n=13) as their first language and with good (university level) command of the other language. Sentences were presented at 65 dB SPL with a background noise of sufficient intensity to mask the sentence. The level of the noise was progressively reduced in 2 dB steps until the subject could adequately repeat the sentence. Normal hearing was assured by pure tone threshold audiometry prior to testing.

The results demonstrated that for both groups the native language sentences were correctly repeated after fewer presentations, i.e., (approximately 3 dB) <u>lower</u> signal-to-noise ratio than the second language sentences ($p<0.001$), <u>even</u> under these "close to optimal" conditions.

The results show that second language message comprehension may be impaired under backgraound noise conditions that are sufficient for adequate comprehension of native language speech. The phenomenon may thus have negative influence upon acquisition of information presented in a foreign language, e.g., influence safety/control operations that are verbally based.

INTRODUCTION

The problem of studying differences between native and second language comprehension is that the second language comprehension threshold inevitably will also mirror second language proficiency and command in the listener. Simple comparisons of native and second language speech comprehension in noise, for some groups of subjects on a (random) sample of sentences may give arbitrary comprehension threshold difference - and thus be of limited general interest.

However, if a significant difference between native and second language speech comprehension thresholds could be demonstrated under conditions where the relevant variables for speech comprehension were controlled, one would be left with the eventual "net effect" of concept - reference coherence upon comprehension of (native and second language) speech -- to which, in practice, the other elements of influence would be added in a given listening situation.

If an effect could be demonstrated under "optimal" conditions, second language speech comprehension would be expected to be significantly impaired in a number of situations in daily life.

ON CEREBRAL STRATEGIES FOR SPEECH PERCEPTION

Language is a means of communication by way of symbolic representation of concepts and thoughts. In speech, a number of characteristic sound patterns (phonemes) are combined to create entities (words, morphemes) that refer to specific concepts. The words are correspondingly combined to communicate information that cannot be accurately expressed by a single word.

The speaker communicates his message by transforming his thoughts into speech according to the rules of the language. The goal of the listener is to derive the communicated message using primarily the acoustic pattern analysis of the sounds uttered by the speaker. Successful communication requires that the words and modes of expression used by the speaker evoke the appropriate associations and refer to familiar concepts in the listener.

One puzzling phenomenon of speech perception is how a person can derive the correct messages from continuous speech - and even follow logical reasoning - without needing intermediate pauses for analysis and adaption of the acoustical input. To accomplish this, the listener must obviously perform some sort of rapid, progressive analysis of the utterance while it is pronounced by the speaker. An explanation is offered by the "analysis by synthesis" model of speech perception [1], where the listener is believed to "guess" (synthesize) the most probable content of the entire utterace - based on the analyzed information available at each moment, consulting "lexicon stores," grammatical rules, and knowledge acquired through previous experience.

The "analysis by synthesis" model implies that the strategy of speech perception will involve comparison: the information progressively presented by the speaker is continuously compared with the listener's expected (guessed, synthesized) completion of the utterance. As the speaker proceeds, the number of probable completions is progressively reduced. Consequently, the listener most often knows (by guessing) the content of the utterance by or before the actual ending, thus being prepared for what follows without delay. Several models of speech perception introduce corresponding concepts of "active listening," "analysis by synthesis," etc.

A consequence of such a model is that speech perception will be a function of the listener's ability to produce rapid and relevant alternatives of sentence completions. Such sentence synthesis must be regarded as a creative, cognitive process involving logical reasoning. Rommetveit [2] found that logical reasoning and cognitive operations in children are improved if one uses referential units that are represented as "discrete, meaningful and familiar" entities in the individual.

The comprehension level needed for operative semantic competence is therefore far beyond the level required in conventional assessment of word comprehension [2].

In children, the acquisition and command of language develops along with, and in close connection with cognitive development. Because of this, one would expect a tighter link between words (references) and concepts in a person's first (naive) language than in a second language, where a new reference code is introduced for access to the already established semantic memory and association network. It is a common observation that true native command of a language appears to be acquired only through practical language performance in childhood - most probably before a certain critical age) somewhat before puberty, after which age the person will characteristically fail to acquire native language command of a second language and most often will be unable to drop the accent and phoneme boundaries/ categorical perception of his first language. This seems to be true even for professional interpreters (author's observation).

If the degree of established coherence between reference and concept influences logical reasoning ability, as indicated by Rommetveit [2] - and speech perception is a function of the listener's ability to synthesize relevant alternatives of message completion during the utterance - second language speech comprehension would be expected to be poorer than native language comprehension of corresponding complexity, even if all words involved appear to be well comprehended.

Normal speech contains superfluous information, far more than essentially needed for communicating the message. This would be expected to compensate for eventual poor second language concept-reference coherence in many situations. However, if the "informational overflow" (redundancy) is reduced below a certain level, the communicated message will not be adequately comprehenced by the listener. This may occur in case of poor signal-to noise ratio registered when a spoken utterance is just comprehended. Regardless of which cues that carry essential semantic information, individuals familiar with the reference code would be expected to be able to perceive the content at a lower signal-to-noise ratio - that means to synthesize the message from fewer informational cues - than individuals with less established concept-reference coherence.

Syntax and semantics both influence sentence intelligibility [3]. Intonational block boundaries have a strong tendency to coincide with, and thus signal, syntactic block boundaries [4]. Using stimuli that are short, regular statements of the type noun + verb + complement/adjunct, syntax and intonation as well as prosody will provide the listener with few clues to sentence comprehension. If one presents tape-recorded, isolated sentences to the same listener in his first and second language, the influence of cognitive capacity, experience, tempo, concept familiarity and non-verbal communication elements would be controlled ("the same man with the same brain") - leaving concept-reference coherence in the native and second language as the variable. In such a paradigm, the syntax of all sentences as well as the contents/semantics must be unknown to the subject, whereas all the words and concepts must be known. Further, a corresponding degree of concept/word familiarity in the two (necessarily) different sets of sentences (one set in each of the two languages) is needed. This can be compensatorily controlled by presenting the same two sets of sentences to two groups of listeners, each being native speakers of one of the two languages involved, and having good command of the other (second) language. If both groups of listeners then comprehend all sentences, while comprehending the sentences presented in their first language at a lower signal-to-noise ratio than the sentences presented in their second language, sentence intelligibility would be demonstrated to be a function of concept-reference coherence, supporting the idea of speech perception as an active, "top-down" process involving more than plain decoding of acoustic information.

If an effect could be demonstrated under "optimal" conditions (with all the sentences read by a true bilingual person with perfect accent/ pronounciation in both languages, using well-educated, normal hearing subjects with good command of their second language as listeners), second language message comprehension would be expected to be significantly impaired in a number of situations in daily life, especially in background noise, even under conditions proved sufficient for native listeners.

METHOD

The comprehension threshold for sentences presented in the first (native) language and the second language were compared for 13 Norwegian adults (males and females) with university degrees and "professor level command" of English, and for 13 English adults (males and females) with university degrees and/or corresponding command of Norwegian. The subjects were recruited from the University of Oslo, The British Council, Oslo and the British Embassy, Oslo (Norway). Normal hearing was confirmed by pure tone threshold audiometry prior to testing.

The stimuli were 10 Norwegian sentences and 10 English sentences, all semanticaly different, but with corresponding syntax. They were short, everday utterances of about four lexical words each, typically noun + verb + complement/adjunct. The sentences were devoid of specific cultural idioms. The phoneme frequencies (occurrence) in each sentence set corresponded to that of the respective language.* The initial word in each sentence gave no clue to the completion. No thematic relationship existed between any of the sentences, which were all unknown to the subjects. The words included were familiar to everybody in both languages.

The sentences were read by a bilingual male adult (with one Norwegian and one English parent, having moved regularly between the two countries since birth) as if occurring in daily conversation. His reading was supervised by university professors with native command of each language. The sentences were then tape-recorded on a full-track Nagra Kudelski tape recorder (Bruel & Kjaer condensor microphone), from which they were copied onto one track of a two-tract Nagra Kudelski tape recorder (on-line), each sentence repeated 10 times with 6 secs intermediate intervals. USASI-noise was recorded on the other tract, starting about 1/2 sec before each sentence repetition and ending about 1/2 sec after the last word of the sentence. The sentence was thus "hidden" in the noise.

During testing, the subject was sitting alone in an easy-chair in a sound-attenuated room facing a loudspeaker which was mounted with the center 140 cm in front of his face (free field conditions, Tandberg TL 5010 loudspeaker, modified by the factory for optimal linearity). The investigator, placed in the adjoining room, could check the subject's position through the window. The two could communicate with each other through a separate intercommunication system. The subject was given a short, standardized, written instruction. When his understanding of the task was verbally confirmed, both tracks of the tape recorder were connected to the loudspeaker (via a Quad amplifier).

Each sentence was first presented with a background noise completely masking it and then repeated with the (USASI) noise level progressively

---

* For the English sentences, one followed the phoneme frequencies given in A. C. Gimson, An Introduction to the Pronounciation of English, 2 ed. London 1970, pp. 148, 219. As no phoneme frequency count has been published for Norwegian, a fairly extensive count was carried out, using newspaper articles (informal interviews) in the type of Norwegian used in the set of sentences.

reduced in 2 dB steps from presentation to presentation. (USASI noise may be described as "synthetic cocktail-party/conversation noise.")

The sentences (signal) were always pressented at 65 dB SPL (sound pressure level, dB rel. to 2 x 10(-5)N/m2 measured free field in the test chamber just in front of the ear of a subject seated as described above). The noise level was 76 dB SPL at the first presentation of each sentence, being lowered in 2 dB steps to 56 dB SPL at the last presentation of each sentence.

The task of the subject was to repeat the utterance verbally in the 5 sec. pause following each presentation. The investigator listened, marking in a scheme how many presentations the subject needed to repeat each sentence correctly, also indicating the kind of error if the subject was close to the solution. The sentences in each of the two languages were presented in fixed order and at the same sound pressure level for all subjects. Half of the subjects in each native language group started with the English sentences, the other half started with the Norwegian sentences. They were informed whether the following sentence would be in English or in Norwegian.

RESULTS

The results demonstrated that for both subject groups, the first (native) language sentences were correctly repeated after fewer presentations - that means at a <u>lower</u> (approximately 3 dB) signal-to-noise ratio than the second language sentences. The difference between the naive and second language repetition thresholds were statistically significant for both subject groups ($p<0.001$) when applying t-test on the mean number of presentations needed for correct repetition of sentences (Table 1a). The same was true when using a criterion that tolerated error in one lexical word <u>or</u> in two grammatical words (Table 2a). Mean sentence repetition thresholds in terms of signal-to-noise ratio are given in Tables 1b and 2b.

DISCUSSION

As all the subjects had normal hearing and the same sentences were presented by tape recorder at the same sound pressure level and at the same signal-to-noise ratio, any recorded difference in sentence repetition faculty must reflect the influence of non-acoustical parameters.

Sentence intelligibility has been shown to decrease with decreasing contextual influence [5]. For instance, ungrammatical phrases with no meaning are more difficult to "shadow" than meaningful sentences [3]. Repetition of nonsense sound pattern will accordingly require better signal-to-noise ratio than is needed for repetition of meaningful sentences.

If one increases the signal-to-noise ratio of an unknown sentence, starting at an unintelligible level as in this experiment, the sentence comprehension threshold will accordingly be reached <u>before</u> the nonsense sound repetition threshold. Consequently, sentence repetition reflects sentence comprehension in the present paradigm.

The influence of cognitive capacity, experience, tempo, concept familiarity and communicational context were controlled by presenting the same two sets of tape-recorded Norwegian and English sentences to the same two groups of listeners. The influence of grammatical knowledge was controlled by the use of short regular phrases. The sentences were devoid of cultural

TABLE 1. CORRECT REPETITION OF SENTENCES

	Norwegian subjects(n=13)		English subjects(n=13)		T-test	
a) number of presentations	mean	SD	mean	SD	value	prob.
10 Norwegian sentences	6.55	0.64	8.55	1.33	4.88	p<0.001
10 English sentences	7.54	0.83	6.31	0.68	4.13	p<0.001
b) signal-to-noise ratio needed (dB)						
10 Norwegian sentences	0.10	1.26	3.90	2.66	4.88	p<0.001
10 English sentences	2.10	1.66	0.40	1.36	4.13	p<0.001

TABLE 2. SENTENCE REPETITION WITH ERROR IN ONE LEXICAL WORD OR IN TWO GRAMMATICAL WORDS

	Norwegian subjects(n=13)		English subjects (n=13)		T-test	
a) number presentations needed	mean	SD	mean	SD	value	prob.
10 Norwegian sentences	5.22	0.61	6.98	1.26	4.53	p<0.001
10 English sentences	6.60	0.77	5.02	0.63	5.73	p<0.001
b) signal-to-noise ratio needed (dB)						
10 Norwegian sentences	-2.60	1.22	1.00	2.52	4.53	p<0.001
10 English sentences	0.20	1.54	-3.00	1.26	5.73	p<0.001

idioms, and the beginning of each sentence gave no clue to the conclusion. All sentences were comprehended by all of the subjects.

The recorded differences between native and second language comprehension thresholds must therefore be ascribed to different degrees of concept - reference establishment/coherence in each listener's native and second language, following the reasoning presented in the introduction.

COMMENTS AND IMPLICATIONS

The results show that individuals need fewer acoustical cues to comprehend sentences presented in their native language than corresponding sentences presented in their second language, even for simple everyday sentences presented under "optimal" conditions to people with good command of their second language. Put another way - the subject's ability to "fill in," guess or synthesize what is hidden in the background noise and arrive at a probable, meaningful message, is better for messages presented in his native language, which is acquired along with concept learning and cognitive development in early childhood.

Interestingly, English and Norwegian speech comprehension thresholds were the same for one subject born in South Africa by Norwegian parents, speaking only English until moving to Norway at the age of ten years, after which they spoke only Norwegian. However, he spoke Norwegian with a heavy accent - indicating different critical periods for the establishment of native competence for different speech/language features.

The results provide experimental support for the relevance of an "analysis by synthesis" element in models of speech perception, demonstrating that adequate speech perception relies upon "active listening" and "top-down" processes which involves creative cognitive functions resembling logical reasoning.

In terms of models of semantic memory organization [6,7], the capacity for relevant sentence synthesis in speech perception would be a function of the size and quality (richness) of the association networks activated by the language (reference code) in question.

Adequate "filling in" for what is hidden in the noise should accordingly improve with increasing number of relevant associations, in good agreement with the present results: speech perception improving with increasing concept - reference coherence/establishment.

If so, concept-reference coherence would also be expected to lead to impaired acquisition of <u>written</u> information, even when all the words presented are known by the reader. Besides, the less efficient access to the concept/association level via the second language would most likely imply slower, less direct signal processing, leading to impaired comprehension of both written and spoken second language beyond a certain (threshold of) <u>tempo</u> (a phenomenon familiar at least to the author!).

Any percept must be regarded as the brain's interpretation of a given sensory input - judged against a background of environment and experience. For the brain, the percept can therefore not be false or correct, only the best (most probable?) interpretation when taking into account the actual circumstances of influence.

A marginal signal-to-noise ratio will leave the listener with few clues to the presented verbal message, increasing the chances of the brain making a wrong "guess" and reducing the chances for the brain to realize that the guess was wrong. Consequently, the brain may stick to the wrong guess - which will <u>appear</u> to be the correct message for the listener, who will behave according to the (wrong) message.

Wrong guesses would be expected to be influenced by the subject's native phoneme system, leading to association networks activated by the most probable <u>native</u> language concept activated by the speech signal. Indications of this were illustrated by the type of error (wrong guesses) registered in some of the subjects in this study.

Such misinterpretation may easily lead to disaster in verbally based safety routines (e.g., in aviation/air traffic control). English is the language generally used in aviation throughout the world. A considerable number of flights, therefore, involve aircrew or air traffic controllers for whom English is a foreign language. The communication is mediated by intercommunication systems with amazingly poor characteristics as regards signal-to-noise ratio and distortion. As one needs a better signal-to-noise ratio to comprehend messages presented in a foreign language, aircrew and air traffic controllers that are non-native speakers of English may accordingly represent a hazard to aviation safety due to increased chances of misinterpretation of lack of comprehension of essential messages.

The English language used in aviation is strongly influenced by (technical) jargon, which should be familiar to all individuals trained for key positions in aviation or air traffic control regardless of native language. This might be regarded to counteract or more or less eliminate an eventual negative effect of second language upon speech comprehension in routine aviation.

However, for reasons of aviation safety, aircrew and air traffic controllers must be capable of understanding unexpected messages which are most likely to occur in critical situations. Under poor listening conditions the advantages of jargon may easily lead to increased problems. Such jargon typically contains only essential information (little or no redundancy) given as standard orders of largely the same sentence length and with standard prosody/intonation pattern. As signals, they will accordingly be grossly identical. The brain, which is biased towards perception of one of the routine commands, will need an extra distinct message and favorable listening conditions to get rid of this bias - if not, the person is likely to be "stuck with his original guess/interpretation [8]. (Examples of this phenomenon were seen in this study, but not frequently, as demonstrated by the low standard deviations obtained - see Tables 1 and 2.) Conditions designed and proved to be just sufficient for native language comprehension may thus leave the foreigner with too few clues for adequate decoding of the message. Corresponding arguments will be valid for a number of conditions involving second language comprehension (in noise/distortion).

The influence of concept - reference coherence upon speech comprehension is a good example of the influence of non-acoustical parameters, and the consequent relevance of a "top-down" approach to the study of speech perception. Another example is the loss of pitch control in singing while preserving pitch control (prosody) in speech, observed during (temporary) selective right hemisphere anaesthesia [9]. In a "bottom-up" approach, studying the subject's ability to analyze some isolated fragment of speech, one may easily activate other analyzing systems in the brain than those relevant for the complex sound analysis in question - so that the results of the study may be irrelevant for the processes one intended to study a part of [10].

The present experiment demonstrated impaired second language speech comprehension even under conditions that may be regarded as close to optimal. Second language speech comprehension would be expected to be even poorer in a number of situations (e.g.,

- poor second language competence in the listener
- poor second language competence in the speaker with foreign accent and consequent errors in phoneme/word pronounciation and prosodic features
- unfamiliar context/theme/comcepts/cultural idioms
- sentences where the last part could be guessed with high probability from the first part
- high speech tempo
- distorted speech (e.g., radio/intercom./reverberation conditions
- noise-induced hearing loss in the listener
- poor auditory discrimination/identification and cognitive faculty in the listener
- second language phoneme boundaries less close to those of the listener's native language than in the case of English/Norwegian),

from what is known of the effects of these parameters upon speech perception in general. However, second language speech comprehension would be expected to be improved if the non-native speaker had the same first language (phoneme pronounciation and prosodic features) as the listener - e.g., in case of English spoken with French accent to French listeners [11].

If one wants to test whether a person's speech comprehension faculty is sufficient for service under certain conditions, the most adequate functional evaluation would accordingly be to examine his comprehension of unexpected messages under (field or simulated) conditions relevant for the situation in question [12].

Used as a test, the present paradigm can serve to compare native and second language comprehension faculty in a subject, for instance to decide which should be considered his first/native language. Besides, the paradigm can be used as a test for speech intelligibility threshold in noise in either language - and to decide the degree of speech comprehension handicap in a given subject, as well as decide whether he has sufficient (second) language comprehension ability for a given operative service - for instance whether he should be allowed continued service with an acquired hearing loss.

CONCLUSION

This study demonstrates that speech perception must be considered an active, "top-down" process that draws heavily upon cognitive strategies and concept-reference coherence; the degree of establishment between the concept level and the reference level in the code (language) used.

Normal speech contains superfluous information, far more than essentially needed for communicating the message. Under poor listening conditions, one needs more acoustical information (better signal-to-noise ratio) to comprehend second language messages than corresponding native language messages, even for comprehension of simple sentences where all words included are well understood.

The phenomenon may lead to impaired acquisition of material presented in a (even well-commanded) foreign language, and may influence safety/control operations that are verbally based, especially when unexpected or complex conditions that are (just) sufficient for native listeners (e.g., air traffic control).

Adequate prophylaxis would include improved listening conditions (reduced background noise and distortion), as well as introduction of specific tests for (second language) speech comprehension under relevant operative conditions. The present paradigm may serve as a model for such tests.

REFERENCES

1. K. N. Stevens and A. S. House, Speech perception _in_: "Foundations of Modern Auditory Theory," J. V. Tobias ed., vol. 2 London/New York (1972).
2. R. Rommetveit, On Piagetian cognitive operations, semantic competence and message structure in adult-child communication, _in_: "The Social Context of Language," I. Markova ed., London (1977).
3. G. A. Miller and S. Isard Some perceptual consequences of linguistic rules _J. Verbal Learn. Verbal Behav._, 2:217 (1963).

4. R. Collier and J. T. Hart The role of intonation in speech perception, in: "Structure and Process in Speech Perception", A. Cohen and S. G. Nooteboom eds., Berlin/Heidelberg/New York (1972).
5. A. N. Stowe, W. P. Harris and D. B. Hampton, Signal and context components of work recognition behavior, J. Acoust. Soc. Am. 35:639 (1963).
6. A. M. Collins and M. R. Quillian, How to make a language user, in: "Organization of Memory", E. Tulving and W. Donaldson eds., New York (1972)
7. E. Tulving, Episodic and semantic memory in ibid. [6]
8. H. M. Borchgrevink, Second language speech comprehension in noise - a hazard to aviation safety, in: "Aural Communication in Aviation" Conf. Proceed. 311, AGARD (1981).
9. H. M. Borchgrevink, Prosody and musical rhythm are controlled by the speech hemisphere, in: "Music, Mind and Brain, The Neuropsychology of Music," M. Clynes ed., New York (1982).
10. H. M. Borchgrevink, Mechanisms of speech and musical sound perception, in: "The Representation of Speech in the Peripheral Auditory System", R. Carlson and B. Granstrom eds., N. Holland (1982).
11. K. Buck (personal communication)
12. H. M. Borchgrevink, Cerebral mechanisms of complex sound perception, Consequences for the functional evaluation of hearing, in: "Hearing and Hearing Prophylaxis," H. M. Borchgrevink ed., Scand. Audiol. Suppl. 16 (1982).

ACKNOWLEDGEMENTS

This projct was supported by the Norwegian Research Council for Science and the Humanities, and the University of Oslo. The sentence material was made by B. Bird, B.A., Dept. of English, University of Oslo, together with T. Fretheim, professor, Dept. of Linguistics and S. Berge, B.A., Dept of English, both presently at the University of Tronhjem. T. Fretheim and S. Berge made the phoneme frequency count for Norwegian. B. Bird chose the subjects for the study and also participated in the analysis of the sentence repetitions performed by the subjects during testing. Audiometry, as well as other technical assistance were provided by G. Flottorp, Ph. D., K. E. Hogstad, M. Sci., J. Havstad, technical engineer, and M. Szalay, technical engineer - all at the Institute of Audiology, National Hospital of Norway, Oslo. K. E. Hogstad also made the statistical analysis.

DISCUSSION

Gerken: One of the problems in the bilingual studies when comparing performance in two languages, it is always difficult in deciding which language is the persons dominant language. I was wondering if you would comment on whether you thought that this experiment might be turned around and converted into an objective test of language dominance..

Brochgrevink: I certainly think so, because language proficiency obviously effect the threshold difference. We have one person raised in South Africa by English speaking, Norwegian parents who move to Norway at the age of 9, then changing to Norwegian speech. He spoke Norwegian with an English accent but he scored exactly like a native on both sentence tests.

Smoorenberg: A comment with respect to the method. Your subjects repeat the same sentence at higher signals to noise ratios. From our experience, when people have responded incorrectly, they tend to stick to that incorrect response. Our experience is that it is better and more reliable to use a new sentence with every presentation.

A PARAMETRIC EVALUATION OF THE EQUAL ENERGY HYPOTHESIS

Donald Henderson and R. P. Hamernik

University of Texas at Dallas
Callier Center for Communication Disorders
1966 Inwood
Dallas, TX 75235, USA

INTRODUCTION

A current issue of debate is whether the effects of impulse/impact noise are the same as the effects of continuous noise. Passchier-Vermeer [1] reviewed several demographic studies and reported that for equal amounts of sound energy, exposure to noises that had impulsive components produced larger amounts of hearing loss than the exposure to continuous noise. A series of laboratory studies, using an animal model of hearing loss, have shown that exposure to impulse noise of 140 dB or greater produces lesion in the cochlea that are probably mechanical in nature [2,3] and the pattern of recovery of auditory sensitivity following the exposure is often complicated; i.e., there is an initial period of recovery of sensitivity, then a reversal to higher levels of loss at 6 to 12 hours post-exposure, then a more gradual return to either a permanent hearing loss or to pre-exposure levels of auditory sensitivity [4,5].

The audiological and morphological differences between the effects of continuous and impulse noise may have important implication for the scientific rationale of noise standards. The Equal Energy Hypothesis (EEH), as proposed by Burn and Robinson [6], assumes that the permanent hearing loss produced by exposure to noise is a function of the A-weighted sound energy of the exposure. This is an attractive idea because there are some data consistent with it [7] and it is simple to apply. Atherley and Martin [8] have proposed an extension of the EEH to cover the effects of impulse noise. It is difficult to assess how appropriate the EEH is for impulse or impact noise in industry, because impulse or impact noise is usually accompanied by background continuous noise. Furthermore, most of the demographic studies of either continuous or impulse noise contain so much intersubject variability [9,10] that it is difficult to evaluate the effectiveness of the EEH or any other theory of hearing loss.

Thus, the following experiments were designed to evaluate the EEH for impact noise in a controlled laboratory setting. Ward et al. [11] have pointed out that there are different forms of the EEH. While this is true and relevant for the establishment of noise standards, this paper is concerned with the generic form of the EEH (i.e., hearing loss is proportional to the total energy of the exposure) and how it applies to impact noise. In order to test the EEH under a number of conditions, experimental animals were all exposed to one of 17 conditions, each with the same amount of acoustic energy. The actual conditions were varied between peak pressures of 107 to 143 dB SPL and rates of 4/sec to 1/16/sec.

METHODS

Subjects. Seventy-five adult chinchillas were used as subjects. The animals were anesthetized (0.1 mg/kg Ketamine) and made monaural by the surgical destruction of the left cochlea. A chronic bipolar electrode was then implanted in the region of the inferior colliculus using procedures outlined previously [12]. The animals were allowed to recover for several days prior to threshold testing.

Audiological Assessment. Auditory evoked response (AER) was used to estimate hearing thresholds [12,13]. Three pre-exposure thresholds were measured at 0.5, 1, 2, 4, 8, and 16 kHz; the mean of three measures was used to establish the pre-exposure thresholds for that animal. After the exposure, the animals were tested at 0.5, 2, and 8 kHz at post-exposure times of 0.25, 2, 8, 24, and 240 h in order to estimate the amount of temporary threshold shift (TTS) and the threshold recovery function. At 30 days post-exposure, thresholds were remeasured at all frequencies in order to estimate the amount of permanent threshold shift (PTS).

Exposures. One or two animals at a time were placed in small separate cages (31 x 51 x 38 cm) located below a loudspeaker and were given free access to food and water. The animals were then exposed to electronically synthesized impact noise. The impact consisted of a burst of broadband noise, whose spectrum was shaped with an equalizer, so that it roughly approximated that of an impact generated by striking a steel plate with a hammer [14,15]. The

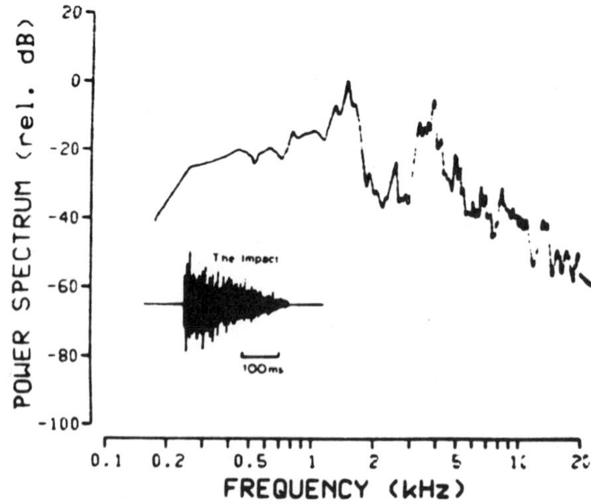

Fig. 1 Relative amplitude of the acoustic spectrum of the impact noise. Analysis was done with a 40 Hz bandwidth. The insert shows the pressure time profile of the noise.

Table I contains the exposure conditions. Two variables were systematically manipulated. Experiments B, C and D were conducted to examine the effect of "rate of presentation," thus the impact was delivered at B=1/sec, C=4/sec and D=1/sec. Within each experiment, the level was varied between 107 to 143 dB (peak equivalent SPL). All the experimental groups were counterbalanced in terms of level, rate and number of impacts, so that each group received the same amount of acoustic energy. Not all the conditions have been completed, but the results, to date, are quite interesting.

TABLE I

EQUAL ENERGY EXPERIMENT

	Level	Rate	Exposure Duration		Rate	Exposure Duration
	107 dB	4/s	5 days		4/s	5 days
	113 dB	1/s	5 days		4/s	30 hr.
(A)	119 dB	1/4s	5 days	(C)	4/s	7.5 hr.
	125 dB	1/16s	5 days		4/s	1.8 hr.
	131 dB	1/64s	5 days		4/s	.47 hr.
	137 dB	1/256s	5 days		4/s	.12 hr.
	143 dB	1/1024s	5 days		4/s	1.8 min.
	107 dB	1/s	20 days		1/4 s	80 days
	113 dB	1/s	5 days		1/4 s	20 days
	119 dB	1/s	30 days		1/4 s	5 days
(B)	125 dB	1/s	7.5 days	(D)	1/4 s	30 hr.
	131 dB	1/s	1.8hr.		1/4 s	7.5 hr.
	137 dB	1/s	.47 hr.		1/4 s	1.8 hr.
	143 dB	1/s	.12 hr.		1/4 s	.47 hr.

electrical signal was generated by multiplying (Analog Devices AD534) the spectrally-shaped noise with the output from an exponential waveform generator. The waveform generator controlled the repetition rate and envelope of the synthesized impact. The signal was amplified and transduced by a loudspeaker located above the animal's head. Fig. 1 shows the waveform and spectrum of the impact. The duration of the impact at a point 20 db down from the peak was 200 ms and the nominal rise time of the signal was 12 ms.

RESULTS AND DISCUSSION

The Effect Of Level

After each of the exposures, hearing loss was monitored at .5, 2 and 8 kHz at various times after the exposure for 30 days. Fig. 2 shows the average temporary threshold shift (TTS) immediately after the exposure for each of the levels at each of the three repetition rates, i.e., B=1/sec, C=4/sec and D=1/sec. The trend of the data is clear: as the level of the impulse is increased, the level of TTS, at each of the test frequencies, increases. The actual rate of increase in TTS with increased level is difficult to state because not all the experimental conditions have been completed. Also, the audiometric test system limits TTS measurements above 70-80 dB. Thus, the level of TTS may even be higher for some of the conditions, i.e., levels of 131 dB and greater.

A perspective on the variability across subjects and groups is provided in Fig. 3. This figure shows the TTS for individual subjects, at each of the three test frequencies, for the seven levels of Experiment C. While the data overlap between groups, the 119 dB impulses may be at a transition point because of the extreme variability at this level (i.e., 15 dB TTS for

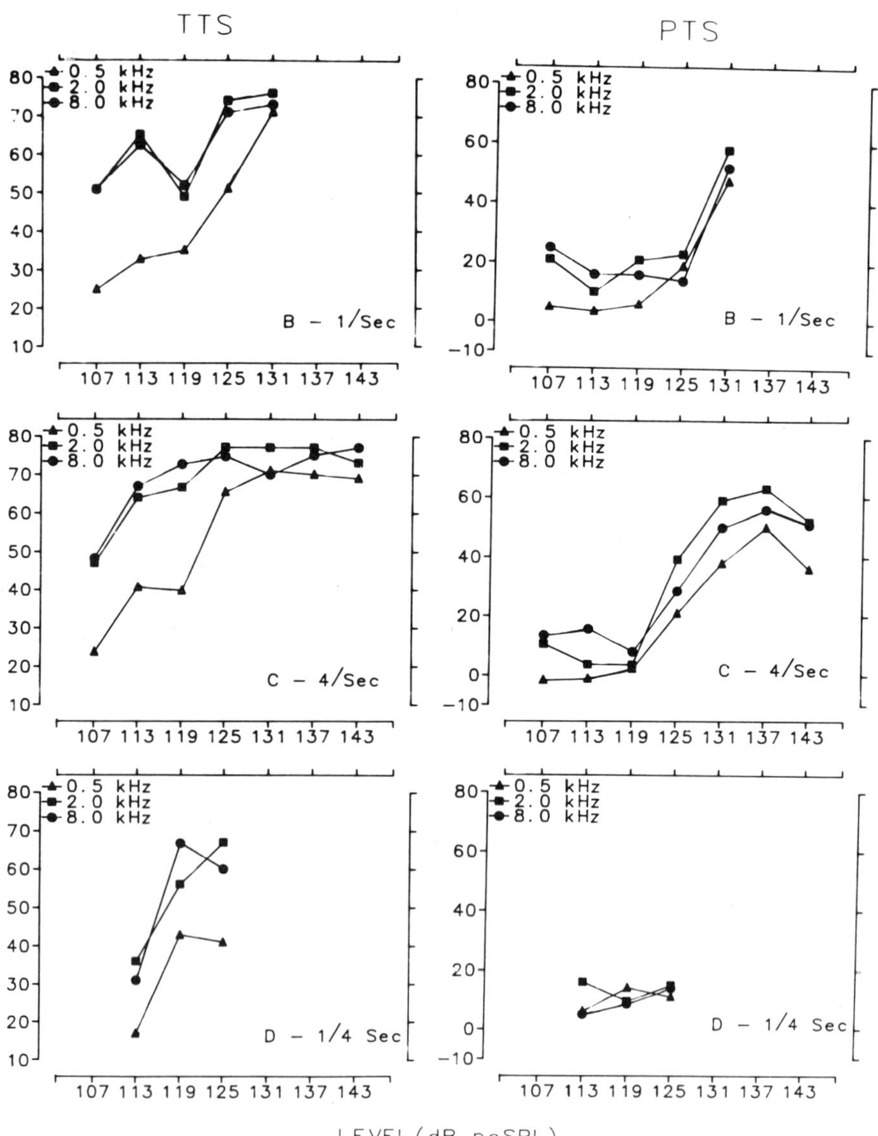

Fig. 2 The average (N=4 or more animals) 5, 2 and 8 kHz. Group B received the impacts at 1/sec; Group C at 4/sec and Group D.

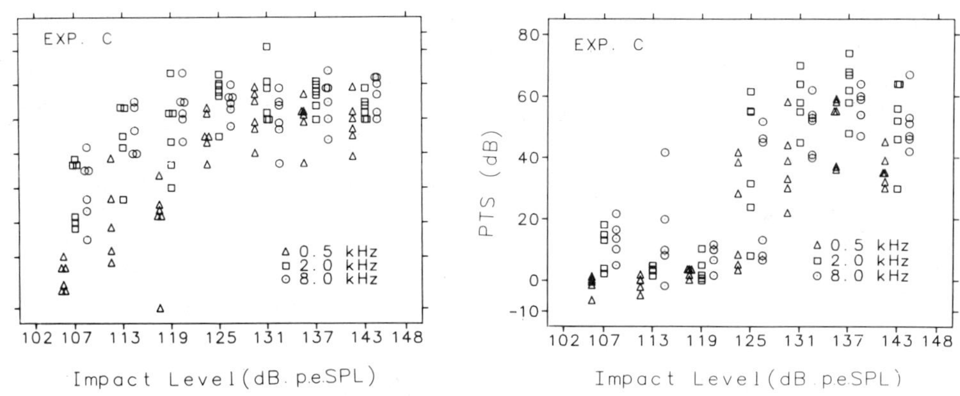

Fig. 3 Individual TTS and PTS for all the experimental subjects of Group C.

one subject at 4 kHz to 85 dB TTS for two subjects at 2 and 8 kHz). By contrast, the higher levels (>119 dB) have relatively homogenous results.

The experimental animals were retested 30 days after the exposure; the hearing loss at that time was defined as permanent threshold shift (PTS). The right side of Fig. 2 shows the average PTS for the three experiments. There is a range in each of the three experiments where there is no significant PTS (107 to 125 for B and D and 107 to 119 for C). Above these levels, however, there is a substantial increase in PTS. The results from individual subjects are quite consistent with the group averages. The right side of Fig. 3 shows the individual PTS for the animals in Experiment C, the 4/sec exposures. Animals in the 107 to 119 dB groups recover or have minor amounts of PTS; in the 125 dB group, there is a large range from normal to 60 dB PTS; above 125 dB, all animals developed severe PTS at all test frequencies. Thus, the transition level of 119 dB seen in the TTS data also appears in the PTS results.

A distinction between the effects of impulse and continuous noise is more a question of degree rather than a dichotomy; i.e., very high levels of continuous noise can cause the same effects as impulse noise, and, conversely, low levels of impulse or impact noise can produce the same effects as continuous noise. If we are concerned with the effects of impulse noise that are different from the effects of continuous noise, then one issue is: what levels produce "impulse" effects? The results of these experiments, as well as other experiments from our laboratory, suggest that, for the chinchilla, the 119 to 125 dB region may be a transition region. In the current experiment, even though all groups were exposed to the same amount of acoustic energy, only exposures of 119 dB or greater provided significant PTS. In an earlier experiment [15], chinchillas exposed to similar impact noise acquired TTS at the rate of 1.5 dB for each dB of impact noise below 119 dB; when the level of the impulse was over 119 dB, TTS increased at the rate of 3.5 dB for each dB increase in the noise. Spoendlin [16] has reported that the cochlear pathology of guinea pigs changes when the level of an impulse is increased over 120 dB, and shows many of the signs of direct mechanical damage. These results suggest that the type of damage in the cochlea is partially the level dependent upon, but it is quite likely that the transition level will vary with the signature of the impulse and the species.

The Effect of Rate

The importance of the rate of presentation can be seen in Fig. 4. The top panels show the TTS and PTS data from the 113 dB exposures. When the rate of presentation was increased from 1 every 4 seconds to 4 per second, TTS increased a minimum of 15 dB at 5 kHz to an average 29 dB at 2 and 8 kHz. However, each of the groups recovered to essentially pre-exposure levels or minimum amounts of PTS. The rate of presentation is more important for the data of the 125 dB exposures. The bottom two panels of Fig. 4 show that both TTS and PTS increases significantly as the rate of presentation is increased. The result is even more surprising, considering at 4/sec the middle ear reflex could be expected to provide some measure of protection.

The rate of presentation is an important but not particularly well understood variable. The greater losses caused by faster repetition rates may be the result of the animals susceptibility changing during an exposure. The biological effects of a single exposure may cause a period of vulnerability in the cochlea, and if another impulse hits the cochlea during this time, then the effects of that impulse will be even greater. Conversely, at the slower rates, the longer periods between impacts allowed for some recovery to occur. This period of vulnerability is seen in a number of quite

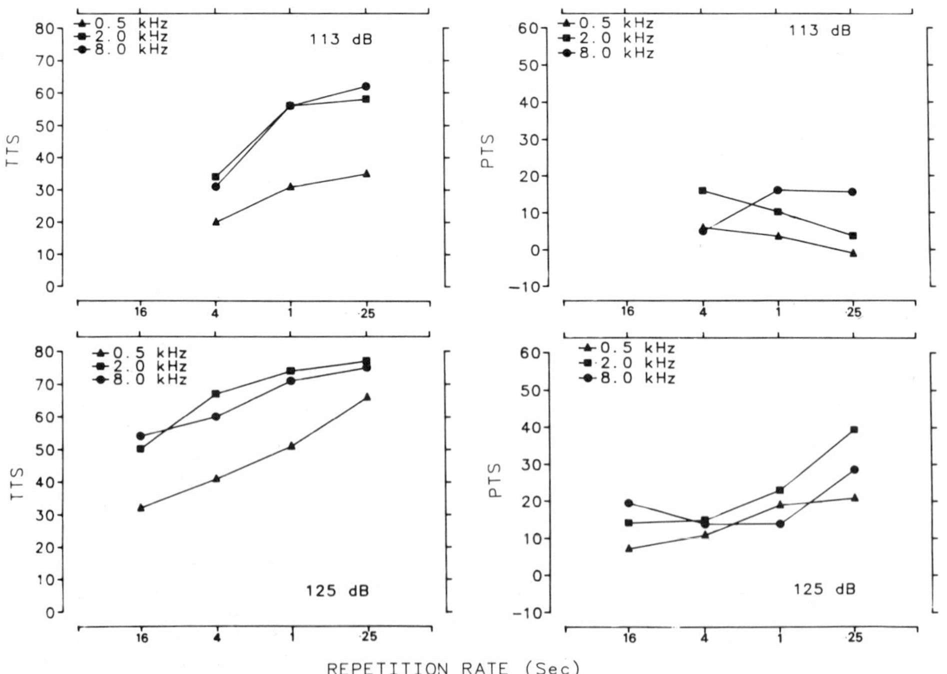

Fig. 4 Average TTS and PTS for subjects exposed to the 113 and 125 dB levels. Data from comparable levels were taken from each of the three experiments and a fourth group was added (1/16 sec) to the 125 level.

different experiments; i.e., Price [17] showed that changes in the cochlear microphonics of cats caused by bursts of noise was directly dependent on the period of time that had elapsed since the last noise exposure. Also, Perkins [18] showed that the amount of TTS, PTS and hair cell loss was greatly enhanced when the rate of presentation of 50 impulses was increased from 1/min. to 1/10 sec. Collectively, these results show that the rate of exposure to a given quantity of acoustic energy can be an extremely important variable in the creation of a hearing loss.

Equal Energy Hypothesis

The experiments were designed to evaluate the Equal Energy Hypothesis. Thus, all the experimental groups had the same total acoustic energy but, distributed with different repetition rates, levels and total numbers of impulse. We have previously discussed the contribution of both level and rate, but perhaps the most significant finding is that exposures with the same acoustic energy can develop widely different levels of TTS and PTS. The auditory system does not react to a noise exposure like a simple integrator - it reacts differently to high and low level impacts, and the rate of energy delivery is an important variable.

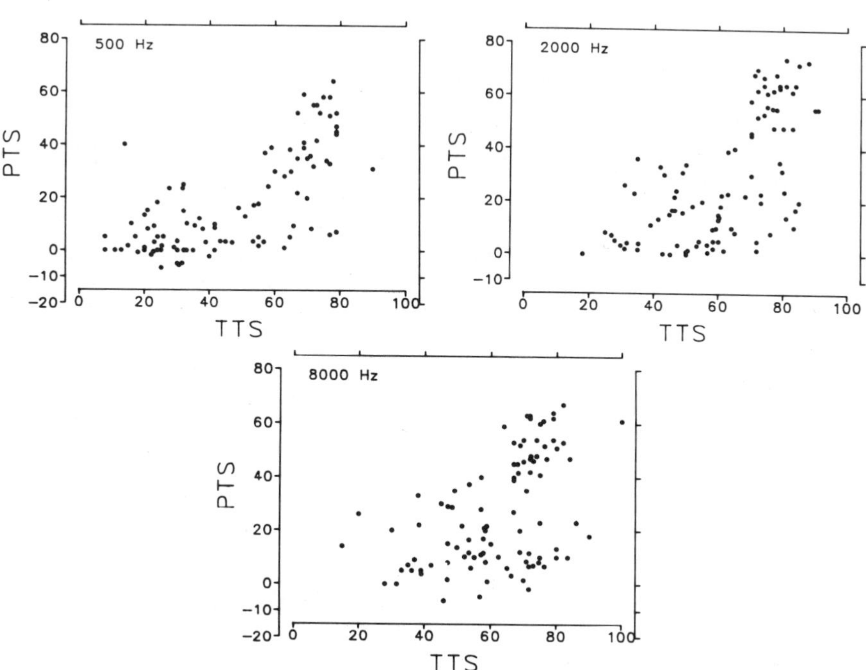

Fig. 5 Scatterplots of the TTS/PTS distribution of all subjects in the three experiments.

TTS AND PTS RELATION

The experimental design used in these experiments allows a perspective on the relation between TTS and PTS. TTS has been assumed to be correlated with PTS, and thus has been used as a dependent variable in many studies of experimentally-induced hearing loss [19]. The confirmation of the TTS/PTS relation is difficult to do in humans because of the difficulty of doing controlled studies in the workplace and the ethical problem of studying the formation of PTS. However, the data from this experiment do provide an interesting perspective on how TTS and PTS convary. The TTS and PTS data from all the experimental groups have been plotted on each of the three graphs of Fig. 4. It is clear that TTS levels below 50 dB do not correlate with PTS, primarily because there is usually no PTS with TTS level of 50 dB and less.

CONCLUSION

These experiments were designed to test the appropriateness of the EEH for impact noise. Chinchillas were exposed to the impact noise of equal energy, but at levels ranging from 107 to 143 dB at rates ranging from 1/16 sec. to 4/sec. Two major trends emerged - at lower levels (< 119 dB), the effect of rate and level were only important for the production of TTS and not PTS, but at levels above 119, faster rates and higher levels produced greater amounts of TTS and PTS. These results do not agree with the EEH. The relationship between TTS and PTS was examined and found that TTS of 50 dB or less did not routinely lead to PTS; TTS of 50 dB or greater after, typically lead to PTS.

REFERENCES

1. W. Passchier-Vermeer, Measurement and rating of impulse noise in relation to noise-induced hearing loss, in: Noise as a Public Health Problem, ed. G. Rossi (Proceedings of the Fourth International Congress) Milano, Italy (1983).
2. R. P. Hamernik, G. Turrentine, M. Roberto, R. J. Salvi, and D. Henderson, Anatomical correlates of impulse noise-induced mechanical damage in the cochlea, Hearing Research 13:229 (1984).
3. R. Hamernik, G. Turrentine and C. G. Wright, Surface morphology of the inner sulcus and related epithelial cells of the cochlea following acoustic trauma, Hearing Res. 16:143 (1984).
4. G. A. Luz and J. D. Mosko, The susceptibility of the chinchilla ear to damage from impulse noise, US Army Medical Research Lab Report #921 (1971).
5. D. Henderson and R. P. Hamernik, Audiometric and histological correlates of exposure to 1-msec noise impulses in the chinchilla, J. Acoust. Soc. Am. 56: 1210 (1974).
6. W. Burns and D. W. Robinson, Hearing and Noise in Industry (Her Majesty's Stationery Office, London, England) (1970).
7. W. Burns and D. W. Robinson, The concept of noise pollution level, National Physical Lab Aerodynamics Div., MPL Aero Report AC 38 (1969).
8. C. R. C. Atherley, Noise-induced hearing loss: The energy principle for recurrent impact noise and noise exposure close to the recommended limits, Ann. Occup. Hyg. 16:183 (1973).
9. W. Passchier-Vermeer, R. van den Berg and R. Leeuw, Measurement of impulse noise at workplaces: relation between oscilloscopic measurements with an ordinary precision sound level meter, Scand. Audiol. Suppl., 12:85 (1980).

10. W. Taylor and P. L. Lord, Noise levels and hearing thresholds in the drop forging industry, Med. Res. Council Project Rep. Grant G972/784C, June, London (1976).
11. W. D. Ward, C. W. Turner and D. A. Fabry, The total energy and equal energy principles in the chinchilla, Proceedings of Fourth International Congress in Noise as a Public Health Issue, ed. G. Rossi, 399-410 (1983).
12. D. Henderson, R. P. Hamernik, C. Woodward, R. W. Sitler and R. J. Salvi, Evoked-response audibility curve of the chinchillas, J. Acoust. Soc. Am., 54:1099 (1973).
13. R. J. Salvi, W. A. Ahroon, J. W. Perry, A. D. Gunnarson and D. Henderson, Comparison of psychophysical and evoked-response tuning curves in the chinchilla, Am. J. Otolaryngol, 3:408 (1982).
14. E. A. Blakeslee, K. Hynson, R. P. Hamernik and D. Henderson, Asymptotic threshold shift in chinchillas exposed to impulse noise, J. Acoust. Soc. Am., 63:876 (1978).
15. D. Henderson and R. P. Hamernik, Asymptotic threshold shift from impulse noise, in New Perspectives on Noise-Induced Hearing Loss, eds. R. P. Hamernik, D. Henderson and R. J. Salvi, Raven, New York (1982).
16. H. Spoendlin and J. P. Brun, Relation of structural damage to exposure time and intensity in Acoustic Trauma, Acta Otolaryng., 75:220 (1973).
17. G. Richard Price, Effect of interrupting recovery on loss in cochlear microphonic sensitivity, J. Acoust. Soc. Am., 59:#3 709 (1976).
18. C. Perkins, R. P. Hamernik and D. Henderson, The effect of interstimulus interval on the production of hearing loss from impulse noise, J. Acoust. Soc. Am. Suppl., 1:57, S62 (1975).
19. CHABA, National Research Council Committee on Hearing, Bioacoustics and Biomechanics, "Hazardous exposure to intermittent and steady-state noise, Report of Working Group 16 (Washington, D.C.) (1965).

DISCUSSION

Per Nilsson: Spoendlin reported the critical intensity to be at 130 dB for 4 minute exposures, but for exposure times of 1 hour, the critical intensity was lowered to 125 dB. We repeated these experiments with guinea pig and found it to be 117 dB for 6 hours. So there appears to be a trading relation between time and intensity, therefore we renamed it a critical level instead.

Pfander: Where is the frontier between TTS and PTS with respect to recovery, because we see recovery up to 1 year?

Henderson: We define PTS as the amount of hearing loss that is left at 30 days. There are probably instances where, at 30 days there is still recoverable hearing, but I think most of our experience leads us to believe that by 30 days, you have most of the recovery taken place.

Trahoitis: If you look at TTS/PTS relation at 500 and 8000 Hz, one could argue you there were tender ears and tough ears. The big difference between the graphs was there may not have been as many samples of the tender ears, i.e., it may be just a sampling problem.

Henderson: All the points that were on the 500 Hz data were also on the 8000 Hz Data because they are the same groups of animal. Perhaps, there is a differences in "tough" and "tender" within parts of the cochlea and there may not be a generally "tough ear" or a generally "tender ear."

Buck: There might be a different mechanism between PTS and TTS because Liberman showed that PTS is likely to be located on the low frequency side and TTS is more located on the high frequency side of the exposure. If there is a correlation between TTS and PTS, it should be at the lower frequencies.

Henderson: Most investigators would now agree that there are clear differences between the processes underlying the audiometric profile of TTS and the audiometric profile of PTS.

Smoorenburg: What will be the best physical measure rigit now, to protect hearing loss once you exceed the critical level?

Henderson: I do not know, what would be the best measure, and the point of these experiments is that there is probably not a simple best measure. For example, there are instances where the Equal Energy Rule works quite well, and other noise conditions where it does not work. Audiometric data from exposures with systematic variation in acoustic parameters will help us design a more effective noise hazard metric. One way of capturing the effects that we showed today would be building a leaky integrator process into a dosimeter.

IMPULSE NOISE HAZARD AS A FUNCTION OF LEVEL AND SPECTRAL DISTRIBUTION

G. Richard Price

U. S. Army Human Engineering Laboratory
Aberdeen Proving Ground, MD 21005-5001 USA

INTRODUCTION

Given an interest in impulse noise, there are many research issues that could be addressed, but for practical application, two of them are especially important. Specifically, they are the roles played by level and spectral distribution of energy. So far as the auditory system is concerned, there must be some internally consistent answers. The practical problem is that the damage-risk criteria (DRC) in use in the world differ in their treatment of these two critical issues. Furthermore, the present research program is producing data that indicate that the current DRCs are fundamentally incorrect and that traditional theoretical approaches don't work.

There is increasing interest in an A-weighted energy measure for rating hazard from all sounds. Such a measure would be easy to use, an important issue in practice. ISO-1999 [1] has proposed it; but has restricted its application to levels below 140 dB. The French Ministry of Defense [2] has recommended use of a criterion based on A-weighted energy (equivalent to 8 hours at 90 dB SPL), provided the peak does not exceed 160 dB. A DRC in use in the Netherlands [3] extends the limit upward so that any exposure to impulses containing the energy equivalent to 8 hours at 85 dB SPL (without frequency weighting) would be acceptable. A problem inherent in upward extrapolations is the possibility that there is some level at which the loss mechanism changes and loss may grow much more rapidly than expected. Whether or not there is such a critical level (CL) and just where it is, should it exist, are obviously important questions.

On the other hand, DRCs in the USA [4-6] have been specifically formulated for use at high levels. They are based on measures of impulse duration and peak level and make no allowance for the frequency content of the energy within the impulse. If the susceptibility of the ear varies as a function of frequency for intense impulses, as it does for continuous sounds, then an absence of a frequency weighting of some sort means that criteria of this type suffer corresponding inaccuracies.

An extended series of studies has been conducted over the years addressing these issues with the intention of providing some quantitative structure to the response of the ear to intense sounds. Salient portions of this ongoing effort will be presented here.

Today there is probably not much disagreement with the idea that with exposure to increasing SPLs, there is some level at which the ear can be disrupted by essentially mechanical forces. Experiments in which cat ears were exposed to spectrally narrow impulses [7] produced results consistent with the argument that the basis for loss was mechanical stress at the level of the organ of Corti. These data have been used as the basis for developing a tentative estimate of this CL for the human ear [8]. The curve in Fig. 1 looks very much like the A-weighting curve, possibly because both reflect the transfer characteristics of the external and middle ears. Although the absolute level is high, nevertheless it is well within a range to which human beings are exposed at home and at work. For a median ear, the level was calculated to be near 140 dB, where the ear is tuned best (about 3.0 kHz). In a normal population, the more susceptible individuals were estimated to be 10 dB or more sensitive than the median. It does not constitute an adequate test of this calculation; but Singleton et al. [9] have reported permanent hearing losses in human ears resulting from one exposure to the ringing of a cordless telephone at about these levels. However, this effort to establish a CL was not definitive because the approach was essentially empirical and was based on data from a specific class of impulse (tone pips and a damped sinusoid). A definitive answer would provide a method of calculating mechanical stress within the organ of Corti given any free field pressure-time history.

Before going further, it would be a good idea to make explicit an additional presumption about a CL. Consistent with the admonition of William of Occam, a very simple model of the stress process is used [10]. Broch [11] has observed that in the study of the fatigue in materials, an approximate mechanical relationship exists between the amplitude of the stress and the number of sinusiodal cycles to failure. Essentially, the number of cycles is inversely proportional to the stress (raised to a power which is characteristic of each material). Thus, the CL is pictured as a range of intensities where mechanical stress becomes the predominant mechanism for loss. As intensities rise, it might be expected that the rate at which damage accumulates will undergo an acceleration when CL is exceeded and at

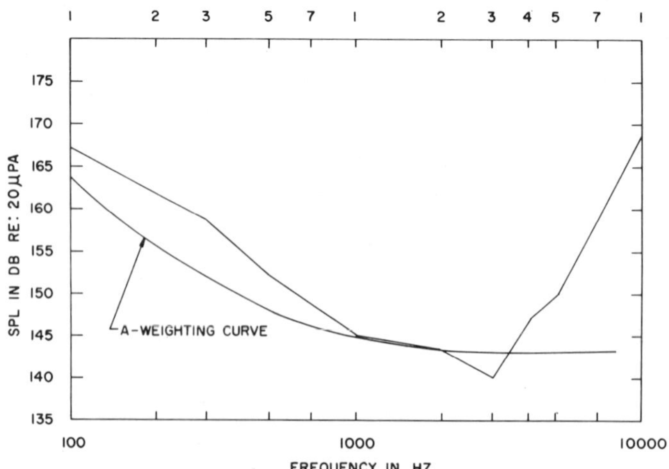

Fig. 1. The free field SPL reaching the critical level for an exponentially damped sinusoid and the median human ear. Also plotted for comparison is the A-weighting curve.

some very high level even one cycle may produce a failure. Once CL has been exceeded, some repair might take place after the exposure, but because it is recovery from mechanical trauma, it will be slower than recovery from something like a metabolic deficit, which is probably characteristic of losses below the CL.

If indeed there is a CL and it implies impending cellular damage, then it follows that it would be risky to tolerate exposures above such a level. Therefore, CL might make a good basis for a criterion of acceptable exposure. The problem now is to establish that such a level exists and to pin it down both quantitatively and theoretically.

It might be added parenthetically that the CL concept is a function of level, regardless of the type of noise involved. So far as CL is concerned, it makes no difference whether the noises are described as impulse, impact, or continuous. Such descriptors doubtless will make a difference when one considers the effects of intermittency, however.

There is considerable practical interest in exposures to gunfire. All gunfire impulses are essentially similar in that they can be approximated by a Friedlander waveform. The impulses differ primarily in their duration which is in turn a function of the amount of explosive producing the impulse. The spectra of such impulses are all similar in shape, the location of the peak reflecting the duration. The proposed shape of CL is shown in Fig. 2 along with a typical weapon impulse spectrum. The observation that the loss threshold is more sharply tuned than the spectrum has led to prediction that no matter where the peak of the spectrum is, the first losses should be seen in the mid-range [8]. The work establishing this is still in process, but it can be said at this point that it appears to be true for both electrophysiological and histological measures of loss [8,12,13].

An important question for noise hazard is whether susceptibility changes as a function of location of the spectral peak. All three possible answers to the question have been advanced. A simple frequency analysis of impulses with the same peak pressure but differing durations shows (as in Fig. 2) that in theory all impulses have the same energy at any point on the high frequency side of the spectral peak (at 3.0 kHz, for instance),

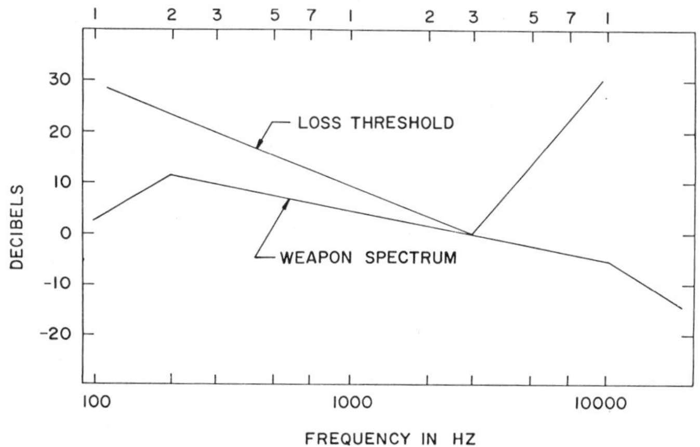

Fig. 2. Spectrum of a typical weapons impulse with a peak at a low frequency. Also shown is the loss threshold from Fig. 1.

and it might be supposed that all impulses should therefore reach a CL at the same peak pressure. However, Price [12,14,15] has hypothesized that at high SPLs the ear acts as though the impulses are distorted cosine waves and, due to the tuning of the ear and/or the limiting effects of middle ear displacement [16], impulses with their spectral peaks at low frequencies might be less hazardous by about 3 dB/oct below 3.0 kHz (for the human ear). It has also been contended (by those who favor an energy measure), that for equal peak pressures, the lower frequency impulses should be much more hazardous because they contain much more energy.

Auditory theory is not well developed for modeling the ear's response to intense sounds; consequently all these viewpoints are extremely tenuous. The middle ear is essentially linear for most stimulation; but at high intensities it amplitude limits [16]. The inner ear is highly nonlinear at even moderately high pressures. Even if this were not true, we are only now coming to an adequate theoretical understanding of intracochlear mechanics (at normal levels). It is, of course, desirable to begin with a firm theoretical understanding and make predictions which can then be tested. However, it is often the case that, even without a good theory, the empiricists make some guesses and gather data anyway.

PROCEDURES

A series of studies was undertaken to test the effect of impulse duration (location of spectral peak) on susceptibility. Specific test procedures have been described in several reports [7,12,17]. In essence, cat ears were exposed to 50 or 60 impulses from a howitzer, a rifle or a primer, which had spectral peaks at about 100 Hz, 800 Hz and 4000 Hz respectively. Hearing sensitivity was tested by signal averaging responses to tone pips at the vertex (wave P5). Hearing was tested at 2.0, 4.0, 8.0 and 16.0 kHz before exposure, immediately afterward, and two months afterward. Animals were lightly anesthetized at the time of testing, sounds were delivered via a closed tube system, and sound pressures were calibrated by a probe microphone near the ear drum. In the case of the howitzer and rifle, exposures were in the free field. Animals were awake and restrained in bags with their ears about a meter off the ground and facing the muzzle of the weapon. Wave forms of the stimuli, typical of such weapons, have been published [8,12]. For each weapon, exposures were made at three different peak SPLs about 5 or 6 dB apart, each animal being exposed only once. The interimpulse intervals were 2-7 seconds and irregular, so as to avoid the possibility of temporal conditioning of the middle ear muscles. Never was an animal observed to react before the arrival of an impulse, which argues against conditioning of a middle ear muscle response. (It does not rule out the possibility of a tonic contraction, however.) Experiments with the primer impulse are still going on; but a sufficient number of ears have been exposed to allow tentative comparisons. In these latest exposures, the animals were lightly anesthetized when exposed in an anechoic chamber.

The measures of sensitivity took about 1/2 hour per ear, and in the case of the howitzer, five animals were exposed at one time. This meant that the first measures were made between 1 hour and 6 hours post-exposure. There was no obvious order of measurement effect. They were exposed in pairs to the rifle impulse and as singles to the primer. As a convention, no ear was exposed to audiometric test stimuli above 90 dB SPL, as a precaution against doing additional damage to the ear. No response at this level was arbitrarily recorded as an 80 dB threshold shift. In addition, impedance measures were made before and after exposures to check on the possibility of direct damage to the conductive mechanism. In no case was any damage seen.

RESULTS AND DISCUSSION

Effect of Spectrum

Experimental results. For all impulses the maximum losses tended to be in the 2.0 to 4.0 kHz region; therefore the data reported here are all for 4.0 kHz threshold shifts, and each data point in Figs. 3, 4, and 5 represents the mean loss for each animal. The losses immediately after exposure to the howitzer impulse are shown in Fig. 3, which combines data from two studies (N=41). Exposures were at peak SPLs between 153 and 166 dB. Losses grew with increasing intensity as expected; it is apparent that even at the highest level some ears showed little loss while other losses were too great to measure. The dotted line is the mean-square regression line, which has a slope of about 2 and predicts zero loss at about 144 db.

The data for rifle impulses are presented in Fig. 4 (N=22). The same general pattern is seen as before: the regression line predicting zero loss at 139 dB SPL, about 5 dB lower than for the howitzer. Other methods of comparing these ears have been used [17] and the difference is always in the same direction. If all 4 audiometric frequencies are used, the howitzer appears to be less hazardous than the rifle by about 9 to 13 dB, depending on the statistical technique.

Fig. 5 contains the latest data on the primer impulses (N=16). The slope of the regression line is steeper than before; but even so it intersects zero loss at about 132 dB. It would appear that this impulse with its spectral peak at about 4.0 kHz is extremely hazardous to the cat ear, much more so than the other impulses.

The practical implication of this result can be seen in the next figures. Fig. 6 portrays the relative hazard of the various impulses as a function of their spectral peak. The primer is arbitrarily set at zero dB and the other impulses are scaled from there. The rifle and howitzer fall close to the -3dB/oct line. In contrast, again using the primer impulse as

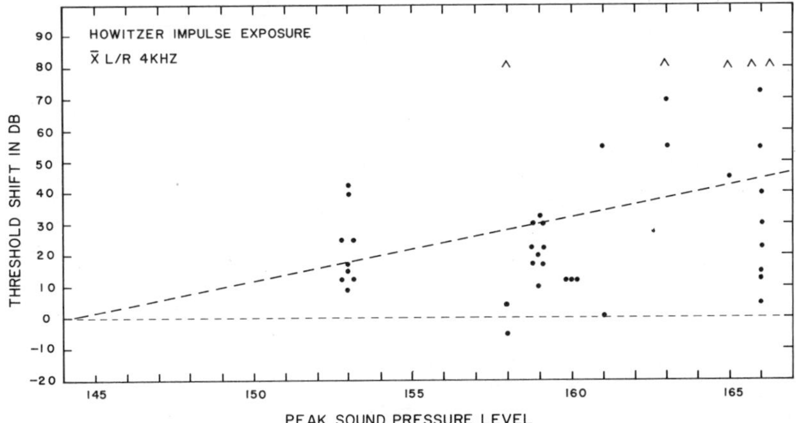

Fig. 3. Threshold shifts at 4.0 kHz immediately following exposure to 50-60 impulses from the howitzer. Each data point is the mean of two ears of each animal. The dashed line is the least squares regression line fitting the data.

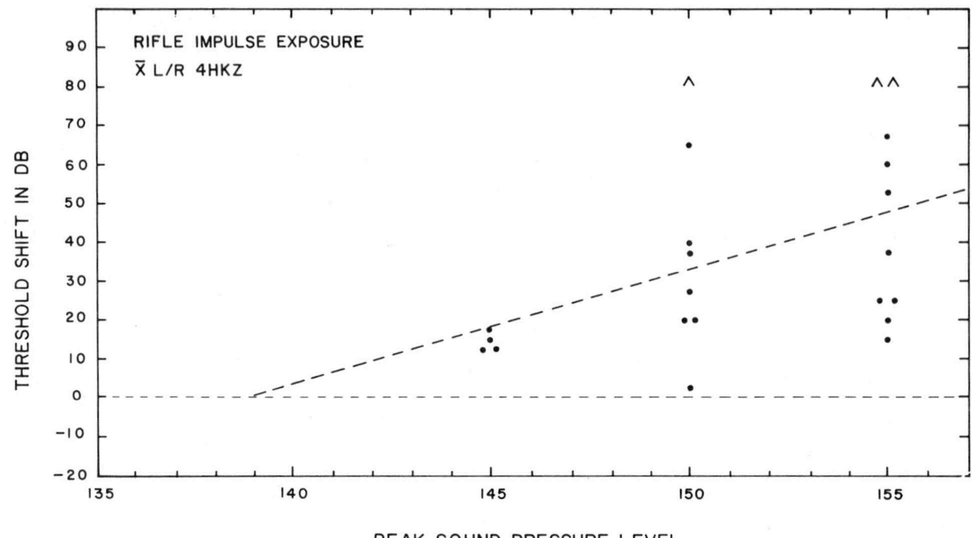

Fig. 4. Threshold shifts at 4.0 kHz immediately following exposure to 60 impulses from a rifle. Each data point is the mean of two ears of each animal. The dashed line is the least squares regression line fitting the data.

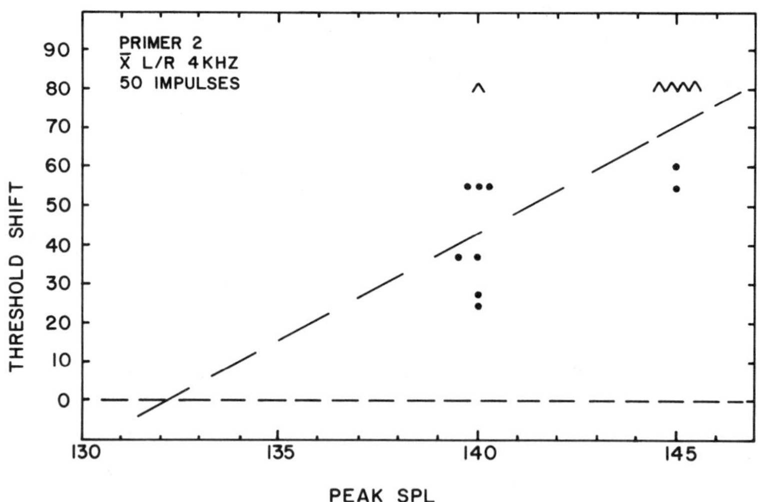

Fig. 5. Threshold shifts at 4.0 kHz immediately following exposure to 50 impulses from a primer. Each data point is the mean of two ears of each animal. The dashed line is the least squares regression line fitting the data.

a starting point, the shaded area indicates the predicted hazard from these same impulses calculated according to the CHABA, Pfander and Smoorenburg criteria. The disagreement is obvious.

Comparison with existing criteria. It is instructive to look at these data in light of each of the present criteria for impulse noise. In making this direct comparison, it should be remembered that the criteria were derived for the human rather than the cat ear. The human is probably less susceptible than the cat; but apart from the fact that the human ear is tuned a little lower in frequency and is less sensitive, the ears of these two species are similar in their basic properties. Thus, while the absolute levels might not be directly transferrable, the general trends should be.

The differing slopes of the regression lines in the previous figures make use of the zero intercept a little questionable. Therefore, in the next comparisons, the SPL producing a 40 dB threshold shift in an average cat has been calculated. As will become apparent later, such a threshold shift implies a permanent threshold shift of almost 20 dB.

Fig. 7 shows the present data plotted on the same coordinates as the CHABA criterion. The contrast in the slopes of the functions is apparent, the CHABA criterion rating hazard just the reverse of the present data. In reality the CHABA criterion does not specifically correct for spectral location. Its downward slope is based on the greater hazard of reverberant impulses, given the same weapon (rifle) [4].

Fig. 8 shows a similar pattern when plotted on the coordinates of either the Pfander or Smoorenburg criteria. These criteria also make no allowance for spectrum. Even though it is not appropriate to make direct comparisons across the two species, it is probably not too far out of line to assume that a mean cat ear is about as susceptible as a sensitive human ear. It is therefore of some concern to note that serious loss in the cat ear can be produced by impulses rated as not hazardous for the human ear. In the mid-range, these criteria might not be stringent enough.

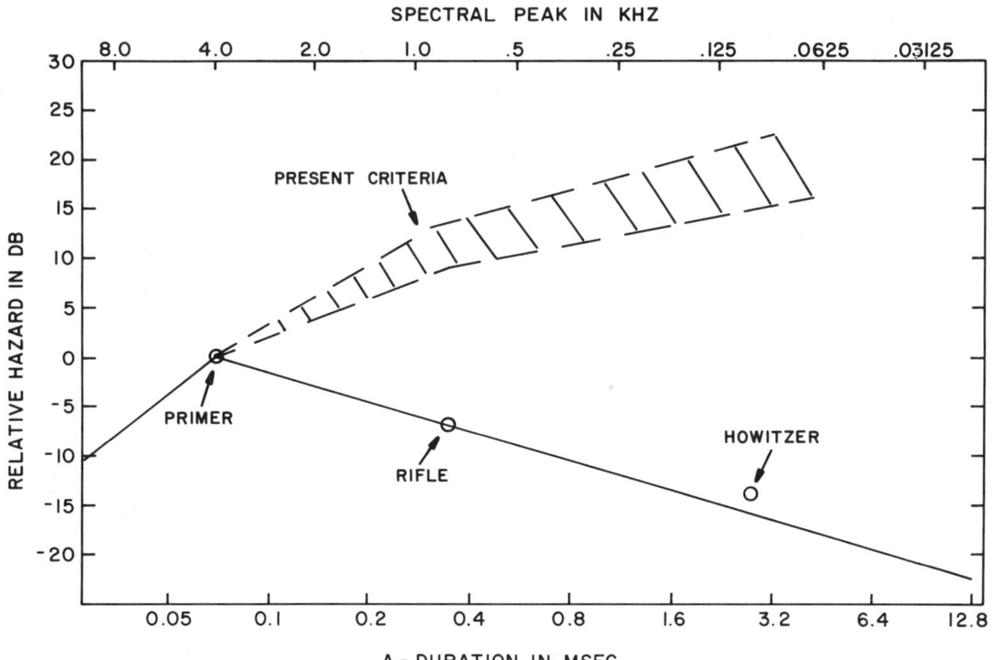

Fig. 6. The relative hazard of the three types of impulse used in these studies. Data points represent the threshold of loss for each impulse. The shaded area is the relative hazard as rated by existing criteria (assuming the primer impulse were just acceptable).

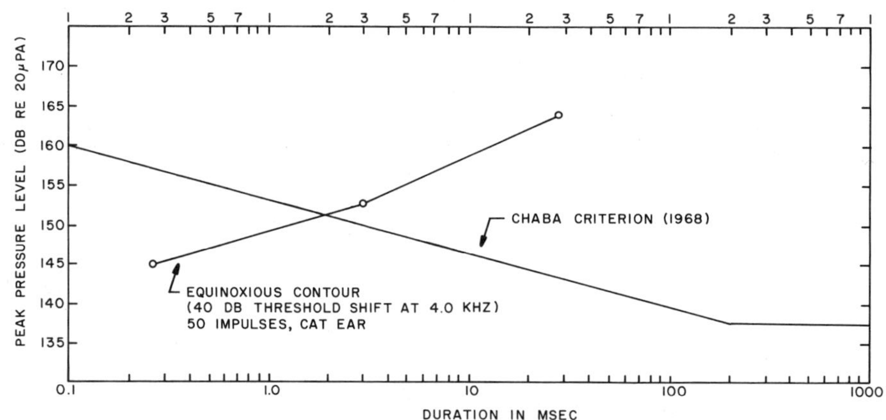

Fig. 7. The exposure producing a 40 dB threshold shift in the cat ear plotted on the coordinates of the CHABA criterion.

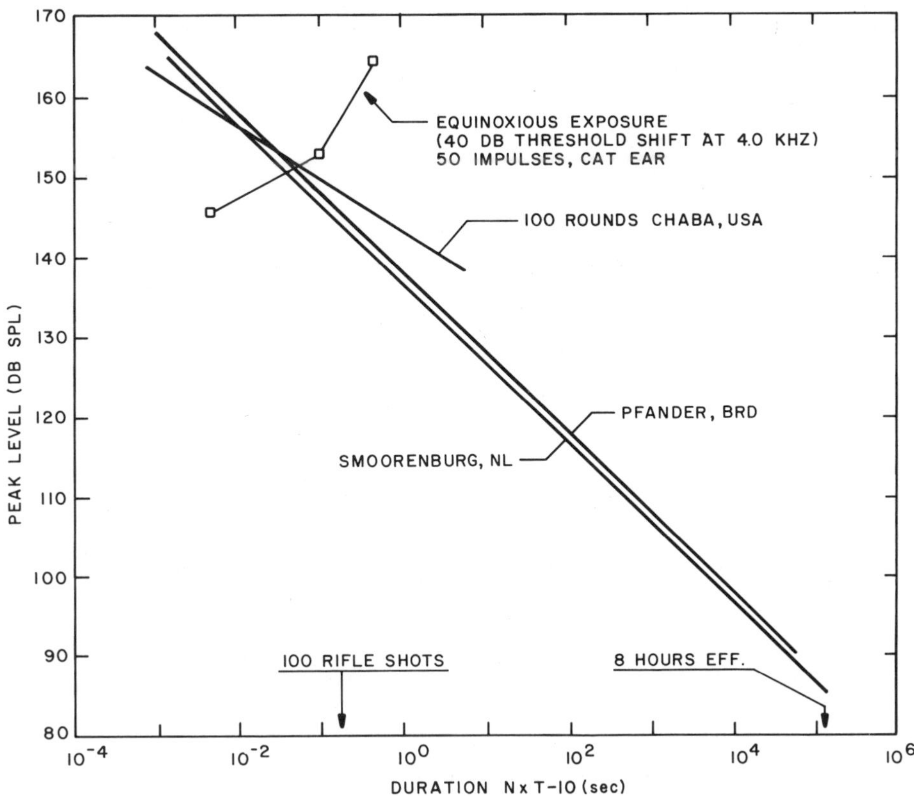

Fig. 8. The exposure producing a 40 dB threshold shift on the cat ear plotted on coordinates with the German and Dutch criteria.

Might A-weighted energy be a good compromise measure? The result is seen in Fig. 9, where the A-weighted energy needed to produce a given threshold shift is plotted. Even when A-weighted, the howitzer required about 400 Joules/M^2, the rifle about 10 Joules/M^2 and the primer only about 0.4 Joules/M^2. If A-weighted energy were a good answer, then the line on the graph should have been horizontal. Instead, the ends of the plot differ by 40 dB! If no weighting had been applied, then the howitzer exposure would have contained about 1200 Joules/M^2 and the other two data points would not have been too different. The effect of A-weighting on rifle and primer is minimal because most of their energy is in the mid-range.

Has a CL Been Exceeded?

A major contention of the CL hypothesis is that loss is primarily the result of mechanical stress which produces damage that is not readily reversible. Thus, threshold shifts measured immediately after an exposure might not fully recover, even when they are not large. With this possibility in mind, the following figures show compound threshold shift (CTS) (threshold shift immediately after exposure) versus permanent threshold shift (PTS) at 4.0 kHz for individual ears. The term compound threshold shift was used because the threshold shift measured immediately after exposure had both temporary and permanent components. Figs. 10, 11, and 12 present data for the howitzer, rifle and primer respectively. The data for 4.0 kHz were plotted because that was where the maximum loss generally

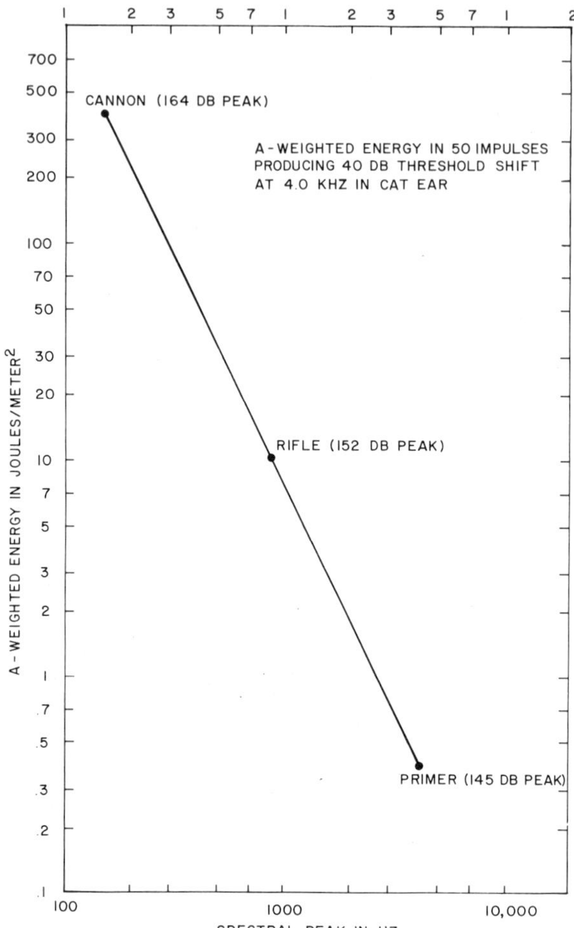

Fig. 9. A-weighted energy in the impulses required to produce a 40 dB threshold shift in the cat ear.

occurred for all impulses; but plots of the same relationship at other frequencies are essentially the same. The product moment correlation coefficient between CTS and PTS in these figures is about 0.8, and the slope of the regresion line is 0.5 or a little higher (implying that about half of CTS will resolve to PTS). The additional point of real concern is tha the intercept of the regression line is near zero for the howitzer exposure, and about 10 or 15 dB for the other exposures. Given the relatively small amount of data, it is premature to say whether or not the howitzer effect is really different from the other two. Also, another mechanism might be operating to produce the effect. Because animals were exposed to the howitzer in groups of five, on the average, measures of threshold shift were made later than for the rifle or primer. Therefore, it may have been that some early recovery did occur and the loss measured for the howitzer, on the average, lacked this early recovery component. But in any event, prudence would argue that any loss measured an hour or so after an exposure of this type should be considered to have permanent components. This finding is consistent with Pfander, Bongartz, Brinkman, and Kietz's [18] emphasis on a prolonged recovery time as being indicative of a dangerous

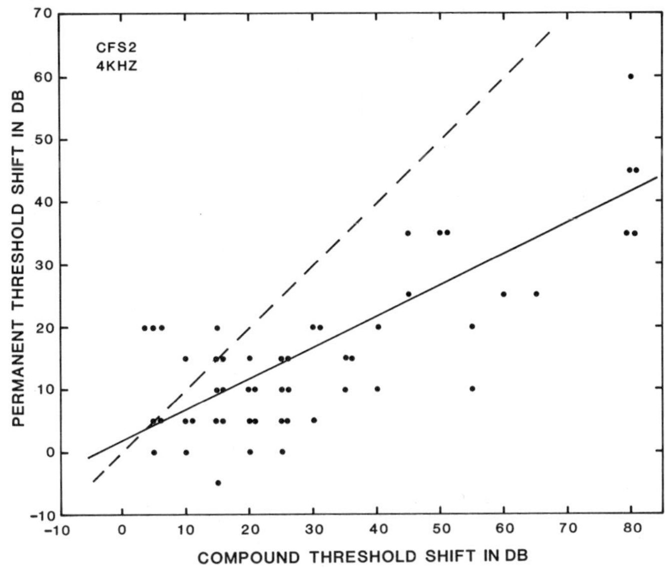

Fig. 10. Scatter plot of CTS vs PTS at 4.0 kHz for ears exposed to howitzer impulses. Each data point represents one ear. The solid line is the least squares regression line fitting the data and the dashed line is plotted along a line of equal CTS/PTS.

The relationship between CTS and PTS is consistent with the premise that a CL has been exceeded for these exposures.

Practical Issues

Before the applications are discussed briefly, a number of caveats should be expressed. As always, it would be desirable to have more data. Further, the data we have on the primer exposure, even within the present study, are only preliminary results. As is always the case with experimental programs that have matured over a long period of time, the data have been collected under slightly different conditions (ear height, inter-round interval, timing of measurements, etc.). It is also unfortunate that the data are available for only one species, even if the cat is a reasonable model of the human ear. Lastly, confidence in the findings would be greatest if a good theoretical model were available that could explain all the results.

If one were to extrapolate these data to human settings, a number of important points emerge. As a premise, it is probably not too far wrong to assume that for the arguments advanced here, the average cat ear is like a susceptible human ear. Therefore, for a Friedlander impulse with its spectral peak at 3.0 kHz, about 0.04 J/M^2 is sufficient energy to reach a threshold of permanent loss for one exposure. That is equivalent to an exposure to as little as 62 dB for 8 hours. It is also true that the peak pressure meeting that condition is about 135 dB SPL. This latest figure is close to that calculated for the human ear earlier [7]. It is difficult to

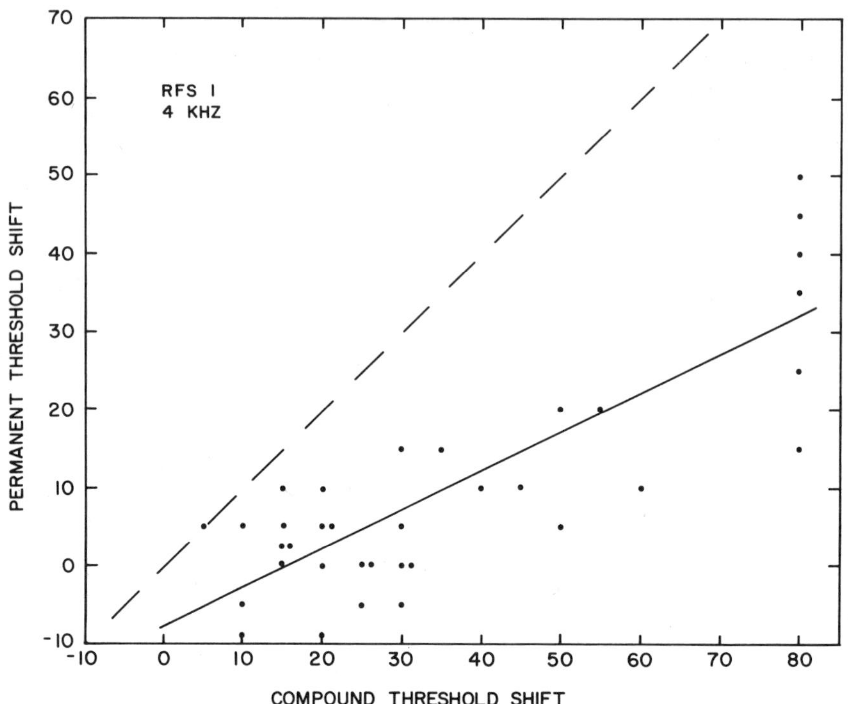

Fig. 11. Scatter plot of CTS vs PTS at 4.0 kHz for ears exposed to rifle impulses. Each data point represents one ear. The solid line is the least squares regression line fitting the data and the dashed line is plotted along a line of equal CTS/PTS.

say whether or not impulses of this type are prevalent outside the laboratory, in part because the short duration makes it difficult to measure accurately. If an impulse like that produced by the primer were measured by a meter on the commonly used "impulse" scale, the meter's relatively long time constant would cause it to under-indicate the true peak by about 20 dB.

It is hard to evaluate the possible effect of exposure to impulses above their respective CLs with respect to their contribution to the overall problem of noise-induced hearing loss. There is no doubt that only a few exposures in a lifetime can produce permanent loss. However, in industrial noise surveys such impulses may not be measured accurately, or because of their rarity may not be included in estimates of noise exposure. Also, the total energy required to do permanent loss is really small compared to other noise sources and so could logically be overlooked. Therefore, the strong possibility exists that current noise standards may tolerate levels that are much too high where the ear is tuned and even when measurements are made, they may underestimate the true exposures by an order of magnitude. Fortunately, there are probably not many noise sources that focus their energy just where it will do the most damage.

A final comment. While there is not time or space available to develop the arguments in detail, as far as I am aware, the concept of a spectrally dependent critical level is consistent with all the weapons noise exposure data that are available. In contrast, none of the existing DRCs appear to be reconcilable with the data. It is perhaps too early to

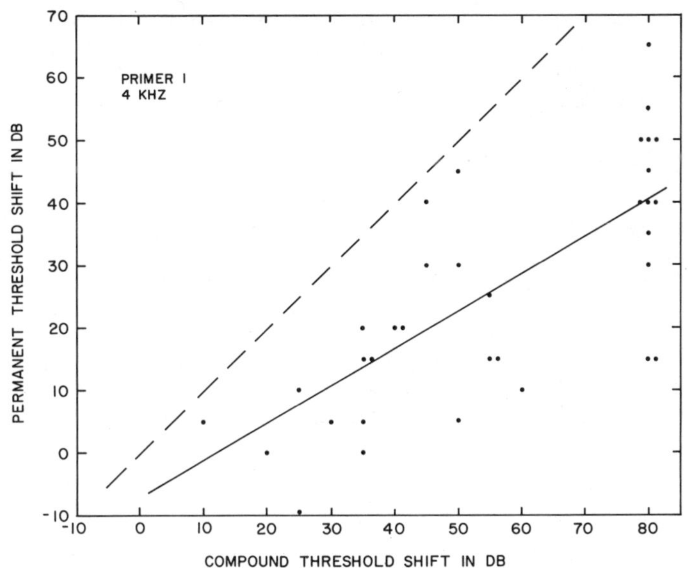

Fig. 12. Scatter plot of CTS vs PTS at 4.0 kHz for ears exposed to primer impulses. Each data point represents one ear. The solid line is the least squares regression line fitting the data and the dashed line is plotted along a line of equal CTS/PTS.

propose a perfect DRC; but it does appear that today we are in a position to do better.

REFERENCES

1. ISO-1999, Acoustics - determination of occupational noise exposure and estimation of noise-induced hearing impairment, Intn'l. Org. for Standardization (1981).
2. Ministry of Defense, Recommendation on evaluating the possible harmful effect of noise on hearing, Technical Coordination Group "Human Factors and Ergonomics", Direction Technique des Armaments Terrestres, 9211 Saint-Cloud Cedex (1982).
3. G. F. Smoorenburg, Damage risk criteria for impulse noise, Rept. 1980-26, Institute for Perception TNO, Soesterburg, The Netherlands (1980).
4. CHABA, 1968, Proposed damage-risk criterion for impulse noise (gunfire), Reprt of Working Group 57, Wash. D.C., NAS-NRC Comm. Hear. Bioacoust. Biomechan. (1968).
5. MIL-STD-1474B(MI), U.S.Army Missile Command, Redstone Arsenal, AL. (1979).
6. F. Pfander, Das Knalltrauma, Springer-Verlag, N.Y. (1975).
7. G. R. Price, Loss of auditory sensitivity to spectrally narrow impulses, J. Acoust. Soc. Am. 66:456 (1979).
8. G. R. Price, Implications of a critical level in the ear for assessment of noise hazard at high intensities, J. Acoust. Soc. Am., 69:171 (1981).
9. G. T. Singleton, D. L. Whitaker, R. J. Keim, F. J. and Kemker, Cordless telephones: a threat to hearing, Ann. Otol. Rhinol. Laryngol., 93:565 (1984).

10. G. R. Price, Mechanisms of loss for intense sound exposures, *in*: Perspectives in modern auditory research: A conference in honor of Dr. E. G. Wever, Amphora, Groton, Conn (1983b).
11. J. T. Broch, Random vibration of non-linear systems, *in*: Safety of structures under dynamic loading, Tapir Publishers, Trondheim, Norway (1979).
12. G. R. Price, Relative hazard of weapons impulses, *J. Acoust. Soc. Am.*, 73:556 (1983a).
13. G. R. Price and D. J. Lim, Susceptibility to intense impulses, *J. Acoust. Soc. Am.* 74:S8 (1984).
14. G. R. Price, A damage-risk criterion for impulse noise based on a spectrally dependent critical level, *Proc. 11th Int'l. Cong. Acoust.* 3:261 (1983c).
15. G. R. Price, Toward a theoretically based DRC for impulse noise, *J. Acoust. Soc. Am.*, 62:S95 (1977).
16. G. R. Price, Upper limit to stapes displacement: Implications for hearing loss, *J. Acoust. Soc. Am.*, 56:195 (1974).
17. G. R. Price, Hazard from intense, low spectral frequency acoustic impulses, Report in preparation (1985).
18. F. Pfander, H. Bongartz, H. Brinkmann, and H. Kietz, Danger of auditory impairment from impulse noise: A comparative study of the CHABA damage-risk criteria and those of the Federal Republic of Germany, *J. Acoust. Soc. Am.* 67:628 (1980).

DISCUSSION

von Gierke: You suggest that A-weighting does not work, but you did not show us the kinds of impulses. If you take the energy in each of the 3-5 kH range, do they show equal damage? For example, on the 3 spectra you showed, they fit one into the other. They have different peak pressure, but they have the same energy in the 3-5 range.

Price: In fact it is worse. That is to say, there is more energy in the cannon in the 3-5 kH region than there is in the rifle or the primer and yes the damage goes just the opposite. None of the physical analysis fits the data. There is a real problem essentially, with exposures to large caliber weapons noise which tend to be much higher, much more intense than exposures to the rifle and so if hearing protection fails, then you are in real trouble.

EXPERIMENTAL STUDIES OF IMPULSE NOISE

Per O. L. Nilsson[1], Jan Grenner[2], Bharti J. Katbamna[2], Sven Rydmarker[2] and Derek E. Dunn[2]

Department of Occupational Audiology,[1]
University of Gothenburg, Sahlgren's Hospital
Gothenburg and Department of Otolaryngology and
Department of Experimental Research,[2]
University of Lund, Malmo General Hospital
Sweden

INTRODUCTION

Based on empirical data from continuous noise exposures, the equal energy hypothesis (EEH) seems to provide a useful approximation of a trading relation between the noise level and the exposure time when the risk for hearing damage is evaluated. The basis for the EEH is discussed by Henderson et al. [1] in this volume. From the EEH, damage risk criteria (DRC) have been derived that relate the risk of hearing loss to noise exposure.

The new international DRC proposal, ISO/DIS 1999 [2], includes impulse noise as a risk criterion. However, investigations indicate that hearing loss does not follow the EEH under all conditions, particularly for impulse noise [3,4]. Even if the EEH is approximately correct, a literal interpretation may erroneously focus the attention of those concerned with noise abatement on reducing only the general sound level.

Impulse noise, however, contains many parameters that separately or in combination may have a different influence on hearing loss. Some of these factors are the rise time, the peak level, and the decay time expressed as the A-duration or the B-, C- or E-duration. Other important factors are the energy content of each impulse, the repetition rate between impulses, the equivalent sound level (Leq), as well as the crest factor. The crest factor is the ratio between the peak level and the equivalent sound level and is thus another expression of the impulsiveness of the noise.

Since experiments in humans may not be performed when there is a risk of permanent hearing damage, we must use animal experiments to study the effects of impulsive noise on the auditory system. Because of our earlier experience with continuous noise experiments in guinea-pigs, we preferred to use this model for our experiments with impulse noise. This chapter discusses the effects of different parameters of impulsive noise on the elevation of the threshold of the compound action potential (CAP) of the auditory nerve.

METHODS

We used pigmented, half-inbred, female guinea pigs with melanotic eyes that were 5 - 6 weeks of age (225-275 gms) at the time of exposure to noise. Five guinea pigs were used for each exposure in all experiments.

All sound exposures were performed in an anechoic chamber. Sounds were directed from above onto a circular, wire mesh cage in which each animal was individually enclosed in a separate sector. The cage was adjusted in the sound field so that the peak sound pressure and the Leq values were within $\pm$ 0.25 dB in each of the five sectors. The sound variables were always adjusted when the animals were not in the cage. Calibration was done for each exposure. In all experiments, we monitored peak sound pressure level, equivalent sound pressure level, frequency spectrum, repetition rate, and exposure duration.

To produce an impulse sound that permitted variation of the height of the pressure peak, duration of the total pulse, frequency content, and the repetition rate of the impulses, we used a click generated by an HP 3312 function generator. Signals were filtered by a Norwegian Electronics 704-017 multi-filter in order to shape the spectra. A Nagra IV SJ tape recorder was used to reproduce the exposure stimulus in the experiments with high frequency content impulses (metal plate blow) because it was not possible to simulate the ringings produced by such impulses with the function generator.

Four to five weeks after the noise exposure, we measured the auditory thresholds electrophysiologically by means of a standardized CAP threshold measurement procedure [5]. In addition, both ears of each animal were prepared for morphologic analysis with electron microscopic or light microscopic studies [6].

For each experimental group of five noise exposed animals, one control animal was used. Data on the control animals were analyzed according to the same procedure as for the experimental animals. Thresholds in the control animals were used as normative data for evaluating the threshold elevation in the experimental animals.

RESULTS

Effect of Leq

In order to investigate the effect of varying the Leq, we conducted a series of impulse noise exposures in which the animals were exposed to increasing energy levels. The repetition rate was varied but the peak level was maintained at the same 131.5 dB SPL for the impulses in all series. Continuous steady state noise exposures were also performed for comparison. In Fig. 1, the results are plotted for both the impulse noise series and the corresponding continuous noise series.

With continuous noise, no threshold elevation was demonstrated for Leq. levels below 102 dB SPL. However, above 102 dB, threshold increased linearly up to 117 dB Leq. By contrast, all impulsive noise exposures consistently caused threshold elevations. This elevation showed a small increase with increases in the Leq in the moderate energy range up to 114 dB Leq for six hours. Above 114 dB Leq, the threshold loss increased dramatically thus defining 114 dB Leq as the critical level. At 117 dB Leq, the CAP threshold shift was about the same as for steady state noise exposures.

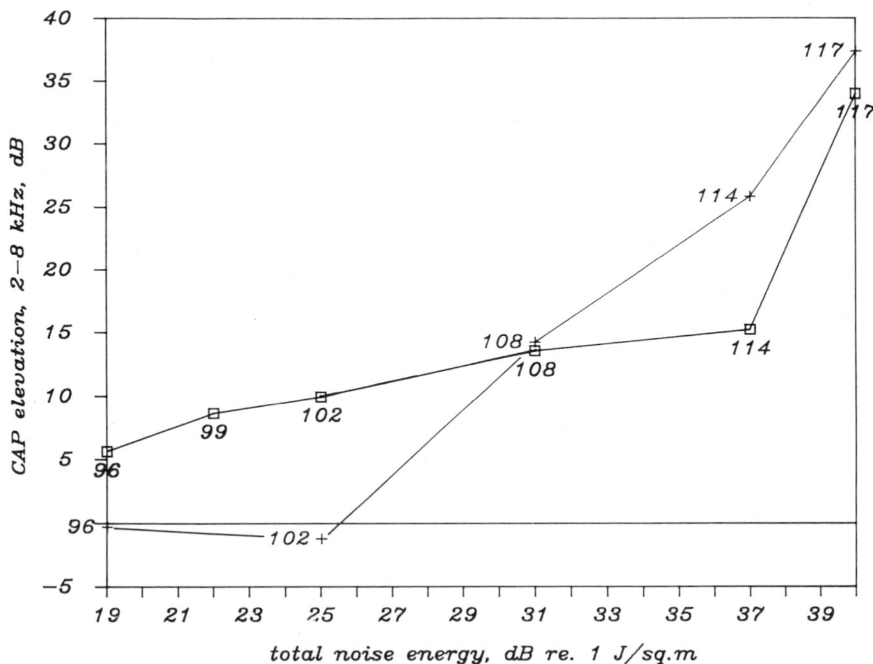

Fig. 1. CAP threshold elevation as a function of the total energy (in dB re 1 J/m^2) of steady state (crosses) and impulse (squares) noise exposures. Each symbol shows the average threshold for five animals. The numbers at the symbols give the Leq level in dB for each group. All groups were exposed for six hours. Peak-level of all impulse noise exposures was 131.5 dB SPL.

These results suggest that the physiological mechanisms underlying impulsive and continuous noise damage may be different. This is in agreement with our previous findings [7] that showed different morphological alterations resulting from the two types of noise exposure. In agreement with the findings of Ward and Turner [8], the critical level for continuous noise seems to be located at the level of zero threshold shift and increases linearly in accordance with the EEH. This finding contrasts sharply with results in the impulse noise series in which all results deviated from normal thresholds and the critical level was located at a higher energy level. This finding therefore indicates the existence of two critical levels in agreement with earlier studies [9-11]. Since the threshold elevation curves for the two noise exposures have different slopes for intensities between 102 and 117 dB, it is incorrect to combine the continuous and impulse noise data in the same DRC.

Importance of Exposure Duration

Fig. 2 shows the effect of changing the total sound energy by successively doubling the exposure time between 3 and 24 hours. We did two series of this kind, one exposed below (at 102 dB Leq) and one above the critical level (at 117 dB Leq). The slopes of these two exposure duration curves are similar, even though the equivalent sound levels (i.e., the impulsive repetition rate) differed. The effect of duration was fairly linear, and the regression lines had the same slope in both series.

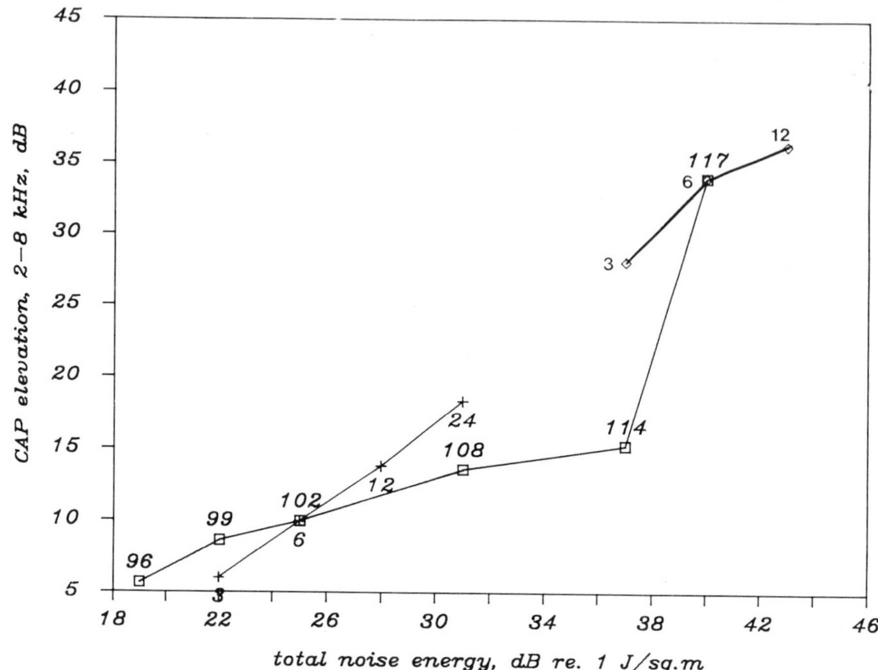

Fig. 2. CAP threshold elevation following impulse noise exposure as a function of total noise energy. At each symbol, which gives the mean value for five animals, the number indicates either exposure time and/or exposure intensity. Exposure intensity for the crosses was 102 dB Leq and for the diamonds, was 117 dB Leq. Squares show the data from Fig. 1 in which the peak level was 131.5 dB SPL, the duration was 6 hours and the repetition rate was varied resulting in Leq values from 96 to 117 dB.

For comparison, Fig. 2 shows the CAP thresholds for the six hour exposures with different Leq values. Below the critical level, the slope of the noise intensity function differed significantly from the slope of the noise duration function. From the regression lines, it was thus possible to calculate the q-value for the trading relation between the time and intensity changes. For changes below the critical energy level, q = 7.85, which means that doubling or halving the exposure time corresponds to a 7.85 dB change in the sound intensity. By contrast, above the critical level, the trading relation was different. A doubling of the time for a 117 dB intensity exposure would change the mean threshold (between 2 and 8 kHz) by about 4 dB, but only a 0.64 dB change in intensity was required to cause the same change in CAP threshold.

It is thus apparent that an EEH with a trading relation of 3 dB (q=3) is not valid. The results also indicate that the trading relation between exposure time and intensity is non-linear with regard to the critical level, which agrees with the Ward assumptions [12].

Importance of Impulse Peak Level

In Fig. 3 results are given for auditory threshold as a function of increasing sound energy. For each exposure, the Leq and the impulse peak level were increased simultaneously. Thus, the crest factor, (the ratio

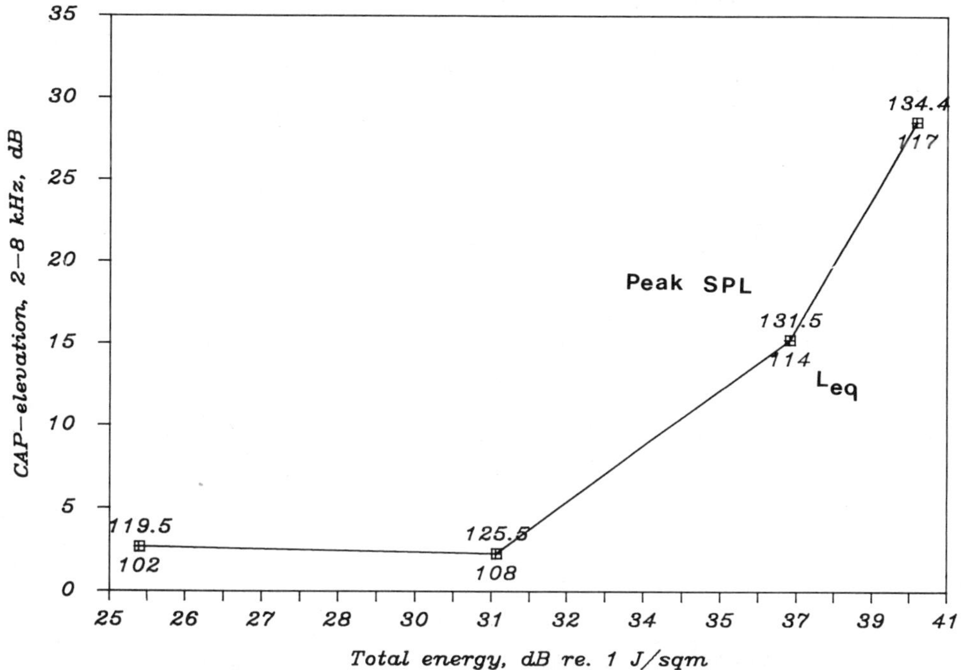

Fig. 3. CAP threshold elevation following impulse noise exposures as a function of increasing total noise energy. Each symbol represents the mean value for each group of five animals. The numbers give the peak sound pressure level and equivalent level at which the groups were exposed.

between the sound peak SPL and the equivalent level) was kept constant in contrast to the impulsive noise exposures shown in Fig. 1. For this impulsive exposure, the results were similar to those found with continuous noise exposure (Fig. 1). For exposures below a peak value of 125.5 dB and a Leq of a 108 dB, there was little change in the CAP threshold. However, above that level, the change in threshold was great. This difference suggests that the main reason for the shape of the impulse noise threshold elevation curve in Fig. 1, may be that a constant sound peak level was used. Consequently the crest-factor must be important to the threshold elevation.

We therefore investigated the influence of changing peak levels. In Fig. 4, the auditory threshold change is given as a function of different peak levels without changes in the other exposure parameters. For different curves, the Leq level, the exposure time, and total energy were the same. Since most energy is located in the peak (energy is proportional to the square of the sound pressure), increasing peak levels were compensated for by a reduction of the repetition rate in order to maintain the equivalent level. As can be seen in the figure, the threshold generally increased with peak level. However, in some instances, threshold was also diminished. While some of these decreases were within the error of measurement, the decreased repetition rate might contribute to an increase in the resting time between impulses and thus to the reduced threshold.

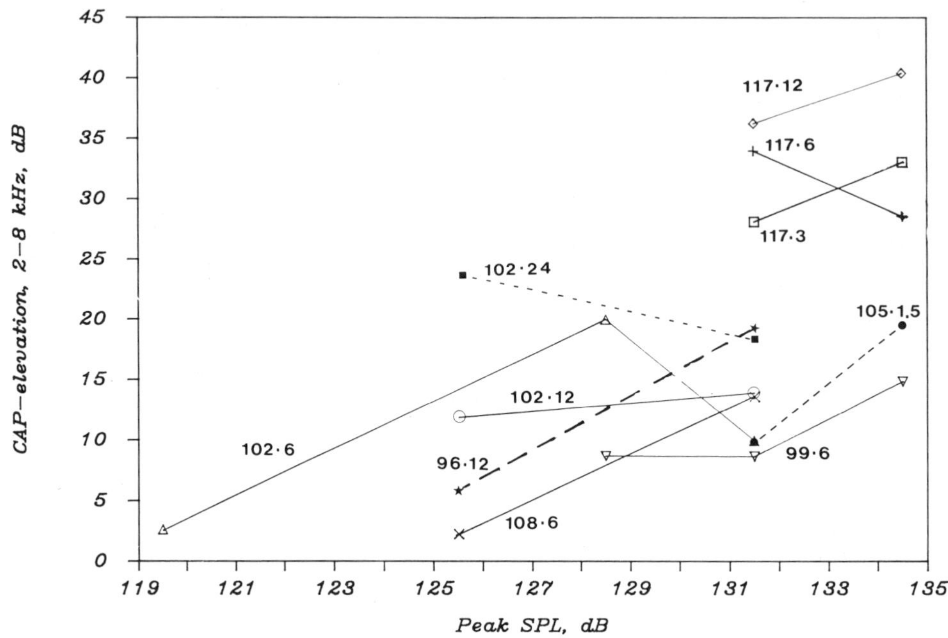

Fig. 4. CAP threshold elevation following impulse noise exposures as a function of peak sound pressure level. For ech curve in the graph, the other parameters of impulse noise were kept constant, thus keeping the total energy exposure constant.

Importance of Crest Factor

Figs. 5a and 5b give the result of the CAP elevation as a function of increasing the crest factor. In about half of the exposures, increasing the crest factor resulted in a reduction in threshold shift (Fig. 5a) and increasing threshold elevation in the rest (Fig. 5b). The reason for this variability is probably that the crest factor is arbitrary in relation to real peak levels. Since all exposures which exceed the critical level cause severe threshold elevation, low crest factors above the critical level would give rise to high threshold elevation. Below the critical level, the situation is reversed. When total energy is low enough, even high crest factors would cause very little change in threshold. Therefore, the crest factor does not have an independent role in determining cochlear damage, but it must be evaluated in connection with other impulse noise factors, such as total energy and critical level. At comparable noise levels, Bruel [13] found that differences in crest factors were related to differences in damage from industrial noise exposures in humans.

Importance of Impulse Spectra

In order to investigate the effect of the spectrum of the impulse, we created another impulse noise by recording a hammer blow on metal. This noise was then compared with the previously mentioned synthetic hammer blow on wood. The sounds were recorded on a Nagra IV SJ tape recorder and replayed on an endless loop. Fig. 6 gives the threshold elevation for all test frequencies for the series exposed to the hammer blow on wood, whereas Fig. 7 gives the corresponding results for the "metal-exposed" animals. Comparison between the figures indicates a more prominent threshold change in the 4 - 10 kHz region for the high frequency metal exposure. Although

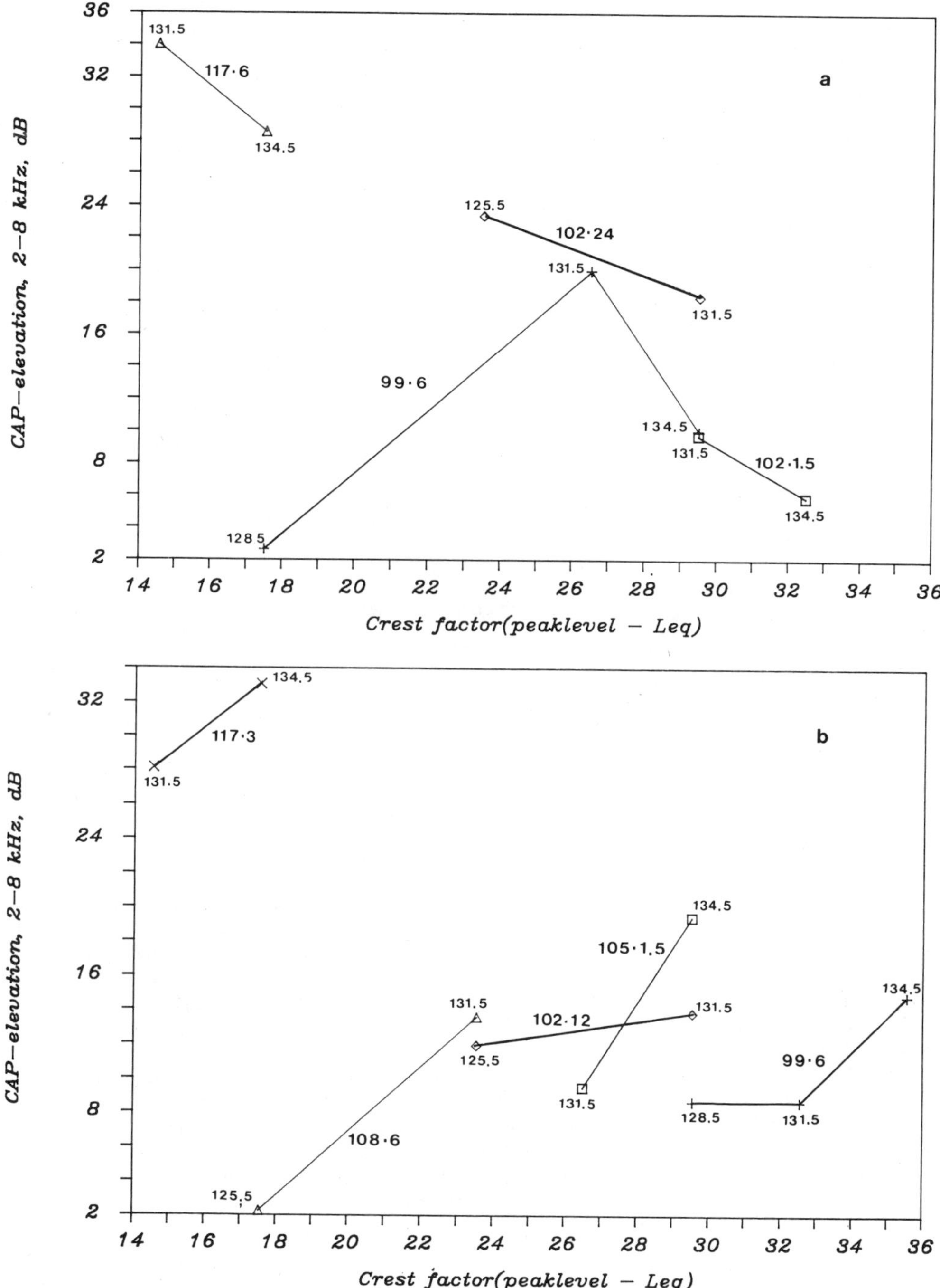

Fig. 5. CAP threshold elevation after impulse noise exposure as a function of crest factor. a). Decreasing threshold elevation as a function of crest factor. b). Increasing threshold elevation with increasing crest factor. Each symbol represents the average for five animals. For each group the numbers indicate the peak SPL and for each series the exposure intensity and time are given.

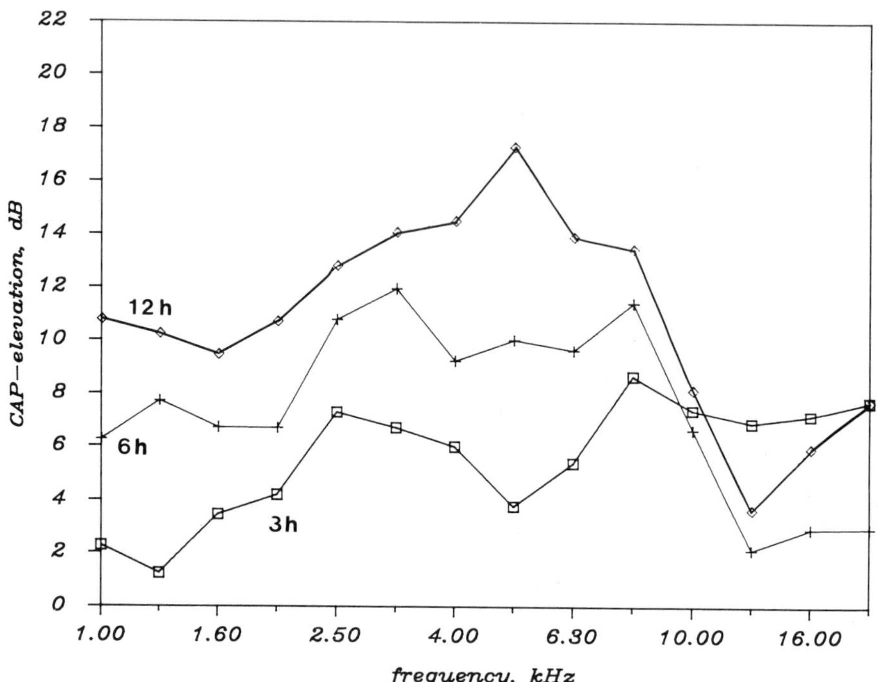

Fig. 6. CAP threshold elevation after exposure to impulsive noise simulating a hammerblow on wood. Each curve represents the average threshold for 10 ears from five animals for three different exposure times of 3, 6, and 12 hours.

mean values for the 2 - 10 kHz frequency range were higher for the metal than the synthetic noise-exposure, the differences were not statistically significant because of great individual variation.

The issue of the noise spectrum and its subsequent damaging effect has been subject to controversy. Burns and Robinson [14], in their investigation of industrial, continuous noise exposures found that spectra with a higher proportion of low frequency noise induced more damage in workers than spectra with high frequencies. Their finding was explained, however, by the error of A-weighting, since the A-filter does not parallel the sensitivity of the ear at high level noise exposures. Contrary to their findings, Passchier-Vermeer [15] found that workers in the metal industry with high frequency impulse noise suffered more hearing loss than workers in the wood industry. When plotting risk criteria for different types of noise, Bruel [3] also found that in industries with high frequency noises, hearing loss was more likely to occur than in low frequency noise. The tendency from our results seems to agree with this conclusion.

Importance of Decay Time

In this experiment one animal group, exposed in the anechoic chamber, was compared to another group exposed to the same impulse noise, but in an ordinary concrete room. In the latter group, the B-duration of each impulse was at last ten times longer and therefore contained much more energy than in the first group. In order to produce the same Leq, the repetition rate was reduced for the latter group. Fig. 8 gives the threshold elevation for the test frequencies of the two groups. The animals exposed in

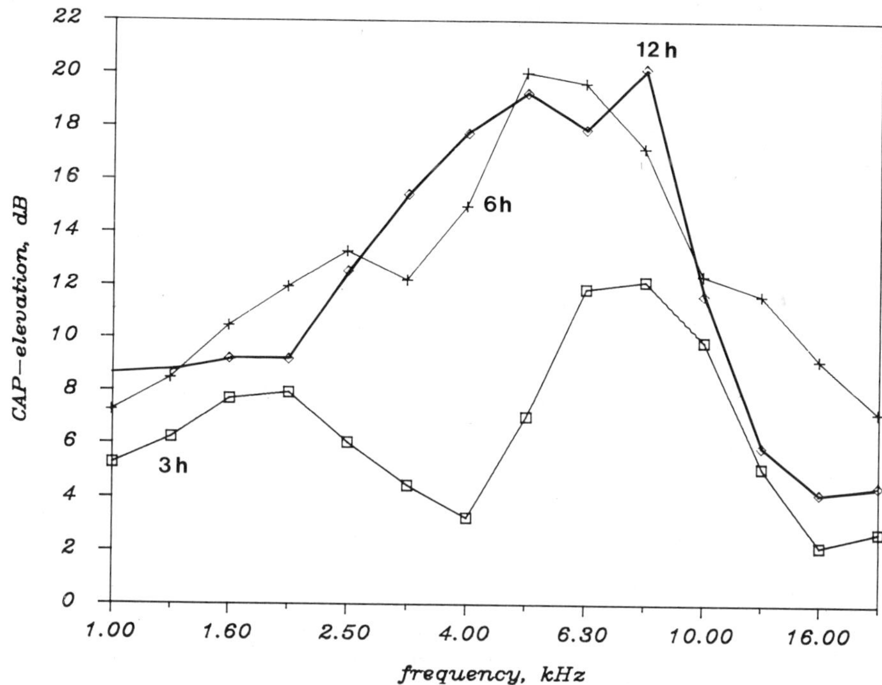

Fig. 7. CAP threshold elevation after exposure to impulsive noise simulating a hammer blow on metal. Each curve represents the threshold average for 10 ears from five animals.

the reverberant room had a much higher threshold elevation than those in the anechoic chamber, and the difference was significant. We therefore conclude that the decay time for each impulse has a very important function in causing threshold elevation. Since both groups were exposed to the same peak SPL, equivalent level, and exposure time, the damaging effect of the longer decay time in the reverberant room was not compensated for by the longer interstimulus interval. It is important to recognize that ordinary noise measurements do not reveal the effect of reverberation on the decay time of the individual impulses, and such differences in decay time may contribute to differences in threshold elevation.

SUMMARY

This chapter discusses the results from a variety of impulse noise exposures in the guinea pig which could be of great importance to humans. The results indicate that a generalizing formula for evaluating the risk of threshold elevation like the EEH may ignore the importance of some impulse noise parameters, but not others. Our experiments verify the existence of a critical level of noise energy which constitutes a definite non-linear change in the input/output function of noise-induced threshold elevation. In addition, the threshold shift caused by impulse noise differs from that caused by continuous steady-state noise. Furthermore, changes in exposure time below the critical level of energy are of greater importance than changes in intensity. At corresponding noise energy levels, the peak sound pressure level has a damaging effect which seems to be of greater importance than the repetition rate. Increasing the high frequency content of the impulse only results in a non-significant tendency to higher damage

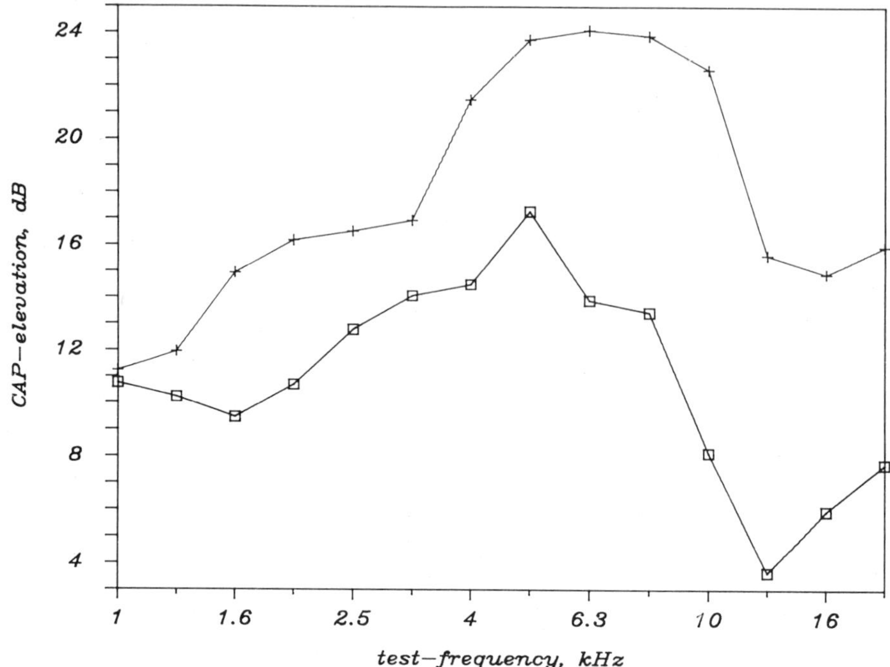

Fig. 8. CAP threshold elevation as a function of impulse noise exposure illustrating the threshold elevation for different test frequencies for two different groups. Crosses represent the average threshold elevation for five animals (10 ears) exposed in the reverberant room and the squares represents values for the animals exposed in the anechoic chamber.

induction as compared to impulses with low frequency content. This difference could perhaps be explained by the frequency sensitivity of the ear of the guinea pig. However, differences in decay time of each impulse seem to be of great importance. Our experiments demonstrated that a ten-fold increase of the B-duration significantly increased threshold.

It must be emphasized that the absolute values from our experiments on auditory thresholds and noise energy cannot be transferred to humans. Nevertheless, we believe that the general conclusions of the effects of different parameters of impulsive noise can be applied to humans also. One important goal for future research is to find methods to verify that humans are subject to similar risks from different impulse noise parameters. Such knowledge could then be used to improve noise abatement programs.

ACKNOWLEDGEMENT

The project was supported by the Swedish Work Environment Fund.

REFERENCES

1. D. Henderson, R. P. Hamernik and R. J. Salvi, A parametric evaluation of the equal energy hypothesis, in: "Noise-induced Hearing Loss: Basic and Applied Aspects," eds., R. J. Salvi, D. Henderson and R. P. Hamernik, Plenum Press, New York.

2. ISO/DIS 1999, "Acoustics - Determination of Occupational Noise Exposure and Estimation of Noise-Induced Hearing Impairment, Draft," ISO (1982).
3. P. V. Bruel, Do we measure damaging noise correctly?, in: "Noise Control Engineering," (1977).
4. W. Passchier-Vermeer, Measurement and rating of impulse noise in relation to noise-induced hearing loss, in: "Proceedings of the Fourth International Congress on Noise as a Public Health Problem," G. Rossi, ed., Ampliphone, Milano (1983).
5. P. Nilsson and J. Grenner, A system for evoked response audiometry in small animals , LUMEDW/(MERM-3005) (1985).
6. P. Nilsson, S. Rydmarker, D. E. Dunn and C. Lindkvist, Methods for morphological evaluation of the inner ear, LUMEDW/(MERM-3007) (1985).
7. P. Nilsson, B. Erlandsson, H. Hakanson, A. Ivarsson and J. Wersall, Morphological damage in the guinea pig cochlea after impulse noise and pure tone exposures, Scand. Audiol. Suppl. 12:155 (1980).
8. W. D. Ward and C. W. Turner, The total energy concept as a unifying approach to the prediction of noise trauma and its application to exposure criteria, in: "New Perspectives on Noise-Induced Hearing Loss", eds., R. P. Hamernik, Donald Henderson and R. J. Salvi, Raven Press (1982).
9. H. Spoendlin and J. P. Brun, Relation of structural damage to exposure time and intensity in acoustic trauma, Acta Otolaryngol. (Stockh) 75:220 (1973).
10. B. Erlandsson, H. Hakanson, A. Ivarsson, P. Nilsson and J. Wersall, Hair cell damage in the guinea pig due to different kinds of noise, Acta Otolaryngol. Suppl. 367:1 (1980).
11. H,. Wagner and H. Berndt, On the overload effect of sound impulses to the inner ear, Arch. ORL 232:179 (1981).
12. W. D. Ward, Effects of impulse noise on hearing, Scan. Audiol. Suppl. 12:339 (1980).
13. P. V. Bruel, The influence of high crest factor noise on hearing damage, Scan. Audiol. Suppl. 12:25 (1980).
14. W. Burns and D. W. Robinson, Hearing and noise in industry, Her Majesty's Stationery Office, London (1970).
15. W. Passchier-Vermeer, Steady-state and fluctuating noise: Its effects on the hearing of people, in: "Occupational Hearing Loss," ed., D. W. Robinson, Academic Press, London (1971).

DISCUSSION

Manninen: Do you have any data on the rate of growth of TTS? Our experience with humans is that TTS grows steadily for about an hour, then the rate plateaus and finally begins to grow again as the exposure continues.

Nilsson: For three different intensity levels, there appears to be a growth up to about six hours. At six hours there may be a plateau.

McFadden: Is it possible that the plateaus you are seeing for durations might be influenced by some biological cycle of the animal rather than a direct effect of the noise?

von Gierke: Don Parker at Miami University and Dave Lim did some experiments with us using guinea pigs. They were exposed to noise during their daily feeding period or slightly before, during and prior to being electrically stimulated. The histology showed no difference whatever in the amount of damage.

Trahoitis: Have you ever used the same stimulation but put in a peak clipper? I am thinking specifically of Henderson and his colleagues work about the interaction or peaks and noise. Perhaps if you used the peak clipper you may get different data for the same nominal exposure.

Nilsson: We have not used a peak clipper, but according to the formula for calculating the energy, the peaks contribute greatly because pressure squared is the quantity measured. So, if you could clip the peak you would assume much less damage.

Stevins: What is the correspondence between the response of guinea pigs and humans to a 90 dB or another equivalent level?

Nilsson: I am not quite sure because we cannot do these kind of experiments in humans.

THE ROLE OF PEAK PRESSURE IN DETERMINING THE AUDITORY HAZARD OF IMPULSE NOISE

James H. Patterson, Jr.[1], Ilia M. Lomba-Gautier[1], Dennis L. Curd[1], Roger P. Hamernik[2], Richard J. Salvi[2], C. E. Hargett, Jr.[2], and George Turrentine[2]

[1]Sensory Research Division, U.S. Army Aeromedical Research Laboratory, Fort Rucker, Alabama 36362-5000

[2]Callier Center for Communication Disorders, University of Texas at Dallas, Texas 75235

INTRODUCTION

Most current Damage Risk Criteria (DRC) for human exposure to impulse noise are written in terms of peak pressure as the primary index of the traumatic potential or hazard associated with exposure to an impulse noise. Since the peak pressure is only one of many parameters of an impulse, there is a question whether a DRC based on peak pressure can reflect accurately the hazard to hearing posed by impulse noise.

The current U.S. Army recommendation on what constitutes hazardous impulse noise is traceable to the 1968 report [1] from the National Research Council Committee on Hearing, Bioacoustics, and Biomechanics (CHABA). The impulse noise limit stated in the CHABA document was based on the scant data available at the time and was defined in terms of peak pressure, A-duration, and B-duration. The authors of the CHABA document recognized the potential shortcomings and included a series of disclaimers which are typified by the statement: "While these curves do not do great violence to the published data on either Temporary Threshold Shift (TTS) or Permanent Threshold Shift (PTS) from impulse noise ... they admittedly represent only a first attempt at a reasonable DRC for exposures to impulse noise. Parameters that are ignored in the present criterion may eventually be shown to be important." This was an open invitation for further refinement of this DRC through additional research. This research has generally not materialized. However, the CHABA document was the basis for the current versions of the two Army documents which restrict noise exposure. The first document, TB-MED-501 [2], "simplified" the original criterion by ignoring durations and setting a conservative limit of 140 dB on the peak sound pressure level (SPL). Consequently, whenever impulse noise exceeds 140 dB peak SPL, TB-MED-501 dictates that hearing conservation measures must be taken. The second U.S. Army document based on the CHABA criterion is MIL-STD-1474B(MI) [3]. This standard specifies noise limits for Army material.

The United Kingdom [4] has adopted a noise limit standard very similar to that of the U.S. Army. The basic parameters used to assess hazards are identical. However, the limiting level is different because of a difference in protection percentages. The Netherlands and West Germany employ standards [5-7] which use a peak pressure criterion as in the U.S. documents, except that the impulse duration is defined differently. Only the French [8] have recently adopted a standard which is not based on peak pressure. They use the A-weighted energy of an impulse in their noise limits.

One of the primary shortcomings of the earlier research was that it focused primarily on peak pressure as a quantifier of impulse noise exposures. Until recently, there has been an almost complete lack of attention to the distribution of acoustic energy across frequencies. In most cases, it is now impossible to reconstruct the energy density spectra of the impulses used in many of the early studies, because the peak measures reported do not contain sufficient information to permit this calculation. The general lack of research in this area has left most of the questions posed by the authors of the original CHABA DRC still unanswered.

The experiments described in this report were designed to determine whether peak pressure is an adequate quantifier for an impulse noise DRC. The general approach was to construct two types of impulse noise waveforms with the same Fourier pressure spectrum [9], but with different peak pressures (i.e., with a different phase spectrum). This makes it possible to compare the hearing loss and injury resulting from impulses which have the same total energy distributed the same way across frequency, but with different peak pressures. In addition, we can compare injury from impulses having the same peak pressure and different energy levels. For the limited range of exposure parameters used in these experiments, this approach provides a test of the sufficiency of using peak pressure as a predictor of auditory hazard.

METHODS AND PROCEDURES

The experiments that are described in this report follow a relatively straightforward paradigm: Pre-exposure measures of hearing are obtained on each animal; the animal is exposed to the impulse noise; following exposure, the animal's hearing thresholds are remeasured at various postexposure times; then, following a fixed period of recovery, the sensory structures of the cochlea are prepared for histological examination. Such a paradigm allows for comparisons to be made among variables, such as (1) the physical exposure conditions, (2) temporary changes in hearing, (3) permanent changes in hearing, and (4) the extent and nature of the cochlear damage.

Subjects

The subjects were monaural chinchillas aged from 12 to approximately 49 months at the start of the study. Each animal was made monaural by surgically destroying the left cochlea. The surgery was performed with the animal anesthetized using halothane gas. The animals were allowed at least one week postoperative recovery time before proceeding with the audiometric training and testing.

Behavioral Testing Procedures

The audiometric instrumentation and procedures have been previously described in detail by Patterson et al. [10]. The chinchillas were tested in a double-grilled cage within a soundproof room. Mounted on the cage was a row of photocells to detect the animal's location and an electronic buzzer which was used as a secondary reinforcer. Standard audio equipment was used to generate and adjust the signal level. The pure tone signals were delivered through an Altec coaxial loudspeaker. The control, duration, and sequencing of events, as well as recording, were accomplished using a microprocessor. The behavior of the animals was monitored on a closed-circuit television.

Each animal received training sessions until it scored 95% correct for three successive sessions. A modified method of limits [10,11] was used to estimate thresholds. Audiograms were taken until the average threshold was within plus or minus 5 dB of the normative data for the chinchilla [11,12] on five consecutive sessions. Then audiograms were obtained until the day of exposure. The last five audiograms before exposure were averaged across sessions to produce the baseline audiogram for the particular animal. The baseline audiogram for each animal was used as a reference for computing the postexposure threshold shifts.

Exposure Stimuli

Two types of impulses were synthesized for use as exposure stimuli. One of these, called the high peak stimulus, is the result of applying a 200-microsecond rectangular pulse to the exposure circuit described below. The second type of impulse, the low peak stimulus, was generated using a procedure described by Patterson and Green [13]. Briefly, a digital impulse was passed through a bank of digital all-pass filters. This produced a signal whose amplitude spectrum is the same as the original impulse, but with an altered phase spectrum and, consequently, an altered time history. To produce the low-peak impulses, 25 elemental all-pass filters were selected from a set of 50 elemental filters. The selection was made by generating several hundred of the combinations of 50 filters chosen 25 at a time and picking the signal with the lowest peak.

The exposure stimuli were synthesized on a PDP 11/34 minicomputer or an SEL Systems 85 and converted to electrical pulses by a 16 bit digital-to-analogue (D-A) converter. The output of the D-A converter was low pass filtered at 5.0 kHz by a Rockland System 816, 8-pole Bessel filter. This signal was amplified through an Altec amplifier and converted to acoustic impulses by an Altec 290D driver. A 10 cm extension throat with 4.8 cm diameter opening was bolted to the driver.

Figs. 1 and 2 show the time history and spectrum of the high peak and the low peak impulse, respectively. These spectra are essentially the amplitude response of the Altec 290D driver. When these two impulses are equated for total energy (and energy spectrum), there is an 8 dB difference in the peak pressures as well as a difference in when the peak of the impulse occurs.

The animal was positioned with the entrance of the ear canal at the center of the driver extension throat. The animal's pinna was taped to a flange on the throat which served to stabilize the positioning of both the ear canal and the pinna. Casual observation indicated that stabilizing the pinna was necessary, since animals would fold the pinna back along the head and possibly close the ear canal.

Each exposure consisted of 100 impulses of the same wave shape (high or low peak) presented at constant intensity throughout. The impulses were delivered at a rate of one every three seconds.

Experimental Design

A total of 36 animals were used in these experiments. They were divided into six groups (six animals/group) and exposed to the impulse conditions presented in Table 1.

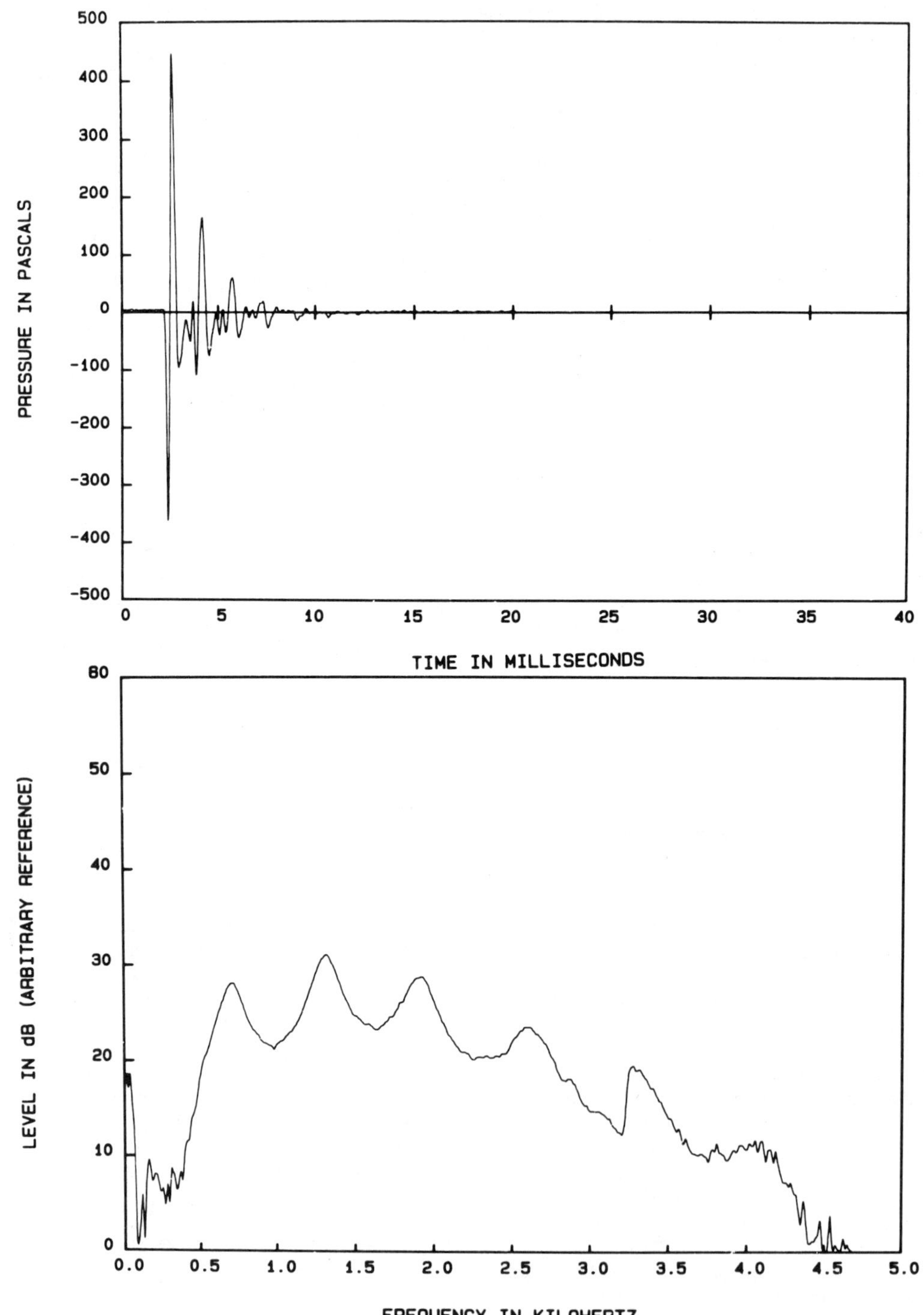

Fig. 1. The high-peak impulse pressure-time waveform (upper) and the frequency spectrum of the impulse (lower).

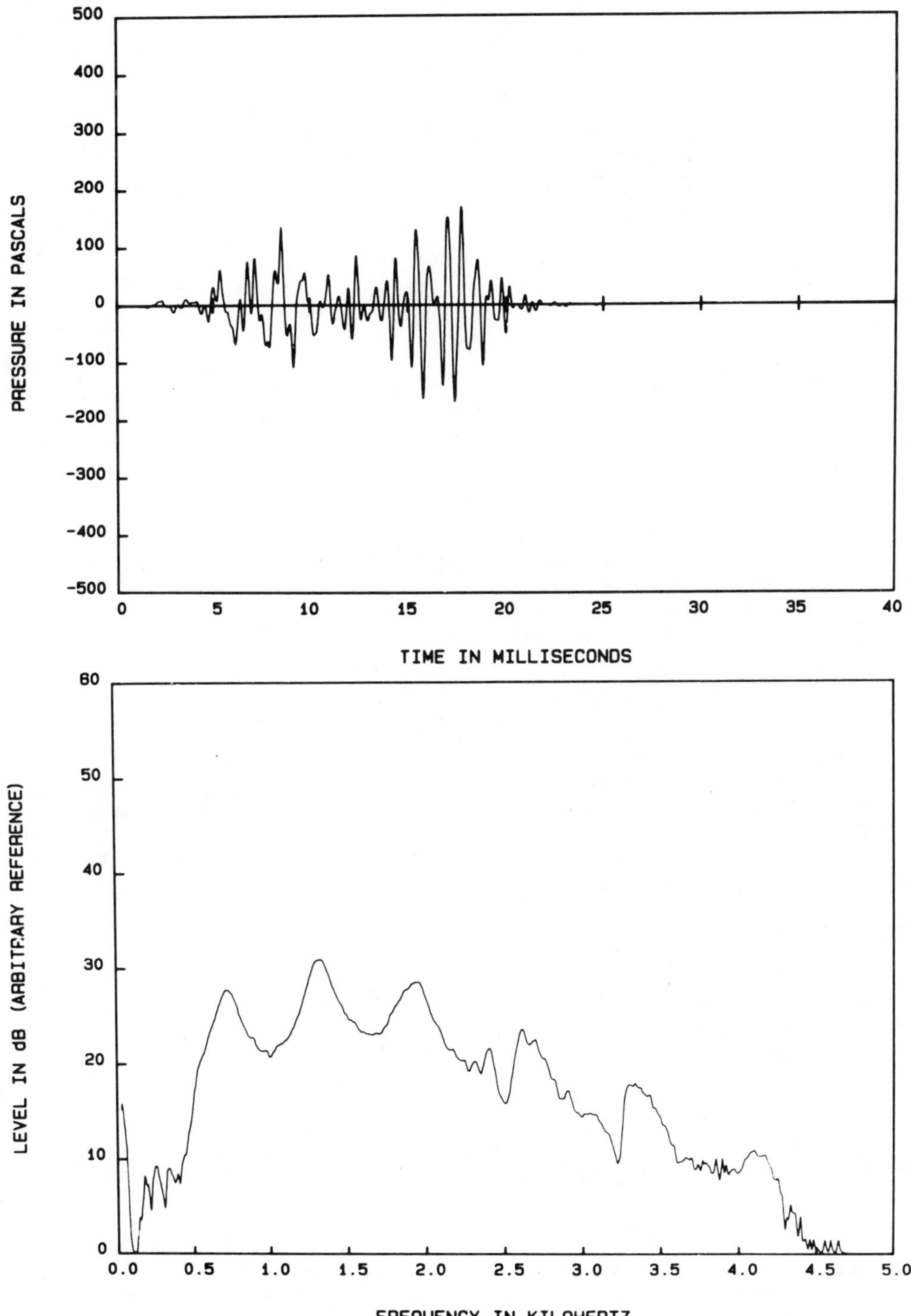

Fig. 2. The low-peak impulse pressure-time waveform (upper) and the frequency spectrum of the impulse (lower).

Table 1. Identification of the Exposure Conditions for the Six Experimental Groups

Subject Group	Stimulus Type	Peak Pressure (dB SPL)	Energy per n t rea Per Impulse (J/M^2)	Total Energy Level of the Exposure (dB re 1 J/M^2)
1	High peak	147	.095	9.78
2	Low peak	139	.097	9.87
3	High peak	139	.015	1.76
4	Low peak	131	.015	1.76
5	High peak	135	.006	-2.22
6	Low peak	127	.006	-2.22

Groups 1 and 2 were exposed to impulses having approximately equal energy, but with peak pressures that differed by 8 dB. Similarly, Groups 3 and 4 and Groups 5 and 6 formed pairs of exposure groups where the energy was equivalent, but the peak pressures differed by 8 dB. On the other hand, Groups 2 and 3 received exposures where the peak pressures were equal, but the energy differed by 8 dB. An attempt was made to match Groups 4 and 5 with respect to peak pressure; however, after gathering preliminary data it was apparent that the high peak stimulus produced virtually no effect at a peak of 131 dB. Therefore, the peak level for Group 5 was set at 135 dB and Group 6 at an equivalent energy level. This arrangement of two wave types crossed with three energy levels fits the analysis of variance model for a two-factor independent groups experiment. In order to analyze all frequencies simultaneously, audiometric test frequency was added as a third factor with repeated measures [14].

Recovery Conditions

Complete audiograms were obtained starting 2 minutes after an exposure (referred to as time t=0) and at postexposure times of 32, 62, 92, 182, and 362 minutes; 24 and 48 hours; and at 6, 9, 13, 16, 20, 23, 27, and 30 days after exposure. Temporary Threshold Shifts (TTS) for each animal were calculated from each postexposure audiogram by subtracting the animal's baseline audiogram. The threshold shifts for each animal obtained at 20, 23, 27 and 30 days postexposure were averaged to produce an estimate of the animal's PTS. These TTS or PTS data were averaged across all animals constituting a particular group to obtain the group average TTS or PTS.

Histology

At 88 to 90 days postexposure, the animals were anesthetized with halothane and then decapitated. Following decapitation, the right stapes was removed and the round window membrane was slit. Each cochlea was fixed by perilymphatic perfusion of 2.5 percent glutaraldehyde in 0.1 M PO buffer and postfixed in 1 percent osmium-tetroxide in 0.1 M PO buffer. Cochleas were washed in buffer, and then dehydrated in ETOH. The entire basilar membrane and stria vascularis were piecewise dissected free from their bony attachments and mounted in glycerin on glass slides for a surface preparation light microscopic analysis [15].

The percentage of missing inner and outer hair cell were determined as a function of distance along the cochlear duct. Baseline normal sensory cell populations were established at octave lengths along the cochlea using a population of 30 normal chinchillas. A frequency-place map established by Eldredge et al. [16] was used to superimpose frequency on the length coordinate of the cochleogram so that audiometric data could be directly related to the sensory cell populations along the length of the cochlea.

RESULTS AND DISCUSSION

Postexposure Threshold Shift

The group average threshold recovery curves at 1.4 kHz for all six experimental groups over a period of 30 days are shown in Fig. 3. The recovery curves at other test frequencies were qualitatively similar. The overall temporal configuration of these recovery curves is similar. In general, each of the recovery curves can be broken into two parts; the early phase $0 < t < 24$ hours (t = postexposure time) and a later phase $1 < t < 30$ days. During the early phase, there is not a consistent pattern to the recovery function, i.e., threshold shifts in general either do not recover or continue to get worse before an orderly recovery period begins. This phenomenon has been described previously [17,18], where it has been referred to as a postexposure growth of TTS. During the later phase, there is an orderly recovery of threshold which follows a time course which is approximately linear in log-time, until a relatively stable plateau is reached at around 25-30 days after exposure. The mean threshold shift at this plateau is defined as PTS. There is, in general, an orderly increase in the amount of TTS across groups of animals as the energy of the exposure increases.

Traditionally, threshold shift measured minutes after exposure (TTSo) has been used as an index of the severity of a noise exposure. For moderate exposures, TTSo is usually the maximum shift observed. However, in situations where the recovery function follows a complex biphasic recovery pattern, a more appropriate measure may be the maximum threshold shift (TTSmax) recorded, regardless of the point in time at which it occurs. In Figs. 4 and 5, the group mean TTSo and TTSmax audiograms are plotted for each experimental group. In both figures, we get an appreciation for the orderly increase in threshold shift across test frequencies for each group as the energy of the exposure increases. The shift across frequency for each group is relatively flat, and increases from approximately 20-30 dB at the lowest exposure level to 80-90 dB at the highest exposure level. It should be noted that TTSmax is greater than TTSo for virtually all test conditions at all frequencies. This is another indication of the growth of TTS following exposure. When the threshold shifts become large, the ability to distinguish between groups on the basis of TTS becomes more difficult.

Within groups having approximately equal energy exposures, there is the tendency in the mean data for the exposures with higher peak pressures to produce greater TTSo and TTSmax. However, in comparing groups with unequal energies, i.e., Group 4, 131 dB low peak exposure with Group 5, 135 dB high peak exposure, the 131 dB exposure consistently produces greater mean TTSo and TTSmax. Such relations between pressure and energy variables hold at the higher levels, but the effects appear less pronounced due to the compressive effect mentioned above.

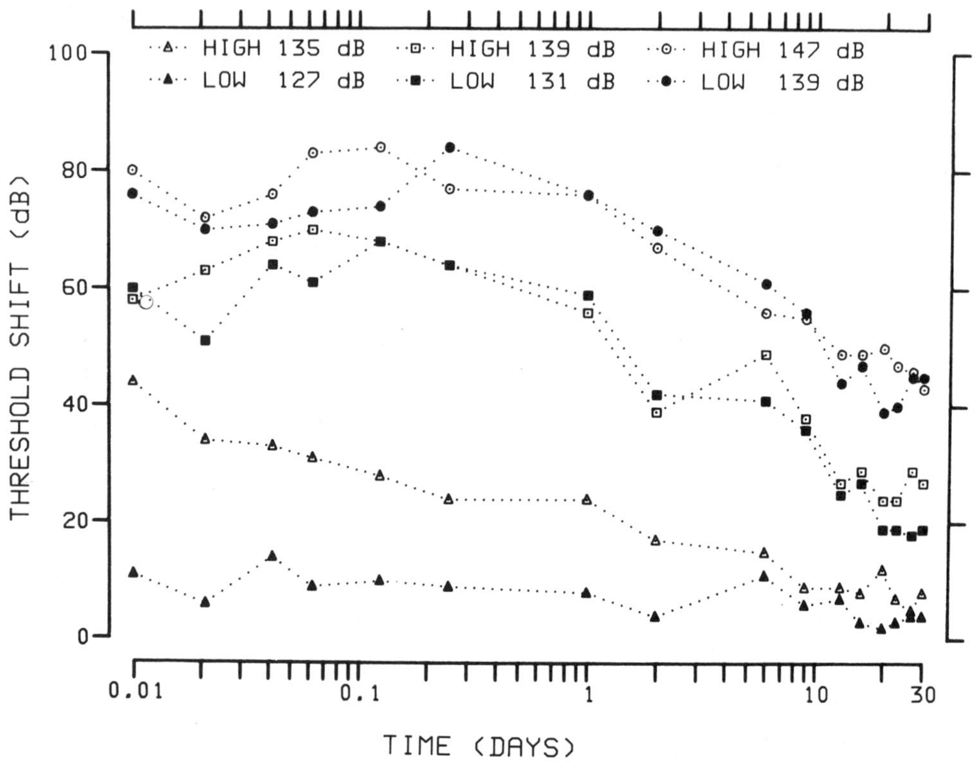

Fig. 3. The group mean threshold recovery curves for each exposure condition at the 1.4 kHz test frequency.

The differences between pairs of exposure groups having equal energies are less pronounced if one considers the TTS data at times t>24 hours. During this late phase of recovery (See Fig. 3), groups with equal energy exposures have similar TTS.

The threshold shift remaining at 20 to 30 days postexposure was used as a measure of PTS. The last four data points on the recovery functions were averaged for each test frequency to estimate the PTS for each animal.

Fig. 6 illustrates the PTS for each exposure group. Within exposure groups, the PTS is relatively uniformly distributed across frequency, producing a flat audiometric configuration. Generally, the PTS is well ordered according to increasing energy of exposure [9,10] with the lowest energy levels producing on the average, less than 10 dB PTS. Moderate energy levels produced on the order of 20 dB PTS, and the highest energy levels produced around 40 dB PTS. This increase of PTS with energy level of the exposure is shown more clearly in Fig. 7 where the average PTS at 1, 2, and 4 kHz is computed and plotted against energy level of the exposure. In addition to the regular increase of PTS with energy level, we also notice that within exposure groups having equal energy, the high peaked waves produce a greater PTS. To determine if this effect was significant, these data were subjected to an analysis of variance [14] with energy level and wave type as the two primary treatment effects. Test frequency was included as a repeated measure factor. Table 2 contains a summary of this analysis, which indicates that not only are energy, test frequency, and the interaction of these two factors highly significant, but that wave type is marginally significant in the production of PTS also.

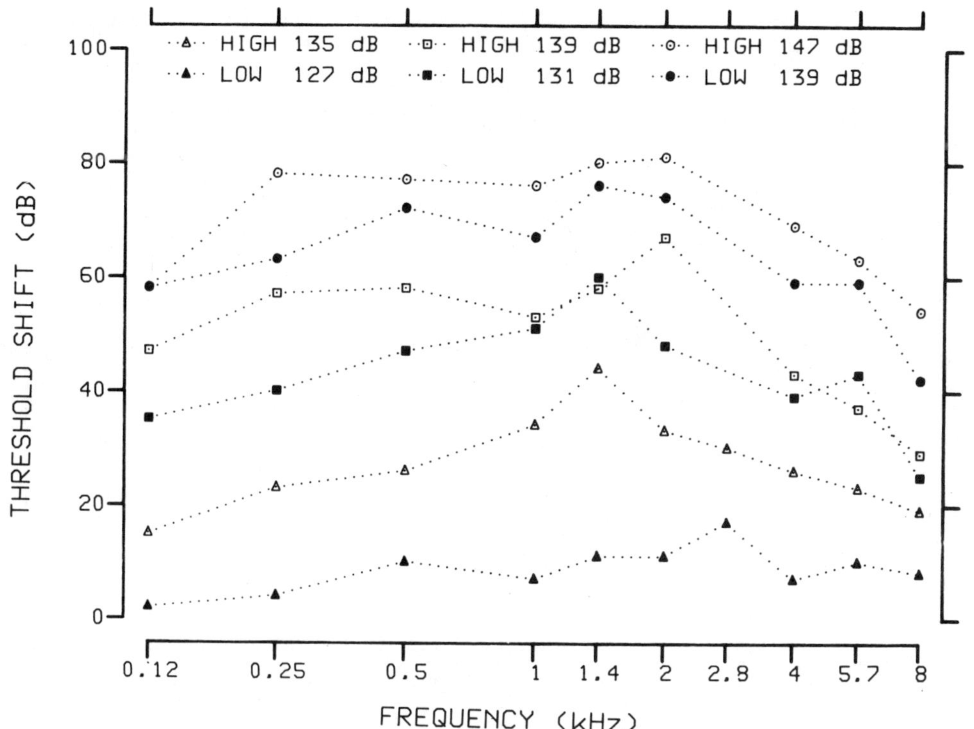

Fig. 4. The group mean temporary threshold shift immediately following the impulse noise exposure (TTSo) for each of the experimental groups at each test frequency.

Table 2. SUMMARY OF THE ANALYSIS OF VARIANCE ON PERMANENT THRESHOLD SHIFT

Treatment	F	DF	P
Wave type	4.26	1/30	<.05
Energy level	82.87	2/30	<.001
Wave type by energy	.08	2/30	>.10
Test frequency	16.7	8/240	<.001
Wave type by frequency	.8	8/240	>.10
Energy by frequency	3.49	16/240	<.001
Wave type by energy by frequency	1.36	16/240	>.10

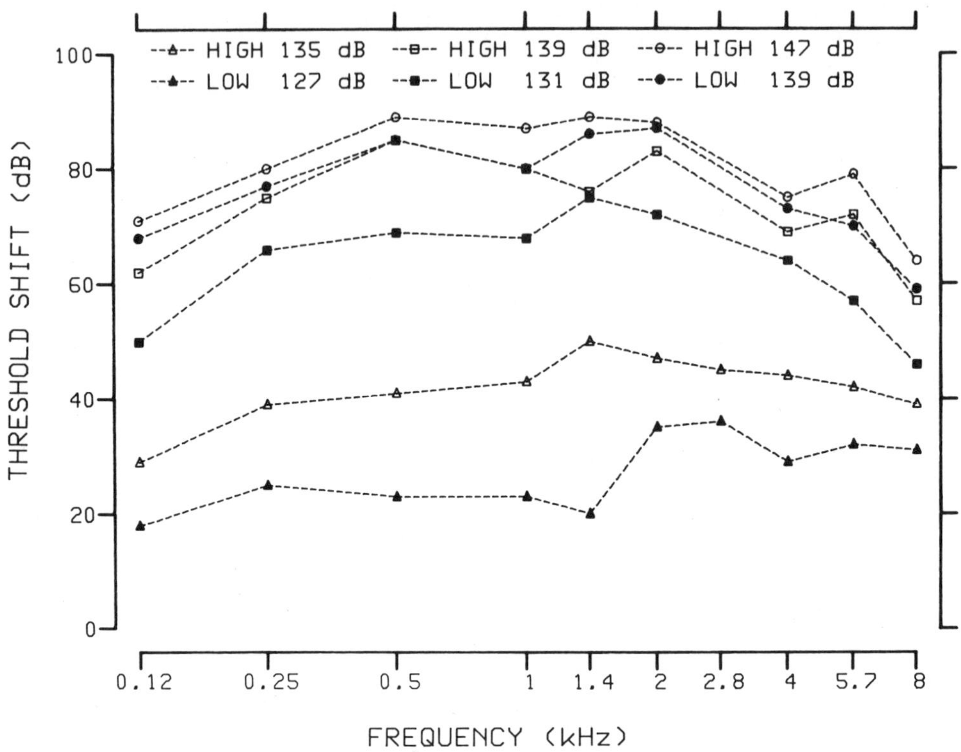

Fig. 5. The postexposure group mean maximum temporary threshold shift (TTSmax) for each of the experimental groups at each test frequency.

Histological Findings

Figs. 8 and 9 show surface preparation micrographs of the organ of Corti from typical chinchillas. These figures illustrate some of the features of the noise damaged organ of Corti that were, more or less, typical of each exposure condition. In general, the two highest energy exposures produced widespread massive damage to the inner and outer sensory cells, supporting Deiter and Hensen cells, and nerve fibers. The remaining four exposure conditions generally produced more localized kinds of lesions. The lesions in the groups exposed to the medium energy levels tended to be restricted to the midregions of the cochlea. The most severe lesions were punctate. Most of the cochleas from the two lowest energy conditions showed comparatively little sensory cell loss, and much of the organ of Corti exhibited a uniform appearance similar to non-noise-exposed animals. In all groups, the appearance of the lesioned organ of Corti (when a lesion occurred) exhibited a similar pattern: a central area of severe loss in which the basilar membrane was devoid of sensory and supporting epithelium. This primary focal lesion was frequently bordered by regions of the organ of Corti with structural elements relatively intact, but with sensory cells showing varying degrees of loss apical or basalward of the primary lesion. The Hensen cells are involved in the formation of the edges of the lesion, and the focal areas of the lesion are covered by cells originating in the area of the Claudius cells and the cells of the inner sulcus. Inner hair

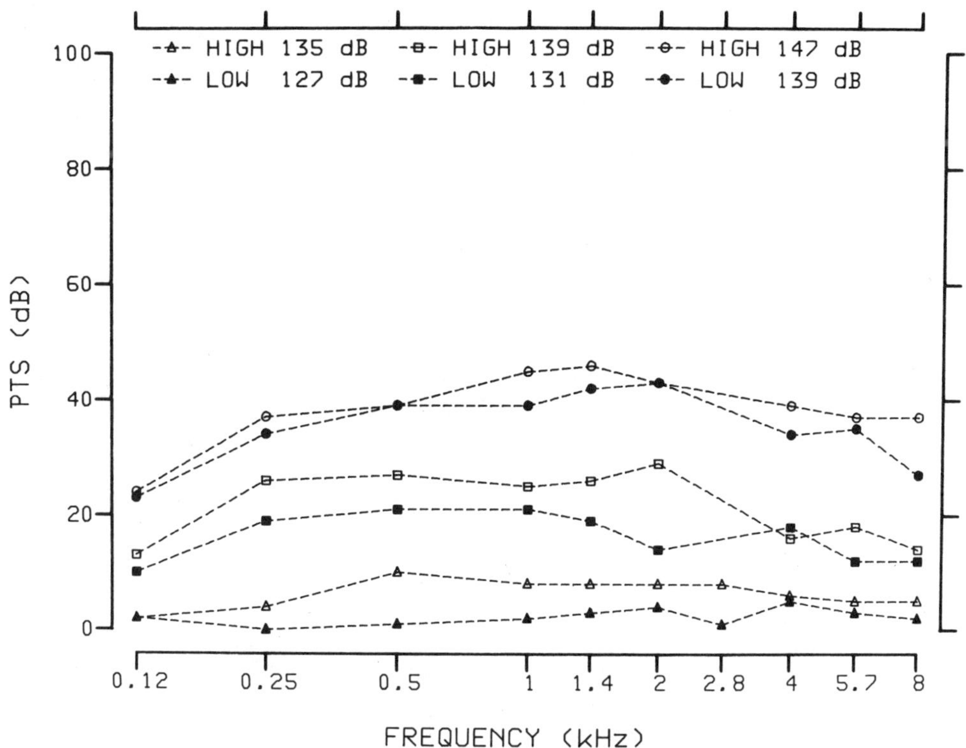

Fig. 6. The group mean permanent threshold shift at each test frequency for each of three six exposure conditions.

cells tend to be missing most frequently when the inner pillar cells have been damaged.

In general, the behaviorally measured hearing losses are reflected in the distribution of sensory cell loss in the cochlea. A summary of the group-averaged sensory cell losses is shown in Fig. 10 for all 6 experimental groups. Each data point represents the average number of sensory cells lost in the particular experimental group within an octave band length of the cochlea centered at the indicated frequency. The octave band-group average sensory cell loss, in percentage, was computed by averaging sensory cell losses within octave band lengths of the cochlea for the individual animals that constitute that particular group, and dividing the loss by the normative sensory cell populations obtained from normal control animals. Fig. 10 should be compared to the mean PTS for individual groups plotted in Fig. 6. Several generalizations can be made from the group mean cell loss and PTS data. As in the PTS data, there is an orderly increase in the mean sensory cell loss, both inner hair cells (IHC) and outer hair cells (OHC), as the energy level of the exposure increases. The sensory cell lesion begins to develop in the 1 kHz region of the cochlea, and with increasing energy levels, spreads systematically towards the base of the cochlea. This effect can be seen clearly in Fig. 10 where all the sensory cell losses from each group are plotted together. The sensory cell losses in Groups 3-6 show a strong peak which is somewhat symmetric around the 1 kHz area. However, the PTS audiograms for these groups are relatively flat, showing approximately a 20 dB hearing loss in Group 3 between 0.25 and 2 kHz. In general, the low-peaked waves, for a given energy level of the

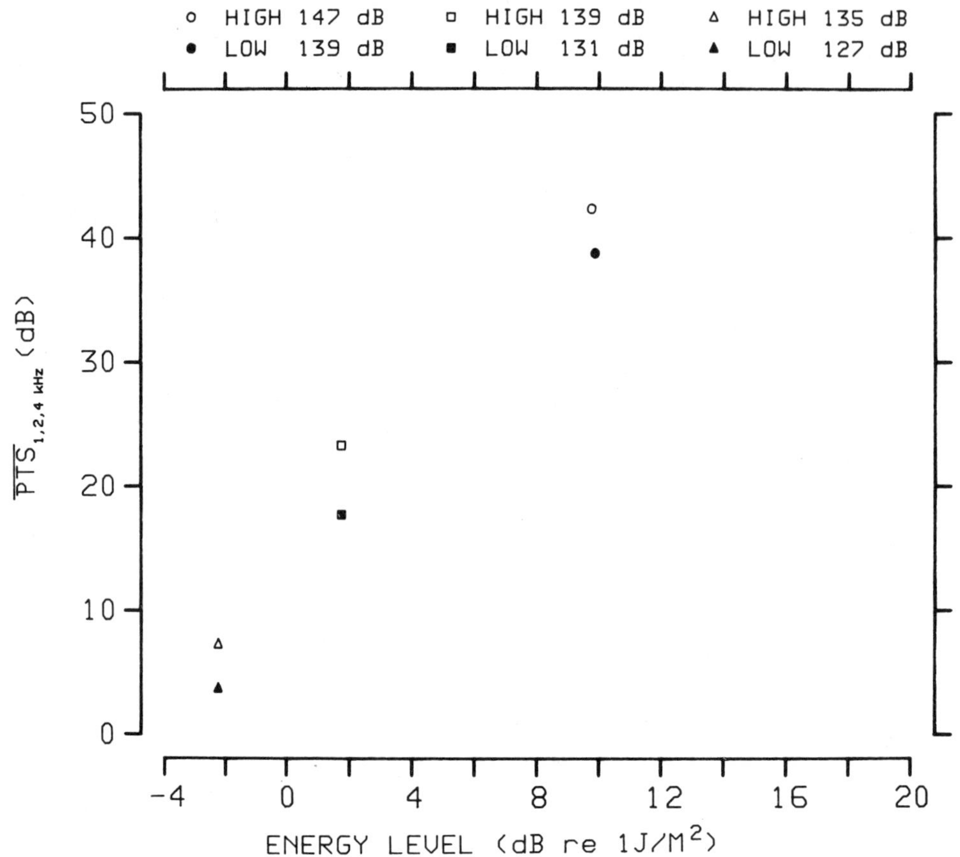

Fig. 7. The mean PTS computed at 1, 2 and 4 kHz (PTS 1,2,4) as a function of the total energy level of the exposure.

exposure, consistently produced less sensory cell loss than did the high-peaked waves. However, the standard deviations in the sensory cell data are large and this effect should be interpreted with caution.

In order to establish the statistical significance of the above observations, the inner and outer hair cell loss data were subjected to analyses of variance with energy level and wave type as the two primary treatment effects. Tables 3 and 4 present summaries of these analyses which indicate that the effects of energy, test frequency, and the interaction of these two factors show significant effects ($P < .01$) in both inner and outer hair cell losses. Wave type and the interaction between wave type and frequency and between wave type, frequency, and energy were not significant at the .05 level for either inner hair cell or outer hair cell losses produced by these exposures.

A maximum hearing loss of about 40 dB is seen in the group exposed to the highest energy level (Group 1). This loss is relatively flat from 0.25 through 8.0 kHz. The mean sensory cell loss for these animals is very severe with a nearly complete loss of OHCs in the basal 70% of the cochlea, and 50% IHC losses throughout the basal one-half of the cochlea. Surprisingly, the low peaked Group 2 animals showed a much reduced loss of IHC compared to Group 1, while the final PTS audiograms for the two groups were quite similar.

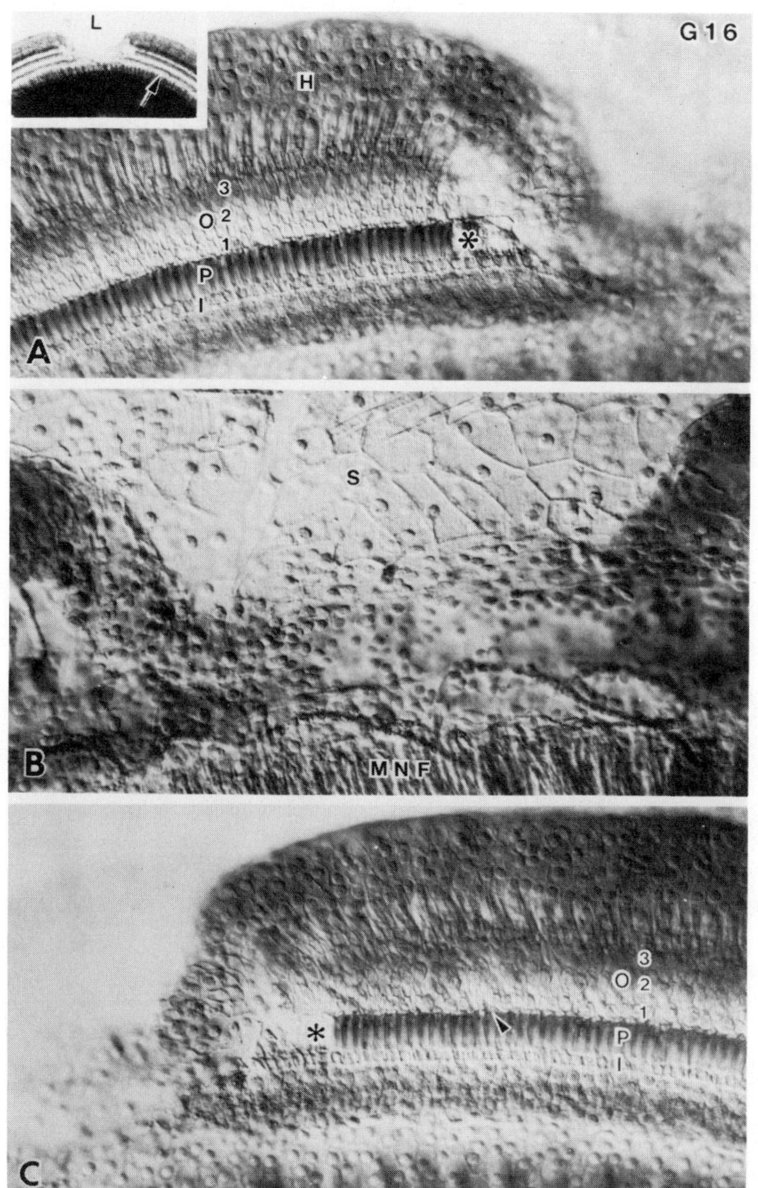

Fig. 8. Surface preparation micrographs showing the region of impulse noise-induced damage in the cochlea of animal G16. (Exposure: 139 dB low peak wave) Inset: low magnification view of the punctate lesion (L); Panels A and C show the abrupt transition from a normal appearing sensory epithelium to a complete loss of all epithelial structures on the basilar membrane. Panel B shows the central area of the punctate lesion illustrating the reepithelialization of the basilar membrane (S) and the decrease in the number of myelinated nerve fibers (MNF). H-Hensen cells; O-Outer hair cells; P-Pillar cells; I-Inner hair cells; *-indicates pillar cell lesions.

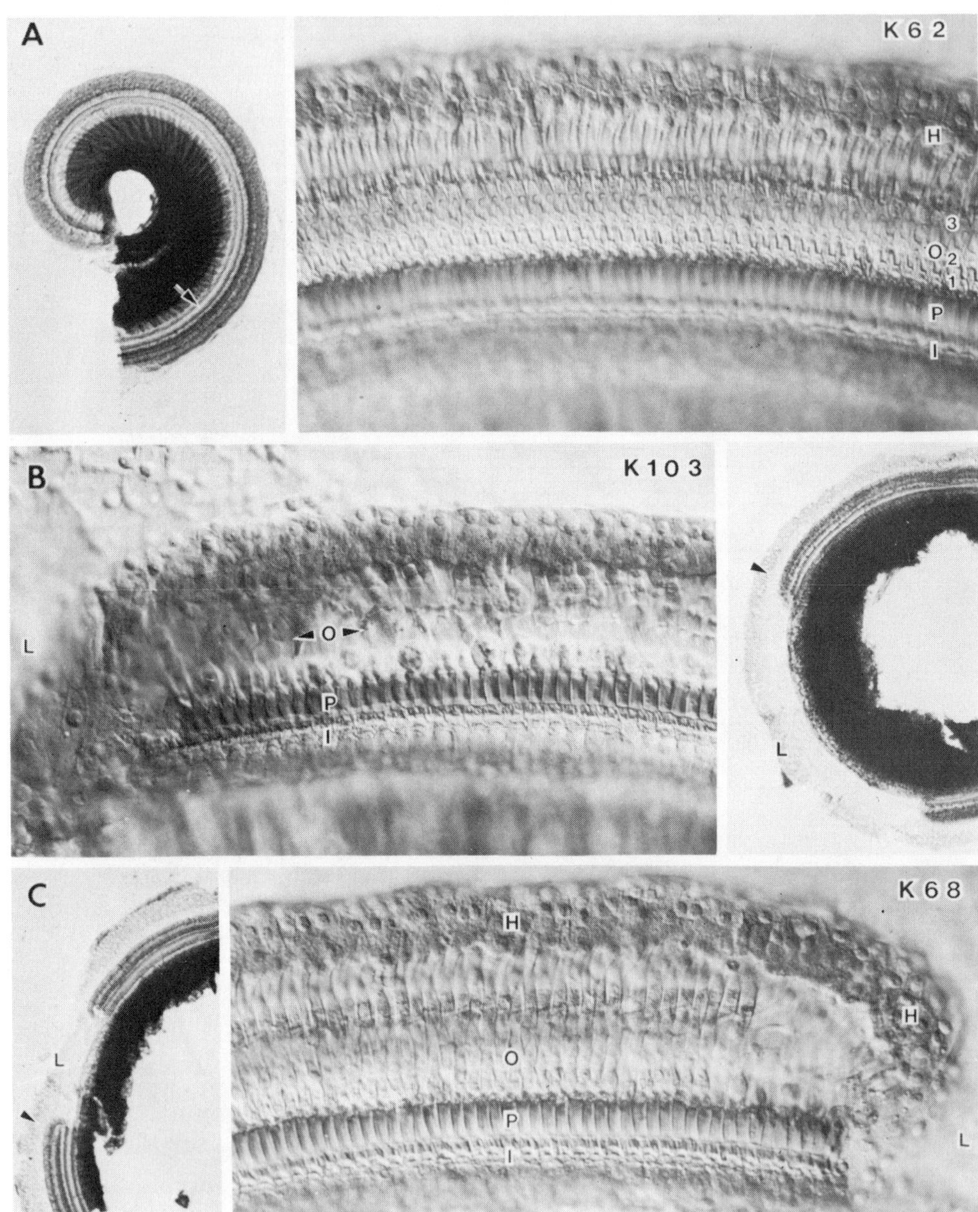

Fig. 9. Panel A shows a normal appearing region of the cochlea from animal K62 (Exposure: 135 dB high peak wave) and a low magnification inset of the apex which shows relatively little sensory cell damage. Panels B and C show punctate lesions from the regions indicated in the insets from animals K103 and K68 (Exposure: 135 dB high peak wave) respectively. H-Hensen cells; O-Outer hair cells; P-Pillar cells; I-Inner hair cells.

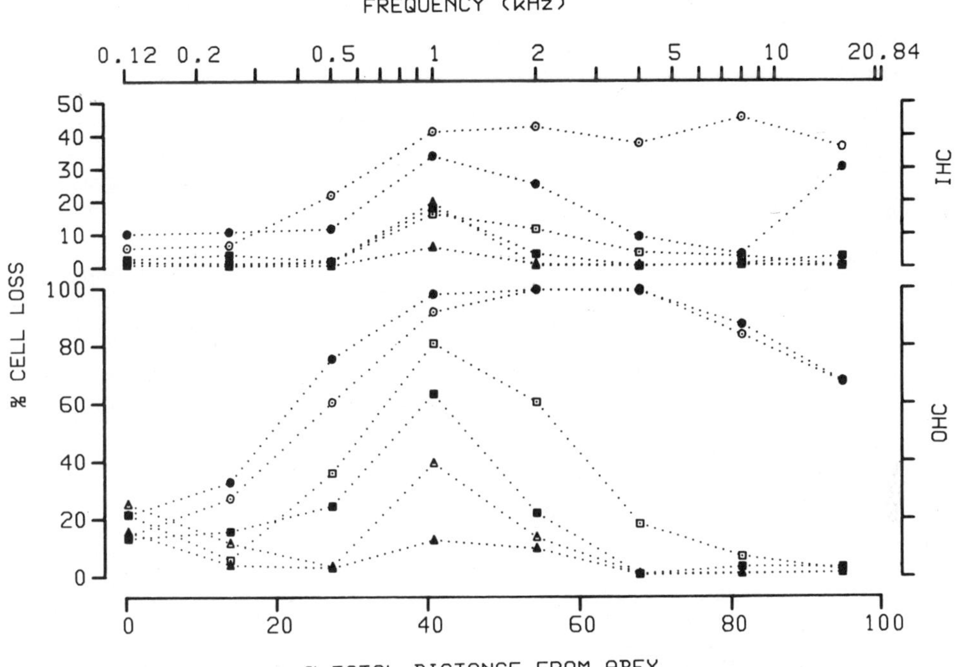

Fig 10. A comparison across all exposure energy levels of the inner and outer hair cell losses computed over octave band lengths of the cochlea at the indicated frequencies.

Table 3. Summary of the Analysis of Variance for Inner Hair Cell Loss

Treatment	F	DF	P
Wave type	3.26	1/30	<0.10
Energy level	21.58	2/30	<0.001
Wave type by energy	1.87	2/30	>0.10
Test frequency	8.12	7/210	<0.001
Wave type by frequency	1.91	7/210	<0.07
Energy by frequency	2.36	14/210	<0.005
Wave type by energy by frequency	1.67	14/210	<0.07

Table 4. Summary of the Analysis of Variance for Outer Hair Cell Loss

Treatment	F	DF	P
Wave type	0.88	1/30	>0.10
Energy level	111.19	2/30	<0.001
Wave type by energy	1.84	2/30	>0.10
Test frequency	40.41	7/210	<0.001
Wave type by frequency	1.19	7/210	>0.10
Energy by frequency	17.72	14/210	<0.001
Wave type by energy by frequency	0.97	14/210	>0.10

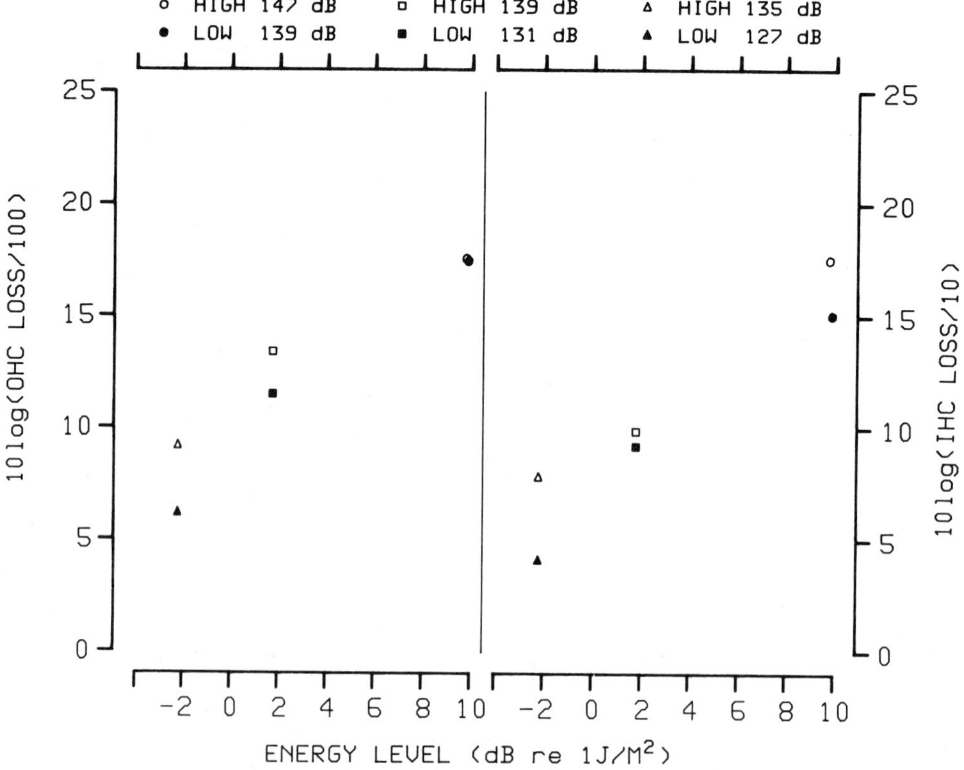

Fig. 11. The group mean total number of inner and outer hair cells lost throughout the entire cochlea, expressed in dB, as a function of the energy level of the exposure.

An alternative way of presenting the sensory cell loss is shown in Fig. 11. The total number of IHCs and OHCs that were missing in the entire cochlea were determined and then converted into a "dB-level" form, for comparison with PTS values. The data points in Fig. 11 were obtained as follows: the total hair cell losses (either OHC or IHC) were found for each animal and the mean for the group determined. The average total number of OHCs and IHCs lost in an experimental group was referenced to 100 or to 10 cells respectively and a dB level was computed according to the following:

$$\text{dB(OHC) loss} = 10 \log (\text{OHC loss}/100)$$

$$\text{dB(IHC) loss} = 10 \log (\text{IHC loss}/10).$$

The rationale for choosing the 100 OHC and 10 IHC cell reference was somewhat arbitrary, but can be justified by noting that a cochlea with losses of 100 OHCs and 10 IHCs scattered throughout the length of the cochlea could be considered a normal cochlea. This assumption breaks down if the sensory cell loss is concentrated in a very narrow region of the cochlea. However, in that case, the lesions would occupy less than 0.25 mm of the cochlea and by our available psychoacoustic testing procedures could probably not be detected. When using these two reference figures to relate sensory cell loss on a dB scale, an average chinchilla cochlea devoid of all OHCs and IHCs would have approximately a 20 dB loss in each case.

Both the IHC and the OHC loss functions in Fig. 11 appear to reach upper and lower asymptotes at similar energy levels. We can estimate by extrapolation that for 100 impulses presented at a rate of 1 per 3 sec, having a total energy of about -6 dB (re 1 J/M^2), the IHC and OHC losses will be negligible and thus the exposure will be safe. Similarly for an energy of more than 10 dB, the cochleas will sustain a near complete sensory cell loss.

CONCLUSIONS

The threshold shift measured within the first few hours after exposure showed a systematic variation with both peak pressure and energy level. The permanent threshold shift measured 20 to 30 days post-exposure, and the loss of sensory cells showed a strong dependence on energy level with a less pronounced dependence on peak pressure. These results indicate that peak pressure is not a sufficient indicator of auditory hazard; however, energy alone is not a sufficient indicator either.

Acknowledgement

A portion of this work was supported by US Army Medical Research and Development Command Contract DAMD 17-80-C-0109.

Disclaimer

The views, opinions, and/or findings contained in this report are those of the authors and should not be construed as an official Department of the Army position, policy, or decision, unless so designated by other official documentation. Citation of trade names in this report does not constitute an official Department of the Army endorsement or approval of the use of such commercial items.

Animal Use

In conducting the research described in this report, the investigators adhered to the "Guide for Laboratory Animal Facilities and Care," as promulgated by the Committee on the Guide for Laboratory Animal Resources, National Academy of Sciences - National Research Council.

REFERENCES

1. Committee on Hearing, and Bioacoustics and Biomechanics, Proposed damage risk criterion for impulse noise (gunfire), Report of Working Group 57, NAS-NRC, Washington, D.C. (1968).
2. Department of the Arm, "Noise and conservation of hearing," Department of the Army, TD-MED-501, Fort Monroe, VA (1980).
3. Department of Defense, "Noise limits for material," Department of Defense, MIL-STD-1474B(MI) Washington, DC, (1975).
4. M. F. Forrest, personal communication, NATO Panel 6 Meeting, Meppen, Germany (1984).
5. G. F. Smoorenburg, Damage Risk Criteria for Impulse _in_: "New Perspectives on Noise-Induced Hearing Loss," R. P. Hamernik, D. Henderson, and R.J. Salvi, eds., Raven Press, New York (1982).
6. F. Pfander, "Das Knalltrauma," Springer-Verlag, Berlin (1975).
7. F. Pfander, H. Bongartz, H. Brinkman, and H. Kietz, Danger of Auditory Impairment from Impulse Noise: A Comparative Study of the CHABA Damage-Risk Criteria and Those of the Federal Republic of Germany, _J. Acous. Soc. Am._ 67:628 (1980).
8. A. Dancer, personal communication, NATO Panel VIII/RSG 6 Meeting, Meppen, Germany (1984).
9. R. W. Young, On the Energy Transported with a Sound Pulse, _J. Acous. Soc. Am._ 47:441 (1970).
10. J. H. Patterson, Jr., I. M. Lomba-Gautier, D. L. Curd, R. P. Hamernik, R. J. Salvi, C. E. Hargett, Jr., and G. Turrentine, "The Effect of Impulse Intensity and the Number of Impulses on Hearing and Cochlear Pathology in the Chinchilla," United States Army Aeromedical Research Laboratory Report No. 85-3 (1985).
11. J. D. Miller, Audibility Curve of the Chinchilla, _J. Acous. Soc. Am._ 48:513 (1970).
12. C. K. Burdick, J. H. Patterson, B. T. Mozo, and R. T. Camp, Threshold Shifts in Chinchillas Exposed to Octave Bands of Noise Centered at 63 and 1000 Hz for Three Days, _J. Acous. Soc. Am._ 64:458 (1978).
13. J. H. Patterson, and D. M. Green, Discrimination of Transient Signals Having Identical Energy Spectra, _J. Acous. Soc. Am._ 48:894 (1970).
14. B. J. Winer, "Statistical Principles in Experimental Design," McGraw-Hill Book Company, New York (1971).
15. H. Engstrom, H. W. Ades, and A. Anderson, "Structural Pattern of the Organ of Corti," Almquist and Wiksell, Stockholm (1966).
16. D. H. Eldredge, J. D. Miller, B. A. Bohne, and W. W. Clark, Frequency-Position Map for the Chinchilla Cochlea, _J. Acous. Soc. Am._ 62:S35 (1977).
17. G. A. Luz, and D. C. Hodge, The Recovery from Impulse Noise-Induced TTS in Monkeys and Men: A Descriptive Model, _J. Acous. Soc. Am._ 49:1770 (1971).
18. D. Henderson, and R. P. Hamernik, Asymptotic Threshold Shift from Impulse Noise, _in_: "New Perspectives on Noise-Induced Hearing Loss," R. P. Hamernik, D. Henderson, R. Salvi, eds., Raven Press, New York (1982).

DISCUSSION

Henderson: In high energy groups there was 100% missing outer hair cells over a large range, but one of the high energy groups had almost normal inner hair cells. Can you comment on what the difference in hearing loss was between the two high energy groups at frequencies with and without outer hair cells?

Patterson: The two high energy groups were almost on top of each other in terms of PTS, although it was only 40 dB. We did not find threshold shifts much bigger than 40-50 dB in these animals.

Neilson: I am not sure if I saw it right, but as I understand the morphology, you had some places where there was a total loss of the organ of Corti and some places where there were hearing cells still intact. Is that in the same ear? Yet the threshold shifts were flat across frequency.

Patterson: The threshold shifts in these aimals, in spite of the rather discreet histological findings, are really very broad band. It is a peculiar finding. I do not have any explanation for it, but it appears to be consistent.

McFadden: The maximum hearing loss could occur about a day after the termination of the noise. Is there some prospect that the successive testing in the interval between the termination of the noise and the 24 hour period may have contributed to it? That is, they have a lot of hearing loss and they presumably were getting exposed to lots of pretty intense pure tones. Does that contribute to that?

Patterson: I do not think so. The peak seems to occur after the successive testing has slowed down, as a matter of fact, around the six hour point.

EFFECTS OF WEAPON NOISE ON HEARING

A. Dancer and R. Franke

French-German Research Institute of Saint-Louis
68301 Saint-Louis, France

INTRODUCTION

"In military spheres, the need for prevention of weapon noise-induced hearing loss is receiving ever-increasing attention. The question as to which impulse noises are hazardous and which are not is frequently raised, and research is being conducted in a number of countries to obtain data relating to these problems. The approach has to be made along two lines: (1) to find a satisfactory method of measuring and expressing the physical characteristics of the noise, and (2) to assess the potential for auditory damage of various noise sources [1]." This statement, made by English and American scientists in 1968, is still up to date.

Measurements of some simple physical parameters of the weapon noises and observations of weapon noise induced TTS and PTS [1-4] led to the pro-posal of damage risk criteria (DRC). A thorough comparative review of these DRC was made by Smoorenburg [5].

These DRC differ from those established for occupational or environmental noise in two respects: a) by the method of measuring the physical characteristics of the noise and b) by the criteria of evaluation of the hearing damage.

a) Weapon noises differ generally from other noises in peak pressure level (which can reach 100 kPa) and duration (the time required for the initial or principal pressure wave to rise to its positive peak and return momentarily to ambient pressure, or A-duration, ranges typically from a fraction of millisecond for light weapons to a few milliseconds for heavy weapons, in the free field). Peak pressure and duration are simple to measure, and have been widely used to define the physical characteristics of weapon noise.

b) Since people are not exposed each time to the same weapon noise and are not generally exposed every day, DRC currently in use are based on TTS experiments. Criteria proposed by CHABA [1] and Smoorenburg [4] correspond to given values of TTS (which is widely assumed to indicate eventual PTS) as a function of frequency not to be exceeded by given percentages of soldiers. Pfander's criterion [2] is based upon the recovery of threshold shifts [5].

If we consider: a) the actual exposure conditions to weapon noises (very often during only a few hours and not every day), b) the actual procedures of measurement of the so-called TTS (it is almost impossible, on the shooting range, to measure the TTS two minutes after the end of the exposure) and c) the possible erratic pattern of the recovery following the exposure to impulse noise [6], the kind of criterion proposed by Pfander seems more fitted to the exposure conditions to weapon noises in the military environment.

The exposure limits of these DRC use both the peak pressure level of the weapon noise and its duration. The relationship between peak pressure level and duration of Pfander's and Smoorenburg's criteria [5] (Fig. 6) corresponds to the isoenergetic principle (i.e. doubling the number of exposures or the duration of the weapon noise corresponds to a decrease of 3 dB of the peak pressure level). In these respect these procedures are nearly identical to those used for assessing the risks due to the exposure to other noises (ISO 1999). But the weapon noise DRC listed before do not take into account the spectral distribution of the acoustic energy: the Pfander's and Smoorenburg's criteria make no distinction between a same amount of acoustic energy due to one shock wave of x.kPa peak pressure and y.ms duration, and n shock waves of the same peak pressure and of (y/n)ms duration, though the acoustic energy in the second exposure condition is located at higher frequencies. These DRC also do not take into account the transfer function which relates the acoustic energy in the free field to the acoustic energy at the input to the cochlea, whereas for occupational and environmental noises, the A-weighting makes allowance for this transfer function.

Nevertheless, people have been well aware for a long time of the importance of the frequency spectrum of the impulses on the effects observed on hearing: "There is evidence that different types of impulse noise produce effects at different frequencies" [1]. But "... while a Fourier analysis can give information regarding the spectral distribution of certain impulse wave forms, in general the spectrum is difficult and time consuming to analyze. For this reason, this parameter has not been included in the DRC..." [1].

It is now much easier to perform a Fourier analysis than 17 years ago. Due to the importance of the parameter "frequency spectrum" in assessing the hazard from exposure to weapon noises (in the free field, in reverberant areas, in case of combined exposures: continuous and impulse noises, with hearing protection...), the French committee on weapon noises (Comite Francais "Bruits d'Armes") following Atherley and Martin [7], Rice and Martin [8] and the recommendations of the workshop on "Impulse noise and auditory hazard" (I.S.V.R., Southampton, 1981) decided to propose to the French army a DRC [9] based upon the measurement of the A-weighted* acoustic energy and the isoenergy principle like DRC for occupational and environmental noises.

This DRC takes into account the previous ones (mainly Pfander's and Smoorenburg's criteria), but it represents a very important improvement as a method for measuring** and expressing the physical characteristics of the

---

* Evidence in favour of the A-weighting, for use with industrial continuous noise, is not compelling but, according to Robinson [10], other standardized frequency weightings fail also to reveal significant advantage.

** Nevertheless, it seems always necessary to obtain a pressure/time relation even if the assessment of the noise is performed in terms of A-weighted energy. Otherwise, errors in measurement are likely to go undetected.

noise and is much more powerful for assessing the auditory hazard in all exposure conditions in the military environment [11].

Now the question is: can we use this DRC in all conditions and are there any limitations to its use?

LIMITATIONS TO THE USE OF THE DRC

As a DRC based upon the isoenergy principle and the measurement of the A-weighted energy is widely used for occupational and environmental noise (ISO 1999), and as this physical procedure seems to provide in many respects a better way to evaluate the auditory hazard due to weapon noises exposures than the previous ones, what could prevent us from using it in all exposure conditions?

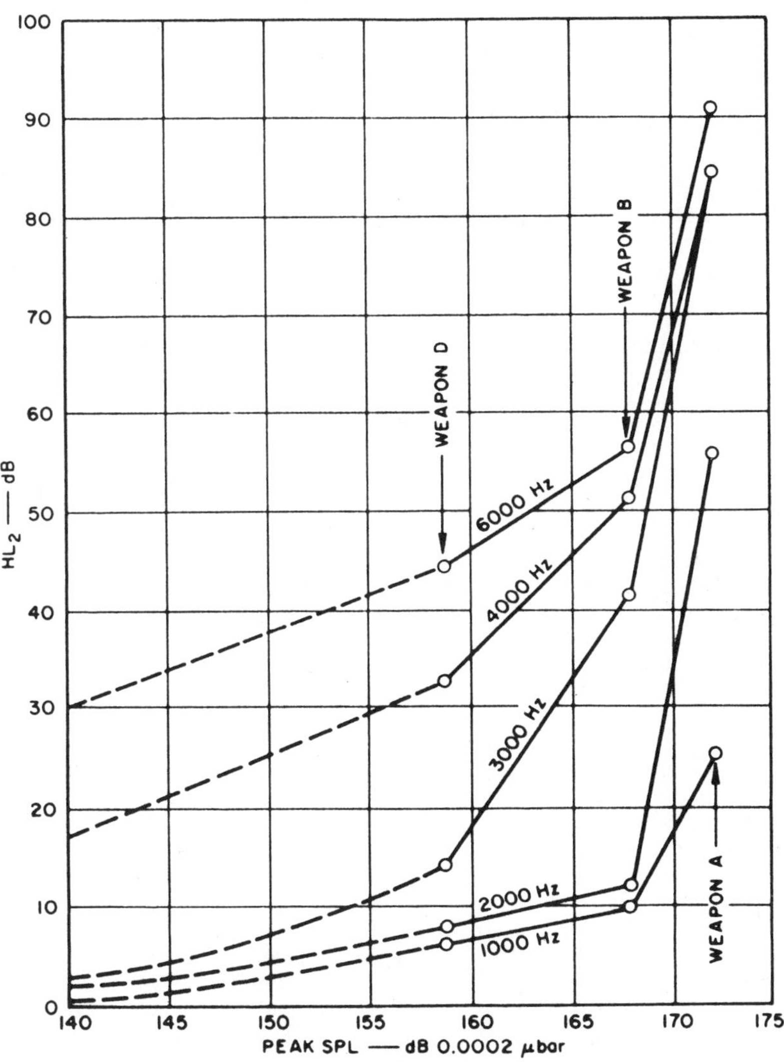

Fig. 1. Hearing level 2 minutes postexposure as a function of peak SPL. 100 trigger pulls, one round per pull, at the rate of one every 5 sec. Parameter is audiometric test frequency [12].

Critical Level

As shown before, the weapon noises differ from other kinds of noise in peak pressure level, which is generally much higher than that reached by occupational noises, and in duration, which is much shorter.

It is possible to think that due to some nonlinear processes the iso-energetic relationship between peak pressure level and duration is no longer valid for very high peak pressure levels. That is one of the reasons why the use of DRC for occupational noise is restricted over a given peak level (145 dB SPL, ISO 1999), and it is the main reason for which the use of DRC for weapon noises was restricted to given peak levels even for very short durations (i.e., 160 dB according to Pfander [2], 140 dB for the US-MIL-STD-1974B-1979, 160 dB for the DTAT-AT-83/27/28 [9]).

Data of Kryter and Garinther [12] for unprotected human ears exposed to four different weapon noises indicate a very rapid increase of TTS over about 167 dB peak pressure level (Fig. 1). These results, as well as those obtained with impulse noises by Ward [13,14], lead Price [15] to emphasize the existence of a "critical level" beyond which the DRC curves based on the isoenergy principle would no longer be valid. This "critical level" could correspond to a change of the type of mechanism by which the auditory injuries occur (this mechanism is probably purely mechanical for the highest levels as indicated by histological observations performed immediately after the end of the exposure [16,17]). The existence of such a "critical level" was confirmed by Dancer et al., [18] on guinea pigs exposed to shock waves of different peak pressures and durations: in this case the "critical level" is located between 148 and 160 dB SPL, depending on the duration (and hence the frequency spectrum) of the shock waves.

For unprotected ears and weapon noises like those produced by firearms in the free field, it seems absolutely necessary to determine a peak pressure level beyond which exposure should be prohibited (whatever the duration of the noise is), even for an energy dose not exceeding the chosen criterion.

Influence of the duration (and of the frequency spectrum) of shock waves

Let us consider two shock waves of the same peak pressure level but of different durations. The longer one contains as much acoustic energy as the shorter at medium and high frequencies but more at low frequencies. Whatever the weighting curve used is, the measured acoustic energy will always be greater for the longer shock wave. All existing DRC will anticipate a larger hazard for the exposure to the long shock wave.

Nevertheless, experiments conducted on two different animal species (cat [19] and guinea pig [18,20] show very surprising results: the longer the duration of the shock wave, the smaller the threshold shifts (Figs. 2 and 3). There is no classical explanation for this phenomenon, though we can think that there exists some kind of interaction between the very low and the medium/high frequency components of the shock wave. The very low-frequency components could limit the medium/high frequency-induced displacements of the middle ear [21] or of the inner ear structures. According to Johnson [22]: "... there is evidence that the infrasonic part of an impulse may ameliorate the effects of the high-frequency components of an impulse." Such an effect was found in a human study on air bag noise inside a test automobile [23,24]: TS from the whole noise (low-frequency component and impulse noise) were significantly smaller than TS from the impulse noise only. Johnson attributes this phenomenon to the loading of the middle ear which could "...attenuate some of the high-frequency sounds that reach the inner ear." On the other hand, studies by Patuzzi et al.

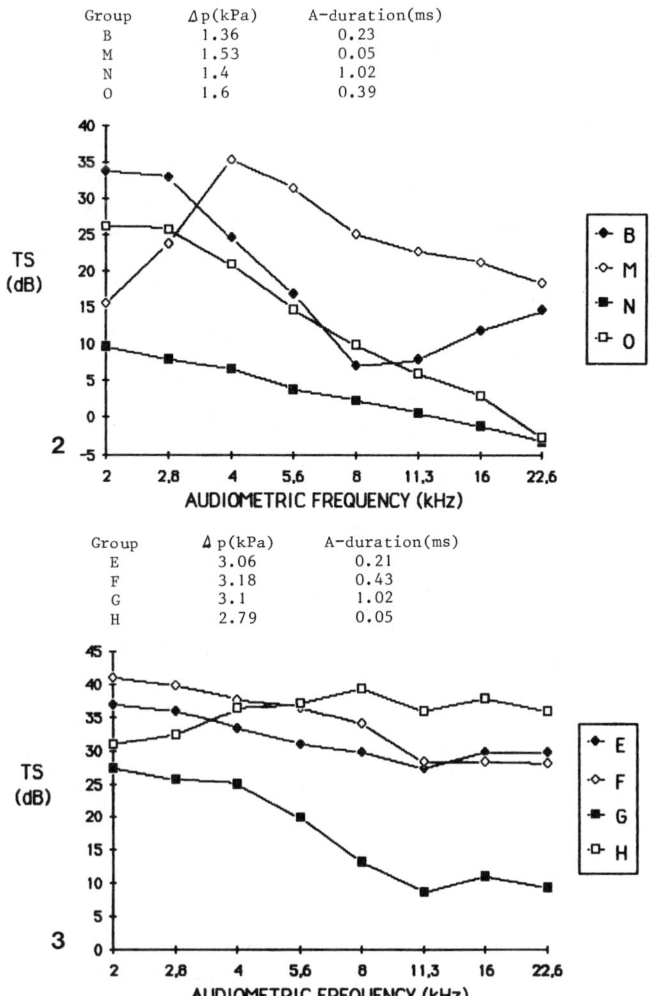

Figs. 2 and 3. TS eight days after the exposure of different groups of guinea pigs to 25 shock waves of a nearly constant peak pressure level (Fig. 2 1.5kPa) (Fig. 3. 3kPa) and of A-durations ranging from 0.05 to 1.02ms.

[25] of "The modulation of the sensitivity of the mammalian cochlea by low frequency tones" show that displacements of the basilar membrane toward scala tympani (induced by low-frequency tones) provide a reduction of the mechanical sensitivity of the basilar membrane. Whatever the exact mechanisms are, these observations are contrary to the predictions of all DRC for weapon noises.

These discrepancies seem very important, especially in the case of exposure to the noise of heavy weapons (which are very rich in low frequencies, and particularly during exposures with hearing protectors. Since a hearing protector provides a good attenuation for medium and high frequencies, but a poor attenuation for low frequencies, the relative importance of the low frequencies versus medium and high frequencies is therefore much higher.

It therefore appears that both the unprotected and the protected ears are more resistant to the shock waves from heavy weapons than current DRC predict.

Influence of the spacing of impulses

No DRC takes into account the influence of the spacing of the weapon noises (problem of the small caliber machine guns for example). This parameter is nevertheless important [20,26,27]. The most noxious duration of the interval between two impulses seems to be of one second: TS are generally much smaller for shorter or longer intervals. For shorter intervals, the mechanism of the decrease of the TS is generally thought to be due to the middle ear acoustic reflex. However, some results from anesthetized and curarized guinea pigs [27] seem to indicate that other mechanisms, probably at the inner ear level, could also be involved.

This problem represents one more difficulty in the formulation and in the use of the DRC.

CONCLUSION

From all these points it could seem not very reasonable to use the DRC listed above. Nevertheless, considering the demand of the military, responsible persons, and the great hazard that weapon noises represent to the hearing of soldiers, researchers were obliged to propose the best available solution.

In our opinion, the DRC developed by the French committee on weapon noise [9] can be regarded as the most appropriate and versatile guideline up to now. Nevertheless, this guideline suffers all the difficulties we have discussed in this paper, and it should be regarded only as a step to a fully reliable DRC.

Since all these difficulties seem to originate from highly non-linear processes occurring only at the very high peak pressure levels and very short durations which characterize weapon noise, the solution can only be found in DRC based upon parametric studies in exposure conditions directly comparable to the real ones.

ACKNOWLEDGMENTS

We are very grateful for the help provided by M. R. Forrest and Dr. Edwards who made corrections of the manuscript and gave us useful comments.

REFERENCES

1. R. R. Coles, G. R. Garinther, D. C. Hodge and C. G. Rice, Hazardous exposure to impulse noise, J. Acoust. Soc. Am. 43:336 (1968).
2. F. Pfander, "Das Knalltrauma," Springer-Verlag, Berlin (1975).
3. F. Pfander, H. Bongartz, H. Brinkmann and H. Kietz, Danger of auditory impairment from impulse noise: A comparative study of the CHABA damage risk criteria and those of the Federal Republic of Germany, J. Acoust. Soc. Am. 67:628 (1980).
4. G. F. Smoorenburg, Damage risk criteria for impulse noise, TNO Soesterberg, rept IZF 1980-26 (1980).
5. G. F. Smoorenburg, Damage risk criteria for impulse noise, in: "New perspectives on noise-induced hearing loss, R. P. Hamernik, D. Henderson and R. Salvi, eds., Raven Press, New York (1982).

6. G. A. Luz and D.C. Hodge, Recovery from impulse noise induced TTS in monkeys and men: a descriptive model, J. Acoust. Soc. Am. 49:1770 (1971).
7. G. R. C. Atherley and A. M. Martin, Equivalent-continuous noise levels as a measure of injury from impact and impulse noise, Annals of Occupational Hygiene, 14:11 (1971).
8. C. G. Rice and A. M. Martin, Impulse noise damage risk criteria, J. of Sound and Vibration, 28:359 (1973).
9. DTAT, Recommendation on evaluating the possible harmful effect of noise on hearing, AT-83/27/28 (1983).
10. D. W. Robinson, The spectral factor in noise-induced hearing loss: A case for retaining the A weighting, J. of Sound and Vibration, 90:103 (1983).
11. A. Dancer, Isoenergy principle and A-weighting in the rating of the hazard of noise exposure in the military environment, in: "Hearing and hearing prophylaxis," Scandinavian Audiology, Suppl. 16:49 (1982).
12. K. D. Kryter and G. R. Garinther, Auditory effects of acoustic impulses from firearms, Acta Oto-Laryngol., Suppl. 211 (1966).
13. W. D. Ward, W. Selters and A. Glorig, Exploratory studies on temporary threshold shift from impulses, J. Acoust. Soc. Am. 33:781 (1961).
14. W. D. Ward, P. A. Santi, A. J. Duvall and C. W. Turner, Total energy and critical intensity concepts in noise damage, Ann. Otol. Rhinol. Laryngol. 90:584 (1981).
15. G. R. Price, Mechanisms of loss for intense sound exposures, in: "Hearing and other senses; presentation in honor of E. G. Wever," R. R. Fay and Goweritch, ed., The Amphora Press (1983).
16. H. Spoendlin, Anatomical changes following various noise exposures, in: "Effects of noise on hearing," D. Henderson, R. P. Hamernik, D. S. Dosanjh and J. H. Mills, eds., Raven Press, New York (1976).
17. R. P. Hamernik, M. Roberto and G. Turrentine, Mechanically induced morphological changes in the organ of Corti, in: NATO Advanced Study Workshop, "Noise-induced hearing loss: basic and applied aspects," Lucca, Italy, September 1985.
18. A. Dancer, M. Lenoir, K. Buck and P. Vassout, Etude de l'influence du niveau de crete et de la duree de bruits impulsionnels, du type bruit d'arme produit en champ libre, sur l'audition du cobaye, Acustica, in press (1985).
19. G. R. Price, Relative hazard of weapons impulses as a function of spectrum, J. Acoust. Soc Am. Suppl. 1:579 (1982).
20. A. Dancer, R. Franke, G. Baillet, P. Vassout and F. Devriere, Influence de la pression de crete et de la duree d'un bruit impulsif (bruit d'arme) sur l'appareil auditif du cobaye, ISL Rept. R109/75 (1975).
21. C. W. Nixon, Human auditory response to intense infrasound, in: "Proceedings of the colloquium on infrasound," L. Pimonow, ed., Centre National de la Recherche Scientifique, Paris (1973).
22. D. L. Johnson, Hearing hazards associated with infrasound, in: "New perspectives on noise-induced hearing loss," R. P. Hamernik, D. Henderson and R. Salvi, eds., Raven Press, New York (1982).
23. C. W. Nixon, Human auditory response to an Air Bag Inflation Noise, Dept. of Transportation, FHA, Wash. D.C., PB-184-837. Clearinghouse of Federal Scientific and Technical Information, Springfield, Virginia (1969).
24. H. C. Sommer and C. W. Nixon, Primary components of simulated air bag noise and their relative effects on human hearing, DOT/USAF Study, AMRL TR-73-52, Wright-Patterson Air Force Base, Ohio (1973).
25. R. Patuzzi, P. M. Sellick and B. M. Johnstone, The modulation of the sensitivity of the mammalian cochlea by low frequency tones, Hearing Research, 13:1 (1984).
26. W. D. Ward, Effect of temporal spacing on temporary threshold shift from impulses, J. Acoust. Soc. Am. 34:1230 (1962).

27. K. Buck, A. Dancer and R. Franke, Effect of temporal pattern of a given noise dose on TTS in guinea pigs, J. Acoust. Soc. Am. 76:1090 (1984).

DISCUSSION

Forrest: We always see a tremendous variation between individuals exposed to the same noise. Some people will show almost no hearing loss, others will show a very large loss from the same noise exposure. Did you find that?

Dancer: No. At 600 Hz ± 1 SD was from 60 to 90 dB TTS. The disastrous thing was that practically every man had a very big loss.

Forrest: Yes, I think that is very interesting because it is not what we find with exposures to heavy weapons. It may be that the blank rounds which you were using are giving a different result or having a different effect from heavy weapons.

Flottorp: The variation between individuals may be due to many differences, but one main difference is the position of the outer ear with the respect to the blast. I have seen people who have been exposed to a rifle shot for many times without getting damaged, but then one shot, at a wrong position and you have a noise resonance which in that is use in the reach you know of 3000 to 4000 Hz. The resonance may add 20 DB to the peak pressure.

CRITICAL PEAK LEVEL FOR IMPULSE NOISE HAZARD: PERMANENT HEARING THRESHOLD SHIFTS IN MILITARY DRILL SQUADS FOLLOWING KNOWN VARIATION OF IMPULSE NOISE EXPOSURE

H. M. Borchgrevink[1], O. Woxen[1] and G. Oftedal[2]

Joint Medical Service of the Norwegian Armed Forces[1]
FSAN, Oslo mil/Huseby. Oslo 1 Norway
ELAB,[2] NTH, 7000 Trondheim, Norway

INTRODUCTION

From 1982 to 1983, new recruits of The Royal Norwegian Guards Ceremonial Drill Squad (n=32, males, 20 yrs), on their own initiative, changed from low horizontal to high vertical rifle positions during ceremonial firing. In addition, they used the more powerful brass Energa 7.62 mm blank ammunition when firing a simultaneous round which ended each of the 20 official ceremonial drill performances distributed over a 3 months period. The soldiers did not use hearing protection during these ceremonies. Permanent noise-induced hearing losses in the 1983 squad were substantially increased (Fig. 1). Apart from this change, routine and training programs were identical. This gave us the unique opportunity to make a retrospectively-designed, controlled study on the effects of known variations of weapon position and impulse noise exposure on permanent noise-induced hearing losses in man. This was accomplished by letting the 1984 Drill Squad (new recruits) go through the drill program with 1982 red blank ammunition and 1983 (vertical) weapon position under audiometric surveillance.

METHOD

The 1982 Drill Squad (new recruits) used red blank 7.62 mm ammunition both for ceremonial firing and for training. Ceremonial firing was performed standing with the gun in a low horizontal position lateral to the right pelvis, with the muzzle pointing forward and the arms stretched downward.

The 1983 Drill Squad (new recruits) changed to a vertical weapon position for ceremonial firing with the muzzle pointing upward and the trigger 40 cm in front of the man's face, arms stretched forward. In addition, on their own initiative, they had changed for each official ceremonial performance to the more powerful brass Energa blank ammunition. On each of 20 performance days, which were randomly distributed over the 3 month drill season, one simultaneous round occurred per day.

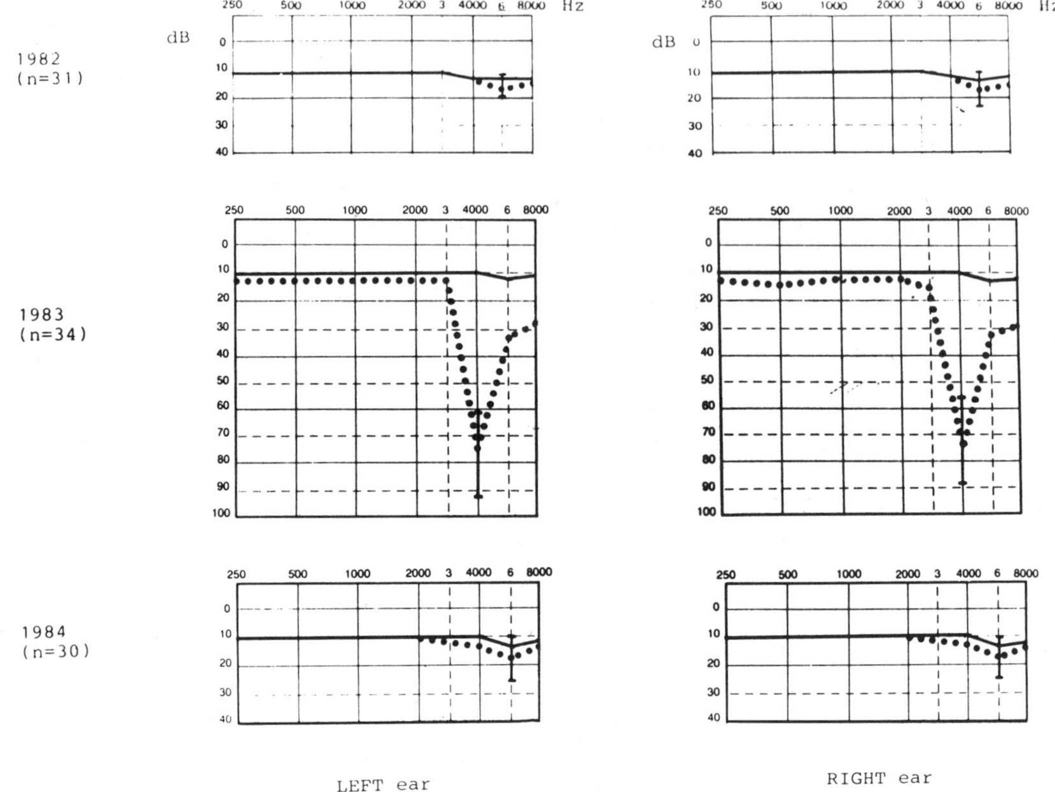

Fig. 1. Audiometry Drill Squads 1982, 1983 and 1984. Mean dB Hearing Thresholds upon entering (-------) and leaving (......) Military Service. Standard deviations shown for 4000 Hz (1983) and 6000 Hz (1982 and 1984).

<u>The 1984 Drill Squad</u> (new recruits) went through the drill program with 1982 red blank ammunition and the 1983 vertical weapon position under audiometric surveillance.

<u>Impulse noise measurements</u> were performed in the field on the ceremonial drill squad's standard asphalt-covered exercise field with hearing protection (E A R-plugs or Silenta mil cuffs per individual choice with proper fit controlled by an audiologist in the field). The field recording equipment consisted of 1+1 Bruel & Kjaer 4136 1/4" microphones, B&K 2619 microphone amplifier, B&K 2807 power supply, SONY PCM-FI transformer, SONY SL-FIE Beta video cassette recorder with SONY L-370-HG cassette and a Hewlett-Packard HP8052A peak meter. Microphone distortion was <2% at 170 dB SPL, and the PCM recorder was low-pass filtered at 20 kHz and overloaded at 176 dB SPL. The recorded signals were analyzed in the ELAB laboratory with the same cassette recorder coupled via a B&K 2606 amplifier to a Wavetek Rockland 5820A analyzer (normal FFT-technique) and the curves were drawn by a Hewlett-Packard HP7470A plotter.

The microphone was placed on the man's left shoulder, 5 cm lateral to the left ear canal, facing upward with a 60° forward tilt. Single rounds were recorded with one man standing alone, 10 m from the recording equipment. Simultaneous rounds were recorded with the 32 men in a 8 x 4 man square ceremonial position, each man placed 2 steps (1 - 1.5 m) from his neighbor. Two microphones were used, one on the center man and one on the assumed least exposed left front wing man.

Audiometry was performed on every member of the 1982, 1983 and 1984 Drill Squads upon entering and leaving military service. For the 1984 squad, audiometry was performed at least monthly during the drill season, as well as before and after impulse noise measurements. All audiometric measures were obtained by the same operator in a Tegner sound attenuated cabinet using a calibrated INTERACOUSTICS AD12 Diagnostic Audiometer according to standard procedure [1].

RESULTS AND DISCUSSION

Audiometry showed that in the 1984 squad, permanent noise-induced hearing losses were as rare as in 1982 (Fig. 1). The effect of horizontal or vertical weapon position was thus negigible, leaving the 20 powerful ceremonial impulse events as the probable source of the substantial permanent threshold shifts in the 1983 squad since all other programs in 1982, 1983 and 1984 were otherwise identical.

Because of the low number of more powerful exposures (20) randomly distributed over a long period (3 months), the high degree of hearing loss observed in the 1983 squad is hardly compatible with an iso-energy concept of impulse noise hazard. Instead, the results favor the presence of a critical intensity level for impulse noise hazard in man beyond which inner ear damage is extensive even after short and infrequent exposure.

This is in line with the conclusions of the Oslo 1982 Noise Symposium [2] where the iso-energy hypothesis was reported to be incompatible with several well-controlled animal experiments using pure tone stimuli [3], different equal-energy impact noise exposures [4], and different presentation patterns of iso-energy impact and continuous noise exposures [5]. The experimental results suggest a critical level exists for hazardous noise.

Impulse noise measurements of single rounds fired with Garand 7.62 mm SL rifles showed that red blank ammunition (1982 and 1984 squads) had peak levels less than 158 dB linear. However, great variation was observed among rounds, with 5 of 10 rounds less than 150 dB linear, both in the low and high weapon positions. Brass Energa blank ammunition (1983 squad) had peak levels of 169-170 dB linear, with the high weapon position (only two rounds were available since that type had been replaced by a new, less powerful model: yellow Energa blank ammunition). Yellow Energa blank ammunition showed peak levels of 160-161 dB linear, with a high weapon position (5 rounds) and 160-162 dB linear, with a low weapon position (5 rounds).

Impulse noise measurements of simultaneous rounds showed that the impulses reached the ear as a rapid succession of largely single pulses, resulting in an increase in impulse duration, but with the peak level similar to that of a single round. Five of 6 rounds of red blank ammunition were less than 160 dB but greater than 150 dB linear, indicating that the 32 simultaneous single rounds compensated for the great SPL variation between individual rounds. The 4 rounds of yellow Energa blank ammunition measured 160-163 dB linear. Simultaneous rounds were only fired with a high (vertical) weapon position. Peak levels were identical in the center and left front wing position for yellow Energa simultaneous rounds, and were lower by 2-13 dB at the left front wing position than at the center position for red blank ammunition, indicating that the noise from the man's own weapon was the main source for the sound reaching that man's ear.

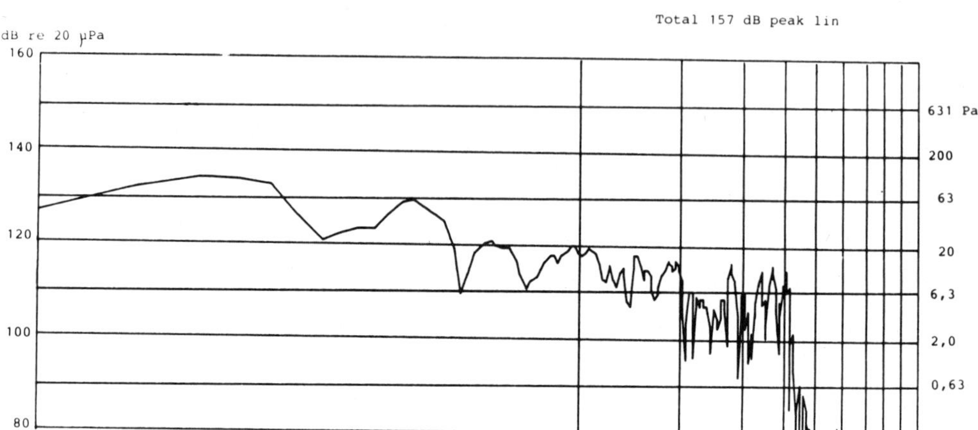

Fig. 2A. Power spectrum distribution of a single round 7.62 mm Garand SL rifle, red blank ammunition, vertical rifle position.

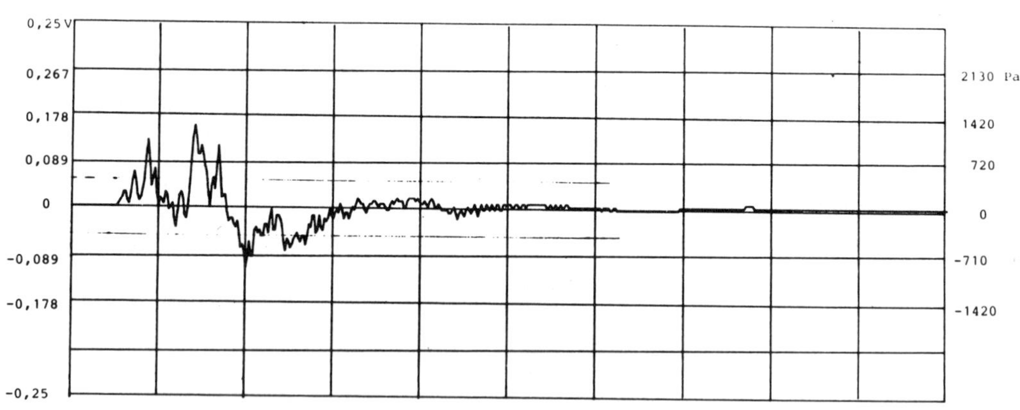

Fig. 2B. Amplitude time history of a single round 7.62 mm Garand SL rifle, red blank ammunition, vertical rifle position.

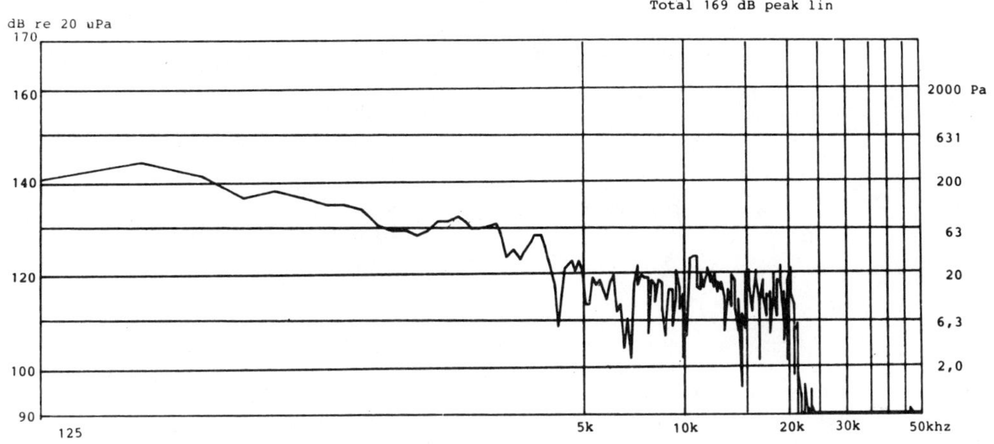

PWR SPECT A : N: NONE P: 125HZ

SPAN: 0. 000HZ -50. 000KHZ SN: - 2dBV FS: - 2. 00dBV 10dB/

Fig. 3A. Power spectrum distribution of a single round 7.62 mm Garand SL rifle, brass Energa blank ammunition, vertical rifle position.

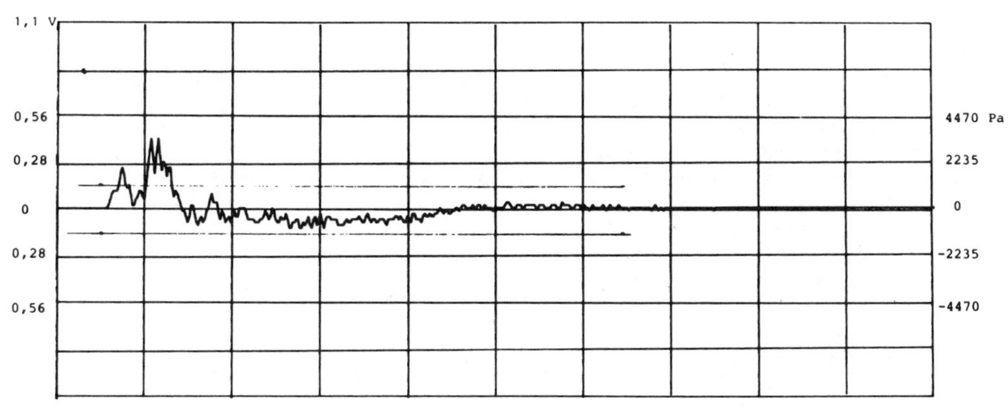

TIME A: 799. 89µSEC/ N: NONE

SPAN: 0. 000HZ -50. 000KHZ SN: 7. 9-01V FS: ±1. 1+00V 2. 8-01V/

Fig. 3B. Amplitude time history of a single round 7.62 mm Garand SL rifle, brass Energa blank ammunition, vertical rifle position.

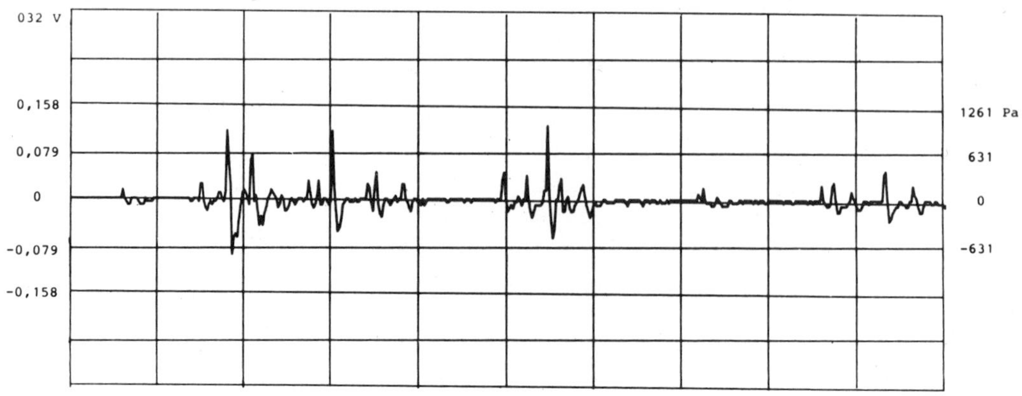

TIME B: 20.00mSEC/ N: PEAK

SPAN: 0.000HZ -2.0000KHZ SN: 2.2-01V FS: ±3.2-01V 7.9-02V/

Fig. 4. Amplitude time history of simultaneous (32 Single) rounds 7.62 mm Garand SL rifle, yellow Energa blank ammunition, vertical rifle position, center man.

Measurement of simultaneous rounds could not be performed with brass Energa blank ammunition as only two single rounds were available (old model). From the above data, there is reason to assume that simultaneous rounds with brass Energa blank ammunition would have given a single round peak level around 170 dB SPL and an increase in duration.

Selected time history and spectral distribution curves are given in Figs. 2A, 2B, 3A, 3B and 4. When the time history curves are studied, neither differences in rise time nor in A, B, C or D-duration (according to [6]) seem to account for the differences between the noise hazard potentials of red blank ammunition and brass Energa blank ammunition. The spectral distribution of brass Energa blank ammunition, however, shows an even slope towards the higher frequencies (and the limits of the 20 kHz low-pass filter), whereas the red blank ammunition shows two rather distinct peaks around 500 Hz and 1 kHz frequencies. The significance of these distributions, in terms of noise hazard, is not known to the authors. It is also hard to state whether the frequency difference in the maximum mean hearing loss in the 1983 squad (4000 Hz) versus the 1982 or 1984 squad (6000 Hz) (Fig. 1) is related to peak or spectral differences between red blank ammunition and brass Energa blank ammunition (Figs. 2A, 2B, 3A, 3B).

CONCLUSION

We feel that the above data indicate that it was the high peak level of 170 dB that caused the substantial permanent noise-induced hearing losses observed in the 1983 squad. This indicates a critical peak level for impulse noise hazard which, in man, lies between 160 and 170 dB linear (at least for impulses with the above frequencies, rise times, durations and repetition rates). If the above noise exposures are replicated in animal experiments, the results may serve to link PTS data in man and various animal species.

REFERENCES

1. H. M. Borchgrevink, Hearing and Hearing Prophylaxis, Proc. Oslo Int. Sympo. Effects of Noise and Hearing, Scand. Audiol. Suppl., 16:65 (1982).
2. H. M. Borchgrevink, Editor's Summary, in: Effects of Noise and Hearing, H. M. Borchgrevink ed., Scand. Audiol. Suppl. 16:122 (1982).
3. B. M. Johnstone D. Robertson and A. Cody, Basilar membrane motion and hearing loss, in: Effects of Noise and Hearing, H. M. Borchgrevink ed., Scand. Audiol. Suppl. 16:89 (1982).
4. D. Henderson, R. J. Salvi and R. P. Hamernik, Is the equal energy rule applicable to impact noise, in: Effects of Noise and Hearing, H. M. Borchgrevink ed., Scand. Audiol. Suppl. 16:71 (1982).
5. K. Buck, Influence of different presentation patterns of a given noise dose on hearing in guinea-pig, in: Effects of Noise and Hearing, H. M. Borchgrevink ed., Scand. Audiol. Suppl. 16:83 (1982).
6. G. Smoorenburg, Damage risk criteria for impulse noise, in: New Perspectives on Noise-induced Hearing Loss, R. P. Hamernik, D. Henderson and R. J. Salvi eds., Raven Press, New York (1982).

CAN TTS BE AN INDICATOR FOR INDIVIDUAL SUSCEPTIBILITY TO PTS?

Karl Buck and R. Franke

Franco-German Research Institute of Saint Louis
St. Louis, France

INTRODUCTION

It has long been agreed that there would be great interest in finding a test which predicts individual susceptibility to permanent threshold shift (PTS). Such tests would allow identification of people who are most likely to develop a noise-induced hearing loss in high noise areas and thereby reduce the number of people who suffer hearing impairment (and save much in compensation costs). Twenty years ago, Ward [1] analyzed about 20 proposed tests of individual susceptibility, and found none of them good enough to be useful.

Since that time, many other publications on this subject have appeared. Most of the procedures were described by Howell [2] in 1982. In this publication he tried to evaluate the whole repertory of proposed tests. The proposed tests can be divided into two major groups, auditory and nonauditory.

Nonauditory Tests

Bonaccorsi [3] showed, in men and guinea pigs, that a correlation exists between the concentration of melanin in the stria vascularis and susceptiblity to noise. Because the concentration of melanin in the iris of the eye is positively correlated with the concentration in the stria vascularis, it follows that dark eyes are correlated with low noise susceptibility. It has also been proposed that there is a correlation between general health and susceptibility. Different studies [4,5] indicate that good cardiovascular function decreases the risk of hearing loss. Overall, however, the relationship between nonauditory factors and susceptibility is sufficiently weak that they do not seem to offer a basis for an effective susceptibility test.

Auditory Tests

There are a very large number of proposed tests, almost all of them using some procedure to determine the sensitivity to temporary threshold shift (TTS). A few of them will be mentioned. Carhart [6] proposed the "Threshold of Distortion Test" as an index of susceptibility to TTS. This test used the level at which pure tone nonlinear combination tones could be heard. The "Threshold of Octave Masking Effect" proposed by Humes et al. [7] is based on a similar principle.

The "Loudness Discrimination Index" was proposed as an early indicator for TTS [8]. This test is based on recruitment, which is usually seen after a subject is exposed to intense noise.

Pederson [9,10] showed that changes in the cochlea due to intense noise alter the slope of the temporal integration function. Thus, Humes [11] proposed that "Brief Tone Audiometry" might be an indicator of susceptibility.

Humes [11] also proposed that "Speech Discrimination in Noise" might be used to detect 'fragile' ears because frequency integration in the ear might be affected long before any TTS could be detected. "Acoustic Reflex Measurement" [12] has also been suggested as a test of susceptibility. It has been proposed that reflex latency, rise time and fall times could give an indication of sensitivity to TTS.

All the auditory tests purport to predict individual susceptibility to TTS, but not to PTS. In fact, most of the tests deal with TTS in humans, and there is no ethical way to induce a PTS in humans for experimental purposes. So the problem for all tests is that there must be a correlation between sensitivity to TTS and sensitivity to PTS if they are to have any practical value.

Relationship between TTS and PTS

Temkin [13], in 1933, first stated the hypothesis that there should be some relationship between TTS and PTS. In the intervening years, discussion has gone on and there is still no definite answer as to whether this relationship exists or not. Burns and Robinson [14] measured the PTS acquired during a worker's previous employment and compared it to the TTS acquired during one working day. They reported that the group of workers which showed a lower initial hearing sensitivity developed less TTS at the end of the working day. They also concluded "that a higher susceptibility to TTS tends to be associated with higher susceptibility to occupational hearing loss, and vice versa." However, there is considerable uncertainity with respect to the hearing thresholds before the work experience, which makes it difficult to interpret these findings unequivocally.

Using the data of Richartz [15], Kraak [16,17] reported a close relationship between TTS integrated over time (ITTS) and PTS. This approach correlates the ITTS (growth and recovery) for a four hour exposure with the PTS due to about one year's exposure to the same noise (measured after several weeks of vacation). Although there are some methodological questions (Richartz's original article was not available), this method shows a surprisingly good correlation between ITTS and PTS.

Kryter et al. [18] postulated that the TTS observed after one working day should approximate the amount of PTS after ten years work in the same environment. The postulate was mainly based on data of others [19-23]. However, these data are mean data for groups and are not applicable to the prediction of individual susceptibility.

Jerger and Carhart [24] exposed subjects to 3 kHz tones at 100 dB for 60 seconds and then measured the time it took threshold at 4.5 kHz to return to within 20 and 10 dB of preexposure levels. The subjects then took a course on jet-engine maintenance where they were regularly subjected to intense noise exposure. Eight weeks after the exposure, PTS was measured. Their results suggest that subjects with a longer recovery time for TTS are more susceptible to PTS. Although there is a trend in their data, the large scatter shows that recovery time is not highly correlated with susceptibility to PTS.

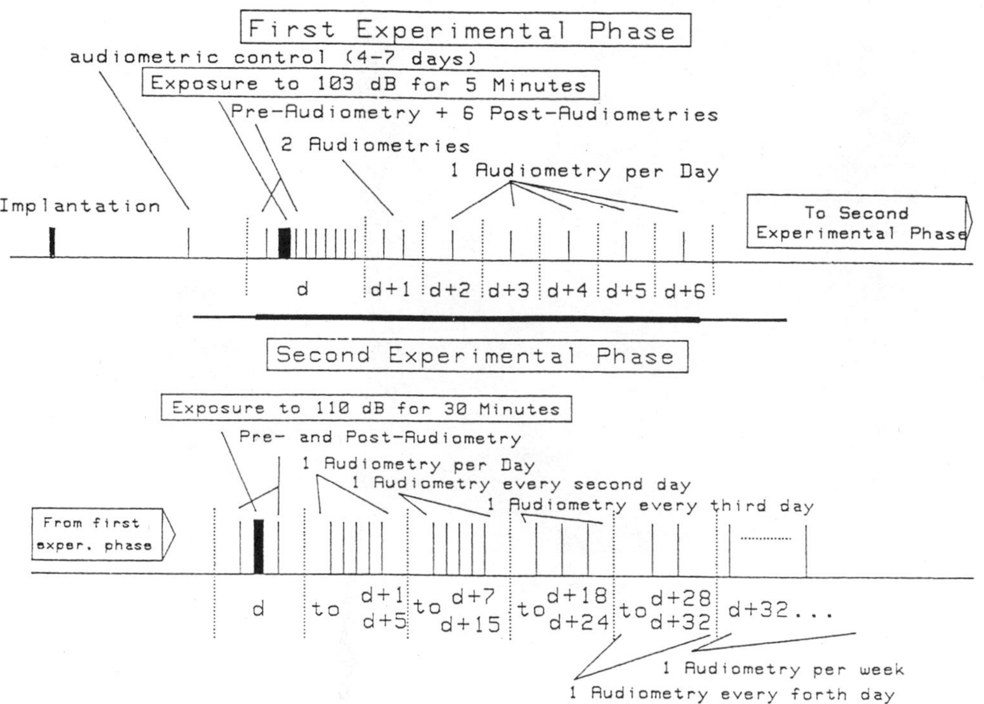

Fig. 1. Testing schedule.

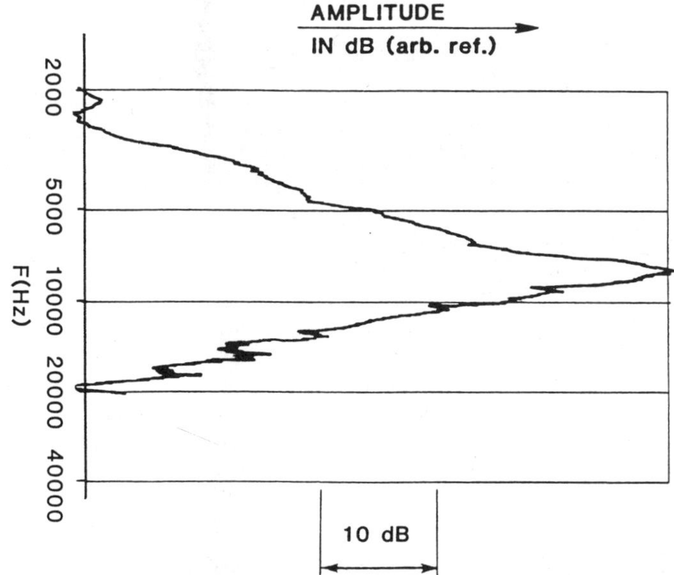

Fig. 2. Spectrum of the noise used to produce TTS and PTS.

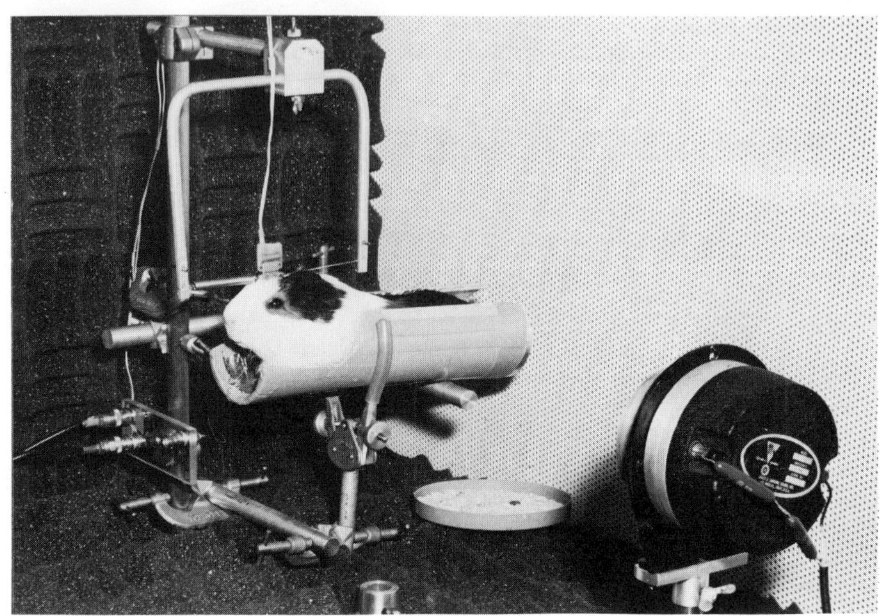

Fig. 3. Animal restraint used during audiometry and exposure.

Pfander [25] did a study in which 100 soldiers were exposed to three different types of noise (two white noises and gunshot). The five soldiers who showed the slowest recovery from the gunshot also showed PTS at the end of the shooting training. Therefore, he suggested that the recovery time of TTS might be the factor characterizing susceptibility to noise.

The foregoing tests show some relationship between TTS (or related factors) and PTS. Unfortunately, they were designed to show the correlation for groups, rather than for individuals. It is possible that a test of susceptibility to PTS based on TTS measures may also work very well for individuals. The literature gives no direct answer to this issue, but rather a lot of inconsistencies. Therefore, we decided to evaluate whether or not it was possible to find some correlation between TTS (or related parameters) and susceptibility to PTS for at least one case.

EXPERIMENT

This experiment was planned to give us maximum data about TTS from the moment at which it was induced until full recovery, and also to provide data from the same animals after the induction of a PTS. The experiment was intended to give us a maximum number of parameters to evaluate the correlation between TTS and PTS in the same animal.

Experimental Plan

In Phase One of the experiment, a TTS was induced in each animal. The exposure (level and time) was chosen so that the maximum TTS was about 25 dB, which insured that only fatigue and not PTS was induced, and that all animals would recover within one week. Ears were stimulated for five minutes with a 103 dB, 1/3 octave band of noise having a center frequency of 8 kHz. Threshold shifts were monitored as shown in Fig. 1.

Phase Two consisted of an exposure intended to produce a PTS (the same noise as before, but at 110 dB for 30 minutes). It was carried out a week later, after all animals had recovered. Fig. 1 also shows the times at which thresholds were monitored in this phase of the experiment.

The noise used to induce TTS and PTS had the same spectral composition (see Fig. 2). The major reason this noise was chosen was that it permitted us to limit threshold shifts to a narrow frequency range. Thus, stable thresholds outside the affected area assured us that the changes measured were in fact due to the exposure and not to instabilities in the preparation. This was important because the animals were tested over a period of about 40 to 60 days. An additional consideration was that a stimulus of 8 kHz is less affected by the acoustic reflex than stimuli at lower frequencies [26].

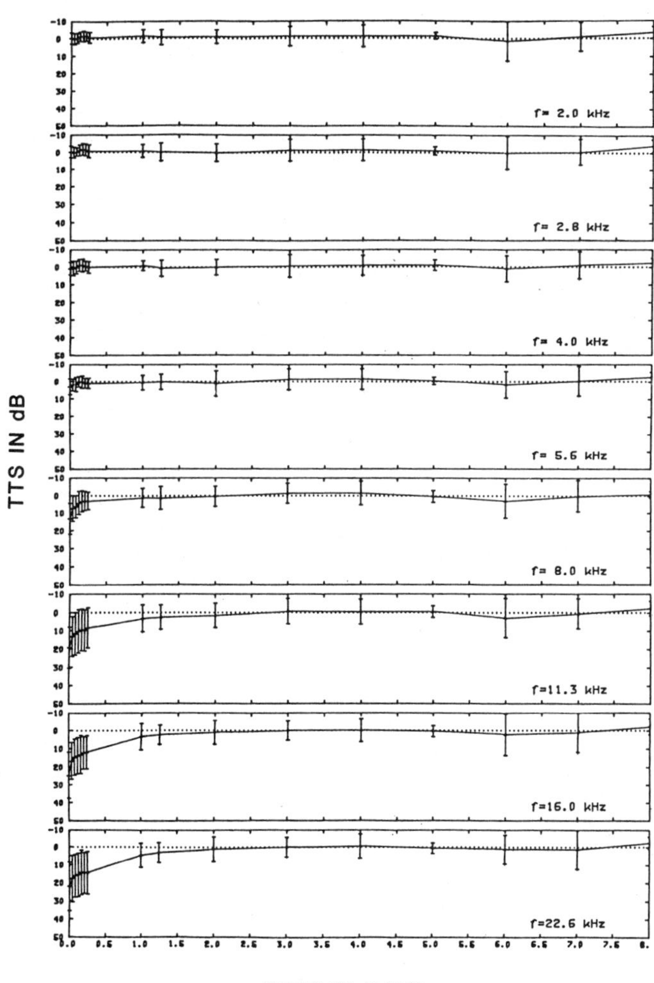

Fig. 4. Mean threshold shift and its standard-deviation as a function of time after exposure to 103 dB for five minutes.

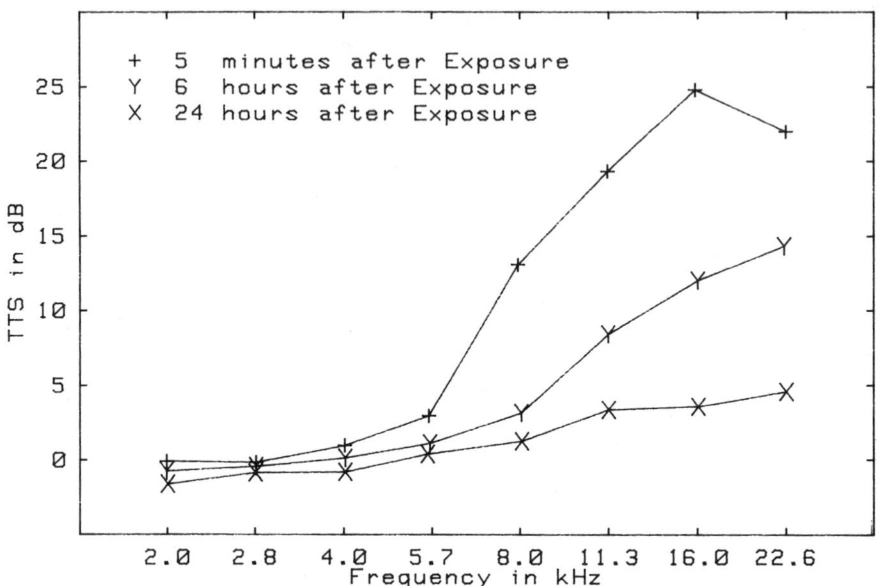

Fig. 5. TTS as a function of frequency at three different recovery times (Mean values of 24 guinea pigs).

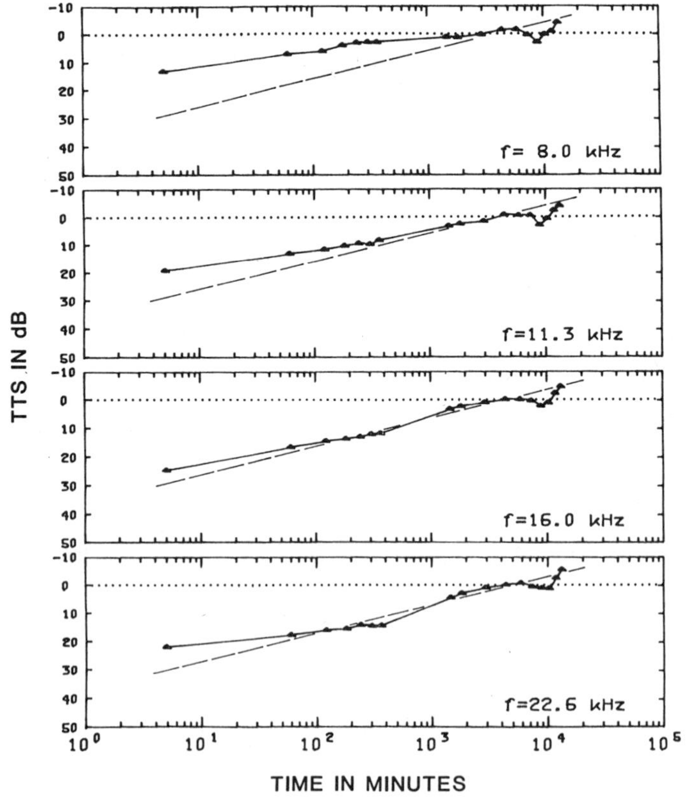

Fig. 6. TTS as a function of time for the four frequencies with the highest TTS. The dashed line shows the recovery function proposed by Kryter [28].

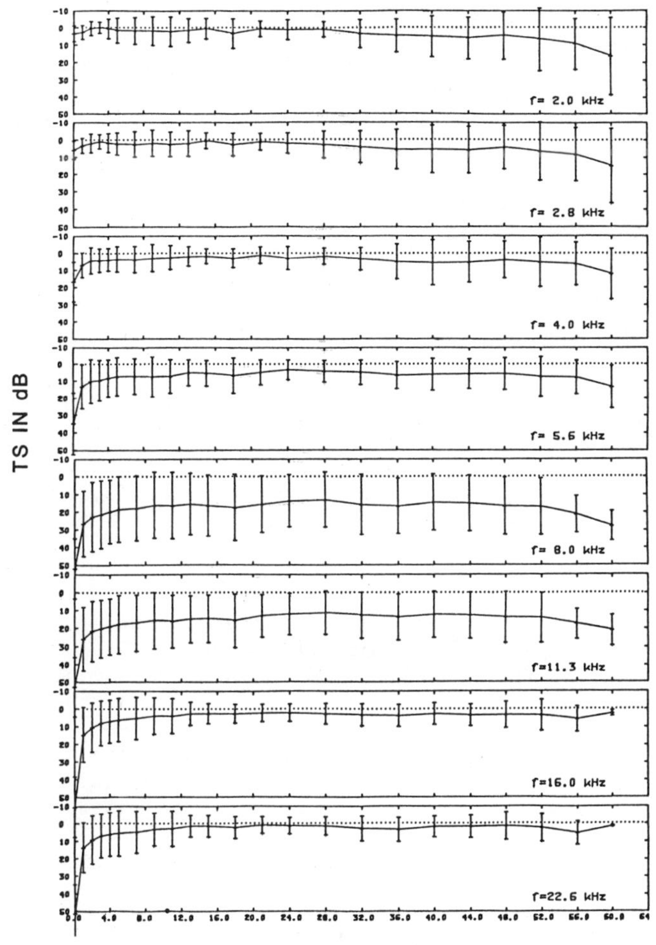

Fig. 7. Mean threshold shift and its standard deviation as a function of time after exposure to 110 dB for 30 minutes.

The threshold measurements were made using an implanted round window electrode [27]. The threshold was measured with "filtered clicks" and defined as the level which was needed to obtain a 3 uV amplitude of the N1 wave of the compound action potential. The threshold measurements and the noise exposure were made with awake guinea pigs in a free sound field. The animal's head was held in a semi-rigid restraint apparatus (Fig. 3); its body was only slightly restrained in a plastic tube, so the animal could move but its head was held in a stable position with respect to the loudspeaker.

RESULTS

TTS

Fig. 4 shows the evolution of the TTS in phase I for all frequencies tested. The data are mean values and standard deviations of a group of

24 animals. For frequencies lower than 8.0 kHz (which is below the noise-band), there was almost no TTS. The standard deviations at these lower frequencies were also smaller than those in the areas where TTS was induced. This figure shows that a fast recovery takes place during the first 6 hours after exposure (linear time scale) and that full (mean) recovery is obtained within three days.

Fig. 5 shows the mean TTS at three different time intervals after stimulation as a function of the frequency. It is clear that the maximum TTS is not located at the same frequency as the maximum energy of the noise, but about one octave higher (for the measurement five minutes after stimulation). The maximum shifted toward even higher frequencies for the 6 and 24 hour curves.

The mean recovery at the four frequencies that showed a shift (8.0, 11.3, 16.0 and 22.6 kHz) is plotted in Fig. 6 (the broken line represents the recovery function given by Kryter [23]. For the frequencies which show the highest TTS (16 and 22.6 kHz), the rate of recovery is quite close to that published by Kryter, but for the frequencies showing less TTS, the slope is not as steep (1.3 instead of 3.0 dB per doubling of time).

Fig. 7 presents the mean threshold shift (TS) in phase II as a function of time. All measured frequencies are displayed. The standard deviations plotted refer to 24 animals after stimulation, and to seven animals at the end of the experiment (60 days after stimulation). This loss in number is due primarily to the interruption of the electrical circuit of the implant (N=12). These problems occurred because of the growth of the animals during the experiment. The other reasons were: otitis media (N=3), lesion of the ear drum (N=1) and one death. This figure also shows some TS for all frequencies immediately after the noise exposure. At this time, TTS and PTS processes are mixed and the maximum value of about 50 dB is found at 16 kHz. The recovery for frequencies below 5.6 kHz and above 11.3 kHz is almost complete after about 15 days. Because recovery is essentially finished at this time, we later refer to these values at "PTS." The figure also shows some TS for low frequencies which becomes greater with time. It seems that this effect also has (at lease in part) to be attributed to the noise exposure, because a study of the reproducibility of the method [29] showed no degradation of sensitivity. This effect could partially be due to microlesions in the ossicular chain during the exposure, which later induce some sclerotic effects in the ligaments.

Fig. 8 shows the threshold shifts at the time of maximal recovery (14 days after exposure) and the 5% confidence interval (measured with 21 animals). Note that frequencies lower than 5.6 kHz and higher than 11.3 kHz show essentially no PTS, whereas thresholds at 8.0 and 11.3 show a TS of more than 15 dB. At 5.6 kHz, the TS is only about 5 dB. As with TTS's, the dispersion of the PTS data becomes much larger when a threshold shift is present. This is consistent with the interpretation that the scatter of the threshold shifts is really due to intra-individual differences in susceptibility, and not to methodological uncertainties.

Individual Data

A set of data similar to those shown in Figs. 4 and 7 were obtained for every animal (the PTS used in data analysis was derived from TS at 14 days because of reasons which were discussed earlier). In the following figures, we try to correlate the TTS or related parameters to the PTS acquired by the same animal in order to see if any of these parameters show some relationship.

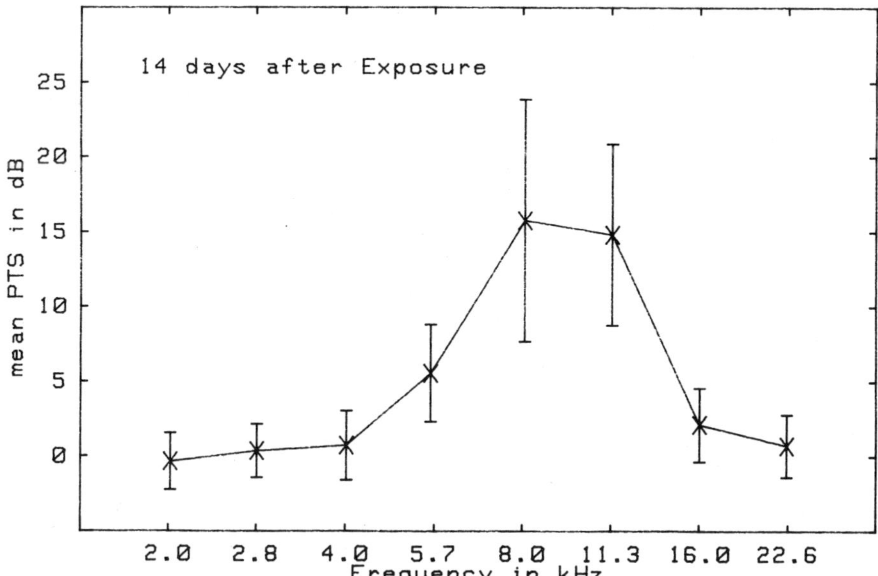

Fig. 8. Permanent threshold shifts as a function of frequency and the 5% confidence interval 14 days after exposure at 110 dB for 30 minutes.

Individual Sensitivity

Fig. 9 shows individual PTS's at 5.6, 8.0, 11.3 and 16 kHz as a function of the initial hearing thresholds at the three surrounding frequencies. There is apparently little or no correlation between initial sensitivity and PTS.

TTS Five Minutes and Six Hours After Noise Exposure

Fig. 10 shows the individual PTS's for the most affected frequencies (8.0, 11.3, 16.0 and 22.6 kHz) as a function of the TTS measured five minutes after the first stimulation (103 dB for five minutes). The PTS's at the three frequencies lower or equal to the TTS frequency are plotted using different symbols. Again, no correlation could be found. Fig. 11 is analogous to the previous one, but the TTS plotted is that measured six hours after noise exposure. Again, no correlation could be found.

Frequency at TTS Max

Fig. 12 shows the maximum individual PTS as a function of the frequency of maximum TTS obtained five minutes or six hours after the end of exposure. No correlation could be found.

Recovery Time of TTS

Fig. 13 shows the individual PTS as a function of TTS recovery time. The recovery time was defined as the time an individual animal needed to recover to within 2 dB of the pre-exposure value. No correlation could be found.

TTS integrated over the frequency range and over recovery time

Fig. 14 PTS_{Max} is plotted as a function of the integral of the TTS (Fig 14a: TTS_{5min}; Fig 14b: TTS_{6hours}) over all measured frequencies. No

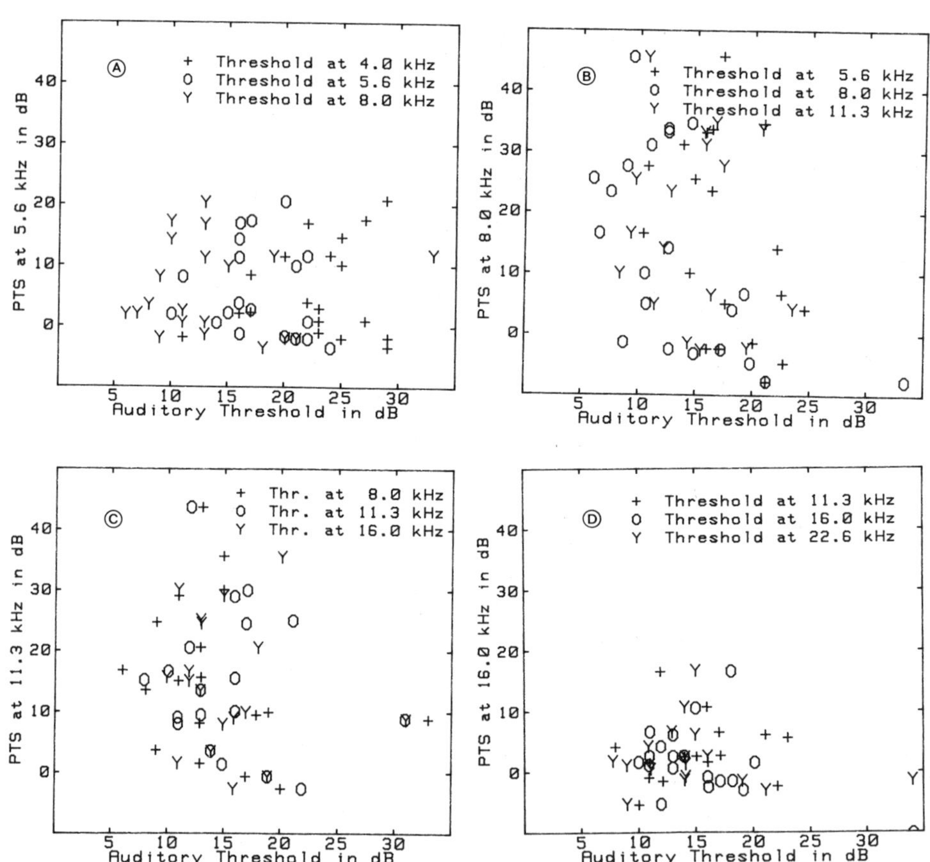

Fig. 9. Scatter diagram of initial audiometric sensitivity and PTS.

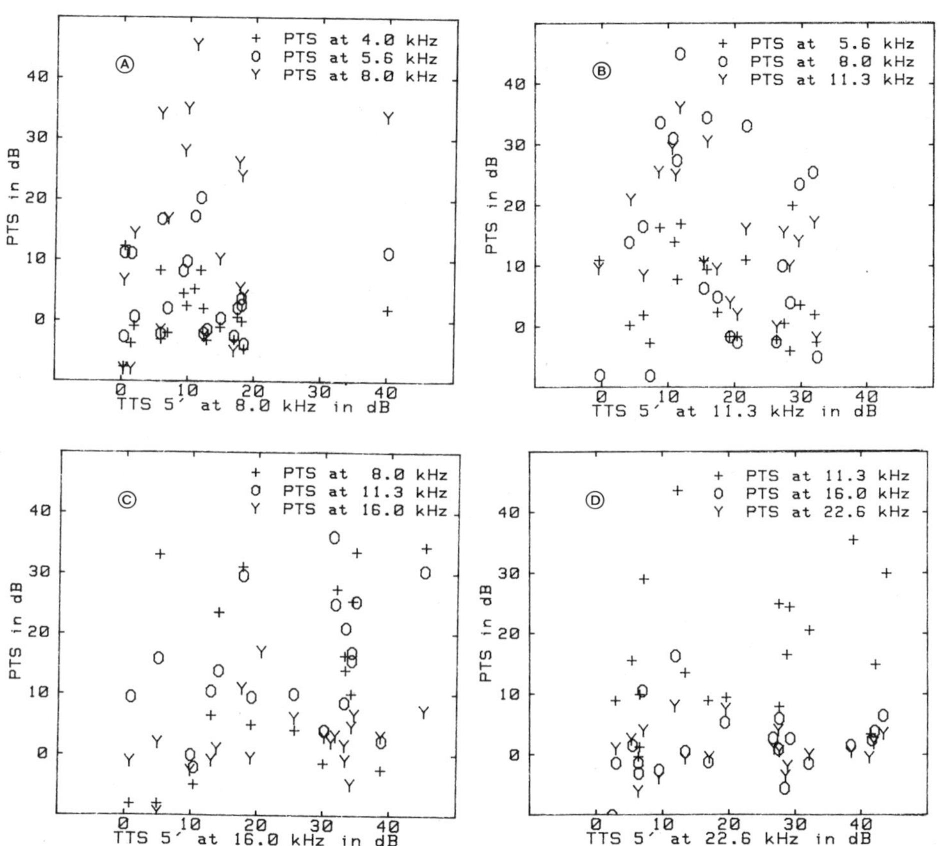

Fig. 10. Scatter diagram showing the relationship between PTS and TTS five minutes after exposure at 103 dB.

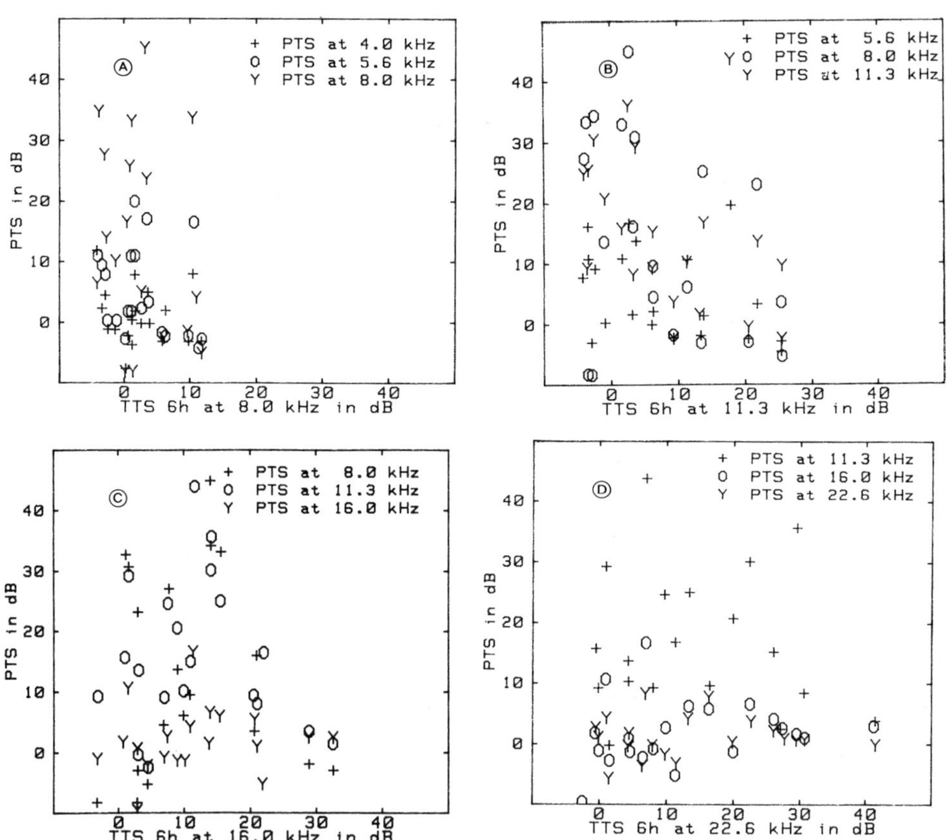

Fig. 11. Scatter diagram showing the relationship between PTS and TTS six hours after exposure.

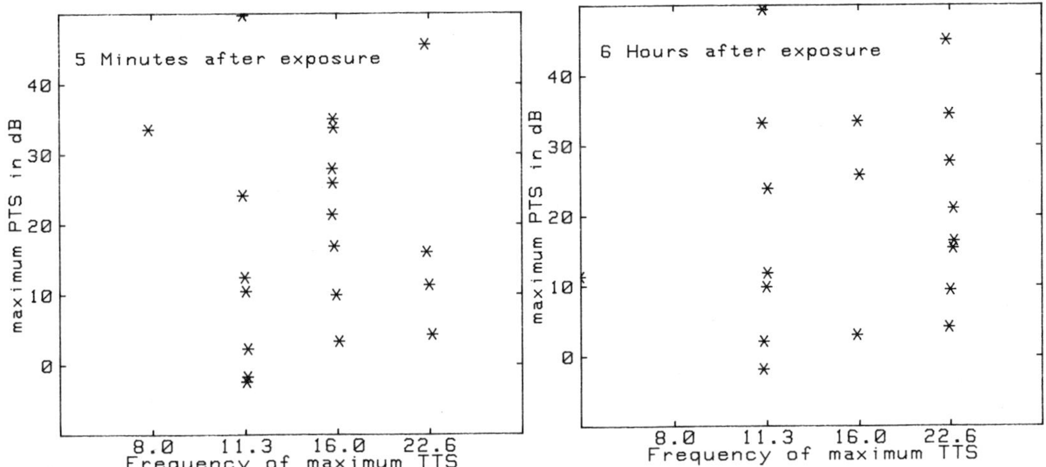

Fig. 12. Scatter diagram showing the relationship between maximal PTS and the frequency of maximum TTS obtained five minutes or six hours after exposure at 103 dB.

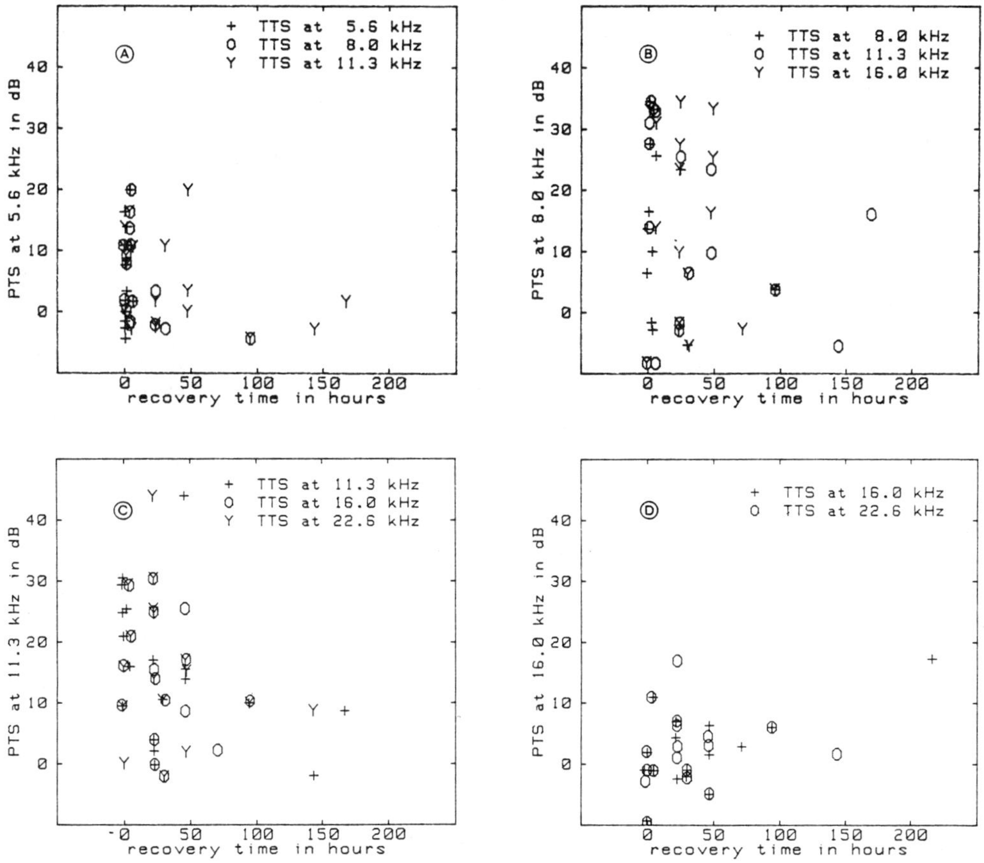

Fig. 13. Scatter diagram showing the relationship between PTS and TTS recovery time at different frequencies.

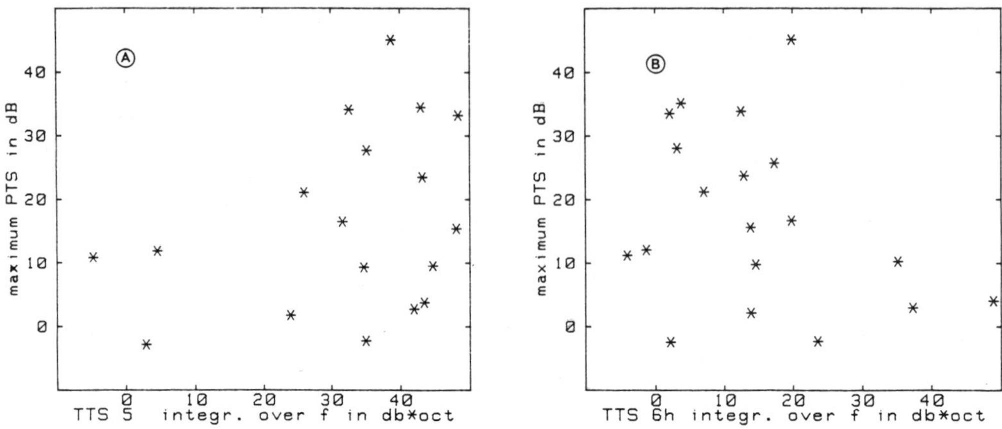

Fig. 14. Scatter diagram showing the relationship between maximum PTS and TTS integrated over the frequencies at five minutes post-exposure or six hours post exposure.

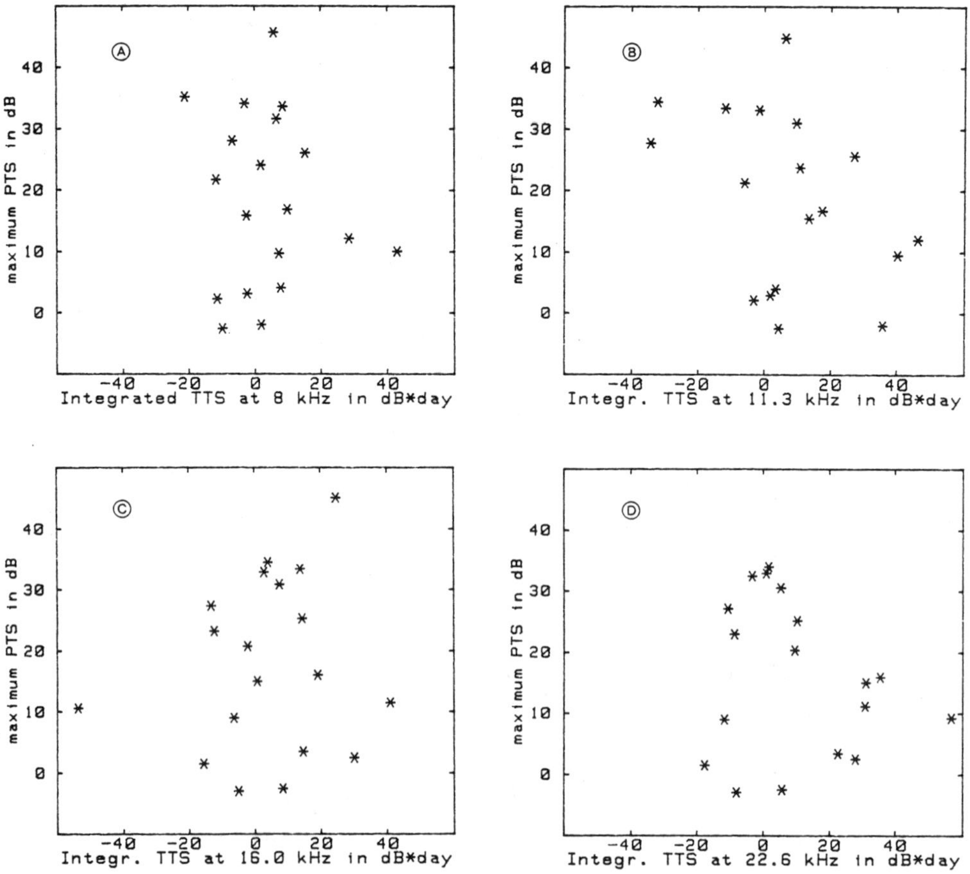

Fig. 15. Scatter diagram of maximum PTS and TTS integrated over recovery time.

correlation could be found. PTS for individuals is plotted in Fig. 15 as a function of TTS integrated over the whole recovery time for four different frequencies (8.0, 11.3, 16.0, and 22.6 kHz). Again, no correlation could be found.

CONCLUSIONS

During the last 20 years, a large amount of work has been done to determine the individual susceptibility to PTS. In general, there have been promising results for group data; however, no conclusive test for individual susceptibility has been demonstrated. As far as just TTS is concerned, there are some interesting approaches, especially tests concerning the temporal evolution of TTS. However, tests predicting susceptibility to PTS by using susceptibility to TTS are likely to be successful only if TTS and PTS are induced by the same mechanisms.

The essentially low correlations between PTS and TTS found in our study seem to indicate that there are different mechanisms involved (or at least for these conditions). Some data for groups of subjects also indicate the same thing. For example, maximum TTS appears at about 16 kHz, one octave higher than the noise stimulus, but the maximum PTS was measured at about 8 kHz (the center frequency of the noise stimulus). This means that TTS is induced in a different part of the cochlea than PTS. Liberman [30] reported that TTS is essentially due to metabolic depletion, evidenced by vacuoles at the base of the hair cells; whereas, it is generally agreed that PTS is the result of structural modification or destruction of hair cells. If TTS and PTS are due to different mechanisms, then susceptibility to PTS should be tested using methods which are more directly related to PTS. Unfortunately, this means that any test which is perfectly reversible might not give enough information about PTS. It follows that a test which induces irreversible changes would be the best "predictor;" but it is doubtful that such a test would ever be practical.

ACKNOWLEDGEMENT

This work has been supported by the "Direction des Recherches Etudes et Techniques," grant DRET 79/353.

REFERENCES

1. W. D. Ward, The concept of susceptibility, J. Occup. Med. 7:595 (1965)
2. K. Howell, "Susceptibility to Noise-Induced Hearing Loss," ISVR Contract Report No. 82/20, London (1982).
3. P. Bonaccorsi, U colore dell'iride cone 'test' di valutazione quantitativa, nell' nemo della concentratione di melamina nella striavasculare, Annali. Lar. Otol. Rhinol. Fraing. 64:725 (1965).
4. G. Jansen, Relation between temporary threshold shift and peripheral circulatory effects of sound, in: "Physiological Effect of Noise," Welch and Welch (ed.), Plenum, New York (1970).
5. S. Rosen, D. Plester, A. El-Mofty, and H. V. Rosen, Relation of hearing loss to cardiovascular disease, Trans. Am. Acad. Ophthalmol. Otolaryngol. 68:433 (1964).
6. R. H. Carhart, Updating special hearing tests in otological diagnosis, Arch. Otolaryngol. 97:88 (1973).
7. L. E. Humes, D. M. Schwartz and F. H. Bess, The threshold of octave masking (TOM) as a predictor of susceptibility to noise-induced hearing loss, J. Audit. Res. 17:5 (1977).

8. G. R. Bienvenue, J. R. Violin-Singer and P. L. Michael, Loudness discrimination index (LDI): A test for early detection of noise susceptible individuals, Am. Ind. Hyg. Assoc. J. 38:333 (1977).
9. C. B. Pederson, Brief tone audiometrie in patients with acoustic trauma, Acta Otolaryngol. (Stockholm) 75:332 (1973).
10. C. B. Pederson, Brief tone audiometrie, Scand. Audiol. 5:27 (1976).
11. L. E. Humes, Review of four new indices of susceptibility to noise-induced hearing loss," J. Occup. Med. 19:116 (1977).
12. B. Hohansson, B. Kylin and M. Langfy, Acoustic reflex as a test of individual susceptibility to noise, Acta Otolaryngol. 64:256 (1967).
13. J. Temkin, Die schaedigung des ohres durch laerm und erschuetterung, Mschr. Ohrenheilk. und Laryngo-Rhinologie, 67 (1933).
14. W. Burns and D. W. Robinson, Hearing and Noise in Industry, HMSO, London (1970).
15. G. Richartz, Untersuchungen zur individuellen laermempfindlichkeit bein menschen, Dissertation, Technische Universitaet, Dresden (1976).
16. W. Kraak, Integration of TTS for permanent threshold shift, in: "Noise as a Public Health Problem," American Speech and Hearing Associated Report No. 10 (1980).
17. W. Kraak, Investigations on criteria for the risk of hearing loss due to noise, in: "Hearing Research and Theory," Vol. 1. J. V. Tobias and E. D. Shubert, eds. Academic Press, New York (1981).
18. K. D. Kryter, W. D. Ward, J. D. Miller and D. H. Eldrege, Hazardous exposure to intermittent and steady-state noise, J. Acoust. Soc. Am. 39:451 (1966).
19. A. Glorig, W. D. Ward, J. Nixon, Damage-risk criteria and noise-induced hearing loss, in: "The Control of Noise: NPL Symposium Number 12," HMSO, London (1962).
20. B. Kylin, Temporary threshold shift and auditory trauma following exposure to steady-state noise, Acta Oto-Laryngol. Suppl. 152:1 (1960).
21. J. C. Nixon, A. Glorig, Noise-induced permanent threshold shift at 2000 cps and 4000 cps, J. Acoust. Soc. Am. 33:901 (1961).
22. N. E. Rosenwinkel and K. C. Steward, The relationship of hearing loss to steady-state noise exposure, Am. Ind. Hyg. Assoc. Quart. 18:117 (1957).
23. W. Rudmose, Hearing loss resulting from noise exposure, in: "Handbook of Noise Control," C. M. Harris, ed., McGraw-Hill Book Co., Inc., New York (1957).
24. J. F. Jerger and R. Carhart, Temporary threshold shift as an index of noise susceptibility, J. Acoust. Soc. Am. 28:611 (1956).
25. F. Pfander, Hoehe der temporaeren schwellenabwanderung (TTS) in audiogramm und 'rueckwanderungszeit' geraeuschund knallbelasteter ohren als test knallgefaerdeter hoerorgane, Arch. Ohr.-Nas.-u. Kehlk.-Heilk. 191:586 (1968).
26. P. Dallos, "The Auditory Periphery," Academic Press, New York (1973).
27. R. Franke, K. Buck, F. Devriere, "Essai d'utilisation de la fatigue auditive comme indicateur de la susceptibilite individuelle au trauma acoustique. Etude chez le cobaue." R 118/84 French-German Research Institute F-68301 Saint-Louis, FRANCE (1984).

DISCUSSION

Oftedal: Have you ever measured the correlation between the individual TTS's from repeated exposures to the same noise?

Buck: No. But it might be a nice experiment to determine if there is some correlation within a single animal.

FIELD STUDIES ON IMPULSE NOISE ANNOYANCE IN THE ENVIRONMENT OF GARRISON FIRING RANGES

Olaf Tech and Heinz Brinkmann

Bundesamt fur Wehrtechnik und Beschaffung, AFB FE IV
(Federal Office for Military Technology Procurement)
c/o Erprobungsstelle 91, 4470 Meppen

INTRODUCTION

Apart from their primary function, namely the firing of projectiles, both small- and large-caliber weapons generate a rather unpleasant side-effect - the muzzle blast. This phenomenon is caused by the propellant gases being suddenly released from the barrel behind the projectile. Directly near the weapon, this muzzle report may present a hazard to life and limb and may also cause damage to material. This limits, to a certain extent, the use of the weapon. Personnel working in the near vicinity of the weapon must wear either protective earmuffs or earplugs. Further away from the weapon, people are (or at least feel) disturbed by the impulse noise.

DESCRIPTION OF PROBLEM

According to 1982 statistics, the Federal Republic of Germany ranges fourth on the list of the most densely populated countries in the world, with 248 inhabitants per km (after Japan with 284, Belgium with 322, and the Netherlands with 400 inhabitants per km2); therefore there are hardly any large areas available which are far removed from populated areas. For this reason it is obvious that the problem of impulse noise annoyance is given particular attention in the FRG.

For the construction of new firing ranges, it is therefore useful to have a forecast model to permit predictions of expected noise levels and to amend the planning for the installation if required. A description of an investigation aimed at garrison firing ranges will be given below.

PROBLEMS RELATED TO MEASUREMENT OF IMPULSE NOISE AND EVALUATION OF TEST DATA

When trying to determine the effect of any given noise on the human body, and to make an objective quantitative assessment on the basis of measured data, the test must be designed to adequately simulate a statistical average of the properties of a "standard ear," excluding any dispersion of data caused by subjective impressions.

The function of the human ear is very complicated, with some details still being unknown; therefore, an instrumented test can only achieve a more or less adequate approximation. How close this approximation is to reality also depends on economic considerations such as instrumentation, time or personnel required. For the practical application of the test, it must be ensured that the same phenomenon may be measured at different times and different locations, but still leading to the same result. The comparability of test results is therefore more important than the degree of "accuracy" in absolute terms.

It is even more difficult to evaluate in fairly general terms the impulse noise, in view of its annoying and disturbing effects on human beings. It is therefore not the objective of this presentation to evaluate impulse noise along those lines, but rather to exclusively present the physically-defined properties of the acoustic phenomenon.

In Germany, a precision impulse sound level meter for the determination of impulse noise levels has been used since the late sixties, gathering comparable data on noise levels, which are relatively true to the acoustic impression on the human ear. For this reason, the results quoted below refer to L_{AI} values, although in recent years the use of L_{AFMAY} for impulse noise is favored both within German and international standardization agencies.

STUDIES

Impulse Noise Source in Open Terrain

The first step to determine the disturbing effect of various noises by measurement is to evaluate the noise source for its objective acoustic emission. In preparation of these measurements, any factors interfering with the noise propagation must be removed as far as possible. The first extensive tests in this field were carried out as early as 1969. The measurements, as summarized by Prof. Burck of the Technische Universitat Munich in his expert report published in WG VI - 3 [1], were taken by a team from Proving Ground 91 at Meppen, members of the former Arbeitsbereich Akustik (department for acoustics). The tests were conducted on a flat and open terrain. Although the tests had been carried out with various small caliber weapons. this presentation will only deal with one noise source, namely the rifle G 3. This rifle was also used for all further field studies as the standard noise source. The resulting test data, which are based on a number of individual parameters, may be presented as directivity diagrams giving the omnidirectional characteristics for distances of 50 and 100 m from the noise source (see Fig. 1). The directivity pattern for the sound radiation of the rifle G 3 is a wide oval shape, with the directional effect in firing direction.

As stated in the expert report (dated 1969), the marked deviation of impulse noise levels registered even at distances of only 50 m, a trend which increases with the distance from the noise source, can obviously not be attributed to variations generated by the noise source itself (at a test point located 100 m from the noise source, the differences in noise level are about 10 dB). As further proof of the above-mentioned statements, radiation characteristics of measurements of the G 3-rifle carried out at short ranges (1 m, 2 m and 5 m) are also shown on Fig. 1. These measurements, aimed at determining the muzzle blast, were carried out in 1977 [2] and 1981 [3] by Meppen Proving Ground. The peak pressure level L was determined after elimination of the ballistic shock wave which may have shown on an oscillogram. The deviation of results lies in this case within a range of less than 1 dB. This demonstrates that the basic features of the radiation characteristics shown at the 50 m or 100 m range are already evident in the short range (1 - 5 m). Only in the direction of fire (0 degrees), and to a minor extent at 45 degrees or 315 degrees to the direction of fire, the N-wave constitutes the dominating noise source, especially around the 100 m circle.

Noise Source in an Open Garrison Firing Range (Type A)

After examining the noise source as to its objective acoustic emission, the effect of the characteristic and firing range-specific environment on the emitted sound phenomena should be investigated. The test to be examined was carried out at the garrison firing range at Haberloh and aimed at determining the effect of the standard design of a garrison firing range type A with blast walls, screens and stop butts, all of conventional design. The Haberloh firing range is situated in a flat terrain surrounded mainly by meadows and boggy ground with low shrubs. Apart from the effect of facilities, there is no additional interference factor caused either by rough terrain features or dense vegetation. It was again the acoustics working group of the Meppen Proving Ground that carried out the measurements, recording simultaneously outputs from eight test

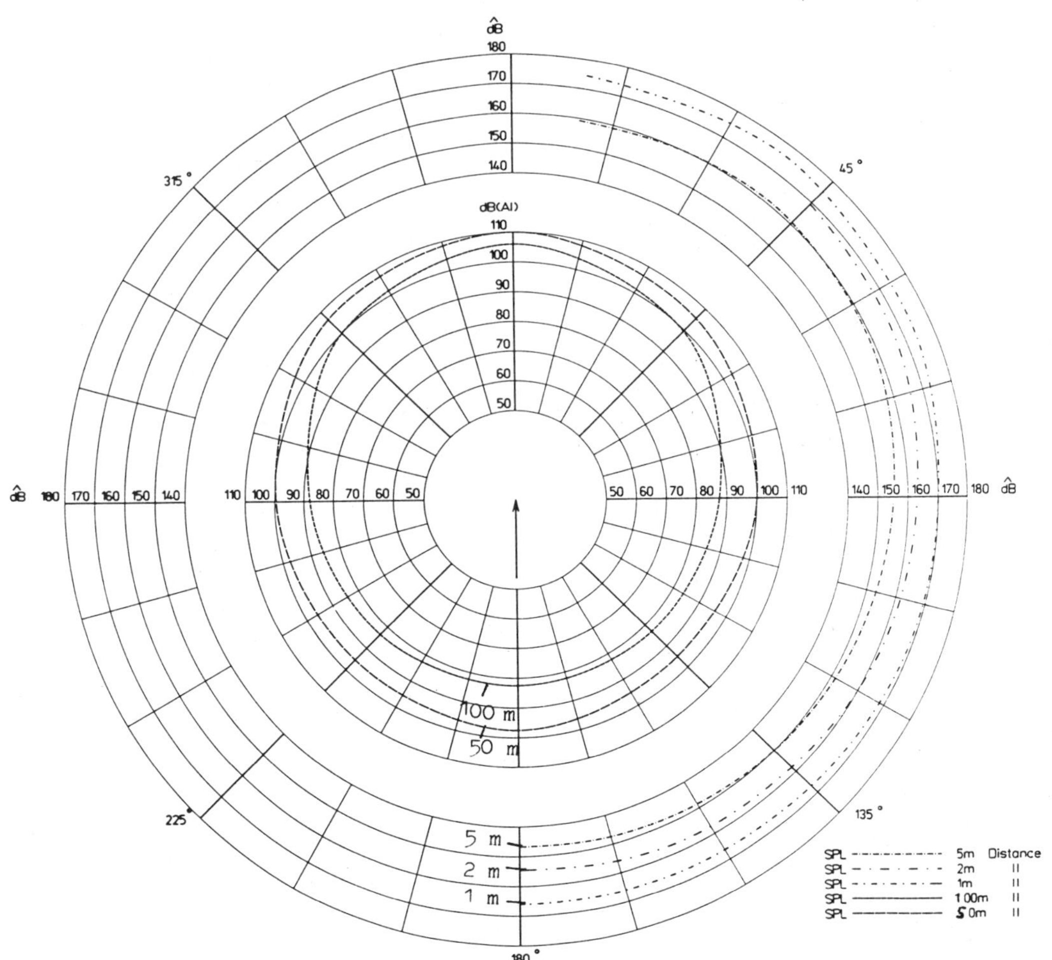

Fig. 1. Directivity Pattern for the Sound Radiation of the Rifle G3

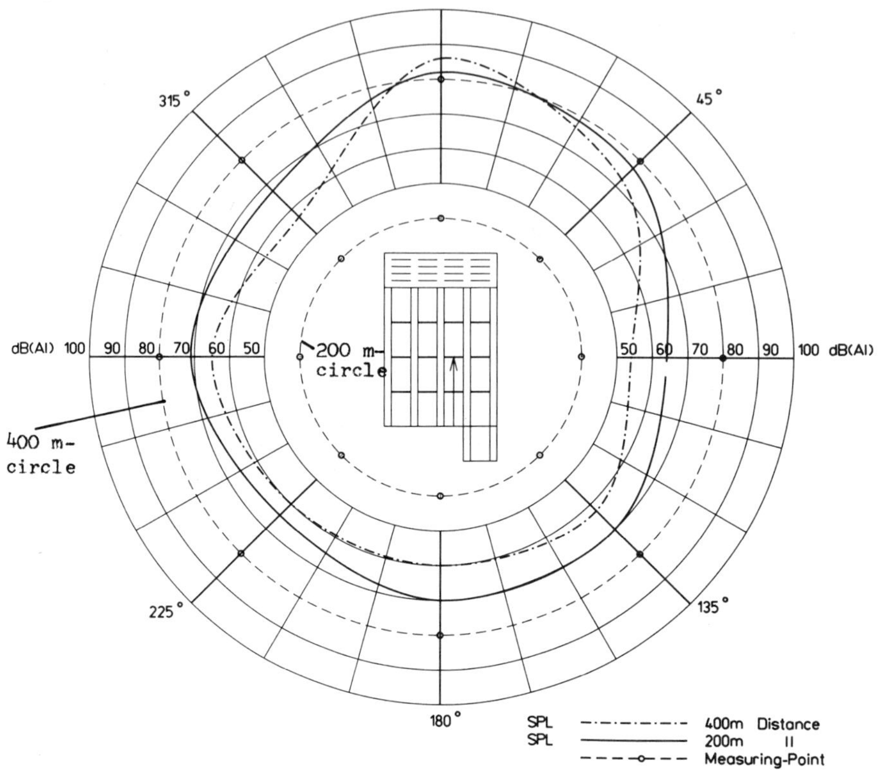

Fig. 2. Circular Sound Emission Pattern of the Garrison Firing Range Haberloh (Type A)

points. The test points were arranged in a circle around an assumed centerpoint of the firing range, with a radius of 200 m or 400 m (Fig. 2). The firing position on rifle range III/150 m being located 25 m away from the assumed centerpoint caused a shift of the measured data of omnidirectional characteristics to one side, because to the right of the firing direction there were two blast walls and to the left, three blast walls between firing position and respective test points [4]. The 200 m test point in firing direction was located directly behind the projectile butt, so that this test point was in the acoustical shadow. For this reason the L -value at the 400 m test point was higher than at the 200 m test point (Fig. 2). A further conclusion of this investigation was the fact that the effects of metereological conditions on the sound propagation have an important influence. Specially, the effect of wind causes a strong dispersion of noise level values. Based on numerous individual measured data, Burck [4] has proposed the following rule of thumb: for tail-wind conditions, an increase of 2 dB(AI) per m/s mean wind speed and for head wind, a decrease of the same order must be taken into account. In October 1970, Burck [5] described the omnidirectional characteristics of a firing range type A, with the noise source being near the center of the range (Fig. 3). This value represents a symmetrically adjusted average of the "Haberloh" test data with the G 3-rifle as noise source. The changes in the omnidirectional characteristics as compared to the radiation characteristics of the G 3-rifle in the open terrain are to be attributed to the firing range-specific features. These measurements, however, offer no basis for generally valid statements which may also apply to other facilities or types of facilities, because of basic differences, such as the number of firing lanes and thus the number of blast walls separating the lanes, as well as the differing arrangement of screens and their location relative to each other. All these features may vary from range to range.

Noise Source on Firing Range with Transverse Screens (Type C)

At the Mainz garrison firing range, a test was carried out in 1983 and 1984 to determine the effect of screens and of metereological conditions on sound propagation. This particular range was chosen because it was a type C firing range situated in a relatively flat terrain with elevations of up to + 10 m and ground depressions of up to - 6 m at a distance of 400 m or - 33 m at a distance 3200 m. The surrounding vegetation consisted mainly of farmland (grain), orchards and vegetable plantations, as well as some woodland. To get a better understanding of the effect of vegetation and different weather conditions, measurements were taken in five test series over one year (June, August, October 1983, January and March 1984). The chosen test points were located at distances of 200 m, 400 m, 800 m, 1000 m and 3200 m from the firing position (at station 150 m). Measurements were taken in eight different directions around the range. The 360 degree measurements, the results of which were to be compared with the previously generated omnidirectional characteristica, were taken at eight test points arranged around a 400 m circle. This 400 m was chosen because the same diatance was used during the earlier measurements and also because it is outside the near-field of the garrison firing range. Some parameters, however, which are required to exactly determine the directional characteristics of a range with transverse screens had not been met. For example, the frequency of occurrence of the different wind directions was not evenly spread over the five test series. Furthermore, the US firing range with its own screens, bordering the Mainz firing range to the South, affected the acoustic events.

Omnidirectional characteristics were generated at each test series, the respective effect of wind being quite obvious [6]; therefore, an average of the directional characteristics for all five test series was computed. An average of the wind properties had also been calculated: wind direction being expressed as a veotorial average, wind speed as an arithmetic average. Using the correction methods described below, the omnidirectional characteristics of the Mainz installation are as shown on Fig. 3. Due to the particular arrangement of the screens and multiple reflexions at the front of one screen and at the back of another, a butterfly-type directivity pattern in contrast to the oval pattern of the "Haberloh range" was generated. The 4-6 dB increase in noise level at 90 and 270 firing lane, where even at the Mainz installation there is no reflexion of the muzzle blast, is probably due to the fact that on both sides there is one blast wall less than that at Haberloh.

With the intention of examining the sound propagation, 10 test points were arranged at 180° degrees. The test points were staggered at distances between + 200 m and + 3200 m as well as between - 200 m and - 3200 m. After one measurement was completed, the measurement axis was shifted by 45°, and the sound propagation measurement was repeated. These symmetrical measurements, along two different measurement beams in opposite directions, allowed an examination of both head-wind and tail-wind conditions. Due to the large number of individual test data to be processed, computer was used, plotting a regression curve through the imputs points and calculating at the same time the appropriate regression coefficients. Head-wind or cross-wind conditions caused a considerable variation of results whereas tail-wind conditions showed a marked trend in the test data. Although the absolute noise level of the individual firings varied considerably, the

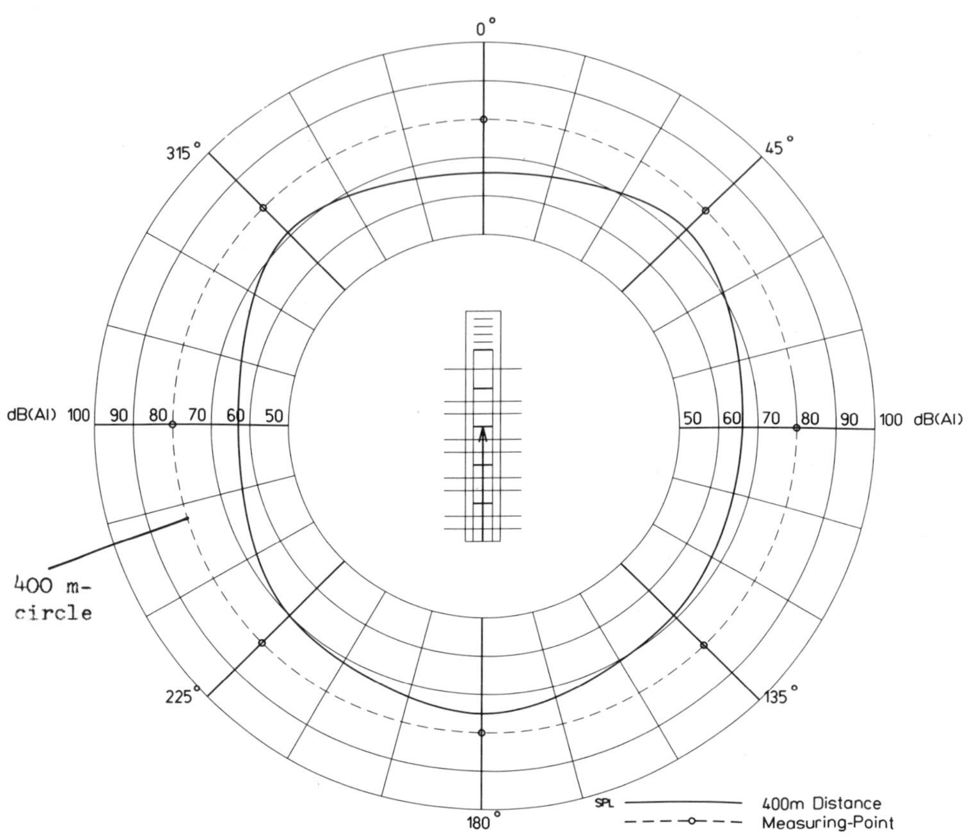

Fig. 3. Circular sound emission pattern of the garrison firing range mainz (type C).

decrease in noise level remained more or less the same. This is confirmed by a very high regression coefficient of approximately 1. The low regression coefficient of the January measurement (0.4 - 0.7) was caused by terrain features and vegetation properties. The test point 1600 m directly opposite the firing direction was located in front of a forest, which obviously caused reflexions and thus affected the test results. Due to the fact that in Germany tail-wind conditions must be considered for any noise-level forecast, this particular condition is of special interest as a subject for investigation.

For the calculation of sound propagation, the 200 m test points were not taken into account, because they are still within the inner boundary of the installation. Only the readings from the 400 m circle may be regarded as reproducible data, since these test points are no longer in the near-field of the range, and because metereological influences are not too marked at this distance.

The correlation between the change of wind speed and the changes of the noise-level reduction shows that the noise-level reduction per duplication of range decreases by 2 dB if the wind speed increases by 1 m/s. In contrast to Burck's [4] findings where the effect of wind on sound propagation had only been examined for a test range of 200 - 400 m, the investigation under discussion has shown that wind speeds up to 1 m/s may be considered as zero-wind condition. This leads to the result of

$$\left(v_{wind}-1\right) \times 2 \text{ dB}$$

for noise-level reduction.

Taking the above-mentioned facts into account, it has been found that under tail-wind conditions, the noise-level reduction per duplication of range is 12 dB.

PRELIMINARY FORECAST MODEL

On the basis of the radiation values recorded over the changing seasons, the following formula has been developed as an algorithm for noise-level calculations.

$$L = L_{400} - \left[40 \times \lg\frac{r}{r_o} - 2 \times (v_{wind}-1)\right]$$

List of symbols used:

L	=	expected noise level in dB (AI)
L_{400}	=	noise level at reference range of 400 m
r	=	examined range in m
r_o	=	reference range in m (400 m)
v_{wind}	=	wind speed in m/s

This function is applicable to tail-wind conditions. Since this is the most critical condition, the expected noise levels in other directions are never higher than the values calculated with the a.m. formula. Using this formula, the noise-level reduction per duplication of range is calculated to be 12 dB. Furthermore, the noise-level reduction decreases by 2 dB per m/s of wind speed with wind speeds above 1 m/s.

Comparing the calculated noise level using the forecast model with the recorded noise levels measured during the various test series, the suggested model proves its worth. The differences are mainly such that the measured noise level is below the calculated levels. A yearly average is presented below:

Tail wind for test beam 45°, v_{wind} = 2,5 m/s.

This leads to a noise-level reduction of 9 dB per duplication of distance.

Distance	400 m	800 m	1600 m	3200 m	
calculated noise level	76 ± 3	67 ± 3	58 ± 3	49 ± 5	dB (AI)
measured noise level	76 ± 3	68 ± 2	57 ± 3	44 ± 3	dB (AI)
L	0	- 1	+ 1	+ 6	dB (AI)

The forecast model is therefore also applicable to other installations, if measured data for the distance of 400 m are available.

REFERENCES

1. W. Burck, Gutachten WG VI - 3 Uber die Storung des Betriebslarms auf die bewohnte Umgebung Teil a) November 1969, Bundesamt fur Wehrtechnik und Beschaffung, Kollenz.
2. H. Brinkmann, NATO-Gewehr-Erprobung, Gefahrdung durch Waffenknall, Test Nr. 2.13.1 Meppen 1977, Bundesamt fur Wehrtechnik und Beschafung, Koblecz.
3. W. D. Wellnitz, Bericht Uber Untersuchungen Schalleistungspegel G 3 AFB - FE IV/ErpSt 91, Meppen 1983, Bundesamt fur Wehrtechnik und Beschaffung, Koblenz.
4. W. Burck, Gutachten WG VI - 3 Teil b) Juni 1970, Bundesamt fur Wehrtechnik uhd Beschaffung, Koblenz.
5. W. Burck, Gutachten WG VI - 3 Teil d) Oktober 1970, Bundesamt fur Wehrtechnik und Beschaffung, Koblenz.
6. H. Hellmann, Me protokoll ErpSt 91 - 2 Nr. 302/1984, Grundsatzmesaungen an der Standortschie anlage Mainz, Bundesamt fur Wehrtechnik und Beschaffung, Koblenz.

DISCUSSION

Stevins

Do you have any idea of the relation between your measurement of the impulse noise and that obtained with an A-weighted equivalent level taken over eight hours?

Brinkman

No, I have not made such a determination for weapons noise.

Forrest

Britain, like most other countries, has a problem with proving ranges. Most of our problem relates to heavy weapons rather than rifles. We have, to some extent, already developed methods of forcasting noise as a function of weather conditions which include windspeed and the presence of temperature inversions. On the whole, with the larger weapons, we tend to find the quantity of interest to be the peak pressure measured linearly. It is the over-pressure in kPa which is related to minor damage to buildings which seems to be heavily related to complaints in the local populace, rather than dBA. Probably dBA is more appropriate to rifles though.

Brinkman

In our experience, if we do not use A-weighting, but rather unweighted impulse levels, then there are greater differences introduced by wind effects.

THE RESULTS OF LONG-TERM FIELD STUDIES ON ACOUSTIC TRAUMATA IN MILITARY PERSONNEL

Friedrich Pfander

Research Commission, FRG Medical and Health Services
Schwachhauser Heerstr.163a, D-2800 Bremen, Germany

INTRODUCTION

In the Federal Republic of Germany, a criterion of exposure limits has been developed on the basis of pre- and post- audiometric results obtained from soldiers participating in firing practice and field studies. The data base has over 10,000 audiometric studies from various field studies, each involving 100 soldiers and the exposures were to many different types of weapons (Fig. 1).

The physical measurement of peak pressure levels and effective durations was compared with the audiometric tests conducted two minutes after acoustic exposure. The results led to noise control regulations for military personnel in the Federal Republic of Germany that require ear protectors to be worn with practically all types of weapons. The protection of 95% of exposed personnel was taken as the basis for the exposure criteria; for the remaining 5%, a recovery from temporary threshold shift (TTS) within two weeks of exposure was considered probable. In addition to TTS [1-9], the recovery time was taken as the standard otological evaluation criterion, because comparative studies on TTS [1] and recovery time have shown that the recovery time is the more reliable evaluation criterion.

In general, these studies indicate that recovery from an audiometrically ascertainable TTS within ten minutes after an acoustic impact may be regarded as unproblematic. Depending on the amount of exposure, recovery times of up to one half hour have been found in 10 to 20% of the personnel tested. Again, these recovery times are within the physiological fluctuation range and can be regarded as unproblematic. TTS recovery times of up to 3 hours can be considered as limits within which physiopathological processes may occur in the cochlea. Recovery times of 24 hours or more indicate a danger of final impairment, particularly if there is any further exposure.

The diagram of exposure limits is designed for daily exposures. During the further course of these studies, there arose the question as to the number of days to which the criterion of exposure limits could be applied. For this reason, we conducted field studies on hearing behavior involving daily exposures in field exercises lasting up to or more than ten days.

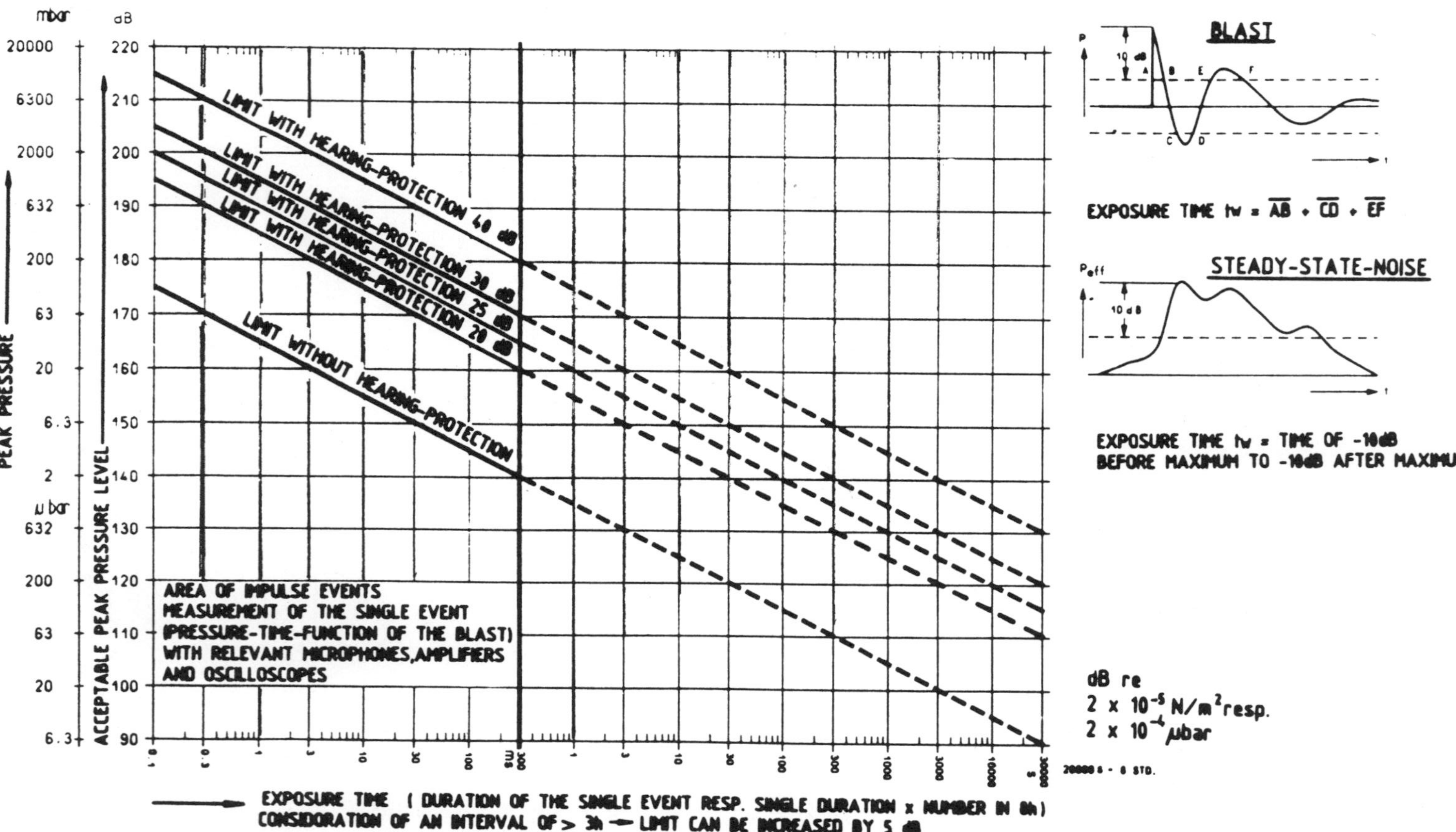

Fig. 1. Damage risk criteria for impulse noise.

In the memorandum by von Gierke, Robinson and Karmy [10] read at the International Workshop on Impulsive Noise and Hearing Damage conducted by the Institute of Sound and Vibration Research at the University of Southampton in October 1981, it was recommended that predictions concerning the risk of auditory deterioration should preferably be based upon statistically significant permanent threshold shifts (PTS) as a function of the effective dose of acoustic impact. Data on temporary threshold shifts (TTS) may be used to supplement these, however, they should be considered as less exact predictions.

Our studies, conducted over many years at regular firing exercises of the Federal Armed Forces, each involving approximately 100 military personnel and various types of weapons, have resulted in very definite indications that the hazard of a permanent auditory impairment in the form of a PTS is indicated by the TTS and, especially, by the recovery time.

The structure of an army, with its frequent changes of location (transfers and limited periods of service), realistically permits a statistical detection of a PTS connected with acoustical noise for only career servicemen and only with good cooperation and great effort.

However, the above-mentioned evaluation criteria pertaining to recovery time from TTS provide reliable indications of the length of time to either recovery or to PTS. Furthermore, in general it can be expected that the greater the TTS, the longer will the ear require for a return to the original auditory condition.

The instantaneous generation of a PTS due to explosions or grenade impacts in the immediate vicinity is generally known in the literature; it therefore constitutes a service-induced disability, especially for war veterans. Fortunately, however, this type of generation of a PTS as a result of an acoustical trauma is a rare occurrence in the peace-time situation of today's army.

The contemporary development of permanent auditory impairment in armies is, in the majority of cases, caused by repeated exposures to impulse or impact noise. A special hazard exists in exercises of longer duration in which ordnance and supervisory personnel are exposed to considerable impacts day after day.

We have just completed audiological tests of soldiers having exposure to the firing of the FH 155/1 field howitzer in open terrain with the M 109 charge, the heaviest so far; peak pressure was 175 to 180 dB. The essential acoustic element in the hazard to hearing ability is to be found in the number of rounds fired. We have found that the recovery time increases after exposure on the second day of firing, whereas the recovery time on the first day of exposure is considerably shorter. These results are examples of an observation that we have made repeatedly in our long-term studies.

In our experience, the duration of the intervals between rounds is not of much significance. In field exercises, these values range from 1-1/2 to 15 minutes, with the duration of the intervals continuously decreasing toward the end of the exercise.

Regarding the question of danger of a permanent auditory impairment developing from an increasing TTS, we have made audiometric controls on a number of career servicemen continuously exposed to acoustic impacts. The instantaneous generation of a PTS as a result of explosions or grenade impact in the immediate vicinity is a situation which frequently occurred during the war, but which can be practically ignored in peacetime, since it is restricted to accidents. The development of a PTS from a TTS with longer recovery times is of practical significance, however.

Here are some examples from a series of tests on career servicemen continously exposed to highly intensive impulse noise:

Sergeant S (Fig. 2)

This pertains to a career serviceman, a sergeant who supervises and controls the training at the firing position and is exposed to numerous traumata from impact noise. Curve No. 1 shows the preliminary audiometry, Curve No. 2 shows the TTS following exposure to 20 rounds. From Curve No. 3, it can be seen that 4 hours after exposure there was a recovery of his hearing ability to its original level. Curve No. 4 indicates the TTS after exposure to charge No. 7. No recovery occurred after 16 hours. There was no change in the curve after renewed exposure. Three months later there was still the same threshold decline. However, after almost one year his hearing ability recovered. This is an example of the fact that the recovery takes longer after exposure, but that recovery is still possible, even after several months.

Private B (Fig. 3)

The preliminary audiometry on 19 September already displayed a threshold decline, indicating acoustic impact. However, it only amounted to 20 dB. After a lengthy period of exposure from driving, there was a distinct worsening of the decline. Finally, after additional long-term exposure due to driving and employment as a cannoneer, the audiogram indicated a further deterioration of the threshold. Three months later, this hearing ability improved again to the level of the preliminary audiometry. If there is any further exposure, this hearing will probably become subject to a PTS.

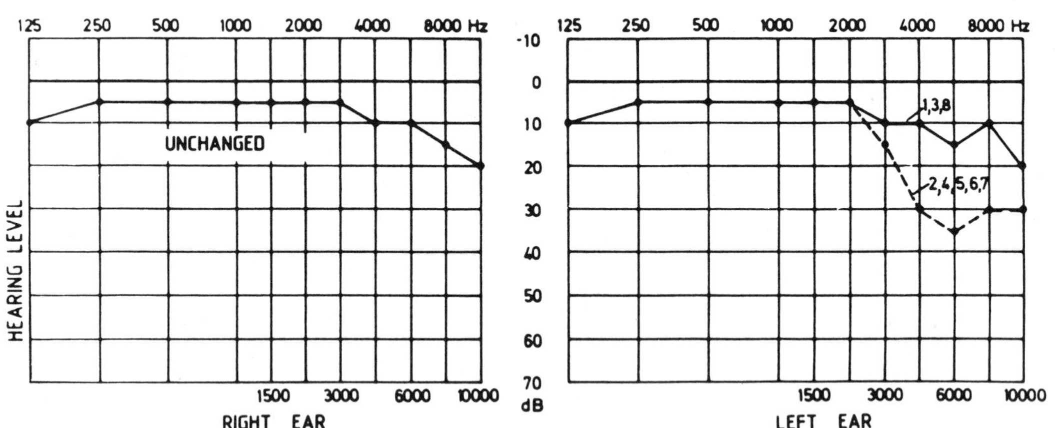

Fig. 2. 1. 21.11.82 Pre-audiometry
2. 22.11.82 TTS$_{2-6}$ after strain caused by 20 rounds FH 155-1/5th charge
3. 22.11.82 TTS$_{4h}$ (4 h after strain)
4. 23.11.82 TTS$_{2-6}$ after renewed strain by 8 rounds FH 155-1/7th charge
5. 24.11.82 TTS$_{16h}$ (16 h after strain)
6. 24.11.82 TTS$_{2-6}$ after renewed strain by 30 rounds FH 155-1/7th charge
7. 21.02.83 Control-audiometry
8. 11.11.83 Control-audiometry

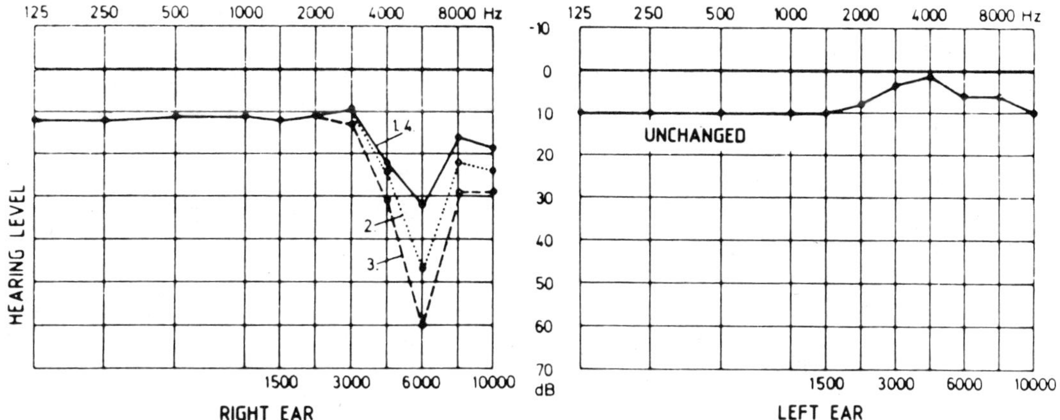

Fig. 3. 1. 19.09.83 Pre-audiometry
2. 21.09.83 TTS after strain due to driving self-propelled Howitzer M110 on 19.09.83 (2.0 hours) and on 20.09.83 (2.75 hours)
3. 29.09.83 TTS after strain due to driving the M110 during 21-29 Sept. (total = 15 hours) and as gunner after 21 rounds/4th to 6 charge
4. 08.12.83 Control audiometry without interim strain

Corporal S (Fig. 4)

This corporal was employed as a cannoneer and gun commander. The preliminary audiometry already indicated a moderate threshold decline in the high frequency range. Continuous exposures resulted in an increase in the TTS. At the last examination, which was conducted almost two months after the conclusion of the long-term exercise, his hearing ability had not yet recovered. A PTS is to be expected.

SUMMARY

Long-term field studies indicate that daily exposure to highly intensive impulse noise increases TTS and prolongs recovery of the ear. Observations on career military personnel who are assigned as training supervisors and frequently exposed to impulse noise traumata indicate that continued exposure may gradually lead from a TTS to a PTS, despite the use of ear protectors. On the other hand, it appears that recovery is possible even after several months of exposure, despite increasing TTS and increasing duration of recovery. The otological experience that hearing damaged by a single acoustic trauma tends to improve (or at least to remain constant) when such exposure no longer occurs, apparently also applies to auditory impairment that has developed gradually, due to multiple exposures to im- pulse noise. The wearing of ear protectors required by the noise control regulation has reduced the proportion of endangered personnel to 5%. How- ever, even these subjects have a tendency to recover from hearing loss once exposure ceases. A service-connected disability due to hearing damage caused by impulse noise should therefore not be regarded as final until several months after the trauma.

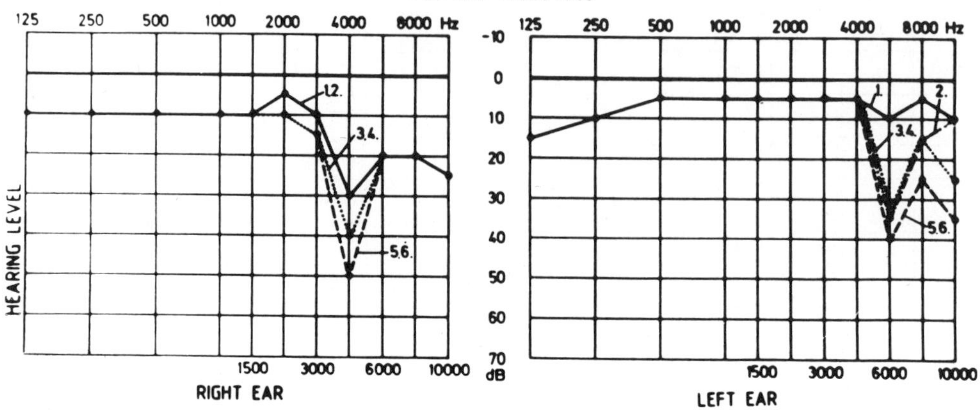

Fig. 4. 1. 21.11.82 Pre-audiometry

2. 24.11.82 TTS_{2-6} after strain caused by FH 155-1, 9 rounds/5th charge on 22 Nov., 8 rounds/7th charge on 23 Nov., 10 rounds/7th charge on 24 Nov.

3. 18.09.83 Renewed pre-audiometry (interim strain with 20 rounds in March 83)

4. 20.09.83 TTS_{2-6} after strain caused by FH 155-1, 3 rounds/3rd charge on 19 Sept., 5 rounds/7th charge on 20 Sept.

5. 29.09.83 TTS_{2-6} after strain caused by FH 155-1, 44 rounds/2nd to 7th charges, 21-29 Sept.

6. 11.11.83 Control audiometry without interim strain

REFERENCES

1. F. Pfander, HNO 13:27 (1965).
2. F. Pfander, Arch Ohr Nas-Kehlk-Heilk 191:586 (1968).
3. F. Pfander, Wehrmedizin 1/2 16-24 (1970).
4. F. Pfander and H. Kietz, HNO, 1340 (1971)
5. F. Pfander, Kampf dem Larm 5 (1973).
6. F. Pfander, Das Knalltrauma. Springer-Verlag-Berlin-Heidelberg, New York (1975).
7. F. Pfander, F., H. Bongartz, H. Brinkmann, and H. Kietz, J. Acoust. Soc. Amer. 67:628 (1980).
8. C. Tremolieress, R. Hetu, and E. A. G. Shaw, Draft report of the scientific adviser to the special advisory committee on the Ontario noise regulation, 1984 National Research Council Canada, Division of Physics. J. Acoust. Soc. Amer., 68:1652 (1980).
9. W. D. Ward., J. Acoust. Soc. Amer.,31:600 (1959).
10. H. von Gierke, Robinson, and Karmy, Results of the workshop on impulse noise and auditory hazard. University of Southampton 1./2., Institute of Sound and Vibration Research Memorandum 618 (1981).
11. W. D. Ward, Selters, and A. Glorig, J. Acoust. Soc. Amer. 33:783 (1962).
12. W. D. Ward, J. Acoust. Soc. Amer., 48:561 (1970).

DISCUSSION

Tyler: Some of the individual results that you showed had a hearing loss in the right ear, others had a hearing loss in the left ear and some had a hearing loss in both ears. Can you comment on the different kinds of situations that produced a unilateral or bilateral hearing loss?

Pfander: We have looked at that question in subjects exposed to rifle fire. The left ear is damaged more than the right ear because the right ear, generally is pointed away from the noise source. For Howitzers, the level of exposure to an ear depends on the location of the individual exposed. We have made measurements all around the cannons and, of course, different hearing losses result because peak pressure can be very different in the various positions. Differences are especially great in confined versus free field firing conditions.

Stevins: Do you have any feeling for the applicability of your results on weapon noise to the kinds of impulse noises one is likely to encounter in industry?

Pfander: The damage to the ear following exposure to weapons noise is probably a result of a mechanical disturbance, while lower level impulses noise trauma in industrial situations may result more from biochemical factors.

Phillips: Are your damage risk criteria based upon the limitation that approximately 5% of your population will incur a prolonged threshold shift from a single (multiple impact) exposure event? Following one exercise, the damage risk criteria would allow up to 5% of those soldiers exposed to have a prolonged temporary threshold loss, is that correct?

Pfander: Yes.

Phillips: I am concerned about the soldiers who had repeated exposures to these noise sources. Presumably, their TTS developed into PTS after some length of time. Predictions based on human experiments are needed which relate TTS in a proportion of the exposed population to consequences of a lifetime or of a career of exposures.

Pfander: While 5% of our subjects are at greater risk, they usually recover in a fortnight.

EFFECTS OF BLAST WAVES ON NONAUDITORY EPITHELIAL TISSUES

James B. Moe, Charles B. Clifford,
and Douglas D. Sharpnack

Division of Pathology
Walter Reed Army Institute of Research

INTRODUCTION

Injuries in mammals exposed to various forms of blast have been recognized for many years, at least as early as the 1920's [1,2]. Classically, blast injury was considered to be an injury resulting from direct exposure to an explosion, originally from highly explosive, conventional type weapons. Later, blast injury was included as one of the potential casualty-producing effects of nuclear weapons [3]. Blast injury was known by a number of terms, including "air concussion," "blast concussion," "wind of shot," "shell concussion," "blast chest," "bomb blast," and "shell shock," in the period before World War II [4], but these terms are seldom used in contemporary reports. A comprehensive report and review of the pathologic changes associated with blast injury was prepared by Chiffelle [5]. This report separated the direct effects, those associated with the blast wave, from indirect effects. Secondary effects are injuries which result from the victim being struck by flying objects energized by the blast. Tertiary effects are injuries which result from the victim being translated and thrown against firm, stationary objectives. Miscellaneous effects are those injuries which occur following exposure to dusts or gases generated by the explosion, direct thermal burns in conjunction with the explosion, and thermal burns resulting from secondary fires ignited by the primary blast [1]. This report will be limited to a consideration of the primary effects of blast on mammalian tissues. Many of the reports on blast injury have focused on the effects of a single, high intensity explosion which produces an acute casualty. Recently, the potential occupational hazards associated with long term exposure to multiple, low intensity blast waves in the military environment have become a cause of concern. Low intensity will be used here to designate blast waves which are below or near the recognized threshold for injury when delivered as a single blast wave. This report will present descriptions and comparisons of the types of non-auditory injury observed in mammals experimentally experiencing these two different categories of exposure. Additionally, "blast waves" in this report refer to the simple, short-duration (a few milliseconds) type.

Single, High Intensity, Short Duration Blast Wave Exposure

The principal military interest in this type of exposure is to derive more effective means of preventing, diagnosing, and treating blast casualties. Of special interest is determining the potential for long-term sequelae in casualties which survive the acute phase of blast injury.

One experiment was designed to compare the nonauditory effects of blast exposure in two large mammalian species, sheep and pigs, and to determine the feasibility of using one of these species for an animal model of human blast exposure.

A total of 10 sheep and 10 pigs were used for the studies. Exposures were accomplished on two days, using 5 animals of each species on each day. Animals were anesthetized and secured in slings in a circular pattern around the blast-generating device at a distance calculated to deliver approximately 75 pounds per square inch (psi) of overpressure. Animals were oriented so that half of the individuals in each species received a left-sided exposure and the other half a right-sided exposure. Animals which died immediately following the blast were necropsied as soon as possible, while those which survived were euthanized and necropsied according to predetermined, scheduled times up to eight (8) hours after exposure. During necropsy, all respiratory and gastrointestinal lesions were assigned a combined severity/distribution/location score, according to a standard scoring system, and photographed. Representative sections of grossly detected lesions and standard sections of the lung were examined microscopically. In the respiratory system and the gastrointestinal tract, injury was reliably produced by a single blast.

In the respiratory system there were various types of gross evidence of injury, usually substantiated by microscopic findings (Table 1). In the larynx and trachea there were petechiae in the mucosa, with more diffuse hemorrhage in the mucosa/submucosa overlying the trachealis muscle. The lungs contained varying amounts of hemorrhage, seen in the least severe cases as ecchymoses or broad strips of hemorrhage, in the subpleural pulmonary parenchyma of the dorsal (posterior) aspect of the diaphragmatic lobes, often following rib-print pattern. In the animals having more extensive involvement, the hemorrhage extended deep into the pulmonary parenchyma, often involving the hilar, ventral, and anterior aspects of the lobes. Standard histologic sections of the perfusion-fixed lungs revealed fibrin thrombi in the bronchi. In all individuals of both species there was microscopic evidence of pulmonary hemorrhage accompanied by pulmonary edema in seven sheep and two pigs. There was morphologic evidence of ruptured pulmonary alveolar septa in six sheep and pigs. The pleura was separated from underlying alveolar parenchyma in both species; this was more conspicuous in pigs where pleural bullae often up to 1.0 cm in diameter were seen at the dorsal (posterior) and ventral (anterior) borders of the diaphragmatic lobes of the lung.

In six sheep there was gross evidence of hemorrhage in the forestomach, most frequently present as focal involvement of the wall of the dorsal sac. The size and depth of involvement was variable, ranging from a few ecchymoses to large transmural hematomas. Although the incidence of ruminal hemorrhage was similar (3/5) in sheep exposed on either side, the subjective severity score (S.S.S.) was much greater (17.8) in those receiving left-sided exposure as compared to right-sided exposure (5.3). In some of the sheep these ruminal hemorrhages appeared histologically to have been of sufficient magnitude to have caused devitalization of the wall and probably would have caused diastrous sequelae in the form of perforation and peritonitis.

There was gross evidence of hemorrhage in the stomach (abomasum) of only one sheep, a right-exposed individual which had mild lesions (S.S.S. = 6.0). Two of the pigs had gastric hemorrhage, one left-exposed (S.S.S. = 8.0) and a right-exposed (S.S.S. = 18.0). Microscopically, hemorrhage was

TABLE 1. Grossly Detectable Effects of Blast Overpressure in Sheep and Pigs.

Lesion	Theoretical Max.	Sheep			Pigs		
		Total	Lt. Exp.	Rt. Exp.	Total	Lt. Exp.	Rt. Exp
Lung Hemorrhage Left Lung	16	7.5[a](1.0)[b]	7.6(1.0)	7.4(1.0)	5.4(1.0)	6.5(1.0)	4.2(1.0)
Right Lung	16	6.2(1.0)	5.1(1.0)	7.4(1.0)	6.2(1.0)	4.2(1.0)	8.1(1.0)
Laryngeal Hemorrhage	5	2.6(0.9)	2.0(0.8)	3.0(1.0)	1.7(1.0)	2.0(1.0)	1.4(1.0)
Tracheal Hemorrhage	15	4.8(0.8)	6.0(0.6)	4.4(1.0)	4.7(0.3)	5.0(0.4)	4.0(0.2)
Ruminal Hemorrhage	36	11.5(0.6)	17.8(0.6)	5.3(0.6)	X	X	X
Gastric Hemorrhage	36	6.0(0.1)	0(0)	6.0(0.2)	13.0(0.2)	8.0(0.2)	18.0(0.2)
Small Intest. Hemorrhage	36	10.0(0.4)	4.0(0.2)	12.0(0.6)	14.9(0.9)	14.0(0.8)	15.6(1.0)
Cecal Hemorrhage	36	11.3(.06)	4.0(0.4)	15.0(0.8)	3.8(0.4)	5.0(0.4)	2.5(0.4)
Colonic Hemorrhage	36	12.1(0.7)	2.3(0.6)	19.5(0.8)	12.1(0.9)	11.8(1.0)	12.5(0.8)

a. Subjective severity score, maximum score on gross is variable for each organ system, mean values determined by Dividing Total Score/No. Affected.

b. Parenthetic figures are proportion of animals affected

most extensive and disruptive in the mucosa and submucosa in both species, and only occasionally involved the muscularis externa.

The small intestine of sheep was grossly affected by exposure to blast in four individuals, whereas nine of the pigs had gross evidence of small intestinal hemorrhage. There was also evidence of the side of exposure as a factor influencing the effects of blast on the small intestine. In sheep, only 1/5 of left-exposed animals, as opposed 3/5 right-exposed, had lesions. Additionally, the left-exposed sheep had milder (S.S.S. = 4.0) lesions than the right exposed (S.S.S. = 12.0). In pigs, severity of small intestinal lesions was quite symmetrical (left-exposed S.S.S. = 14.0, right-exposed S.S.S. = 15.6) and of somewhat greater magnitude than observed in sheep. Therefore, the small intestine of sheep were somewhat protected by the rumen or other anatomic structures from the effects of left-sided blast, while pig small intestines were more uniformly affected. As was the case in the stomach, small intestinal hemorrhage was most severe in the mucosa/submucosa in both species, although hemorrhage extended to the muscularis externa in one sheep and six pigs.

In the cecum of sheep there was evidence for preferential involvement associated with right-side exposure where 4/5 of the individuals had moderate (S.S.S. = 15.0) lesions, while only 2/5 receiving left-sided exposure were affected, and had mild (S.S.S. 4.0) lesions. In pigs, 2/5 of the animals receiving exposure on either side had hemorrhagic ceca and these were rather mild (left S.S.S. = 5.0, right S.S.S. = 2.5). Microscopically, predominantly-submucosal/mucosal hemorrhage extended through the muscularis externa in 2/5 of the right-exposed pigs and appeared to present genuine risk of serosal perforation with additional time.

Evidence of hemorrhage in the colonic wall was identified in 7/10 of the sheep and 9/10 of the pigs. While the pigs showed relatively similar involvement, regardless of side exposed to blast, the sheep exposed on their right side had markedly more extensive and serious hemorrhage (S.S.S. = 19.5) in the colon than those which received left side exposure (S.S.S. = 2.3). Histologically, there was dissecting hemorrhage which extended to the serosa in one sheep and two pigs, including some individuals which were clinically normal up to eight hours after blast exposure.

Other lesions attributable to blast exposure were observed in various organ systems. Air emboli were present in the meningeal vessels and in the coronary arteries of five sheep. Capsular hematomas or lacerations were evident in the spleens of two sheep and four pigs. External manifestations of blast included mild contusions in the skin, epistaxis, and hemorrhage from the mouth.

From these observations, the following conclusions were drawn:

1. The response of the respiratory system was quite similar in sheep and pigs with only minimal evidence of a tendency for greater severity on the blast-exposed side.
2. Blast injury in the forestomach was more severe in left-side exposed sheep.
3. The small intestines of sheep were less severely affected in the left-side exposed sheep than right-side exposed sheep or in pigs exposed on either side. If sheep are to be used as models for small intestinal injury, the exposure should be right-sided.
4. Large intestinal injury was common in both species, except for left-exposed sheep.
5. Throughout the intestinal tract, injuries were of a type that suggested substantial potential for long-term complications.

6. Based solely on pathological data, either sheep or pigs are acceptable host models for study of high level (LD_{50}) blast, provided adequate consideration is given to anatomical variations in the sheep.

Multiple, Low Intensity, Short Duration Blast Wave Exposure

These studies [6] were part of a long-term comprehensive effort to determine the risk of occupational injury to operators and crew members of military weapons systems. There was considerably less scientific information in the literature regarding the biological effects of multiple, low intensity exposures to blast waves than for single, high intensity exposures. Therefore, it was necessary to do basic quantitative and qualitative studies of response to multiple exposures to short duration blast waves. The principal area of concern was the range of overpressure generated in the vicinity of crew operators of extended range artillery systems, especially in the range of 3.5 pounds per square inch (psi). The highest overpressure delivered to crew operator positions of weapons firing extended range ammunition is approximately 3.5 Psi, therefore, a decision was made to monitor the effects of exposure at this and higher overpressures.

The primary objectives were:

1. To determine whether exposure to 50 consecutive blasts with peak overpressure of 3.5, 7.5 and 15.0 resulted in damage to the respiratory system of sheep.
2. To determine the relative sensitivity of various parts of the respiratory system to blast-induced injury.
3. To establish gross and microscopic pathology to serve as bases for later comparison with radiography and various biochemical tests as tools for detecting and evaluating lung injury induced by blast overpressure.
4. To survey other organs and tissues for evidence of blast-related injury under field conditions.

A total of 98 sheep was used for this study. Each sheep was restrained in a specially-designed stand, given a sedative dose of ketamine hydrochloride, and provided hearing protection via placement of ear plugs. Stands were positioned in an array around an artillery weapon to receive appropriate levels of blast overpressure (15,7.5,3.5 and 0.5 psi) as determined by previous pressure monitoring. During test firing, sheep receiving less than 0.5 psi were in stands approximately 50 meters from the muzzle of the weapon, serving as range control animals which were subjected to similar preparatory, transportation and sensory stresses as those receiving 3.5, 7.5 or 15 psi. Barn control sheep were those which were prepared in the same manner as other sheep, but were not transported to the range. During the firing, sheep were observed closely to determine their behavior and prevent postural artifacts. Pressures at each position were monitored during the firing. Blood samples were collected from the sheep, via catheters, before, during, and after the blast exposure period. At necropsy, the lungs were weighed, examined, and photographed. The lungs were then perfused enmasse with 10% neutral buffered formalin instilled at a pressure of 25 cm H_2O. Necropsy was performed within eight hours of blast exposure (immediate) except for half of the sheep exposed to 7.5 psi and half the range controls which were necropsied 22-24 hours post-exposure (delayed). Necropsy was delayed in these groups to determine whether any lesions progressed or resolved with time. Because there were no perceptible differences between immediate and delayed groups, data are combined in this report.

Gross pathologic changes in the lungs were interpreted in regard to the probability of representing blast-type injury and scored from 1 (essentially normal) to 4 (probably blast-type injury). A system was devised for assigning a subjective severity/intensity score for various histopathologic lesions in the lung, whereby a subjective severity score (S.S.S.: 1=minimal, 2=mild, 3=moderate, 4=marked, 5=severe) was assigned for lesion in each section. These scores for each section were then totaled and divided by the number of lung sections examined for each animal to arrive at a mean S.S.S., e.g., mean hemorrhage score. Additionally, the proportion of sheep affected of sections affected were calculated for selected lesions. Lungs and trachea from two sheep which had been exposed to one blast at 50 psi were handled and examined in a similar way for purpose of reference.

There was no evidence in the data obtained of hemorrhage, edema inflammation or focal atelectasis in the pulmonary parenchyma of sheep exposed to 7.5 or 15 psi when compared to controls or those exposed to 0.5 or 3.5 psi (Table 2). Analysis of dorsal subpleural sections revealed no increased incidence of extent/severity of surface-related hemorrhage with increased blast overpressure. Epithelial stripping, often associated with mucosal hemorrhage, was observed in the stem bronchi of five sheep in the 15 psi group.

The predominant laryngeal lesion observed was hemorrhage, seen grossly as petechial ecchymotic foci in the mucosa of the epiglottis or vestibule. Although laryngeal hemorrhage of varying severity was seen to some extent within each group, there was a trend toward higher incidence starting at the 3.5 psi group, continuing at approximately the same level through the 7.5 psi groups (Table 3). There was a markedly increased incidence of hemorrhage (14/15) at the 15 psi level of exposure. Edema followed an incidence pattern similar to, but slightly lower than, that of hemorrhage in the larynx. In the 15 psi exposure group, edema was subjectively viewed as being more severe than in lower exposure groups. In a few of the larynxes having the most severe hemorrhage and edema, the epithelium of the lateral walls of the vestibule, anterior to the arytenoid cartilages, was slightly elevated. Epithelial stripping, expressed as loss of superficial layers of the ciliated respiratory epithelium, was seen in the larynx of only one sheep, a member of the 7.5 psi group.

Tracheal lesions are listed in Table 4. Tracheal hemorrhage, present in one range control sheep, and two sheep exposed to 3.5 psi, increased slightly in incidence in the 7.5 psi group, then occurred universally in the 15 psi group. Hemorrhage generally occurred as petechial to ecchymotic (0.1- 1.0 cm diameter) focal zones in the submucosa of the trachea. These zones of hemorrhage often extended throughout the wall of the tracheas, involving all layers, especially in affected sheep in the 7.5 and 15 psi groups. There was seldom any evidence of significant elevation of the epithelial lining and in no case was there a visible reduction in airway lumen diameter. Severity of hemorrhage, judged subjectively, was more severe in the higher pressure groups. Edema was less prevalent than hemorrhage in tracheas of blast-exposed sheep. Epithelial stripping was evident in the trachea of at least one sheep in every group receiving 3.5 psi or more exposure to blast overpressure. Half of the sheep exposed to 15 psi had evidence of stripping of tracheal epithelium in close association with underlying hemorrhage.

In the gastrointestinal tract there was a trend toward higher incidence of hemorrhage with increasing overpressure in rumen, small intestine and large intestine (Table 5). The abomasum was seldom involved. Moreover, there was a definite increase in severity of ruminal hemorrhage with increasing overpressure. In the control groups of sheep and those exposed to 3.5 psi, ruminal hemorrhage was mainly mild, occurring as paintbrush zones in the superficial layers on the serosal surface. Rumens of the

TABLE 2. Incidence of Lung Lesions in Sheep Exposed to Multiple (50) Blast Waves

Overpressure in psi[a]	Exposure Group (psi) None (Barn Control)	0.5 (Range Control)	3.5	7.5	15	50[a]
No. Examined	9	29	15	30	15	2
Hemorrhage No. Affected (microscopic)	8	21	10	21	13	2
Proportion of Sheep Affected	.89	.72	.67	.70	.87	1.00
Proportion of Sections Affected	.21	.25	.20	.22	.34	1.00
Subjective Severity Score ($\bar{X}$ all std. trim sections)	.33	.28	.29	.32	.48	3.46
Edema Proportion of Sheep Affected (microscopic)	.11	.17	.13	.10	.13	1.00
Proportion of Sections Affected	.006	.024	.008	.024	.012	.128
Bronchial Epithelial Stripping (microscopic) Proportion of Sheep Affected	0	0	0	0	.33	1.0

[a]All multiple exposures, except for 50 psi group, which received only 1 blast.

TABLE 3. Incidence of Laryngeal Lesions in Sheep Exposed to Multiple (50) Blast Waves

	Exposure Group					
Overpressure in psi[a]	None (Barn Control)	0.5 psi (Range Control)	3.5psi	7.5psi	15	50[a]
No. Examined	9	28	15	30	15	0
Hemorrhage						
No. Affected (microscopic)	1	2	4	6	14	---
Proportion of Sheep Affected	.11	.07	.27	.20	.93	---
Subjective Severity Score ($\bar{X}$ of Those Affected)	2.0	1.0	1.5	.17	2.5	---
Edema						
No. Affected (microscopic)	0	1	2	1	9	---
Proportion of Sheep Affected	0	.04	.14	.07	.60	---
Epithelial Stripping						
Proportion of Sheep Affected (microscopic)	0	0	0	.03	0	---

a. As in Table 2.

TABLE 4. Incidence of Tracheal Lesions in Sheep Exposed to Multiple Blast Waves

	Exposure Group					
Overpressure in psi[a]	None (Barn Control)	0.5 psi (Range Control)	3.5 psi	7.5 psi	15	50[a]
No. Examined	9	.28	13	28	14	2
Hemorrhage						
No. Affected (microscopic)	0	1	2	9	14	1
Proportion of Sheep Affected	0	.04	.15	.32	1.00	.50
Subjective Severity Score, ($\bar{X}$ of Those Affected)	---	2.0	1.0	2.6	2.8	2.0
Edema						
No. of Sheep Affected (microscopic)	0	0	1	0	2	0
Epithelial Stripping						
No. of Sheep Affected (microscopic)	0	0	1	2	7	1

a. As in Table 2.

TABLE 5. Incidence of Gastrointestinal Lesions in Sheep Exposed to Multiple (50) Blast Waves

	Exposure Group				
Overpressure in psi	None (Barn Control)	0.5 psi (Range Control)	3.5 psi	7.5 psi	15
No. Examined	9	29	15	30	15
Ruminal Hemorrhage Proportion Affected	.33[a]	.17	.33	.47	1.00
No. with Hematomas	0	0	0	2	12
Small Intestinal Hemorrhage Proportion Affected	0[b]	.03	.07	.07	.20
Subjective Severity Score, ($\bar{X}$ of Those Affected)	0	1.0	2.0	2.0	4.0
Large Intestinal Hemorrhage Proportion Affected	0	.03	.13	.10	.60
Subjective Severity Score, ($\bar{X}$ of Those Affected)	0	1.0	2.5	2.0	3.8
Abomasal Hemorrhage Proportion Affected	0	0	0	.03	0
Subjective Severity Score, ($\bar{X}$ of Those Affected)	0	0	0	2.0	0

a. All incidence figures reflect combined gross and microscopic observations.

b. All proportions are of sheep examined.

sheep which received 7.5 psi had hemorrhages that were a few centimeters in diameter and extended through the entire thickness of the wall from mucosa to serosa, forming hematomas in two sheep in this group. Hemorrhage was severe in rumens of sheep in the 15 psi group, frequently existing as hematomas, 10 cm or more in diameter. These hematomas dissected the ruminal wall and caused intra-peritoneal hemorrhage and spillage of ingesta. Hemorrhage in the rumen was in the dorsal sac region in most cases, corresponding to the normal location of the gas pocket. Hemorrhages were present in the small intestine of a single animal in the range control, 3.5 and 7.5 psi groups and 3 animals in the 15 psi group. In the large intestine, (both cecum and colon) hemorrhage was seen more frequently in those regions where the lumen was physiologically distended with gas and liquid. Small and large intestinal hemorrhage were noticeably more severe at 15 psi than at lower overpressures.

The incidences of hemorrhage in larynx, trachea, and rumen were roughly parallel at low-levels of exposure, but steadily increased through the 7.5 psi exposure groups, with dramatic increases in incidence at 15 psi (Fig. 1). These data are statistically significant (.05) for relationship between increasing blast overpressure and increasing incidence of hemorrhage in these three tissues, when analyzed by Chi square test for trend. Lung wet weight to body weight ratios were not altered in sheep exposed to blast overpressure. Radiologic and biochemical examination failed to provide correlates for the pathological changes observed.

Incidence and severity of pathologic changes in various tissues of sheep exposed to weapon-generated blast overpressure indicated gradations of sensitivity amongst various systems of the body. There was parallel incidence of hemorrhage in larynx, trachea and rumen (forestomach) of these sheep. In all three locations there were slightly higher incidences of hemorrhage in sheep exposed to 3.5 psi and 7.5 psi, with nearly universal incidence of hemorrhage in those exposed to 15 psi. Of these most common lesions, ruminal hemorrhage was the most biologically significant, especially at the 15 psi level of exposure. Laryngeal and tracheal hemorrhages, although occasionally extensive, were interpreted as not having posed significant threat to airway-aptency. Stripping of the superficial layers of the respiratory epithelium in the larynx, trachea and stem bronchi was a blast-associated phenomenon, occurring most frequently in the 15 psi exposure group.

The alveolar parenchyma of the lung appeared to be quite resistant to blast-associated damage in the range of exposure 3.5 to 15 psi. There was no discernible evidence of a trend for greater incidence of severity of hemodynamic, reactive or physical changes in alveolar parenchyma of the lung in any of these exposure groups, when compared to background incidence of similar changes in control animals.

Studies of Blast Wave Injury in a Small Species

Recent experiments have been designed to confirm the previously-described observations in a small species and to determine the basis of these pathological changes. For these studies, rats were exposed to either 1, 2, 4, 8, 9.7, 16, or 22.5 psi, repeated 20 times with approximately 5 minutes intervals between blast exposures. Appropriate controls were included to allow assessment of the effects of animal handling and tissue dissection.

Results are summarized in Table 6. From these subjective observa tions, quantified according to a standardized set of predetermined criteria, it is possible to estimate that the threshold for light microscopic injury to the lung parenchyma of the rat is between 9.7 and

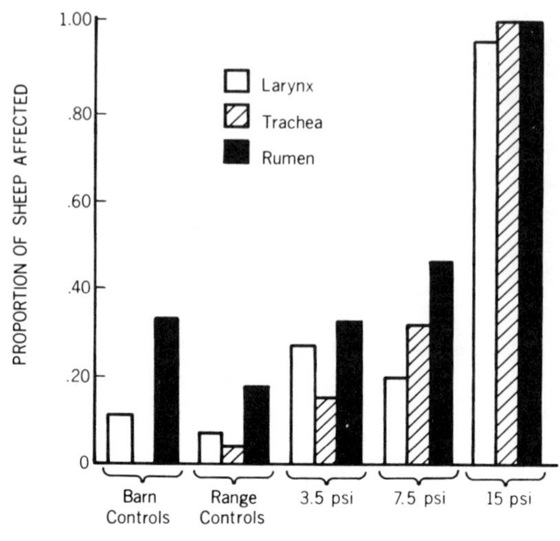

Fig. 1. Incidences of hemorrhage in larynx, trachea, and rumen of sheep exposed to multiple blasts at varying intensities.

16.0 psi. Injury tended to affect a greater proportion of the rats with higher overpressures and severity was judged subjectively to be somewhat greater for both edema and hemorrhage.

Epithelial stripping in the trachea, detected by scanning electron microscopy, was confidently identified only in rats exposed repeatedly to 9.7, 16, or 22.5 psi (Table 6). Affected areas were seen as foci of epithe- lial denudation with adherent aggregates of fibrin and erythrocytes. There was no attempt to grade the severity of these stripping lesions.

The results of the rat studies were in general agreement with the threshold data generated for other small species of mammals. The epithelial stripping and pulmonary parenchymal injuries also seem to have similar thresholds in the rat. The biological implications of pulmonary hemorrhage and edema, as well as focal epithelial stripping, are uncertain. There is potential for hemorrhage in the air spaces to be organized and lead to pulmonary fibrosis, with serious affects on pulmonary function. Focal denuding injuries of the airway epithelium can be repaired, with complete restoration of morphologic features and apparent function [7]. Additional research is needed and planned in two critical aspects of injury resulting from repeated low intensity blast exposures in rodents. 1) Dynamics of the recovery/repair phase; and 2) Effects of additional repeated exposures, over a period of several days on previously injured tissues.

CONCLUDING COMMENT

Recent experiments with animals exposed to various levels of blast intensity are in agreement with much of the previous information relating to experimental blast exposure of mammals. Results from more basic pathologic studies have provided a basis for proceding with more definitive experiments on the biodynamics of nonauditory blast injury. An encouraging note which has arisen from these, and much earlier, studies has been the

TABLE 6. Incidence of Pulmonary Lesions in Rats Exposed to 20 Blasts at Various Intensities

	Exposure Group						
	0	1-2	4	8	9.7	16	22.5
No. in Group	12	8	6	6	6	6	6
Lung (Light microscopy)							
Alveolar Hemorrhage							
No. of Rats Affected	1	0	1	0	0	4	5
Subjective Severity Score, ($\bar{X}$ of Rats Affected)	1.0	0	1.0	0	0	1.2	1.9
Edema							
No. of Rats Affected	0	0	0	0	0	2	5
Subjective Severity Score, ($\bar{X}$ of Rats Affected)	0	0	0	0	0	2.0	1.6
Trachea (Electron microscopy)							
Epithelial Stripping							
No. of Rats Affected	0	0	0	0	1	3	6

similarity in types of injury which occur following exposure of various species to blast. There seems to be, however, some interspecies variation in susceptibility to blast injury which must be considered when interpreting experimental data. The similarity of the pathological changes in mammals experimentally exposed to blast waves to lesions in humans wounded by blasts in hostile actions supports the validity of using animals, when necessary, to investigate the biological effects of various types of blast. Sheep are currently being used as the predominant large mammalian species for more definitive experiments, especially in the respiratory system. Domestic swine may be preferable for gastrointestinal injury. In addition to ultrastructural and morphometric examination, future pathologic studies should focus on noninvasive functional and biochemical tests. Ideally, results from these experiments will provide a generic basis for risk assessment using in vitro systems, mathematical estimates, and computer modeling.

ACKNOWLEDGEMENT

This research was conducted in compliance with the Animal Welfare Act, and other Federal statutes and regulations relating to animals and experiments involving animals and adheres to principles stated in the _Guide for the Care and Use of Laboratory Animals_, NIH publication 85-23.

REFERENCES

1. J. S. Stapczynski, Blast injuries, _Ann. Emerg. Med._ 11:687 (1982).
2. D. R. Hooker, Physiological effects of air concussion, _Am. J. Physiol._ 67:219 (1924).
3. C. A. de Candole, Blast injury, _Canad. Med. Ass. J._ 96:207 (1967).
4. C. J. Clemedson, Blast injury, _Physiol. Rev._ 36:336 (1956).
5. T. L. Chiffelle, "Pathology of Direct Air-blast Injury," Tech. Prog. Rep., Lovelace Foundation for Medical Education and Research, Albuquerque, N.M. (1966).
6. C. B. Clifford, J. B. Moe, J. J. Jaeger, and J. L. Hess, Gastrointestinal lesions in lambs due to multiple low-level blast overpressure exposure, _Mil. Med._ 149:491 (1984).
7. K. P. Keenan, J. W. Combs, and E. M. McDowell, Regeneration of hamster tracheal epithelium after mechanical injury, _Virochows Arch._ (Cell Pathol.) 41:193 (1982).

DISCUSSION

Phillips: You mentioned a couple of times that the injury to non-auditory structures are not encountered in normal occupational exposures. I think it is important to realize that the kind of lesions that were shown here are not the common occurance and do not occur in any of the occupational exposures that are allowed by present U. S. Standards or any of the other labor standards.

Moe: That is correct. We feel that the current standards provide a protective effect of 2 to 4 times.

Pfander: In our studies of soldiers that were shooting the Carl Gustav cannon, the peak pressure was 182 dB. Laryngoscopy on these individuals did not reveal any laryngeal hemorrhages, and they voiced no complaints. However, Mr. Brinkmann who was also exposed to several shots complained of chest pressure during the evening. We also exposed mini-pigs to the same blast pressure and saw hemorrhages on the pleura. However, we discovered that this was an artifact of the method of sacrifice, i.e., electroshock. In your experiment, how were the animals killed?

Moe: Our animals were anesthesized with barbituates and then exsanguinated. Our feeling is the same as yours about the Carl Gustav armed with the long range ammunition. There is no effect that we can determine on biological systems at the 3.5 PSI repeated exposure level. Not only is this the worst case exposure level, but 50 shots with the long range ammunition is far outside U.S. operational guidance for that particular type of ammunition. Dr. Phillips gave a risk assessment statement on this and our feeling was that there was no significant biological risk from operating this weapon with repeated firing of the long range ammunition. Incidently, eardrum rupture was essentially universal in those animals exposed to the 74 PSI peak.

NONAUDITORY EFFECTS OF REPEATED EXPOSURES TO INTENSE IMPULSE NOISE

Y.Y. Phillips,[1] A. Dancer,[2] and D.R. Richmond[3]

[1]Division of Medicine, Walter Reed Army Institute of Research Washington, D.C. 20307; [2]Physiology Group, Franco-German Institute, Saint-Louis, France; [3]Life Sciences Division Los Alamos National Laboratory, Los Alamos, NM 87545

ABSTRACT

Exposure to intense impulse noise can cause injury to all of the air containing structures of the body. While the ear is the most sensitive organ, the upper respiratory tract (URT), the lungs, and the gut can be damaged by air blast. This nonauditory injury has been studied as a consequence of weapon effects research. The development of light, long-range artillery and powerful shoulder-fired antitank weapons has increased the intensity of impulse noise to which soldiers are exposed. Hearing damage is recognized as a military occupational health hazard, and the advent of louder weapons has raised the possibility that nonauditory injury might become a limiting safety concern. Animal research was begun in Europe and the United States in an attempt to define that new hazard. Anesthetized sheep and swine were necropsied after being exposed to a variety of impulse conditions. It was readily demonstrated that with repeated exposures, nonauditory injury could build-up at relatively low overpressure levels. In these experiments, groups of six animals each were exposed to 20 blasts of equal peak pressure (P: 68 kPa) but varying positive phase impulse (I: 63, 110, 145, 184 and 222 kPa-msec). In a complementary study, groups of the same size were exposed to 20 blasts of similar I (136 kPa-msec) but variable P (26, 48, 69, 115, 126, and 262 kPa). These experiments showed that damage occurred in the URT, the gut, and lung with both increasing frequency and severity as either I was increased with constant P or as P was increased with constant I. The URT was most sensitive, with at least minor petechial hemorrhage being evident in the larynx whenever injury to the gut or lung was present. URT injury often occurred in the absence of injury to other organs. Nonauditory injury from Friedlander waves is determined by the interaction of number of exposures, P, and I. URT petechiae are the first gross evidence of injury and can be used to define limiting conditions for exposure.

INTRODUCTION

The pressure wave from an explosion exerts a direct damaging cussive effect on structures, including the human body. This primary effect of a blast wave has been recognized as the cause of injury to air-containing organs since the First World War [1,2]. Airblast, irrespective of associated fragments or gross body displacement, may damage the lungs, the gastrointestinal tract (gut), the upper respiratory tract (URT), and the ear [3,4]. Injury to the ear may range from frank rupture of the tympanic membrane with ossicular disruption to subtle biochemical or ultrastructural changes in the neurosensory apparatus [5]. The latter, reflected clinically as a decrease in hearing sensitivity, is a widely recognized military occupational health hazard which occurs even in peacetime training. The pathophysiology of this auditory injury is the principle subject of this symposium. The development of light, long-range artillery and mortars and powerful shoulder-fired rockets has increased the intensity of impulse noise to which soldiers are exposed. This has raised the possiblity that injury to nonauditory structures may become a limiting concern, particularly where the ears are well protected [6,7].

The potential for primary blast to cause combat casualties has been the subject of military medical research. Work in Sweden [8], France [9], and the U.S. [3,4] has centered on the injurious potential of exposure to a single intense blast as is produced by large quanities of high explosives or nuclear weapons. Injury assessment has centered on mortality or gross internal hemorrhage. Consideration of both the peak pressure (P) and positive phase duration (T_a in Fig. 1) has been shown to be necessary to define the injury potential of a blast wave [3,4,8,9]. In contrast to the strong blast which may produce combat casualties, the blast overpressure that affects a soldier whenever he discharges his own weapon is of much lower intensity, is likely to be repeated many times in a short period and is a hazard in the peacetime training environment.

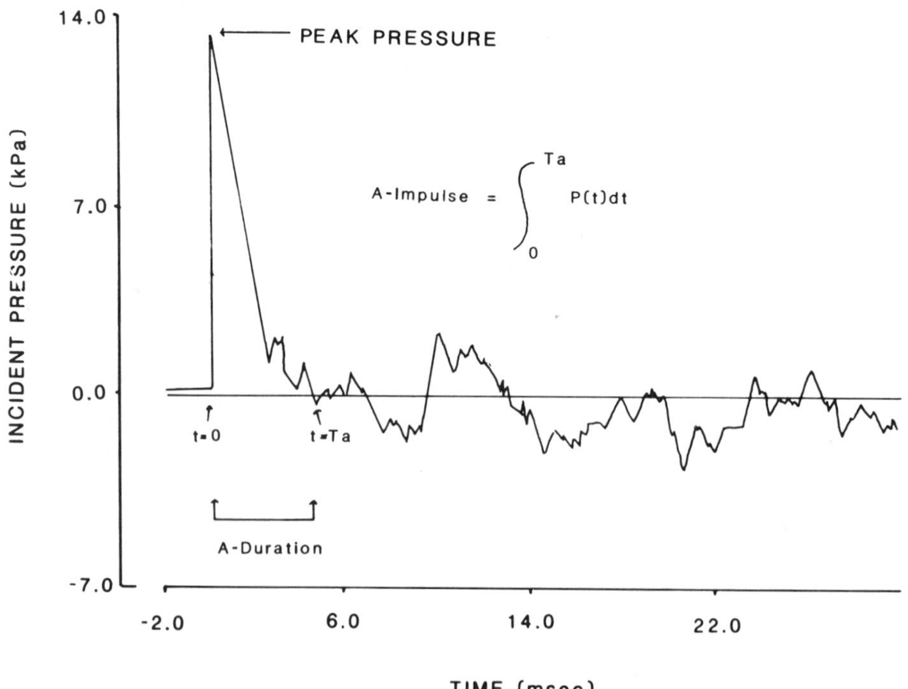

Fig. 1. Typical Friedlander type blast wave characteristic of blast overpressure from weapons fired away from reflecting surfaces. A-duration (T_a) is time from arrival of blast wave to first return to ambient pressure.

Table 1. Airblast Injury Scoring Scheme for Assessing Nonauditory Injury at Gross Necropsy

Injury Level	Gastrointestinal Tract	Upper Respiratory Tract	Lungs
Slight	Contusions, 1 cm^2 or less, isolated.	Petechiae, hyperemic areas.	Ecchymosis
Moderate	Submucosal contusions 1 to 5 cm^2	Ecchymosis, small, submucosal contusions.	Hemorrhages, isolated focal.
Severe	Submucosal contusions, multiple, greater than 5cm^2, hematomas, rupture.	Submucosal contusions, multiple, dark; edema and hematomas.	Extensive areas of confluent hemorrhage extending deep in parenchyma.

The first studies to consider the effect of the number of exposures on nonauditory injury were those carried out at the Franco-German Institute at Saint Louis (ISL) [10,11]. They showed that mortality and morbidity from pulmonary lesions in rats and pigs were clearly related to both blast strength (as measured by peak pressure with a constant duration) and the total number of exposures. Independent studies carried out at the Lovelace Biomedical Research Foundation have also indicated that lethality for large animals for a blast of given strength is a strong function of the number of exposures [12]. Work done by the Walter Reed Army Institute of Research (WRAIR) exposing large animals to very intense muzzle blast from large caliber weapons demonstrated an effect of peak pressure on injury to the gut, the URT and the lungs in the setting of a large number of repetitions [6]. The work detailed in this report was undertaken in an attempt to better define the important blast parameters and target organ sensitivities for non-auditory injury from repeated exposures to intense impulse noise.

METHODS

Adult, mixed breed sheep of both sexes weighing 25-50 kg were sedated with intramuscular Xylazine. Individual sheep were suspended in loose net slings from a metal frame with their right sides oriented towards the blast source. Shaped blocks of TNT weighing from 0.5 to 30 kg were used and the distance from animal to explosive was varied to obtain the desired blast strength. The explosives were suspended over a concrete pad and 20 charges were detonated at 1 to 3 minute intervals. Pressure measurements of the blast waves were made using piezoelectric transducers (Susquehana ST-4). Transducer signals were amplified and recorded on magnetic tape. Paper records were obtained using a fiberoptic light beam oscilloscope and descriptive parameters (peak pressure and duration) of the shock wave were read graphically.

Following exposure, the animals were transported to a laboratory where they were euthanatized with a massive intravenous bolus of Nembutal. A complete gross necropsy was performed within an hour after exposure.

Injury was scored in accordance with the scale in Table 1. Comparisons of the degree of injury in each organ system at different levels of blast were made with chi-squared analysis. One degree of freedom was obtained by comparing no injury with any degree of injury as an indication of incidence or by comparing the incidence of mild or no injury to that of moderate or severe injury as an indication of severity. Significant differences were noted where $p<0.05$.

In what is termed the "iso-peak pressure study" (Table 2), the peak pressure of individual blast waves was kept as constant as possible at 68 kPa and the A-impulse was varied from 63 to 222 kPa-msec by increasing A-duration from 2.3 to 8.6 msec. Groups of 6 animals were exposed simultaneously to 20 consecutive blasts. In a complementary experiment called the "iso-impulse" study (Table 2), the A-impulse was held relatively constant for 20 blasts at about 136 kPa-msec for groups of animals, and the peak pressue was changed from 26 to 262 kPa by varying the A-duration from 11.7 to 1.8 msec.

It can be demonstrated that for triangular approximations for the initial positive phase of a Freidlander wave (Fig. 1), the positive phase energy is proportional to A-impulse duration times peak pressure [13]. The results of the iso-peak pressure study can then be interpreted as indicating increased damage for increased total delivered energy (or impulse). A similar effect is evident in calculating relative energies for the iso-impulse study. To examine this dose effect further, a third experiment was performed in which peak pressure (P) was held constant and A-impulse (I) and number of exposures (N) were varied such that accummulated impulse (NxI) and accummulated relative energy (NxPxI) were the same at two levels (Table 3).

RESULTS

Table 2 summarizes the blast wave parameters and necropsy results for the iso-peak pressure (iso-P) and iso-impulse (iso-I) studies. The variability of peak pressure (P) is smaller in the iso-P study than that of the A-impulse (I) in the iso-I study. The difference in I in the latter case is mitigated by the fact that the lowest impulses are found at the highest peak pressures where the observed injury was greatest. If the I at these levels of P were increased, we would have seen even more injury.

For the iso-P study there was no grossly detectable lung injury at the relatively low P. There was laryngeal injury present for all conditions with a significant build-up in severity with increasing I. Gastrointestinal injury was not present at the lowest I. However, gut damage increased significantly in both incidence and severity as I was increased.

For the iso-I study, lung injury was not present at the lower P conditions; however, incidence and severity increased significantly as peak pressure increased above 115 kPa. There was a significant increase in both incidence and severity for both gut and URT injury with increasing P. Both occurred at lower P than that seen for gross lung injury.

Figs. 2-4 summarize the work above and include data from other experiments [14]. Also included on those figures are the results obtained by researchers at ISL exposing small pigs to 16 repeated exposures of 2 msec duration and variable peak pressure [11]. The figures illustrate the interactive effect of P and I on injury incidence and severity for all three target organ systems in the setting of repeated exposures.

Table 2. Iso-Peak Pressure and Iso-Impulse Studies of Nonauditory Injury

PEAK PRESSURE (kPa)	A-IMPULSE (kPa-msec)	A-DURATION (msec)	LUNG[a]	URT[a]	GUT[a]
68 ± 3[b]	63 ± 3	2.3 ± 0.1	6/0/0/0	1/5/0/0[m]	6/0/0/0[m,q]
64 ± 4	110 ± 8	4.3 ± 0.2	6/0/0/0	0/4/2/0	4/2/0/0[m,s]
69 ± 6	145 ± 8	5.8 ± 0.8	6/0/0/0	0/2/4/0[n]	2/4/0/0[m,r]
69 ± 3	184 ± 18	6.8 ± 0.8	6/0/0/0	0/3/3/0[n]	2/2/0/2[r]
69 ± 7	222 ± 23	8.6 ± 0.9	6/0/0/0	0/4/2/0	0/2/0/4[n,r,t]
262 ± 18	127 ± 10	1.8 ± 0.1	0/0/0/6[n,r]	0/0/0/6[n,r,v]	0/0/0/6[n,r]
126 ± 10	143 ± 10	3.8 ± 0.3	0/5/0/0[m,r]	0/0/1/4[n,r,v]	0/0/0/5[n,r]
115 ± 6	139 ± 10	3.6[c]	6/0/0/0[m,q]	0/1/5/0[n,r]	1/0/0/5[n,r]
69 ± 6	145 ± 8	5.8 ± 0.8	6/0/0/0[m,q]	0/2/4/0[n,r]	2/4/0/0[m,r]
48 ± 5	153 ± 15	8.5 ± 1.3	6/0/0/0[m,q]	0/4/2/0[r,u]	6/0/0/0[m,q]
26 ± 2	132 ± 10	11.7 ± 0.8	6/0/0/0[m,q]	6/0/0/0[m,q]	6/0/0/0[m,q]

Grossly observed non-auditory injury in sheep exposed to 20 repeated blasts. In first 5 rows, peak pressure was held relatively constant at 69 kPa and A-impulse was varied. In last 6 rows (9th identical to 3rd row) the A-impulse is held relatively constant between groups and the peak pressure is increased. a: Denotes injury observed in the lungs, upper respiratory tract (URT) and gut. Columns 3-6 show the numbers of animals scored by the scheme in Table 3 as having injury levels of none/slight/moderate/severe (see Table 1). b: Values are reported as mean +/- one standard deviation. c: Data not recorded, value is estimated. Animal groups with injury score superscripts of n have a more severe degree of injury in the same organ system than those with m and those with v have more severe injury than those with u ($p<.05$). Groups with superscript r have a greater incidence of injury in the same organ system than those with q and those with t have a greater incidence than those with s ($p<.05$).

Table 3 details the results of the summated impulse (sum-I) portion of the study. Two groups of 6 animals were exposed to the same sum-I of 2300 kPa-msec with the same P (68 kPa) by halving the number of exposures in the group with the largest I. None of the animals showed lung injury and there was no difference in laryngeal injury between the two exposure groups. Gut injury was more severe in the group with the larger I, with 2 animals having moderate injury, but the difference was not statistically significant. At the higher sum-I value of 4600 kPa-msec, the same trend is

Table 3. Summated Impulse Study for Repeated Blasts.

PEAK PRESSURE (kPa)	A-IMPULSE (kpa-msec)	NUMBER	SUMMATED IMPULSE (kPa-msec)	LUNG[a]	URT[a]	GUT[a]
68	230	10	2300	6/0/0/0	0/5/1/0	3/1/2/0
68	115	20	2300	6/0/0/0	0/4/2/0	5/1/0/0
68	230	20	4600	6/0/0/0	0/4/2/0	1/0/5/0[b]
68	115	40	4600	6/0/0/0	2/4/0/0	5/1/0/0[b]

Grossly observed, non-auditory injury in sheep exposed to a variable number of blasts with the same peak pressure. The impulse of the individual blasts was varied so as to obtain similar summated impulses (number of exposures times impulse per exposure).
a: Denotes injury observed in the lungs, upper respiratory tract (URT), and gastrointestinal tract (gut). Columns 5-7 show the number of animals having injury levels of none/slight/moderate/severe (see Table 1).
b: Groups differ in injury severity ($p<.01$) and incidence ($p<.05$).

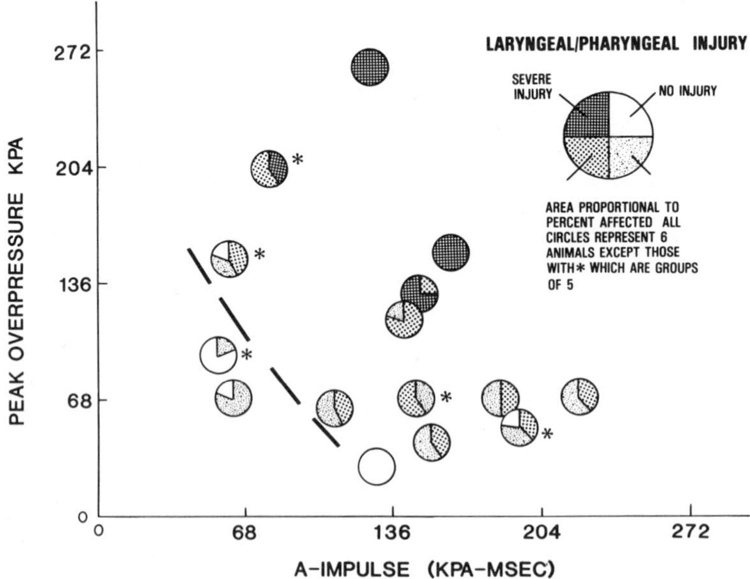

Fig. 2. Incidence and severity of upper respiratory tract injury in sheep and pigs as a function of peak pressure and A-impulse for 20 consecutive exposures.

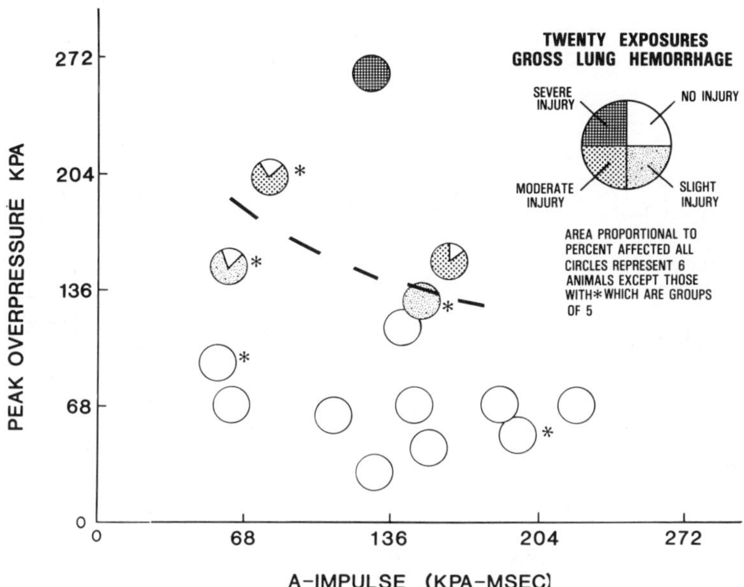

Fig. 3. Incidence and severity of lung injury in sheep and pigs as a function of peak pressure and A-impulse for 20 consecutive exposures.

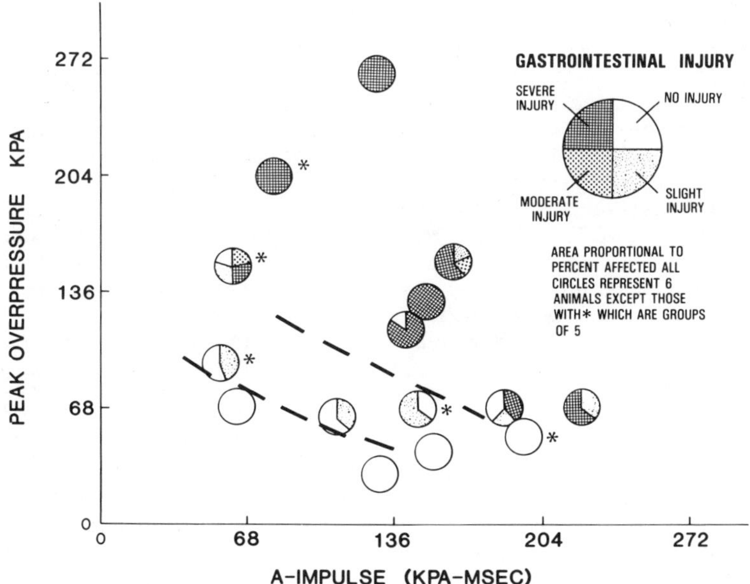

Fig. 4. Incidence and severity of gastrointestinal tract injury in sheep and pigs as a function of peak pressure and A-impulse for 20 consecutive exposures.

evident, with more severe injury being present at the condition with the lowest number of exposures but higher individual blast I. The difference in gut injury severity and incidence was statistically significant.

DISCUSSION

The interactive effect of peak pressure (P) and A-impulse (I) is evident for injury severity and incidence for all three organ systems (Table 2 and Figs. 2-4). The larynx is most sensitive, with at least minor petechial hemorrhage being present in the larynx whenever injury to the gut or lungs is present and often occurring in the absence of other injury. Laryngeal petechiae or small hemorrhages do not present a serious risk of morbidity, whereas contusions in the bowel or lung may pose the risk of incapacitation or worse. Laryngeal injury in the sheep appears to be a sensitive indicator of other organ involvement (i.e., all with gut or lung injury have laryngeal injury), but is not specific (i.e., many have laryngeal injury only). Laryngeal damage is not predictive of the severity of non-laryngeal injury (e.g., only slight laryngeal injury may occur with severe gastrointestinal injury). The vast majority of the data comes from sheep [6,13,14]. Corroborative experiments performed by ISL and WRAIR using the pig as a large animal model have shown a similar buildup in gastrointestinal injury in the absence of significant lung damage [15]. Laryngeal injury in pigs also occurred, but did not appear to be as sensitive as laryngeal damage in the sheep.

Based on the results described above, it seems likely that given a three-dimensional space with axes of number of blast repetitions (N), (P), and (I), a surface defining the threshold of injury could be described (Fig, 5). The plot of P versus I for any N is parabolic in nature, a characteristic shared by many structural damage criteria [16,17]. On one side of this surface each point would correspond to conditions (N,P,I) at which at least laryngeal injury would be expected to occur in some animals. The farther the point from the surface (on the injury side), the greater the likelihood and/or severity of injury. Gastrointestinal and pulmonary injury would occur at more severe conditions. Any point on the noninjury side of the surface would describe conditions (N,P,I) which would not result in consequential injury to any nonauditory structure. Thus, the occurrence of trivial laryngeal injury in a sensitive model (the sheep) could be used to assess risk when the exposure is defineable in these easily measured acoustic parameters. Knowledge of this injury boundary would allow for a safety assessment to be made for occupational exposure for any weapon system which generates simple Friedlander blast overpressure. Exposure conditions (N,P,I) would either be on the 'safe' side of the boundary, and thereby associated with little or no risk of non-auditory injury, or on the 'unsafe' side entailing a risk to exposed individuals.

The relationship between injury and blast parameters (N,P,I) described above is entirely empirical and one would like to be able to deal analytically with some measure of accummulated dose to predict an effect. Total impulse or energy delivered is a logical model. For triangular approximations of the initial positive phase of a Friedlander wave, A-energy is proportional to A-impulse times peak pressure [13]. The iso-peak pressure study can then be interpreted as indicating increased damage for increased total delivered impulse and hence delivered energy. A similar effect is evident in calculating relative energies for the iso-impulse study. To examine this further, a series of experiments were performed in which P was held constant and I and N were varied so that accumulated impulse (NxI) and accumulated relative energy (NxPxI) were the same at two levels (Table 3).

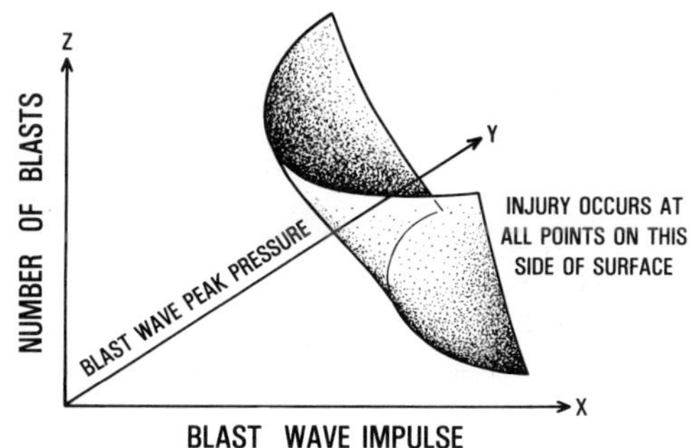

Fig. 5. Hypothetical three-dimensional representation of an iso-damage surface for nonauditory blast injury as a function of peak pressure, A-impulse, and number of exposures.

Groups of six sheep exposed to the same accumulated A-impulse for the first (10, 68, 230 N,P,I) and second (20, 68, 115 N,P,I) conditions showed no lung injury and no difference in laryngeal injury. However, gastrointestinal injury appeared to be worse in the condition where the individual blast had greater I. This was borne out in comparison of the third (20, 68, 230 N,P,I) and fourth (40, 68, 115 N,P,I) groups where the difference in gut injury was significant. Indeed, the animals in the first group (10, 68, 230 N,P,I) had more gastrointestinal injury than those in the fourth group (40, 68, 115 N,P,I), despite having received only half the accummulated A-impulse. It is evident that nonauditory injury is dependent not only on the total energy or impulse delivered, but also on the characteristics of each "packet" of energy.

It must be stressed that there is no evidence that any impulse noise exposure permitted by the present military noise exposure standards of NATO member nations presents any risk of nonauditory injury. Laryngeal and chest examinations performed on 103 soldiers after firing four rounds of the Karl Gustav 84 mm MAW (peak pressure 22-36 kPa with A-duration < 2 msec) showed no blast related abnormalities [18]. Fifty-nine soldiers also failed to show any evidence of laryngeal, pulmonary, or gastrointestinal injury after firing 12 rounds of top zone charge from the 155 mm howitzer (peak pressure 24 kPa, A-impulse, 62.7 kPa msec) [19]. These observations lend credence to the predictions of human safety for these circumstances based on animal data. The prevention of nonauditory injury for soldiers must depend upon keeping exposure conditions below some threshold level. The only known means of protecting nonauditory structures is through the use of rigid armor or barriers. Both human and animal studies indicate that standard ballistic vests offer no protection from blast [20,21].

The work described above has dealt exclusively with free field Friedlander blast waves (Fig. 1). The P and I of such waves effectively define both the power density spectrum and the duration of blast exposure. Use of either A-duration or A-impulse is equivalent when considering Friedlander waves, as either value plus peak pressure defines the other. The relationship breaks down when considering the complex pressure-time histories in reverberant conditions. Strong complex waves are found in such places as the cabs of self propelled artillery and in emplacements or enclosures where antitank rockets are fired. At present there is no systematic way to judge the nonauditory hazard of such environments. Studies by Clemedson et al. of Sweden [22], WRAIR [23], and ISL [24] have indicated that consideration of peak pressure alone or peak pressure and A-impulse can underestimate injury. However, attempting to weight the total positive impulse or total energy in the blast wave can greatly overestimate the hazard. A more basic understanding of the biophysical interaction of the human and animal body with the complicated pressure environment is necessary before we can deal with complex waves in a generalizable fashion. Until that time, complex wave environments will have to be assessed on a case by case basis and some empiric large animal exposures may be necessary to estimate risk.

REFERENCES

1. D. R. Hooker, Physiological Effects Of Air Concussion, Am. J. Physiol., 67:219 (1924).
2. H. Desaga, Blast Injuries in: "German Aviation Medicine World War II," U.S. Government Printing Office, Washington, DC (1950).
3. T. L. Chiffelle, R. K. Jones, D. R. Richmond, E. G. Damon, "The Biologic and Pathologic Effects of Blast Injury," Technical Report on Contract DA-49-146XZ-055 (1966).
4. C. S. White, R. K. Jones, E. G. Damon, E. R. Fletcher, and D. R. Richmond, "The Biodynamics of Airblast," Report DNA 2738T (1971).
5. F. G. Hirsch., Effects of Overpressure on The Ear, A Review, Annals of the N.Y. Acad. of Sci., 152:147 (1968).
6. C. B. Clifford, J. B. Moe, J. J. Jaeger, and J. J. Hess, Gastrointestinal lesions in lambs due to multiple low-level blast overpressure exposure, Military Medicine, 149:491 (1984).
7. R. G. Price, Relative hazard of weapons impulses, J. of the Acoust. Soc. Amer. 73:556 (1983).
8. A. Jonsson, "Experimental Investigations on the Mechanisms of Lung Injury in Blast and Impact Exposure," Linkoping University Medical Dissertations, No. 880 (1979).
9. P. Rigaud, "General Effect of Shock Waves On The Living Organism (Report To the Galf of May 29-30, 1970)," ISL NB 2/71, St. Louis, France, Mar. 2, 1971.
10. P. Vassout, G. Parmentier, A. Dancer, "Influence due nombre d' expositions a unde onde de choc forte sur les lesions pulmonaires et les taux de mortalite chex le rat," Rapport Bericht Institute Franco- Allemand de Recerches de Saint Louis, Saint-Louis, France, (1978).
11. P. Vassout, G. Parmentier, and A. Dancer, "Etude des effects d' unde onde de choc forte sur le porc: Influence du nombre d' expositions," Rapport Bericht Institut Franco-Allemand de Recerches de Saint-Louis, Saint-Louis,France (1981).
12. D. R. Richmond, J. T. Yelverton, E. R. Fletcher, "The Biological Effects of Repeated Blasts," Topical Report DNA5842F, Defense Nuclear Agency, Washington, DC, 30 April 1981.
13. Y. Y Phillips, J. J. Jaeger, A. J. Young, "Biophysics of Injury From Repeated Blast," Proceedings of Tripartite Technology Coordinating Program Panel W-2, Muzzle Blast Overpressure Workshop, May 1982.
14. D. R. Richmond, Annual Report on USAMRDC Contract 82-PP2800 (1983).
15. P. Vassout, A. Dancer, D. R. Richmond, Y. Y. Phillips, "Effets biologiques des ondes de choc fortes: influence de la duree des ondes dans le cas d expositions repetees. Notice S-N 911/84 Institute Franco-Allemand de Recerches de Saint Louis, Saint Louis, France (1984).
16. O. T. Johnson, "A Blast-Damage Relationship," Brl Report 1389, September 1967.

17. D. J. James, K. J. Burdett, "The Response of the Human Ear to Blast, Part 1: The Effect on the Ear Drum of A 'Short' Duration, 'Fast' Rising, Pressure Wave," Joint AWRE/CDE Report No. 0 4/82 (1982).
18. F. Pfander, H. Brinkman, Report to NATO Panel VIII, RSG-6, "Effects of Impulse Noise," May 1983.
19. J. H. Patterson, "Direct Determination of the Adequacy of Hearing Protection For Use With The Viper Anti-Tank Weapon and the M198 Howitzer," Proceedings of Tripartite Technology Coordinating Program Panel W-2, Muzzle Blast Overpressure Workshop, May 1982.
20. A. J. Young, J. J. Jaeger, Y. Y. Phillips, J. T. Yelverton, D. R. Richmond, The influence of clothing on human, intrathoracic pressure during airblast," Aviation Space and Environmental Medicine, 56:49 (1985).
21. Y. Y. Phillips, T. G. Mundie, J. T. Yelverton, D. R. Richmond "Cloth Ballistic Vest Alters Response to Blast," Fifth International Wound Ballistics Symposium, Gothenburg, Sweden, June 1985.
22. C. J. Clemedson, A. Jonsson, "Estimates of Medical Risks for Personnel, Firing with Recoilless Weapons from Bunkers," Forsvarets Forskningsanstalt, FOA Report A 20012-D6, March 1976.
23. D. R. Richmond, J. T. Yelverton, E. R. Fletcher, Y. Y. Phillips, "Biologic Response to Complex Blast Waves," Ninth International Symposium Military Applications of Blast Simulation (MABS 9), September 1985.
24. P. Vassout, G. Evrard, A. Dancer, "Etude comparee chez le porc des effets extra-auditifs d' ondes de choc fortes en fonction des conditions d' exposition: champ libre ou ambiance reverberante," Notice S-N 911/84 Institute Franco-Allemand de Recerches de Saint Louis, Saint Louis, France (1983).

DISCUSSION

von Gierke: In your last study, the 20 exposures were all on the same day, but what is the interval between successive exposures?

Phillips: For the volunteers, we will allow one set of exposures in any 24 hour period.

von Gierke: Yes, but do you use the same volunteers again at a higher level?

Phillips: Yes, the next day.

Alberti: I note that you expose the animals sideways. Is there any difference if they've got their backs or fronts to the explosion as far as the larangeal or pharangeal damage?

Phillips: Yes, our animals are all oriented right side on in accordance with the way we've done things, for gastrointestinal injury. We've not noticed any difference in left or right side with upper respiratory tract injury. Casualty level blast studies have shown decreased injury by orienting the streamlined portions of ones body to the blast source. I would not expect a big effect. If you are familiar with sheep, they have rather a pendulous neck with a very anteriorly located trachea that is very much below the surface. We see the injury principally on the side of exposure on the membraneous portion of the trachea and in the larynx. As a matter of fact, in the sheep the most sensitive injury probably turns out to be tracheal petechia.

Alberti: Are there any good human studies of severe exposure effects? I know for example that there is a very detailed study of the effect on the ear of a bomb explosion in a Belfast restaurant as a result of a terrorist attack.

Phillips: There is a great deal of autopsy work from war casualties. We talked to the people, Graham Cooper and Bob Mayerd, who wrote the article to which you are referring. Those exposures are so much higher than what we are talking about now, that they are not really applicable. The physical response of people is quite predictable and similar to that of the experimental animals, i.e., the species difference is probably a pure mass difference.

Alberti: Is the human upper respiratory track and larynx as much at risk as in your experimental animals?

Phillips: We think not. The only direct evidence we have of that is some of the work of Dr. Pfander, where individuals had been examined after exposure to the Carl Gustaf. We have also examined the larynx of volunteers exposed to the 198 mm howitzer. However, those circumstances are again below the predicted threshold levels. We will be examining them in an incremental fashion as exposure level increases. We will stop them if we find such changes.

Stevins: It would be very interesting if during these trials you could record the A-weighted energy. Also, do you plan to compute the D-weighted energy?

Phillips: We will have the full data records, and we will be recording or calculating all of the parameters used in the standards of the various member NATO countries.

McFadden: How do you get the volunteers?

Phillips: We get them by requesting volunteers for participation. The Army has a very tough criteria, more so than civilian institutions. We must satify a very rigorous scientific peer review and human use review. Individuals can back out with no prejudice at any time.

Brinkman: If I understood you correctly, you would like to get a damage risk criteria in terms of impulse A-duration and peak pressure?

Phillips: What we are saying is that is the structure of the study. The way in which the data are interpreted, is to a degree open. I would suggest that the over pressure from large weapon systems can be characterized in that paradigm. Now whether or not those are really the important characteristics for auditory injury is not going to be clear.

Brinkman: Do you plan to use only Friedlander waves or will you also look at sources such as mortars?

Phillips: Mortars generate waves similar to Friedlander waves. There are reflctions on all of these blasts so they are not absolutely pure Friedlander waves. That is why we prefer to deal with the A-impulse and peak pressures as opposed to duration. We are primarily interested in essentially single sources, i.e., without environmental reflections as occurs with mortars and with howitzers in the open. At a later time we can perhaps deal with more complex waveforms.

EXPERIMENTAL AND ANALYTICAL STUDIES OF BLAST WAVE EFFECTS ON MAJOR ORGAN SYSTEMS OF THE BODY

J. H. Stuhmiller

Fluid Dynamics Division
JAYCOR
P.O. Box 85154, San Diego, California 92138 USA

ABSTRACT

Evidence of acute nonauditory injury in animals from intense blast overpressure (BOP) exposure and the possibility of chronic injury from BOP in the crew area of conventional weapons has prompted the need for detailed biomechanical models to assist the U. S. Army in defining damage risk criteria (DRC) for humans. The methodology uses mathematical models and computer codes to construct a causal, verifiable connection between the external blast environment and the local tissue stresses. Direct, in vitro observation of the damage process and measurement of the tissue strength leads to the determination of critical stress thresholds for damage that define the mechanical conditions producing injury.

Load distribution on a torso model exposed to blast waves of 3-30 psi peak pressure were used to validate gas dynamics calculations of the blast-body interaction and to develop a preliminary blast load relationship. A finite element model (FEM) of the thorax cross section of the sheep has been constructed and parametric calculations varying the material properties has revealed that the only sensitive quantities are the density and compressibility of the lung parenchyma and the effective shear modulus of the thoracic cavity. All of the material properties of the lung required for the thorax model have been measured for a variety of species and the ability of the lung parenchyma to support a low speed compression wave has been directly observed. Comparison of the FEM predictions against the currently available animal data on intrathoracic pressure response have been satisfactory and the variation of ITP under iso-impulse conditions agrees well with data.

A perfusion technique has been developed that allows in vitro investigation of the mechanical origins of injury to the gastrointestinal tract. The results strongly point to the role of local gas bubbles in the gut sections that lead to large motions and stresses in the neighboring gut walls and eventually cause injury.

INTRODUCTION

Interest in the lethality of the blast following a nuclear explosion prompted several animal studies in the 1960's that identified the circumstances in which death would occur [1,2]. Although there was no need to define the conditions of incipient or chronic injury, the results clearly showed that the soft, air-filled organs (lungs, gastrointestinal tract, larynx, and tympanic cavities) are damaged. Research into the mechanisms of injury have continued since then at several laboratories around the world [3-5,7,8].

In the past decade, there has been interest by the U.S. Army in blast injury at occupational exposure levels. Several weapon systems, notably self-propelled howitzers and shoulder-fired anti-tank rounds, are of such power that the crews and troops using them are exposed to pressure fields of unprecedented magnitude. Although it is certain that such exposures are not associated with acute injury, they do approach the exposure limits set by military standards. The limits are based on experience with safe conditions, rather than on known injury thresholds. To extend these boundaries for training purposes, it is necessary to establish the conditions under which subtle or chronic injury will not occur.

A common procedure for determining human risk is to make comparisons with similar animal exposures. The uncertainty of this procedure arises from the extrapolation of results between species. Body weight, size, orientation, internal organ arrangement, and other anatomical factors must be considered in interpreting test results. Furthermore, large numbers of animals must be used to produce statistically significant averages and to overcome variations in individual animals. As the number of blast conditions to be studied increases, the total number of animals, as well as the cost and duration of the testing, grows dramatically.

One way of reducing the amount of animal testing required is to use mathematical models. In the simplest applications, mathematics is used to fit a smooth curve through some test conditions in order to extend the results to other conditions. This approach may not correctly predict results outside of the range already tested and cannot address extrapolation to other species.

A more satisfactory model results from incorporating the mechanics of the process and physiology of the animal. Such a model was proposed as an adjunct to the animal testing at the Lovelace Inhalation Toxicology Research Institute (ITRI) [6]. The lung was represented by a gas-filled volume, the chest wall by a piston, and the rigidity of the skeletal system by an opposing spring. When the pressure history of the blast wave is applied to the external surface of the piston, the piston accelerates inward, compressing the gas until it is finally brought to rest by the combined action of the gas pressure and the force of the spring. The various parameters of the model were calibrated to reproduce the peak internal pressures seen in the test animals. It was also proposed that the parameters would scale with total body mass of the animal according to certain geometric rules.

This model is able to correlate, and to some extent explain, a limited range of internal pressure data for simple waves. Still, it is not capable of answering the hazard questions discussed earlier. First of all, the parameters of the model are not directly related to measurable physiological properties; instead they have been chosen to give the best agreement with internal pressure data. Therefore, although one may speculate as to their origin, one cannot confidently judge how they would change between species. Secondly, there is no connection made with the mechanism of injury. While large internal pressures undoubtedly indicate a more hazardous environment, the location and severity of injury cannot be inferred from such a model.

There is another kind of model of the thorax that has taken the physiological details into account. Borrowing from the techniques of structural engineers, detailed models of the skeletal system of the chest have been produced that use measurable, mechanical properties of the bone and incorporate all of the connections and linkages. These models have been quite successful is studying the blunt trauma of automobile crashes, where the body is thrown into a solid object. The injury of interest in a crash is bone fracture, so that no modeling of the soft tissue is included. In blast exposure, however, skeletal deformation is relatively small and serves only to transmit motion to the compliant organs inside where the damage process take place. Therefore, although the ambiguity of the description is removed, the models do not address the problem of interest.

The work summarized in this paper has expanded upon these ideas to construct a model of the thorax that contains a structural description of the hard and soft tissues. Supplemented with field measurements of load distribution and laboratory measurements of tissue properties, the model predicts the detailed motion of the thorax and indicates the magnitude and distribution of stresses that may be linked to damage. The detailed work and results are documented in Reference 13.

A parallel effort in our laboratory has been studying the mechanisms of gastrointestinal injury [9]. Field studies with test animals have shown that GI injury has a lower threshold of occurrence and may be the limiting process in occupational safety. Biomechanical modeling of the phenomena is in its exploratory phases as more quantitative data is being collected.

SUMMARY OF RESULTS

Blast Loading Description

In order to determine the load distribution on a subject in a blast field, model tests were conducted at ITRI and calculations were made with JAYCOR's EITACC computer code. From this work we found that load impulse can be a multiple of the free-field impulse, depending on the wave intensity, and that the spatial and temporal distribution of the load can be reasonably predicted by computational models for the occupational level exposures.

Structural and Material Description

The animal chosen for field test exposures was the sheep. The sheep has a thorax size and construction that is similar to man and has been the test animal in previous blast investigations so that a body of data already exists. The first step in the structural determination was to review the available anatomical literature and select typical dimensions and orientations of organs. The primary difference is that sheep have large, multiple stomachs that have a considerable air content. It was important to establish early in the investigation what effect this difference might have on the cross-species inferences.

Next, the structural analysis method called finite element modeling was applied [10]. The object to be studied is divided into contiguous blocks, called elements, with shapes that fit natural boundaries. The continuous, differential laws of mechanics are transformed into algebraic equations for the position, velocity, and stress at points within each element. More accuracy (and complexity) results from using more points per element. The properties of the material enter as parameters that are determined by conducting particular experiments. The more complete the description of the material, the more parameters that must be determined.

Finally, to advance the model one time-step requires solving thousands of equations for thousands of unknowns. There are a variety of numerical algorithms available and a trade-off between cost and accuracy of the solution must be made.

There are four types of choices to make in performing a finite element analysis: size of the element, number of points within the element, complexity of the material description, and the numerical solution technique. For this project we used the FEAP computer code [11], which employs the Newmark method of solution. Each element contained four nodal points with a bilinear interpolation scheme. The material was assumed to be of a linear viscoelastic type, requiring that seven parameters must be determined for each substance. Finally, the size of elements was chosen to be small enough to resolve the phenomena of interest, yet resulting in a mathematical problem that can be solved at reasonable cost.

In order to determine if the gas content of the sheep stomach would significantly influence measurements taken within the thorax, a finite element model was constructed of the entire sheep torso. Three-dimensional blocks were used of a size sufficient to capture the major organs (Fig. 1b). In this model, the inertia of the rib cage, skeletal muscle, and diaphragm were incorporated at the appropriate nodal points, thus reducing the number of elements required.

A blast loading, corresponding to cases in which field data was available, was applied to the model surface and the subsequent intrathoracic pressure (ITP) time histories were compared with data. Two extreme cases had the rumen filled with all water and with all air. The difference in the predictions of ITP was judged to be slight and no greater than that due to uncertainty in the data or material constants. Other calculations using this model, however, showed that the element size was too large to capture the behavior of more rapid events. Based on these results, it was decided to develop a separate thorax model with sufficient resolution to follow the phenomena of interest.

From the earlier collection of anatomical data, a sheep cross-section was selected that corresponds to the approximate location where intrathoracic pressure measurements are made. Based on that view, a two-dimensional finite element model was constructed that captured the geometric arrangement of four distinct parts: skeletal muscle, rib, lung, and a water-filled organ such as the heart (Fig. 1c and d).

There are several approximations that must be taken into account when using and interpreting a two-dimensional representation of a three-dimensional body. First, the motion should be primarily in that plane. Since the thorax of a sheep or man is somewhat cylindrical, and since it was previously shown that the motion of the diaphragm has only a small influence on the thorax, this assumption is reasonable. Second, the internal arrangement of the organs varies with the cross-section location and with individual, so that the results are only typical, rather than specific. It is likely that intrathoracic pressures, which are taken in a region removed from the lung boundaries, will be less affected by the choice of cross-section. Third, the cross-section view at some locations cuts across the diaphragm, showing thoracic and abdominal organs in the same plane. Since we know these two regions are not strongly connected dynamically, the region has been modeled as an equivalent water-filled organ. Finally, the rib cage adds stiffness to the chest wall through forces that do not originate in the plane being analyzed. Studies were made to determine the best way to include this effect and it was concluded that modifying the rigidity of the muscle/bone region to a value intermediate between muscle and bone produced the most satisfactory result. This point is discussed in more detail in the section on thoracic response.

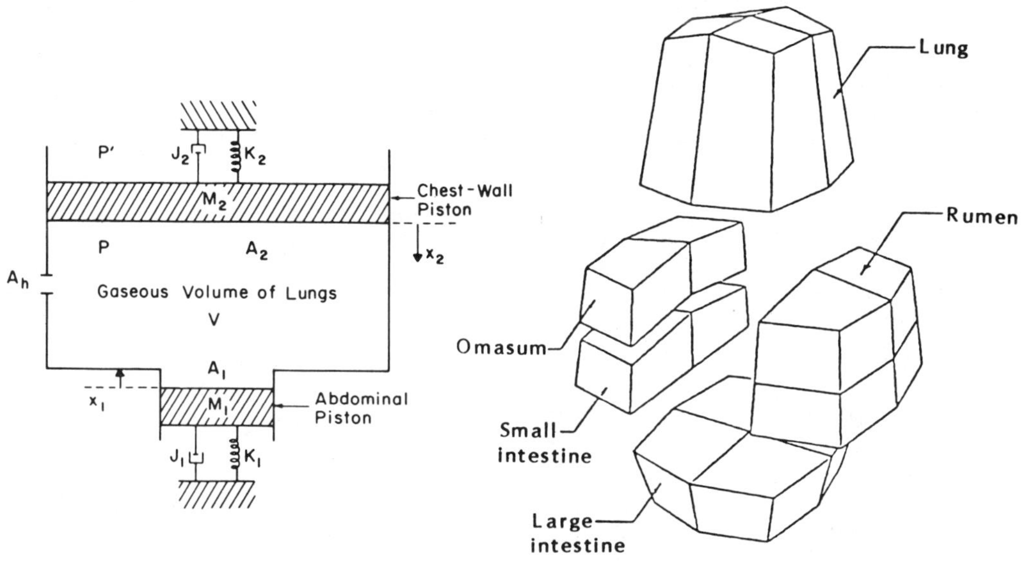

(a) Lumped parameter model (b) Three-dimensional finite element model

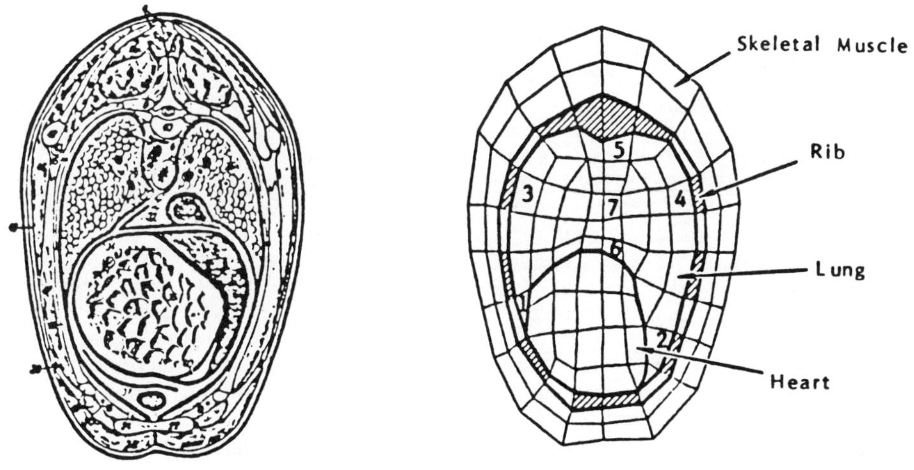

(c) Anatomic cross-section view (d) Two-dimensional finite element model

Fig. 1. Various models of a sheep thorax

Material Properties Determination

The properties of the lung parenchyma have the greatest influence on the thorax response, the evolution of intrathoracic pressure, and the nature of damage to the tissue itself. Because of its central role, a special effort was made to determine its properties precisely. The experiments were conducted in the Bioengineering Laboratory at the University of California, San Diego under the direction of Professor Y. C. Fung [12]. There, special instrumentation was used to determine the viscoelastic properties of the lung tissue and of the whole lung, and to conduct dynamic experiments on wave propagation through the parenchyma.

Thoracic Response

To use the finite element model described in the previous section, it is necessary to provide values for the seven material parameters for each of the four body material chosen to represent the thorax. Those parameters can be summarized by the relations

$$\text{Mass density} = \rho$$
$$\text{Bulk modulus} = K_o + K_1 * \exp(-t/\lambda)$$
$$\text{Shear modulus} = G_o + G_1 * \exp(-t/\beta)$$

Only a few of the 28 parameters have been measured directly, so before elaborate tests were devised and performed, calculations were made to determine which of the parameters are important to predicting and understanding the data currently available, that is, intrathoracic pressure time histories. Data from a particular field test was chosen to be the basis of comparison. In this test, an animal was exposed to two blast waves separated by about 7 msec. Each parameter of the model was varied systematically and in combination with others, and the predictions compared with the measured data.

The results can be summarized as follows. None of the viscoelastic parameters (K_1, λ, G_1, or β) had significant influence on the predicted ITP. Any differences observed were small compared with the deviation of the prediction from measurement, and were small compared with the effects of varying other parameters. Next, it was found that the elastic properties of the rib and heart elements had little effect on the predictions, provided they were chosen reasonably close (within an order of magnitude) to the known physiological values. The mass density of the rib, muscle, and heart are well known and reasonable variations (tens of percent) were not significant. The only truly sensitive parameters were the mass density and bulk modulus of the lung, which have been well measured in the experiments described earlier, and the effective shear modulus of the muscle layer (see Fig. 2a for a summary).

It was mentioned earlier that one approximation introduced by a two-dimensional representation is that out-of-plane forces, such as those due to the rib cage, cannot be mechanistically modeled. If the shear modulus of muscle, $G_o=10^4$, were used in the model, the model would predict unnaturally large distortions and produce ITP results completely unlike measurement (Fig. 2b). If, on the other hand, the muscle layer is assigned a shear modulus that will give the two-dimensional chest the kind of stiffness actually observed, then the ITP predictions are much more reasonable. This parameter can be independently determined through experiments measuring the displacement of the chest wall under loading.

With the material parameters determined, comparison was made with field test data for sheep exposure to blast. For each case, the measured free-field blast wave was translated into a loading distribution based on

Organ	Parameter						
	ρ	K_0	K_1	λ	G_0	G_1	β
Lung	Sensitive	Sensitive					
Rib	Insensitive	Insensitive			Insensitive		
Muscle	Insensitive	Insensitive			Sensitive		
Heart	Insensitive	Insensitive			Insensitive		

Sensitive

Insensitive in physiological range

Can be neglected

(a) Sensitivity studies have shown which material properties are important for gross motion and ITP.

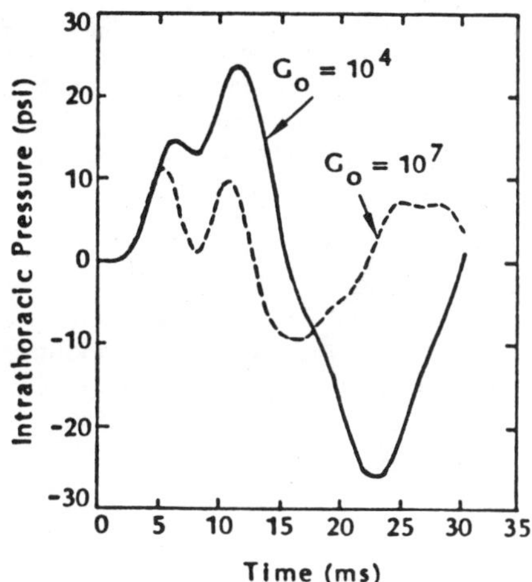

(b) The rigidity of the rib cage must be incorporated into the shear modulus of the thoracic material.

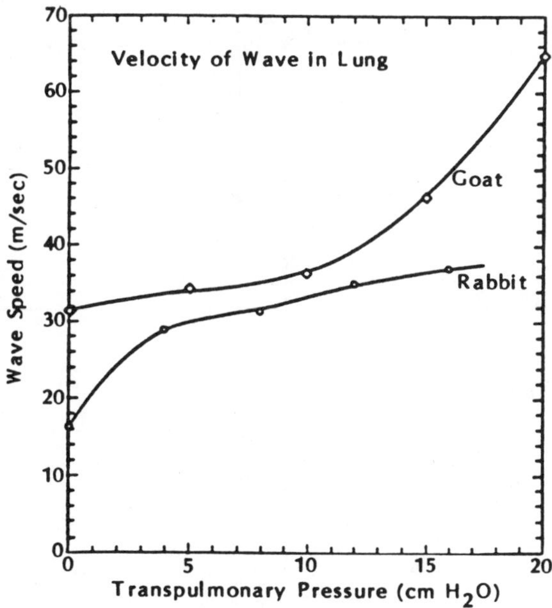

(c) Measured values of wave speed in the lung are consistent with the separately determined elastic moduli and mass density.

Fig. 2. Material properties of the finite element model.

the findings of the torso tests and calculations. When multiple blasts were involved, the loading was simply repeated at the appropriate time interval.

Fig. 3a compares prediction and measurement for a 16 lb TNT charge that produced a single peak blast wave with a peak pressure of about 12 psi. The agreement is considered to be within the uncertainty of the blast conditions, instrument response, and particular animal anatomy. Similar results were obtained for other single blast conditions. After the initial peak, the predictions show continuing reverberation that arises from not including damping processes in the material description.

Fig. 3b compares the results for an exposure to two blast waves with peak pressure of 40 psi separated in time by 7.6 msec--this was the case used in the sensitivity study. The agreement is also good, although the reverberation is more pronounced. The peaks are rounded off due to the finite spatial size of the elements and the negative phase is significantly overpredicted because constant material properties are being used.

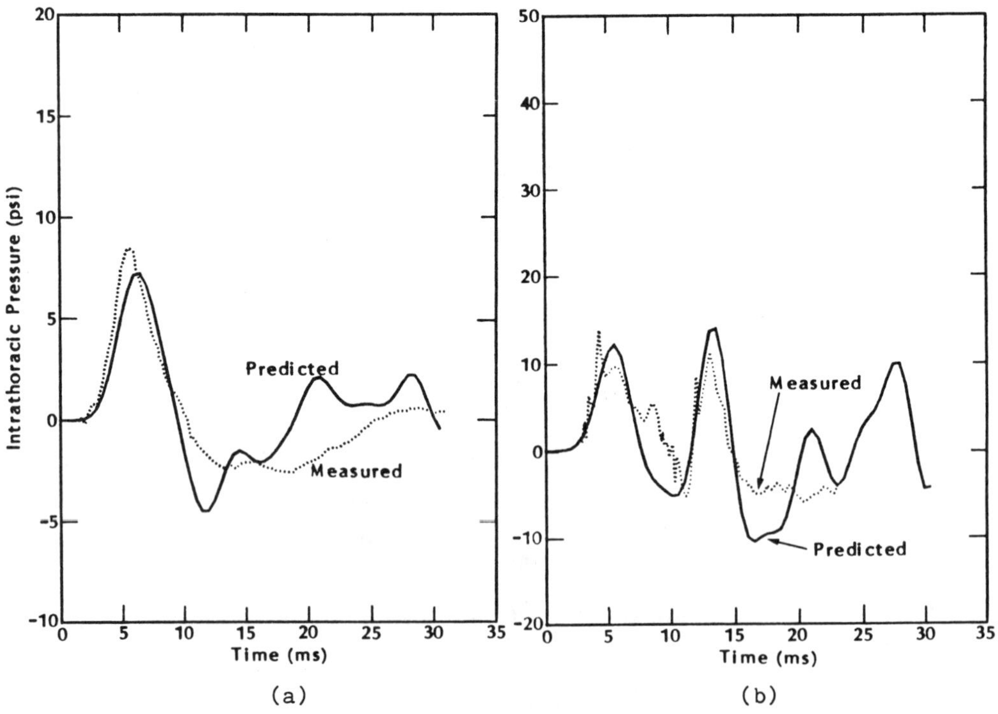

Fig. 3. (a) Exposure to a single peak blast due to a 16 lb TNT charge and (b) exposure to two 40 psi blast waves spearated in time by 7.6 msec.

The dominant feature of the calculated lung pressure distribution is the propagation and reflection of relatively slow waves, predicted by the model to be about 30 m/sec. This phenomena arises in the model because of the combination of highly compressible, yet moderately dense lung material. In a parallel effort in Professor Fung's laboratory at UCSD, the propagation of parenchyma waves due to direct blast exposure was observed and measured. The results varied somewhat with species and transpulmonary pressure, but fell in a range about 30-40 m/sec (Fig. 2c). These results not only support the qualitative nature of the model predictions, but confirms that the dominant material properties for describing lung dynamics are the mass density and the elastic bulk modulus.

Correlation with Lung Injury

A series of tests have been conducted in which sheep were exposed to single blast waves of constant, positive impulse, as measured by a side-on pressure gauge. By varying the test conditions, a range of peak pressure and duration combinations were achieved. The tests showed that the maximum ITP varied with the peak pressure, despite the fact that the waves were iso-impulse, and that the severity of injury increased with the maximum ITP. The finite element model produced the same qualitative trend as the data (Fig. 4). In contrast, the lumped parameter model indicates that peak ITP is nearly constant over the pressure range.

This result is the most encouraging evidence that blast injury can be predicted using an engineering model. The prediction is dependent on the entire causal chain described in the Introduction. First, based on the torso study, the loading on the body increases as the peak pressure of the wave increases. Next, the stress in the lung is amplified by the slow wave speed of the parenchyma. Finally, the location of the esophageal measurement corresponds to a geometric focusing point of the compression waves.

Gastrointestinal Injury

Simulated blast overpressure was generated in a water-filled test chamber to study the gastrointestinal injury mechanism. High speed movies and pressure transducers were used to determine the physical and phenomenological aspects of blast injuries.

To help understand the injury-loading relationship, bursting strengths for each part of the large intestine were measured under static pressurization. There appears to be no well-defined differences in bursting strengths between male and female, nor among the various weight adult rabbits. The results show that ascending colon has the highest values followed by caecum, transverse colon, and descending colon. The strength per unit thickness, however, decreases systematically along the GI tract from caecum to descending colon.

One of the crucial issues of using isolated GI tract for blast injury testing was whether adequate blood supply was provided to the test sections during the test. A perfusion technique using the test rabbit's own cardiopulmonary system as the source of blood supply was developed. Fluorescein tracer showed that, except for a two inch descending colon section near the caudal mesentery artery, the GI tract was well perfused. The approach appeared to be a viable one, and was adopted for all subsequent tests.

Correlation between surface deformation and pressure-time history across the intestinal wall at the bubble site was established. For a given test configuration and blast pressure, the bubble pressure signal and the surface deformation were found to oscillate at a frequency several times higher than the input blast signal. Furthermore, pressure signals inside

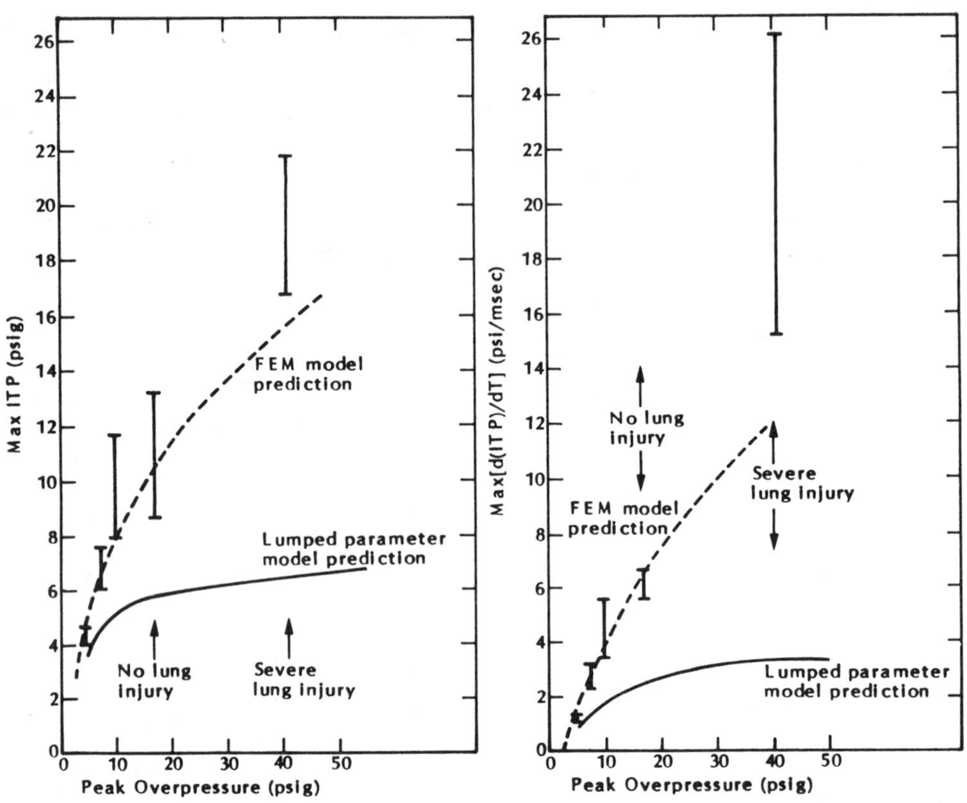

Fig. 4. Iso-impulse study comparison of the FEM model prediction with WRAIR experimental results.

the bubble and along the outer surface indicate that a pressure differential across the intestinal wall was developed during blast. The high differential pressure and high rate of surface deformation were found to correlate well with the initiation of GI injury.

REFERENCES

1. D. R. Richmond, E. G. Damon, E. R. Fletcher, I. G. Bowen, and C. S. White, The relationship between selected blast wave parameters and the response of mammals exposed to airblast, Ann. NY Acad. Sci. 152:103 (1968).
2. T. L. Chiffelle, R. K. Jones, D. R. Richmond, and E. G. Damon, The biologic and pathologic effects of blast injury, technical report on contract DA-49-146-XA-055 (1966).
3. A. J. Jonsson, Experimental investigations on the mechanisms of lung injury in blast and impact exposure, Linkoping University Medical Dissertations No. 80 (1979).
4. C. S. White, R. K. Jones, E. G. Damon, E. R. Fletcher, and D. R. Richmond, The biodynamics of airblast, Report DNA 2738T (1971).
5. H. E. Von Gierke, Response of the body to mechanical forces - an overview, Ann. NY Acad. Sci. 152:172 (1968).
6. I. G. Bowen, A. Holladay, E. R. Fletcher, D. R. Richmond, and C. S. White, A fluid-mechanical model of the thoraco-abdominal system with applications to blast biology, Report DASA-1675 (1965).

7. J. T. Yelverton, D. R. Richmond, E. R. Fletcher, Y. Y. Phillips, J. J. Jaeger, and A. J. Young, Bioeffects of simulated muzzle blasts, "Proceedings of the Eighth International Symposium on Military Application of Blast Simulation," Spiez, Switzerland, June 1983.
8. Y. Y. Phillips, J. J. Jaeger, and A. J. Young, Biophysics of injury from repeated blast, "Proceedings of Tripartite Technology Coordinating Program Panel W-2," Muzzle Blast Overpressure Workshop, May 1982.
9. J. H.-Y. Yu and E. J. Vasel, Experimental study of the correlation between gastrointestinal injury and blast Loading, Final Report under Contract DAMD17-83-C-3221 (1984).
10. O. C. Zienkiewicz, The Finite Element Model, 3rd Ed., McGraw-Hill, New York (1977).
11. R. L. Taylor, and J. L. Sackman, Contact-Impact problems, U. C. Berkeley Report No. SESM-78-4 (1978).
12. Y. C. Fung, M. R. Yen, and Y. J. Zeng, Characterization and modeling of thoraco-abdominal response to blast waves - Volume 3: Lung Dynamics and Mechanical Properties Determination, Final Report to WRAIR under Contract DAMD17-82-C-2062 (1985).
13. C. J. Chuong, and J. H. Stuhmiller, Characterization and modeling of thoraco-abdominal response to blast waves - Volume 4: Biomechanical Model of Thorax Response to Blast Loading, Final Report to WRAIR under Contract DAMD17-82-C-2062 (1985).

HEARING IN FISHERMEN AND COASTGUARDS

Alf Axelsson, Ingmar Arvidsson, and Tomas Jerson

Dept. of Audiology and Occupational Audiology
Sahlgrenska hospital, Gothenburg, Sweden

SUMMARY

Both fishermen and coastguards have a very peculiar working pattern which deviates considerably from that of the regular industrial worker. Instead of 8 hours work followed by 16 hours rest 5 days a week, fishermen and coastguards frequently work for several days with continuous high noise exposure. Also, during sleep they are exposed to high sound levels from the ship engine. In addition, they are exposed to other unfavorable work environment factors such as heave of the sea, whole body vibration, rapid climatic variations, sleep deprivation, work at night, etc. It is quite possible that noise is more deleterious to hearing under such unfavorable conditions. The hearing examination of a large number of fishermen and coastguards showed quite poor hearing, particularly among those at a fairly young age. It is assumed that the major etiology of this poor hearing status is work-related noise exposure, possibly in combination with other interactive ototraumatic factors. In particular leisure time shooting activities performed by 24 and 28% of fishermen and coastguards respectively appear to have contributed to the poor hearing status. Repeated annual hearing check-ups, improved ear protection, and technical noise abatement on board these vessels could improve the hearing of people in these professions considerably.

INTRODUCTION

Maritime workers such as fishermen and coastguards have a working pattern which differs significantly from most other professions. They do not work the regular 8 hours with an interval of 16 hours rest during 5 days a week, but they are more or less continuously exposed to occupational hazards up to one week at a time. During this time they seldom have the possibility of noise-relief. Instead, they spend all their time on board with the engines at work. The vessels are small and the sound levels relatively high in most places on board. This implies that maritime workers are exposed to high sound levels during long periods at a time. In addition, there are a number of interacting effects which might increase the risk of noise-induced hearing loss (NIHL), e.g., vibrations, large temperature variations, physical work load, sleep deprivation, heave of the sea and noise during sleep etc. [1-7]. Very little is known about the development of NIHL under such different exposure conditions. Since the exposure time exceeds the normal 8 hours, 5 days a week, the international standards are not applicable. The damage risk criteria consequently are different. In the WHO-document "Environmental health criteria 12: noise" equivalent sound level Leq for 24 hours sound exposure is limited to 70 dB(A). Inter-governmental Maritime Organization (IMO) suggests 80 dB(A) Leq for 24 hours exposure.

During the past ten years, we have been consulted by a large number of coastguards and fishermen with NIHL. However, there is only limited information concerning noise levels on board vessels like these and about hearing conditions [8-14]. Consequently, it appears to be of interest to examine these two categories of maritime workers concerning their hearing and sound levels on board.

MATERIAL AND METHODS

Fishermen

On the west coast of Sweden, there are 1586 registered professional fishermen. Our sample of this population consists of 529 (33%) randomly selected fishermen who were offered a hearing test, either at the department of occupational audiology or in a mobile van which visited most of the fishing ports along the west coast. All tests were performed by an audiometric technician in a small sound-treated booth placed in the van, using an audiometer (Madsen TBN 80) with earphones (TDH 39). The hearing threshold was established at frequencies 250 - 8000 Hz with an ascending technique and the audiometer calibrated according to ISO 389. All those tested were first examined with otoscopy and on suspicion of middle ear pressure deviations, a tympanogram was taken. The use of the mobile van made it easy to select silent hearing test places with low background noise. Fishermen had avoided noise exposure at least 24 hours before the hearing test. In TTS-measurements, 16 fishermen were tested before and after noise-exposure [7] with sweep-Bekesy-audiometry (Demlar 120). In evaluating the audiograms, only cases with a "typical" noise-dip and a predominance of high-tone hearing loss were regarded as possibly noise induced. The statistic evaluation used was the T-test with a significance level of 95%.

Coastguards

From the different districts in Sweden, 423 coastguards (99% of all Swedish coastguards) were investigated in the same mobile van using the same test booth under the same audiometric conditions. The hearing was screened at 20 dB HL at frequencies 250 - 8000 Hz. For those who failed the hearing screening level at 20 dB HL, the exact hearing threshold below 70 dB HL was established using ascending technique. Those with a hearing threshold of more than $\geq$ 70 dBHL were treated as having a hearing level of 65 dBHL.

History

For both fishermen and coastguards, a careful history was taken analyzing different ototraumatic factors such as hereditary hearing loss, noise during childhood and teenage years, noise during military service, previous noisy jobs, noise conditions on board the actual vessel, subjective note of hearing loss and other symptoms, etc. Also, an analysis was made concerning other previous diseases, accidents and leisure time activities.

Sound level measurements

In all rooms on board fishing and coastguard vessels detailed, measurements of peak sound levels, frequency spectra and equivalent sound levels were performed. Individual noise-dose measurements were also performed using portable noise-dose meters.

RESULTS

Fishermen

Conditions on board. Typically, except for the skipper, all members of the crew performed all kinds of activities. For 55% of the fishermen, a fishing tour lasted 3-5 days without breaks and for 45%, approximately one day. The catch was predominantly herring, whitefish, crayfish, and shrimp. 40% of the fishermen considered themselves to be exposed to high noise levels on board. In spite of this, ear protectors were used only occasionally, and in such cases more or less exclusively in the noisiest place on board, the engine room. Next to the engine, the herring sorting machine was regarded as the noisiest machine on board.

Sound level measurements. The measurements showed hearing-damaging sound levels in all engine rooms in those 8 fishing vessels measured. In most of the engine rooms the maximum permissable exposure time, according to Swedish regulations, was 2-5 min., with a maximum of 10 min. per day. Concerning other spaces on board only, fishing vessels with the sleeping quarters forward showed acceptable sound levels ranging between 65 and 80 dB(A) with short duration maxima of 90 dB(A). Measurements of individual noise-dose analyzed on board one of these vessels showed an equivalent noise-dose of 84 dB(A) over 16 hours, including short visits in the engine room. For fishing vessels with the sleeping quarters astern the sound levels were higher in most spaces with levels from 75 to 95 dB(A). Individual noise-dose measurements showed equivalent sound levels of 88 dB(A) during the continuous exposure of one working week (50-100 hours). Two small coastal fishing vessels were measured; these showed hearing-damaging sound levels at normal pace, and dosimetry with portable noise-dose meters showed an equivalent sound level of 89 dB(A) over 8 hours. Our impression is that these noise levels are typical for the noise situation in the Swedish fishing fleet.

Most fishermen run a considerable risk of being exposed to hearing-damaging sound levels on board. The risk is especially high on board steel trawlers with the sleeping quarters astern, and with a herring sorting machine in the hold. Measurements of infrasound never showed levels exceeding "dangerous" levels. A compilation of the sound levels measured are shown in Fig 1. The sound levels on board are often somewhat lower during the transfer to the haulage area, since most noise sources are turned off then, such as radio communication and the herring sorting machine. In addition, the main engine is usually not used at full speed.

Hearing. Of the 529 fishermen who were offered to be examined, 360 (68%, all male) were hearing tested (Table I). There were no indications that the nonparticipants differed from the population as a whole in terms of hearing, professional or leisure time activities, etc. of the 360 fishermen: 6.1% had noted a family history of hearing loss which could be of a hereditary kind; 10.6% had suffered head trauma; 6.4% had hypertension; 2.2% had high blood lipids; 4.7% remembered an event corresponding to an acute acoustic trauma; 12.8% had suffered from other illnesses which might have affected their hearing.

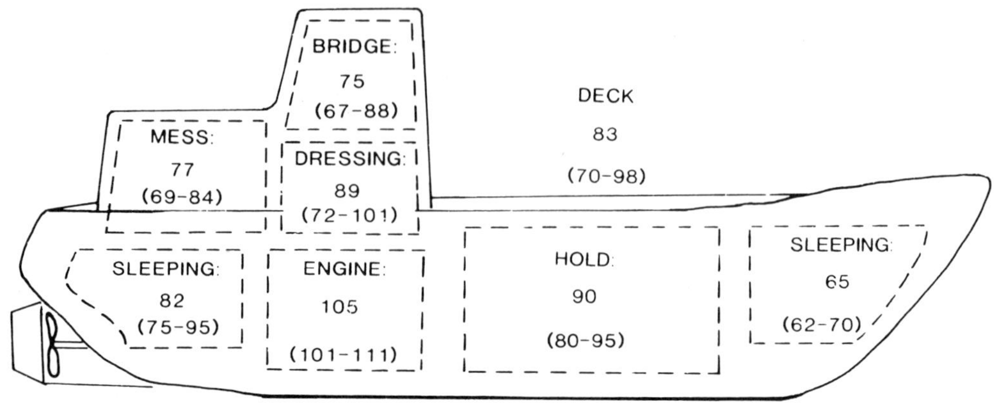

Fig. 1. Sound levels on board a typical fishing boat - dB(A)

TABLE I. Present material

	Fishermen	Coastguards
Number tested	360	423
Age, average years	40	39
Actual profession, average years	22	15
Previous other noisy professions	27%	61%
Average years	1.9	
Leisure time shooting, hunting	24%	28.5%
Fishermen previous/years		14%/6 years
Seamen previous/years	5%/8 years	29%/5 years
Marine corps previous/years		17%/4 years
Industry previous/years	22%/6 years	10%/5 years

The "average" fisherman was 40 years old and had worked for 22 years as a fisherman, had done 11 months of military service, had worked 2 years in other professions than fishing, had noticed hearing loss for 2 years, and had participated in hunting or other leisure time shooting activities for 3 years. He worked on a vessel which was 24 meters long with an engine of approximately 600 HP and with 4.3 other fellow fishermen on board. Of the 360 fishermen, 65% had only had this occupation.

There were no indications that fishermen had been more exposed than others to acoustic trauma during childhood or to more shooting during military service. The relatively high incidence (24%) of hunting and leisure time shooting is probably greater than can be expected for the male population on an average. Ear protectors were only used occasionally.

Hearing tests. The mean hearing threshold for the different age groups of fishermen is shown in Fig. 2. The worst pure tone threshold is found at 6 kHz, which already in teenage years is the least good hearing frequency. The older the fishermen, the more high-tone hearing loss with a typical NIHL configuration. The high frequency pure tone average (3,4,6 kHz) in relation to exposure time as a fisherman is shown in Fig. 3. Linear regression analysis shows a mean loss of 0.9 dB/year during the first 25 years as a fisherman. For the following 15 years the high frequency average decreases 0.4 dB annually. For those who had been fishing more than 40 years, the high frequency pure tone average decreases 1.5 dB annually. The individual results at 6 kHz for fishermen is shown in Fig. 4. In this figure, they are compared to an otologically normal population

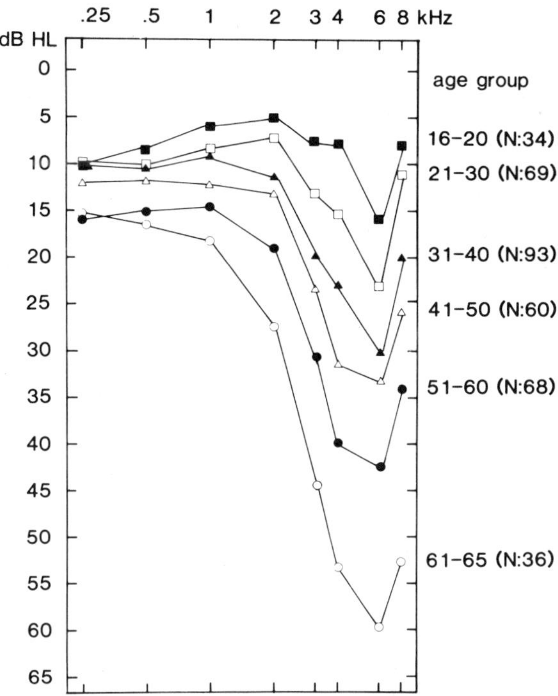

Fig. 2. Fisherman - Mean audiogram for different age groups, left ear

(ISO 7029). When compared to this norm, 31% of fishermen exceed P95 in the left ear at 6 kHz (Fig. 4, Table II). Corresponding figures for the different test frequencies are shown in Table II. Fishermen exceed the expected 5% of individuals with poorer hearing "than expected" at almost all test frequencies.

Temporary threshold shift (TTS). TTS in those 16 fishermen where noise-dose and TTS were measured are presented in Table IIIa. TTS only exceeded 15 dB in three ears, in spite of high noise doses and long exposure times. Maximum TTS in approximately half of the cases occurred at frequencies below 3 kHz. This finding is interesting concerning the very low frequency sound emitted from the fishing vessels. In summary, in those 16 fishermen where the hearing threshold was established immediately before and after the fishing trip, in spite of equivalent noise doses between 84 and 92 dB(A) measured over many hours, the TTS was very limited.

Factors contributing to hearing loss in fishermen. There was no indication that those fishermen who also had been exposed to other noisy professions on an average had poorer hearing than those who exclusively had worked as fishermen. The analysis of the actual fishing technique showed that 42 coastal fishermen, who were often working in small open vessels, had poorer hearing in the left ear than the average, probably due to their position in the back of the vessel close to the outboard engine.

An evaluation of hearing in relation to the machine power showed that fishermen working on boats with the least powerful engines had poorer hearing at 2-8 kHz in the left ear. A number of other parameters were also tested in order to differentiate hearing loss. This analysis showed that hunters and leisure time shooters (24%) had significantly worse hearing at 3, 4, 6 and 8 kHz in the left ear and at 6 kHz in the right ear than others.

TABLE II. Percent fishermen and coast guards exceeding P95 (ISO 7029)[1]

Frequency kHz	Ear	Fishermen %	Coastguards %
0.25	Right	4.7	2.1
0.5	"	6.9	4.0
1	"	8.3	3.3
2	"	10.3	5.7
3	"	22.5	17.3
4	"	18.9	23.2
6	"	21.9	30.8
8	"	9.7	13.7
0.25	Left	6.7	2.6
0.5	"	6.1	2.4
1	"	7.5	3.1
2	"	12.8	7.1
3	"	26.7	20.9
4	"	26.7	26.3
6	"	30.6	36.0
8	"	12.2	17.1

Individual audiograms for the fishermen treated as screening audiograms with minimum threshold 20 dBHL and maximum 65 dBHL.

[1]P95 = the level that 95% of an "otologically normal" population are expected not to exceed. "Otological normal" = a population without noise exposure, ear diseases, etc.

TABLE III a. Temporary threshold shift (TTS) in fishermen.

Individual initials	Type of vessel	Noise-dose dB(A)	Measured over hrs	TTS worst frequency right ear dB	kHz	left ear dB	kHZ
JH	small vessel	89	8	+15	8	+5	0.25
DB	herring trawler	92	65.5	+8	0.5	+14	8
PAO	"	92	65.5	+7	4	+25	1.5
TH	"	90	66.0	+6	6	+10	1
JA	prawn trawler	84	16	+6	8	+2	1.5
FL	"	-	16	+7	1.5	+6	8
BAB	"	-	16	+11	1.5	+13	6
RH	"	-	16	+5	2	-3	8
MO	herring trawler	88	60	+10	1	+5	0.5
DOA	"	88	85	+	3-4	+20	1.5
TB	"	88	91	+5	4	+5	2-8
TC	"	94	97	+10	1.5	+5	6
PAA	"	98	81	+30	0.5	+15	0.25-1
SC	"	86	82	+5	3-4	+15	3
UB	"	88	74	+10	1	+10	0.5-6
JB	"	90	65	+10	1,6	+5	1-2

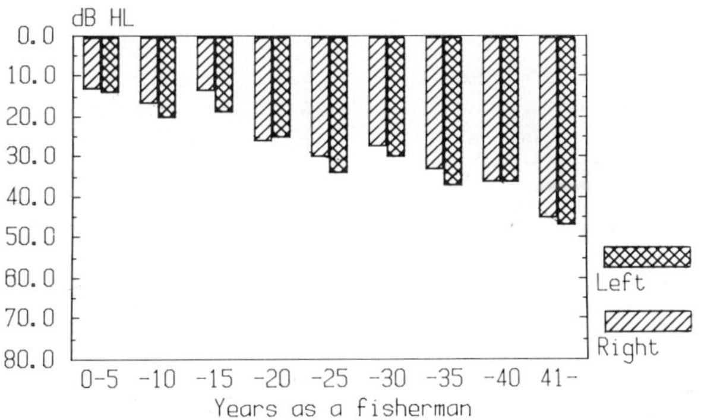

Fig. 3. Average threshold 3-6 kHz

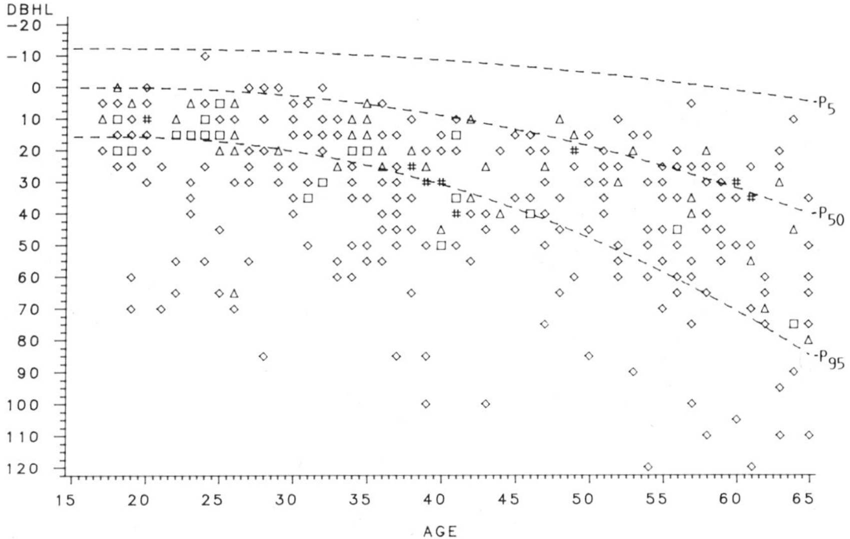

Fig. 4. Fishermen: Individual hearing threshold at 6 kHz left ear in relation to age, compared with P5, P50 and P95 according to ISO 7029.

Those who reported previous acute acoustic trauma (5%) had significant poorer hearing at test frequencies 1.5, 2, 4, 6 and 8 kHz. Fishermen who had hypertension did not differ in terms of hearing threshold from those with normal blood pressure. Those fishermen reporting a possible hereditary hearing loss (6%) had significant poorer hearing than others at 0.25-2 kHz in both ears and 8 kHz in the right ear. The compiled hearing results are shown in Table IV. Normal hearing on both ears was found in approximately 24%. Another 20% of the fishermen had one normal ear and one with a slight NIHL, and 23% slight NIHL in both ears. At least 15% of the fishermen had severe NIHL in at least one ear.

COASTGUARDS

Conditions on board. On the coastguard vessels there were 3-5 members in the crew. These vessels have strong engines (500-3000 hp) in order to be able to move at high speed. The ear protection used has been less than satisfactory; mostly, ear protectors were used only in the engine room. There are several noise sources other than the engine on board. Most of them are found in the wheel house. Particularly noisy are the communication systems with coastguard authorities, military radio stations, sea rescue service, police air crafts, etc. The most typical coastguard raid is either 24 hours or 4 days. In contrast to fishermen, coastguards have more occasions to rest and sleep without high sound levels from the engines.

On an average, the coastguard had been employed in this profession for 15 years (13-17 years). As many as 39% had not been exposed to noise in other professions before the employment as coastguards. Of those 61% who reported previous noisy jobs, the majority had been working in one or several jobs with relation to maritime professions (Table I). Since use of weapons is mandatory in this profession, target practice was, on an average, performed 4 times a year, with a mean total of 150 shots. Leisure time shooting was practiced by 28% on an average of 13 times a year, with an annual average of 340 shots.

Sound level measurements. Sound level measurements and portable noise-dose meter measurements on coastguard vessels showed sound levels which are indicated in Fig. 5. Similar to the fishing vessels, the sound levels frequently exceeded hearing-damaging levels and were most conspicuous in sleeping quarters. The measurements were performed during regular service, sometimes during bad weather with pronounced heave of the sea and strong winds. Under these circumstances both vibrations and sound levels from communication radio systems appeared to increase the sound levels. In several of the coastguard vessels, resonances were registered from the propeller shaft caused by the gear box of the engine. Sound level measurements indicated that pure tones were sometimes emitted during such conditions, making the sound levels even more harmful to hearing. On the bridge, particularly the three to five different radio communication systems decide the sound levels, since the radios are turned up to a high volume in order to mask the background sound levels from the engine, wind, etc.

Hearing tests. The individual hearing status is shown in Table IV. Approximately 1/3 of the coastguards have normal hearing in both ears. Another 20% have one normal ear and one with a slight NIHL, and another 20% a slight NIHL in both ears. Approximately 10% of the coastguards have severe NIHL in at least one ear.

Temporary threshold shift (TTS). TTS was established in 13 coastguards on 33 occasions. The equivalent noise-dose varied between 79 and 97 dB(A) over 2-86 hours (Table IIIb). It can be seen that the TTS exceeded 15 dB in three ears only. The TTS was most pronounced at frequencies below 3 kHz in 18/66 ears. Similar to fishermen, TTS occurred at fairly low frequencies in many instances; however, it was much less pronounced than in fishermen. This, of course, might be due to different noise patterns on board, suggesting that coastguard vessels have more high frequency components in the noise than on board fishing vessels.

Factors contributing to hearing loss in coastguards. In general, the work environment and conditions are similar for fishermen and coastguards. However, as already shown, the engine in the vessels used by coastguards are much more powerful than those generally used by fishermen. Similar to some fishermen, coastguards sometimes used small boats with outboard motors, particularly when entering ships to be searched. These outboard engines are between 18 and 200 hp and regularly emit equivalent sound levels of 90-100 dB(A). However, the exposure time to this noise probably

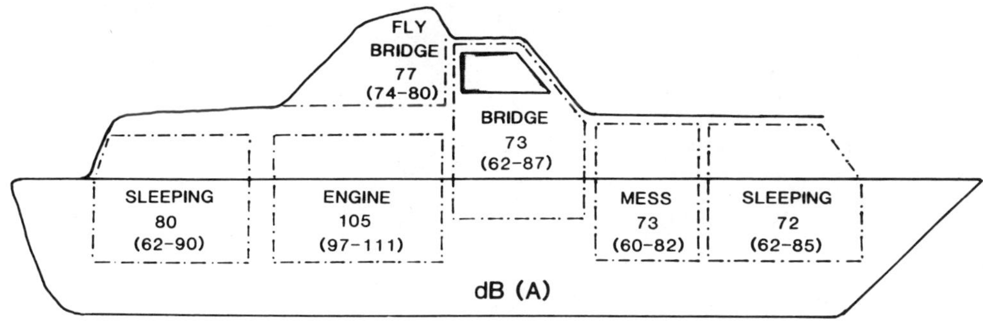

Fig. 5.

TABLE III b. Temporary threshold shift (TTS) in coastguards

Individual initials	Type of Vessel	Noise-dose dB(A)	Measured over hrs	TTS worst frequency right ear dB	right ear kHz	left ear dB	left ear kHz
GA	Patrol boat	85	22	20	2	15	6
GA	"	87	7	10	8	15	6
GA	"	82	22	10	8	15	6
BA	"	87	22	5	4	5	0.25
BA	"	82	7	10	3	5	6
RE	"	82	22	5	6	5	6
RE	"	79	22	15	2	10	6
RE	"	85	7	20	3	10	2
RE	"	87	22	5	2	10	4
AA	Patrol boat	82	22	5	0.5	10	1
AA	"	84	21	5	0.5	10	6
EE	"	81	22	5		5	6
EE	"	79	21	5	4	10	3
KK	"	82	22	10	8	10	4
KK	"	83	21	10	2	5	4
GE	Aircraft	95	2.0	10	4	10	2
GE	"	96	2.5	10	4	5	2
GE	"	95	2.0	5	8	5	2
BF	"	97	2.0	5	3	10	0.5
BF	"	96	2.5	10	6	5	4
BF	"	96	2.0	10	6	10	4
RL	Cruiser	-	-	5	8	10	6
RL	"	84	86	10	6	10	6
RL	"	87	78	10	3	15	2
KE	"	-	-	10	8	5	3
KE	"	83	86	15	4	0	
KE	"	85	78	10	4	10	6
AJ	"	80	86	10	1	15	4
AJ	"	85	78	15	2	10	6
JL	"	92	86	30	6	5	2
JL	"	-	78	10	8	15	6
DF	"	85	86	5	4	15	6
DF	"	85	78	5	6	10	0.5

TABLE IV. Individual hearing results

	Fishermen		Coastguards	
	N	%	N	%
Normal hearing both ears	85	23.6	138	32.6
One normal + one slight NIHL	70	19.4	84	19.9
One normal + one moderate NIHL	3	0.8	4	1.0
One normal + one severe NIHL	1	0.3	4	1.0
Slight NIHL both ears	84	23.3	85	20.0
One slight + one moderate NIHL	12	3.3	31	7.3
One slight + one severe NIHL	15	4.2	14	3.3
Moderate NIHL both ears	14	3.9	23	5.4
One moderate + one severe NIHL	11	3.1	10	2.4
Severe NIHL both ears	29	8.1	13	3.1
Other combinations	36	10.0	17	4.0
	360		423	

Normal = $\le$ 20 dB (all test frequencies)
Slight = $\le$20 dB 0.25-2 kHz
25-60 dB 3-8 kHz
Moderate = $\le$20 dB 0.25-2 kHz
$\ge$65 dB 3-8 kHz
Severe = $\ge$25 dB 0.5-2 kHz
$\ge$40 dB average 3-8 kHz

is limited in time (in general, less than one hour). Ear protectors are typically not used under these conditions. One of the reasons for not using ear protectors under these circumstances, is the use of portable handheld two-way radios.

Similar to fishermen, quite a few coastguards (28%) are regular hunters or participate in leisure time shooting activities. Under these conditions ear protector use is probably much better than in their normal working environment. At certain times the shooting activities may be quite substantial, particularly when killing oil-polluted birds. A relative risk analysis of the high-frequency, pure tone average (3, 4, 6 kHz) showed that those participating in hunting and leisure time shooting activities run 1.5 times higher risk of hearing loss than other coastguards, i.e., there appears to be a slight risk of increased hearing loss for these coastguards.

DISCUSSION

The present material comprises a substantial number of fishermen and coastguards working in Sweden. The analysis for both groups considering hearing was similar. However, the analysis of results and questionnaire was somewhat different for the two groups. The present investigation shows that there is a considerable number of hearing-impaired fishermen and coastguards in all age groups, with fairly rapidly deteriorating hearing with age. A careful analysis of possible factors contributing to such a sensorineural high-tone hearing loss reveals that, in many cases, certain factors such as hereditary hearing loss, previous noise exposure in other professions, skull trauma, ear disease, and in particular leisure time shooting, might have contributed to the high frequency of noise-induced hearing loss (NIHL). Both groups, the fishermen in particular, are characteristic in that they have held few other jobs and the predominance of noise exposure is from small vessels.

Sound level measurements on board both fishing vessels and coastguard vessels showed high and often dangerous sound levels. Considering the fact that the exposure time is quite different from the regular 8 hours for the industrial worker followed by 16 hours "ear rest," obviously damage risk criteria may be different with the actual long duration exposure for both fishermen and coastguards. The International Maritime Organization (IMO) has recommended an equivalent continuous maximum sound level of 80 dB(A) over 24 hours. According to IMO recommendations, the maximum permissable sound level in the engine room is 110 dB(A), on the bridge 65 dB(A), in the sleeping quarters 60 dB(A), in the mess 65 dB(A), and on deck 85 dB(A). Most of our measurements on board fishing vessels and coastguard vessels exceed the IMO recommendations.

Consequently, it is appropriate to conclude that the confinement for many hours at a time in this enclosed environment with exposure to high noise levels contributes to the high frequency of NIHL. It is also characteristic for both types of professions that there are many other possible interacting factors which might contribute to the NIHL, at least theoretically. Some of these have been confirmed in previous investigations, others have been suspected. It is well known that vibrations, either local hand-arm vibrations or whole-body vibrations, may increase the risk for NIHL when they occur simultaneously with exposure to high sound levels. It is also well known that a long-standing exposure for many hours/days to high sound levels increases and enhances the risk for NIHL.

Both fishermen and coastguards are exposed to noise for days at a time with high sound levels which are easily transmitted to all areas on board. Other possible characteristics which might contribute to the rapid development of NIHL are simultaneous noise exposure and heavy work load, work at night, sleep deprivation, sleep in high-sound levels, rapid climate variations, and heave of the sea. It remains to be more closely investigated how these individual factors interact with noise for the development of NIHL.

A surprising and interesting finding for the fishermen was that hardly any temporary threshold shift (TTS) was found in spite of noise-dose meters showing ototraumatic levels over long equivalent periods of time. For coastguards, the equivalent noise dose frequently exceeded 85 dB(A), and more or less regularly exceeded 80 dB(A). In spite of this, the TTS measured immediately after returning with a ship very seldom exceeded 15 dB at the most TTS-sensitive frequency in the individual coastguard. Apparently, this seeming contradiction between exposure to high sound levels on the one hand and a lack of substantial TTS on the other is an important and interesting field for future research concerning the relationship between noise dose, TTS, and permanent threshold shift. In previous short term experiments [15,16], 2 kHz narrow-band noise presented at 105 dB SPL for 10 min. resulted in a 10-15 dB TTS more or less regularly. According to the equal energy principle, 105 dB for 10 min. is equivalent to 83 dB during 24 hours. Then it is surprising that noise levels of 85 dB(A) for more than 25 hours did not result in "dangerous" TTS amounts when fishermen or coastguards were tested immediately after coming ashore. One explanation may be that the TTS differs for the extreme low frequency noise emitted by these vessels or that a possible TTS could have "healed" during the comparatively lower sound levels while returning to port. (From the two populations it seems that the TTS otherwise would appear for this type of noise at equivalent sound levels of over 90 dB(A) and >24 hours).

Fishermen constitute an interesting professional group. Characteristically, they have only held this profession. They are often part owners of the vessel. In Sweden they have not been embraced by the regular occupational insurances. They appear to be individuals with great self-confidence and have a poor attitude toward use of ear protectors. Once this type of hearing examination with follow ups has been instituted, as well as better ear protector use, the hearing situation for fishermen may improve.

For coastguards the conditions are somewhat different. The Department of Occupational Audiology has tested the hearing of all Swedish coastguards during the last 7 years with annual check-ups. During the first check-ups we registered a considerable hearing decrement. From 1979 to 1981 a moderate hearing deterioration (>15 dBHL on 1-3 test frequencies) was found in approximately 12% of the coastguards and a severe hearing deterioration (>20 dBHL at one or >10 dBHL at four frequencies) in approximately 5% of the coastguards. The very poor hearing status in the early examinations has improved considerably. As is well known, the personal influence of the hearing tester on those tested emphasizing even slightly increased impairments in pure tone thresholds, leads to better ear protector use, and subsequent less decrement in hearing. Further, technical noise abatement certainly can be improved on these vessels. Clearly the engine could be better isolated as well as the propellers. The use of skewback propellers has proven to diminish sound levels on board considerably. Further, sleeping quarters in both types of vessels should be kept apart from the engine room noise.

As a spin-off effect of our hearing examination in fishermen and coastguards, another project with the object to diminish sound levels on board has recently been instituted. With improved technical noise abatement, regular hearing check-ups, personal influence, and advice given to those exposed with an emphasis on better ear protection, there is reason to believe that audiological problems for those working in these professions can be improved substantially.

REFERENCES

1. R. S. F. Schilling, Trawler fishing: an extreme occupation, Proc. Roy Soc. Med. 59:405 (1966).
2. A. Okada, H. Miyake, K. Yamamura, Temporary hearing loss induced by noise and vibration, J. Acous. Soc. Amer. 51:1240 (1972).
3. K. Rodahl and Z. Vokac, Work stress in long-line bank fishing, Scand. J. Work Environ. & Health 3:154 (1977).
4. K. Rodahl and Z. Vokac, Work stress in Norwegian trawler fishermen, Ergonomics 20:633 (1977).
5. A. Ekelin and K. Gunther, "Arbetsmiljon i fisket," Rapport 79:7, Ergolab, Stockholm (1979).
6. H. Goethe, E-G Schmidt, D. Majunder, Belastungen der Schiffsbesatzungen durch Vibrationen, ZBL Arbeitsmed 31:156 (1981).
7. L. Lund-Iversen, Noise and hearing conditions on board Norwegian motor torpedo boats and submarines, Acta Otolaryng. (Stockholm) 47:50 (1957).
8. S. Quist-Hanssen, Noise-induced hearing loss amongst engine room personnel on board Norwegian merchant ships, Acta Otolaryng. (Stockh) Suppl. 196 (1964).
9. H. Firestone, Coastguard launches new hearing conservation program, Occupational Health and Safety 47:334 (1978).
10. R. P Menyakin, V. I. Poperetskaya, Occupational changes of the organ of hearing and balance in fishermen and sailors, Vestn Otorinolaringol. 42:39 (1980).
11. E. G. Schmidt, Larmbelastungen der Besatzungen von Schiffen, Zbl Arbeitsmed 30:212-17 (1980).
12. A. Lovik and F. Pettersson, Stoyforhold pa norske fiskefartoyer, ELAB rapport STF44 A81119 (1981).

13. A. Lovik and F. Pettersson, Horselmaling av fiskere, ELAB rapport STF44 A82122 (1982).
14. S. Soderqvist, Sammanstallning av bullernivan i Generaltullstyrelsens fartyg. Tekniskt meddelande 6.313.01, IFM Akustikbyran (1979).
15. F. Lindgren and A. Axelsson, Human noise experiments using a temporary threshold shift model (1986).
16. H. Dengerink, F. Lindgren, A. Axelsson and J. Dengerink, The effects of smoking and physical exercise on temporary threshold shift, Am. Ind. Hyg. Assoc. J. In print (1985).

DISCUSSION

Salvi: The lack of TTS in your results may not be too surprising. Some data on asymptotic threshold shift measured in animals indicates that the amount of hearing loss resulting from these long duration noise exposures was dependent upon the preexisting hearing loss. The animals that already had a hearing loss developed only a small increase in TTS. Preexisting hearing losses could perhaps explain the lack of TTS in your data.

Axelsson: The subjects that we selected for this study, in general, were persons that had good hearing.

Alberti: That was a very interesting paper, with much broader implications than just for fisherman off the coast of Sweden. We have the same problems in our country in the shipping, airline and chemical industries. Workers are exposed for very long periods of time, not just for 8 hours a day. Break periods are variable. How do we specify the acceptable noise levels? I have no idea. Also, I do not think we need to look for many other stressors than just the prolonged noise exposures.

von Gierke: I just wanted to say something in connection with Salvi's comments. The asymptotic TTS data on humans were obtained primarily in response to the military and aviation requirements for exposures that last more than 8 hours or even 24 hours a day. We have no criteria for such continuous long term exposures. It would be interesting to compare your PTS data with what you would predict from Leq weekly equivalent noise exposures based on the dosmetry you did. Just looking at the data, I would agree with what Dr. Alberti said. Namely, that probably one does not have to look for any other factors; the noise exposure alone will explain the hearing loss.

INTERACTIONS BETWEEN DIFFERENT CLASSES OF NOISE

Olavi J. Manninen

The Academy of Finland, Department of Public Health
Faculty of Medicine, University of Tampere
Box 607, SF-33101 Tampere, Finland

INTRODUCTION

Some results on the combined effects of environmental factors have been published recently in a book based on the reports delivered at the First International Conference on Combined Effects of Environmental Factors [1]. Despite the recent publications, our knowledge of the temporary changes in hearing due to complex exposure situations is still very scarce.

The purpose of the following experiments was to study how the temporary hearing threshold in controlled laboratory conditions produced by noises with different intensities and frequency ranges is affected by physical or mental work and how whole body vibrations or different temperatures interact with noise. The results above are meant to illustrate how cardiovascular changes are connected to changes in the temporary hearing threshold.

MATERIAL AND METHODS

The results are drawn from five different experiments. The experiments were conducted in a special exposure room, which has been described in more detail in earlier publications [2-6].

In all experiments, the duration of the test was 105 minutes. It consisted of a control period of 30 min., of three consecutive exposure periods of 16 min. each, of a measuring period of 4 min. after each exposure period, and of a recovery period of 15 min.

The experiments were based on a random block design (Experiments I-III) or on a factorial experimental design (Experiments IV-V).

Experiment I

Fourteen (14) healthy, volunteer male students (28 ears) were exposed. The cutoff frequencies for the noise bands employed were 1 and 2 kHz, 1 and 4 kHz, 1 and 8 kHz and 0.2 and 16 kHz. The intensity of each noise band was 90 dB. Vibration was sinusoidal 5 Hz signal along the Z-axis with an acceleration (rms) of 2.2 m/s^2. During these experimental sessions, the average dry bulb temperature was 20.0°C (see also Manninen [3]).

Audiometric Measurements

The hearing threshold values were determined with a pure tone audiometer, using the ascending technique. The hearing thresholds of both ears were measured in the same way each time at frequencies of 4000 and 6000 Hz, and exactly 2 min. after the cessation of the exposure (TTS_2).

Cardiovascular Measurements

Cardiovascular changes were described by heart rate (HR), systolic blood pressure (SBP) and haemodynamic index (HDI). The haemodynamic index characterizes cardiovascular activity and oxygen consumption of the myocardium of the subjects. To make the index, the product of the heart rate value and the systolic blood pressure value was divided by 1000. The heart rate (beats/min.) was determined manually from an ECG band during each measurement, exactly 10 s after the end of the pre-exposure, exposure and post-exposure periods. Systolic blood pressure was measured with a sphygmomanometer operating on the ultrasound principle. Blood pressure was measured 40 s after the end of the pre-exposure, exposure and post-exposure periods.

Analysis of the data

The subjects acted as their own controls during the experiments. Before the analysis of the results, the values obtained after the 15-min. control period were deducted from the values obtained after the exposure and post- exposure (recovery) periods. The hearing threshold values for each ear were regarded as observation units for audiometric measurements (hence 28, 26, 22, 144 and 216 ears), whereas observation units for HR, SBP and HDI determinations were the number of subjects (i.e., 14, 13, 11, 72, and 108).

The statistical significance of the differences between paired and unpaired means was determined using two-tailed Student's t-tests. Statistical significance of the main effects of and interactions between various factors was examined with the aid of variance analyses.

RESULTS

Of the four noise band conditions, that with a bandwidth of 1 to 2 kHz caused a significantly smaller increase in hearing threshold than the others (Fig. 1). With a higher cutoff frequency, when the upper frequency limit of noise was heightened (from 2 to 4 kHz), the TTS_2 of test subjects exposed to a noise increased very rapidly. By further broadening the band by three octaves towards the higher frequencies (from 1 to 8 kHz) or to both higher and lower frequencies (to 0.2 to 16 kHz) simultaneously, the hearing threshold changes were still clearly observable at 4 and 6 kHz. When subjects were exposed simultaneously to sinusoidal 5 Hz vibration and to such broad bandwidth noise, their TTS_2 values increased 1.4 times (first exposure), 1.2 times (second exposure), and 1.5 times (third exposure) more at 4 kHz than due to exposure to such broad bandwidth noise alone.

Correspondingly, systolic blood pressure increased during the first, second and third exposures especially, due to mere noises with bandwidths of 1-2 kHz, 1-4 kHz and 1-8 kHz (Fig. 2). By contrast, a broadband noise with the cutoff frequencies of 0.2 and 16.0 kHz tended to decrease the SBP values slightly during all exposure periods. The means of the SBP values also decreased due to mere sinusoidal 5 Hz vibration as compared to the resting values prior to the exposure.

When the subjects were exposed simultaneously to noise and vibration, all combinations resulted in decreased blood pressure values after the first

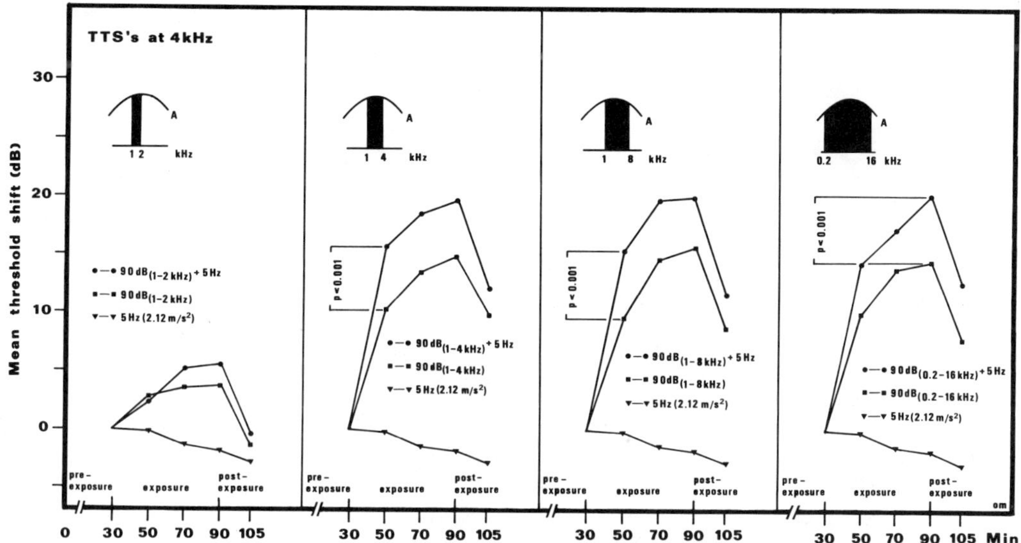

Fig. 1. Arithmetic means ($\overline{X}$) of the TTS_2 values at 4 kHz when subjects were exposed to stable noise of varying bandwidth, to whole body vibration alone, or to simultaneous noise and vibration (n=28 ears).

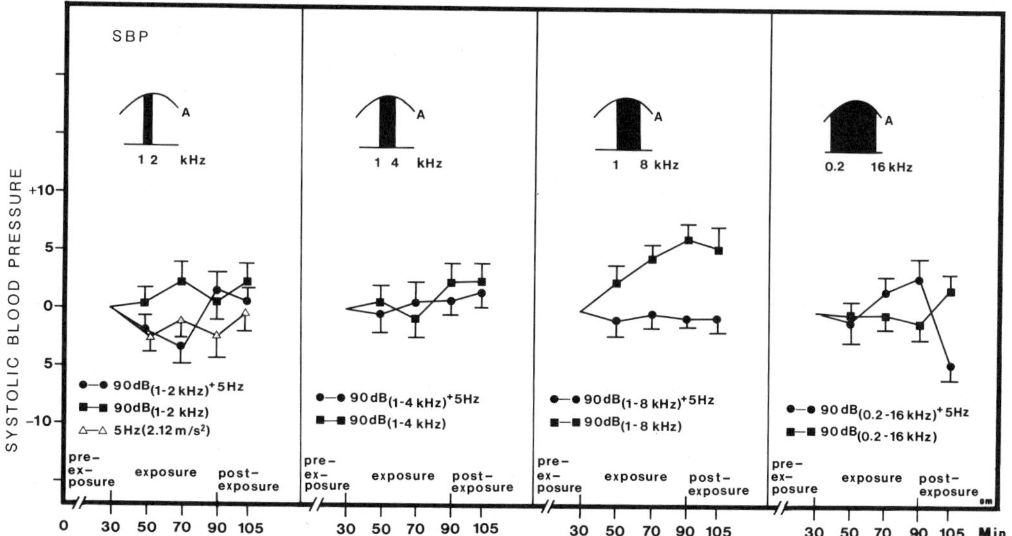

Fig. 2. Arithmetic means ($\overline{X}$) of the SBP values and half of the standard error of the means (SEM) when subjects were exposed to stable noise of varying bandwidth alone, to whole body vibration alone, or to simultaneous noise and vibration (n=14 subjects).

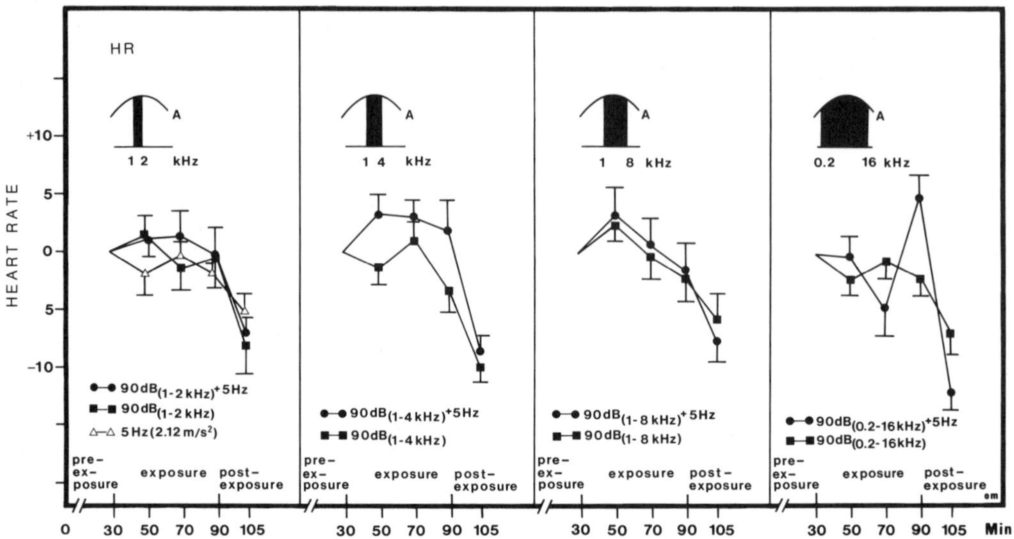

Fig. 3. Arithmetic means ($\overline{X}$) of the HR values and half of the standard error of the means (SEM) when subjects were exposed to stable noise of varying bandwidth alone, to whole body vibration alone, or to simultaneous noise and vibration (n=14 subjects).

period of exposure as compared to the resting values. After the second and the third exposure period, the SBP values were highest as compared to the resting values when the cutoff frequencies of the noise in the combination were either 1 and 4 kHz or 0.2 and 16 kHz.

Fig. 3 shows that mere noises with the cutoff frequencies of 1 and 2 kHz or 1 and 8 kHz increased heart rate; noises with the cutoff frequencies of 1 and 4 kHz or 0.2 and 16 kHz decreased heart rate during the first period of exposure. During the second and the third exposure period, average HR values were (with one exception) lower than the resting values prior to the exposures. Mere vibration also tended to decrease heart rate.

Those combinations of noise and vibration where the cutoff frequencies of the noise were 1 and 2 kHz, 1 and 4 kHz or 1 and 8 kHz increased the HR values during the first and the second period of exposure. However, the very combination to increase the HR values most during the third successive period of exposure, consisted of a sinusoidal vibration and a broadband noise.

Experiment II

Thirteen (13) healthy, volunteer male students (26 ears) were exposed. The cutoff frequencies for the noise bands employed were 2 and 4 kHz, 4 and 6 kHz, 6 and 8 kHz, 4 and 8 kHz, and 0.2 and 16 kHz. The intensity of each noise band was 90 dB. Vibration was sinusoidal 5 Hz signal along the Z-axis with an acceleration (rms) of 2.12 m/s^2. During these experimental sessions the average dry bulb temperature was 19.7°C (see also Manninen [3]).

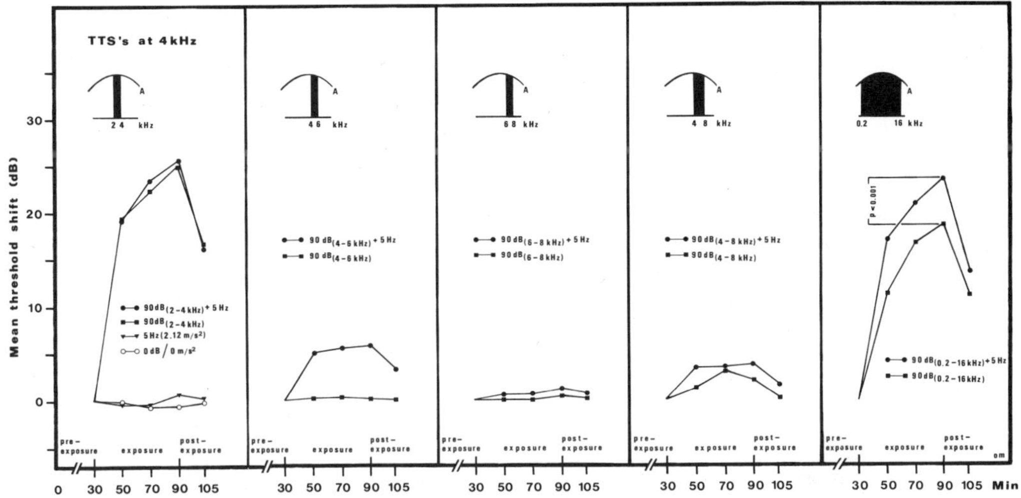

Fig. 4. Arithmetic means ($\overline{X}$) of the TTS_2 values at 4 kHz when subjects were exposed to stable noise of varying bandwidth alone, to whole body vibration alone, or to simultaneous noise and vibration (n=26 ears).

On the basis of these mean changes, we may conclude that the most important exposure combination during all the successive periods of exposure was the combination where the frequencies of the noise were 1 and 4 kHz. It increased the TTS_2 values, as well as the SBP values and the HR values. During the last period of exposure, a combination of vibration and a broadband noise (0.2-16 kHz) gained more importance. After this exposure combination, too, the TTS_2 values, the SBP values and the HR values increased significantly, as compared to the values measured prior to the exposure.

In the second experiment, the mean TTS values at 4 kHz were at their highest when the subjects were exposed to noise with a bandwidth of 2 to 4 kHz (Fig. 4). The threshold shifts were slightly smaller due to noise with the 0.2-16 kHz bandwidth. For each of the two exposure bands, the average threshold values gradually increased during successive exposures. The additional effect of vibration in raising the hearing threshold could be observed when the exposure combination included vibration and the broadest band noise (i.e., noise with a bandwidth of 0.2-16 kHz).

Fig. 5 shows again that the SBP values increased during the first exposure period when the subjects were exposed to mere noises with the cutoff frequencies of 4 and 6 kHz, 6 and 8 kHz, or 4 and 8 kHz. The only kind of noise to increase the SBP values during both the second and the third exposure period, was one with the cutoff frequencies of 2 and 4 kHz. During the third period, noises with the cutoff frequencies of 4 and 6 kHz or 4 and 8 kHz also increased the SBP values.

Out of all exposure combinations used in the study, only a combination consisting of a sinusoidal vibration and a noise with the cutoff frequencies of 2-4 kHz increased the SBP values during all three successive exposure periods. A combination of broadband noise (bandwidth 0.2-16 kHz) and vibration also increased the SBP values after the second and third exposure period. The SBP values also increased after the third exposure period in all cases except the one where the cutoff frequencies of the noise were 4

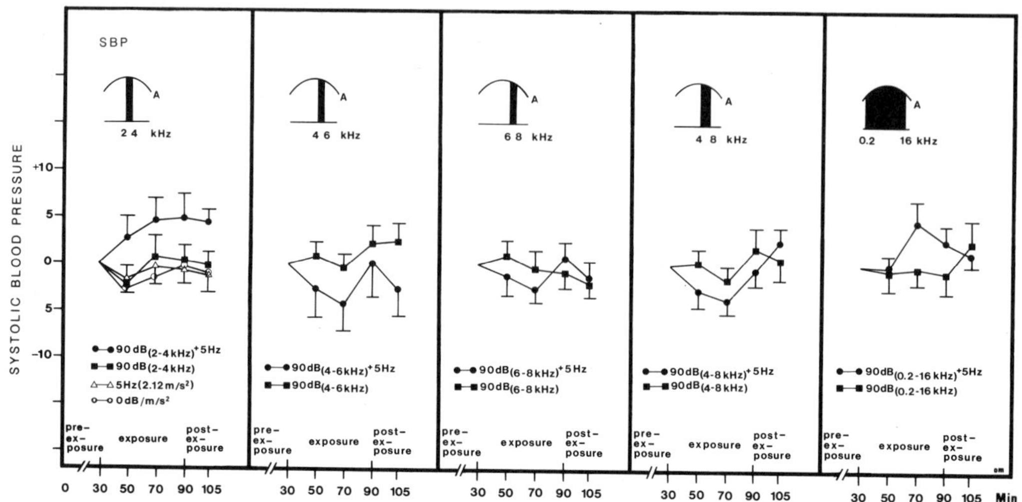

Fig. 5. Arithmetic means ($\overline{X}$) of the SBP values and half of the standard error of the means (SEM) when subjects were exposed to stable noise of varying bandwidth alone, to whole body vibration alone, or to simultaneous noise and vibration (n=13 subjects).

and 8 kHz. As compared to mere noises, a simultaneous exposure to noise and vibration seemed to accelerate the increase in SBP values when the cutoff frequencies of the noise were 2 and 4 kHz or 0.2 and 16 kHz.

As in the previous study, the HR values decreased during all three exposures when the subjects were exposed to mere broadband noise (Fig. 6). Other kinds of noises increased the HR values during the first and the

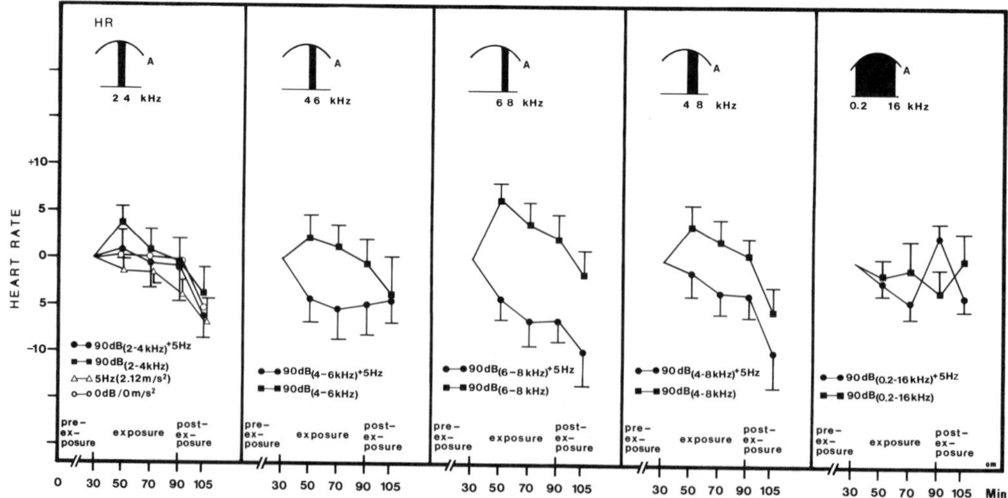

Fig. 6. Arithmetic means ($\overline{X}$) of the HR values and half of the standard error of the means (SEM) when subjects were exposed to stable noise of varying bandwidth alone, to whole body vibration alone, or to simultaneous noise and vibration (n=13 subjects).

second exposure period, and noises with the cutoff frequencies of 6 and 8 kHz or 4 and 8 kHz increased the HR values during the third exposure period as well. During the first exposure period, the only combination to increase the HR values was one where the cutoff frequencies of the noise were 2 and 4 kHz, and during the third exposure period the HR values increased only due to a combination where the cutoff frequencies of the noise were 0.2 and 16 kHz.

The most essential differences between the results of the first and the second experiment were that in the first experiment mere noises most often decreased the HR values, and in the second experiment they most often increased it. When combined with vibration, the noises usually increased the HR values in the first experiment, whereas in the second experiment they usually decreased the HR values. In interpreting the results, it should be noted that the noises used in the first experiment (except the most broadband noise) were limited above 1000 Hz and their bandwidths were set at 1000 Hz, 4000 Hz and 8000 Hz. In the second experiment, the bandwidths were 2000 Hz and 4000 Hz (except the most broadband noise), and the lower cutoff frequencies of each band were 1000 Hz higher. As regards changes in the SBP values, there were no differences between the results of the first and the second experiment.

Changes in heart rate, in turn, seem to reflect in changes in temporary hearing threshold: the more heart rate increased due to noise or simultaneous noise and vibration, the higher increase in temporary threshold. The increase in temporary hearing threshold is further accelerated if systolic blood pressure remains relatively high or increases with heart rate. This observation is supported by the results which concern the effects of the most broadband noise or this noise and sinusoidal vibration on heart rate, systolic blood pressure and temporary hearing threshold.

<u>Experiment III</u>

Eleven (11) healthy, volunteer male students (22 ears) were exposed. The cutoff frequencies for the noise bands employed were 0.2 and 16 kHz. The intensity of noise was either 75 dB, 85 dB or 95 dB. Vibration was sinusoidal 5 Hz signal along the Z-axis with an acceleration (rms) of 2.12 m/s^2. The subjects were always exposed to noise and vibration in pairs, at dry bulb temperatures of both 20°C and 30°C (see also Manninen [4]).

The means of the TTS_2 values at 4 kHz increased correspondingly as the intensity of the noise was raised from 75 to 85 or to 95 dB (Fig. 7). The increase in the hearing threshold was usually strongest during the first exposure period. The means of the TTS_2 values were higher at 30°C than at 20°C. On the other hand, the more intensive the broadband noise to which people were exposed in addition to vibration, the greater the influence of the ambient temperature. A 75 dB noise did not cause much change in TTS_2 values, even with simultaneous exposure to vibration at either temperature.

Fig. 8 shows mean changes in haemodynamic index when the subjects were exposed to simultaneous noise and vibration at two different temperatures. As was previously stated, the haemodynamic index can be used to evaluate changes in heart rate and systolic blood pressure at the same time.

The HDI values were at lowest and decreased with exposure when the dry bulb temperature was 20°C and the subjects were exposed to a relatively low level noise (75 dB) and 5 Hz vibration. The same combination at 30°C caused a decrease in the HDI values during the second and third exposure, too. When the intensity of the noise in the combination was raised from 75 to 85 and 95 decibels, the means of the HDI values also increased. The means of the index scores were highest when the subjects had been exposed to a 95 dB

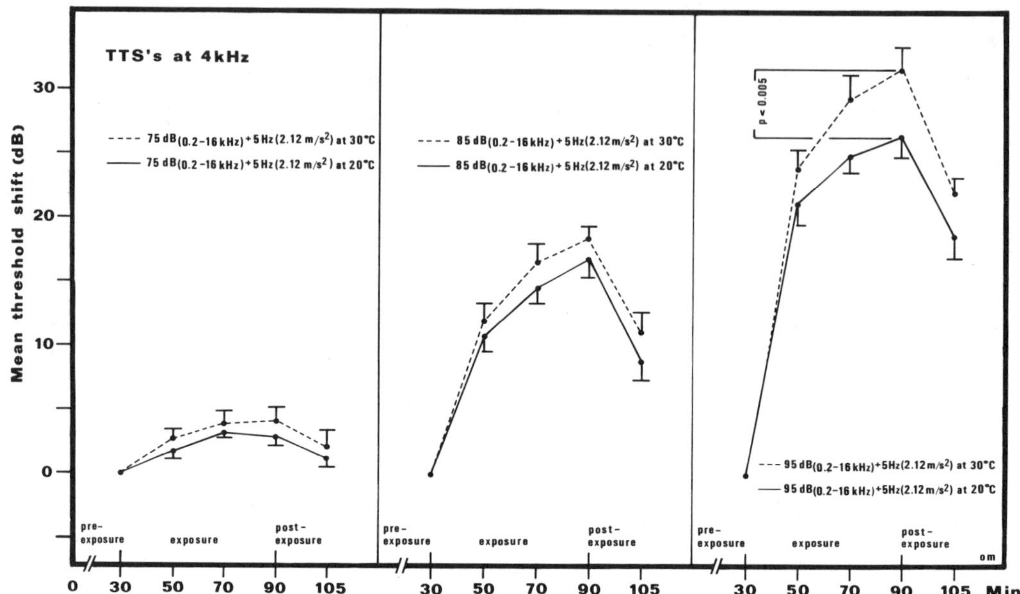

Fig. 7. Arithmetic means ($\overline{X}$) of the TTS_2 values at 4 kHz when subjects were exposed to different exposure combinations (n=22 ears).

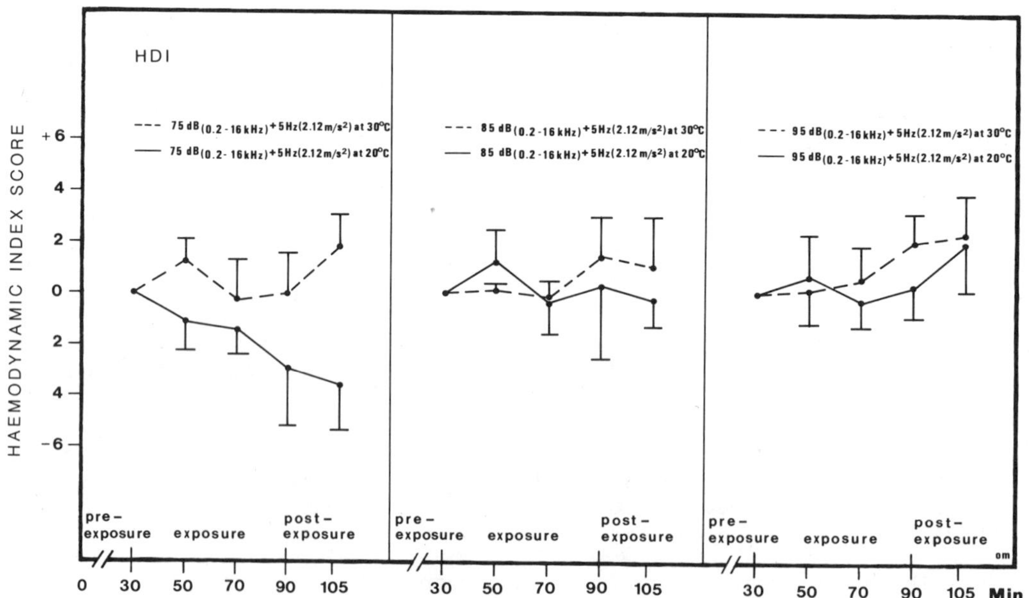

Fig. 8. Arithmetic means ($\overline{X}$) of the HDI values and half of the standard error of the means (SEM) when subjects were exposed to different exposure combinations (n=11).

broadband noise and 5 Hz sinusoidal vibration at 30°C. The values of the TTS_2 at 4 kHz were also highest at this combination (compare results shown in Fig. 7 to results shown in Fig. 8). It is also worth noting that the means of the index scores remain relatively high even after the recovery period.

Experiment IV

Seventy two (72) healthy, volunteer male students (144 ears) were exposed. The cutoff frequencies for the noise bands employed were 0.2 and 16 kHz. The intensity of noise was 90 dB. The noise categories were no extra noise, noise of 90 dB, and noise of 90 dB with simultaneous sinusoidal vibration at a frequency of 5 Hz along the Z-axis (rms acceleration 2.12 m/s^2). The exposure combinations were comprised of two dry bulb temperatures, either 20°C or 30°C. Two different physical work loads were used, corresponding to power outputs of 2 W and 8 W (see also Manninen [2]).

Table 1 gives the arithmetic means of the TTS_2 values and standard errors of the means determined for 4 kHz. The broadband 90 dB noise and the 5 Hz sinusoidal vibration had a particularly clear combined effect on the TTS values when the subjects were working at the 2 W power output at both 20°C and 30°C. With the same power output and the same dynamic muscular work at 20°C, the TTS values were on average 1.1 times (first exposure), 1.4 times (second exposure) and 1.2 times (third exposure), and at 30°C, 1.1 times (first exposure), 1.3 times (second exposure) and 1.2 times (third exposure) higher than when noise was the only influencing factor. At four times the above workload (i.e., 8 W) noise and vibration were not found to have the same combined effect.

Table 1. Arithmetic means ($\bar{X}$) and standard errors of the means (SEM) of the TTS_2 values at 4 kHz by exposure combinations as a function of duration of exposures (n=144 ears).

Noise level		Dry-bulb temperature			
		30°C		20°C	
		Work load		Work load	
		2W $\bar{X}$±SEM	8W $\bar{X}$±SEM	2W $\bar{X}$±SEM	8W $\bar{X}$±SEM
No noise	1[a]	-0.4±0.4	0.4±0.8	0.0±0.6	0.8±0.6
	2	0.0±0.0	0.8±1.0	0.8±0.8	0.8±0.6
	3	0.8±1.0	1.0±1.0	-0.4±0.8	1.3±0.9
	4	0.4±0.4	0.0±0.6	-0.4±1.0	0.8±1.0
Noise of 90 dBA	1	14.2±1.6	14.2±1.7	12.1±1.4	12.1±2.8
(0.2-16 kHz)	2	16.3±1.9*	17.9±1.3	15.0±0.9**	16.3±3.2
	3	17.9±1.7	20.8±5.1	17.1±0.8	17.5±2.9
	4	11.3±1.4	14.6±1.6	10.0±1.1	9.5±2.4
Noise of 90 dBA	1	15.4±1.6	14.2±1.9	13.8±1.8	12.5±2.4
(0.2-16 kHz) and	2	20.4±1.5*	18.8±1.8	20.8±2.0**	16.7±2.3
vibration of 5 Hz	3	21.7±1.6	20.8±2.3	20.0±2.1	18.3±2.0
(2.12 m/s^2)	4	12.3±1.8	11.7±1.7	10.0±2.3	12.9±1.7

[a] 1 = 1st exposure, 2 = 2nd exposure, 3 = 3rd exposure, 4 = post-exposure; **p<0.01, *p<0.05

Table 2 shows that when the subjects were doing mere physically demanding dynamic muscular work at 30°C the means of the HDI values were higher than at 20°C. The same tendency was visible when the subjects were doing similar but four times lighter dynamic muscular work (work load 2 W). When the subjects were exposed to a noise and not only temperature, the means of the HDI values changed in two ways. When the subjects were doing heavy work at a high temperature (30°C), noise reduced the means of the HDI values significantly. At ten degrees lower temperature (20°C), when the subjects were doing physically demanding work, noise tended to increase the means of the HDI values. When they did light work, noise increased the means of the HDI values during the first two exposure periods, especially at 30°C.

When the subjects were exposed to a simultaneous noise and 5 Hz whole body vibration while doing physically demanding muscular work at 20°C or 30°C, the HDI values were considerably lower than when they were only doing heavy work or were exposed to mere noise at these temperatures while doing heavy work.

The results of three-way analyses of variance showed that work had a statistically very significant single effect on the variation in the HDI values during every period of exposure (F-values 33.43-13.67; df=1,60; $p<0.0001$), albeit the effects of work grew milder from the first exposure period to the third successive exposure period. During the first exposure period, work and noise had a significant combined effect on the variation in the HDI values at the level of 10% (F-value 2.45; df=1,60). Temperature affected the variation in the HDI values most during the third exposure and recovery period.

Table 2. Arithmetic means ($\bar{X}$) and standard errors of the means (SEM) of the HDI values by exposure combinations as a function of duration of exposures (n=72 subjects).

Noise level		Dry-bulb temperature			
		30°C		20°C	
		Work load		Work load	
		2W $\bar{X}$±SEM	8W $\bar{X}$±SEM	2W $\bar{X}$±SEM	8W $\bar{X}$±SEM
No noise	1[a]	-1.1±1.0	5.0±2.0	0.1±0.2	4.9±1.4
	2	-1.4±1.1	4.6±2.8	0.4±0.3	4.2±1.0
	3	0.6±0.8	5.9±2.9	0.4±0.3	4.9±1.3
	4	-0.3±0.5	-0.3±0.2	-0.0±0.1	0.1±0.2
Noise of 90 dBA	1	0.6±0.3	3.1±1.2	0.1±0.1	5.2±2.0
(0.2-16 kHz)	2	0.1±0.4	4.7±2.3	-0.1±0.3	4.1±1.9
	3	-0.3±0.4	3.1±1.6	0.1±0.2	6.6±4.3
	4	-0.6±0.3	0.0±0.3	-0.1±0.2	0.6±0.4
Noise of 90 dBA	1	0.2±0.4	2.5±1.3	0.4±0.2	2.0±1.0
(0.2-16 kHz) and	2	-0.1±0.1	2.7±2.2	0.0±0.1	2.8±1.5
vibration of 5 Hz	3	0.1±0.1	3.1±2.1	0.6±0.3	2.1±1.2
(2.12 m/s^2)	4	-2.3±2.1	-0.2±0.2	0.5±0.3	-0.1±0.2

[a] 1 = 1st exposure, 2 = 2nd exposure, 3 = 3rd exposure, 4 = post-exposure

Table 3. Arithmetic means ($\overline{X}$) and standard errors of the means (SEM) of the TTS_2 values at 4 kHz by exposure combinations as a function of duration of exposures (n=216 ears).

Vibration level		Dry-bulb temperature					
		30°C			20°C		
		Noise level			Noise level		
		No noise, no competition	Noise of 90 dB(A), no competition	Noise of 90 dB(A) and competition	No noise, no competition	Noise of 90 dB(A), no competition	Noise of 90 dB(A) and competition
		$\overline{X}$±SEM	$\overline{X}$±SEM	$\overline{X}$±SEM	$\overline{X}$±SEM	$\overline{X}$±SEM	$\overline{X}$±SEM
No vibration	1[a]	-1.3±1.1	15.0±2.5	15.8±1.6* **	0.8±1.0	13.8±2.4	17.1±2.3
	2	-0.4±1.1	18.3±2.1	20.8±1.9	1.3±1.1	15.8±2.9	20.0±2.2
	3	-0.8±1.7	16.3±2.6	19.2±1.7*	-1.7±1.7	17.9±3.2	20.8±2.3
	4	0.8±1.3	12.1±2.3	14.2±1.9	-2.1±1.7	11.7±2.9	12.9±1.7
Vibration frequency of 5 Hz (2.12 m/s^2)	1	0.4±1.7	18.8±2.7	21.7±1.9*	0.0±1.9	17.5±3.2	12.5±1.7
	2	-1.7±1.3	21.3±2.9	24.2±2.0	-2.1±1.7	21.3±3.1	17.5±1.8
	3	-1.7±1.8	20.8±2.8	25.0±1.8	-5.8±2.3	21.3±4.1	15.0±2.1
	4	-1.7±1.7	14.6±3.0	17.5±1.1	-2.1±2.1	18.3±3.0	9.2±1.8
Vibration frequency of 2.8-11.2 Hz (2.12 m/s^2)	1	2.1±3.2	17.5±2.2	22.1±1.5**	-0.4±1.7	15.4±2.1	13.3±1.8
	2	2.1±2.9	19.6±2.1	25.8±2.7	0.8±1.3	16.3±2.1	17.1±2.7
	3	-0.8±2.8	20.8±2.3	25.8±2.0*	0.4±1.1	15.8±2.2	15.8±3.0
	4	0.0±2.6	***12.5±1.3	19.6±2.0***	2.5±1.8	11.7±2.1	11.3±2.0

[a]1 = 1st exposure, 2 = 2nd exposure, 3 = 3rd exposure, 4 = post exposure; ***$p<0.01$, **$p<0.025$, *$p<0.05$

Table 4. Arithmetic means ($\overline{X}$) and standard errors of the means (SEM) of the HDI values by exposure combinations as a function of duration of exposures (n=108 subjects).

Vibration level		Dry-bulb temperature					
		30°C			20°C		
		Noise level			Noise level		
		No noise, no competition	Noise of 90 dB(A), no competition	Noise of 90 dB(A) and competition	No noise, no competition	Noise of 90 dB(A), no competition	Noise of 90 dB(A) and competition
		$\overline{X}$±SEM	$\overline{X}$±SEM	$\overline{X}$±SEM	$\overline{X}$±SEM	$\overline{X}$±SEM	$\overline{X}$±SEM
No vibration	1[a]	-0.5±0.3	0.1±0.2	0.7±0.4	0.1±0.1	-0.1±0.1	0.4±0.3
	2	-0.1±0.2	-0.2±0.2	0.7±0.5	0.0±0.1	0.3±0.2	0.5±0.4
	3	-0.0±0.2	-0.0±0.2	2.8±1.0	0.0±0.1	0.2±0.1	1.2±0.5
	4	0.0±0.2	0.1±0.1	0.5±0.5	0.2±0.1	0.1±0.1	0.0±0.1
Vibration frequency of 5 Hz (2.12 m/s^2)	1	-0.1±0.1	0.7±0.3	0.3±0.6	0.1±0.1	0.1±0.1	-0.5±0.5
	2	0.2±0.1	0.5±0.3	0.1±0.1	0.1±0.4	0.1±0.1	-0.2±0.4
	3	0.0±0.2	0.3±0.3	0.1±0.1	0.2±0.2	0.6±0.3	0.1±0.9
	4	-0.2±0.2	0.5±0.3	0.0±0.1	0.0±0.3	-0.2±0.1	-0.7±0.5
Vibration frequency of 2.8-11.2 Hz (2.12 m/s^2)	1	0.2±0.2	0.1±0.2	-0.0±0.3	0.3±0.1	0.1±0.1	0.6±0.6
	2	-0.0±0.1	-0.2±0.2	0.1±0.5	0.1±0.2	0.0±0.1	0.6±0.5
	3	0.3±0.3	0.1±0.2	1.9±1.0	0.4±0.3	0.0±0.1	0.0±0.6
	4	0.2±0.2	-0.5±0.7	-0.4±0.3	-0.2±0.5	-0.3±0.2	-0.4±0.2

[a]1 = 1st exposure, 2 = 2nd exposure, 3 = 3rd exposure, 4 = post exposure

Experiment V

One hundred and eight (108) healthy, volunteer male students (216 ears) were exposed. The cutoff frequencies of the noise bands employed were 0.2 and 16 kHz. The intensity of noise was 90 dB. The noise categories were no extra noise and no competition, noise of 90 dB and no competition, and noise of 90 dB related to competition about the fastest reaction time. The vibration categories were no vibration, sinusoidal vibration at a frequency of 5 Hz, and stochastic vibration in the frequency range of 2.8 to 1.2 Hz. The (rms) acceleration of the two vibrations was 2.12 m/s^2. The dry bulb temperature was either 20°C or 30°C (see also Manninen [7]).

Competition, associated with noise of 90 dB, seemed to increase the means of the TTS values at 4 kHz more than noise alone (Table 3). This result manifested itself at both 20°C and 30°C. Stochastic vibration seemed to exacerbate the increase in TTS_2 values at 4 kHz at 20°C and sinusoidal vibration at 30°C, especially in those cases where the subjects competed and were exposed to noise. On the other hand, the means of the TTS_2 values were significantly higher at 30°C as of the effects of sinusoidal and stochastic vibration when the subjects competed and were exposed to noise.

The results in Table 4 indicated that the HDI values were highest when the subjects were exposed to 90 dB noise at 30°C in a competitive situation (X=2.8) or to noise and stochastic vibration in a competitive situation (X=1.9). When the subjects were exposed to noise in a competitive situation at 20°C, the means of the HDI values were third highest (X=1.2). Table 4 shows further that sinusoidal vibration increased the HDI values at 20°C and 30°C when the subjects were exposed to noise but were not competing. The effects of stochastic vibration differed from the effects of sinusoidal vibration: it increased the HDI values when the subjects were exposed to noise while competing.

CONCLUSIONS

The results point out that there is a consistent association between changes in systolic blood pressure, heart rate and haemodynamic index values and changes in temporary hearing thresholds in complex exposure situations. Apart from the frequency range and bandwidth of the noise, there are other factors that also affect the intensity of this kind of association, such as whether the subject is simultaneously exposed to a whole body vibration, at what temperature the exposure to noise and vibration takes place, and under what degree of physical and mental load the subject is during the simultaneous exposure to noise, vibration and temperature. Furthermore, my newest findings show that the duration of the exposure and the characters of the vibration have special effects on the observed changes in hearing threshold and in cardiovascular activities [8]. And not only the spectral characters of the noise but also the frequency, acceleration and bandwidth of the vibration as well have a bearing on what kinds of combined effects (e.g., simultaneous noise and vibration) have on temporary hearing threshold [9]. An exposure period of one hour can be regarded as a sort of a boundary value, after which changes in the body functions will vary in cycles; i.e., depending on the criterion variable, the functional changes may periodically become deeper or less pronounced with exposure. This means that, to ensure better reliability of the observations, we should in the future direct more attention to the effects of complex exposure combinations and to longer periods of exposure.

One interesting point, in view of the direction of further studies, is that the temporary increase in the values of haemodynamic index was related to an increase in temporary hearing threshold during certain exposure combinations. We know from earlier studies that the product of heart rate and blood pressure correlates rather strongly with deteriorated contraction of the heart muscle and arrhythmia. It has also been observed that patients suffering from the coronary disease feel chest pain above all when their oxygen intake exceeds a certain critical index value as a result of physical or mental strain. The results presented here, in turn show that noise, vibration and temperature increase the value of this index and thus increases the oxygen consumption of the heart muscle. This naturally means that a certain combination of noise, vibration and temperature contributes to the emergence of coronary symptoms and spells as well as to the deterioration of the sense (hearing) and performance of people exposed to these factors.

ACKNOWLEDGEMENTS

These experiments belong to a research program being carried out under the direction of the author and financed by the Academy of Finland. The author expresses his gratitude to Mr. Veikko Ritvaniemi, Mrs. Ritva Manninen and Miss Paivi Suojanen for their assistance during this study.

REFERENCES

1. O. J. Manninen, Combined effects of environmental factors, Proceedings of the First International Conference on the Combined Effects of Environmental Factors held in Tampere, Finland, 22-25 September 1984. The International Society of Complex Environmental Studies (ISCES), Keskuspaino Central Printing House, Tampere, Finland (1984).
2. O. J. Manninen, Combinations of noise, vibration, temperature, and physical work and temporary threshold shift of hearing, Nordic Council Med. Res. Rep. 33:588 (1982).
3. O. J. Manninen, Studies of combined effects of sinusoidal whole body vibration and noise of varying bandwidths and intensities on TTS_2 in men, Int. Arch. Occup. Environ. Health 51:273 (1983).
4. O. J. Mamninen, Simultaneous effect of sinusoidal whole body vibration and broadband noise on TTS_2's and R-wave amplitudes in men at two different dry bulb temperatures, Int. Arch. Occup. Environ. Health 51:289 (1983).
5. O. J. Manninen, Hearing threshold and heart rate in men after repeated exposure to dynamic muscle work, sinusoidal vs stochastic whole body vibration and stable broadband noise, Int. Arch. Occup. Environ. Health 54:19 (1984).
6. O. J. Manninen, Complementary studies on human reaction to complex exposures, in: "Combined effects of environmental factors," O. J. Manninen, ed., Proceedings of the First International Conference on the Combined Effects of Environmental Factors held in Tampere, Finland, 22-25 September 1984. The International Society of Complex Environmental Studies (ISCES), Keskuspaino Central Printing House, Tampere, Finland (1984).
7. O. J. Manninen, Cardiovascular changes and hearing threshold shifts in men under complex exposures to noise, whole body vibrations, temperatures and competition-type psychic load, Int. Arch. Occup. Environ. Health (in press 1985).
8. O. J. Manninen, Bioresponses in men after repeated exposures to single and simultaneous sinusoidal or stochastic whole body vibrations of varying bandwidths and noise, Int. Arch. Occup. Environ. Health (submitted for publication 1985).

9. O. J. Manninen, A. Ekblom, Single and joint actions of noise and sinusoidal whole body vibration on TTS2 and low frequency upright posture sway in men, Int. Arch. Occup. Environ. Health 54:1 (1984).

DISCUSSION

Axelsson: These are complicated methods and experiments that require controls for each of the variables studied. Would you comment on your experimental design and how it provided for systematic control conditions?

Manninen: Basically, there are two different ways to conduct this type of study. As I showed, part of these studies were conducted using a randomized block design. The other part was based on a factorial experimental design. The data in the figures that I showed are relative data, i.e., all the subjects acted as their own controls. The time period between repeated exposures in those experiments using the random block design was at least 48 hours.

Dengerink: Looking at your figures, it appeared to me you had some very large TTS's on the order of 20-30 dB. That seems very large in comparison to what we often observe in human subjects, certainly with the short time exposures we use. Was that the TTS measured after a single exposure, or, since your experimental design often included repeated exposures, was the TTS the average from an individual?

Manninen: The TTS was an average values from individuals.

von Gierke: Those are very challenging findings at these low levels and I am particularly surprised about the large differences you get in TTS with changes in temperature. Do you measure TTS at times greater than 2 min. after exposure? At the early postexposure times, it is possible that what you are measuring is not a true sensory TTS, but rather the results of an increased circulation? It may be that at a higher temperature you get a higher physiological noise in the middle ear and that this noise can more or less simulate a raised threshold. Such an effect might disappear if you measure TTS 15 minutes or so after exposure.

Manninen: Yes. I agree with you, but for these experiments we used primarily TTS measured two minutes after exposure.

SOME ISSUES ASSOCIATED WITH INTERACTIONS BETWEEN OTOTOXIC DRUGS AND EXPOSURE TO INTENSE SOUNDS

Dennis McFadden

Department of Psychology
University of Texas
Austin, Texas, USA 78712

INTRODUCTION

Certain commonly-used drugs can produce hearing loss having many of the same physiological and psychophysical features as hearing loss induced by exposure to intense sound. Until quite recently, little research had been done on the question of possible interactions between drug-induced hearing loss (DIHL) and exposure-induced hearing loss (EIHL), and the vast majority of what had been done concentrated on drugs which themselves cause permanent threshold shift (PTS) [1-3]. In recent times, however, some studies have been done with drugs which are themselves responsible only for _temporary_ hearing loss, and the results of this work have raised the need for specialists working in the area of EIHL to consider again some logical and practical problems they have struggled with in the past. My goal in this chapter is to raise some of these problems for discussion, in the context of a brief review of our recent research on the interactions between EIHL and hearing loss induced by salicylates.

By way of introduction, let us agree that there are just five logically possible outcomes in an experiment that studies drug/exposure interactions.

(1) Beginning with the most severe, the drug-plus-exposure condition might yield a total hearing loss that _exceeds_ the sum of the separate DIHL and EIHL--a classical synergistic effect.

(2) Second most severe is that the total hearing loss might _equal_ the sum of the separate DIHL and EIHL--what might be called perfect additivity.

(3) The total hearing loss may be a less-than-perfect addition of the separate effects, but still exceed the EIHL alone.

(4) The total hearing loss might equal _either_ the DIHL or EIHL, whichever is greater (or lesser)--that is, there is no true summation of effects, but rather a disjunction of them.

(5) The fifth logical possibility is that the drug might provide some _protection_ against the exposure, so that the total hearing loss is less than either the DIHL or EIHL, and in the limiting (if somewhat fanciful) instance of this, the combined agents would yield no total hearing loss.

Here we will use the term interaction to describe all of these cases (even though some might argue that the perfect-additivity case is not, in the technical sense of the word, an interaction), and the first three possibilities will be characterized as potentiations.

It is tempting to try to distinguish between those potentiating effects that are direct and those that are indirect. For example, a drug which itself has no direct effect on the auditory system might sufficiently modify (say) the action of the middle-ear muscles such that greater TTS or PTS could result. However, a distinction between direct and indirect effects would surely become impossible to maintain once one entered the interdependent realm of the micromechanics of the cochlear partition, so we will not attempt to distinguish direct from indirect effects here. There is a related issue, however, which does demand due consideration--we will call it the <u>sites of action</u> problem. It is logically possible for each of the five logical possibilities described above to occur in at least two ways--either the drug and the exposure could both maximally affect the same neural or structural elements, or they could each operate primarily at different sites. Logically, drug/exposure experiments do not really differ from exposure/exposure experiments in this regard, for it is intuitive that a second noise exposure following hard on the heels of a first might begin to alter features of the cochlear environment <u>in addition to</u> those altered by the first exposure--e.g., some biochemical mechanism might be altered during the second exposure which escaped damage during the first. However, the different-sites issue seems more troublesome in regard to drug/exposure experiments, for there, the two agents logically need not overlap at all in their sites of action. As we shall see illustrated in the case of aspirin/exposure interactions, the single-site and different-site alternatives can give rise to quite different interpretations of drug/exposure data, so it is unfortunate that there are such strict limits on the ability of a psycho-physical experiment to separate the two possibilities.

In passing, we should note that possibilities 4 and 5 above appear to require that the drug act--directly or indirectly--at the same sites as the exposure, since protection against an exposure ultimately must involve a blocking or reversal of the detrimental physiological effects of that exposure.

SALICYLATES PLUS EXPOSURE TO INTENSE SOUNDS

Having briefly introduced some of the conceptual issues we shall be dealing with, it is now time for a brief summary of our studies on the interactions of non-steroidal, anti-inflammatory drugs, and exposure to intense sounds. Since the research predating ours has been reviewed elsewhere[4], we shall not repeat it here. All of our drug experiments have the same preliminary procedures. Following medical screening and careful documentation of each subject's absolute sensitivity at a number of test frequencies, subjects were given daily 10-minute exposures to a 2500-Hz tone. Exposure intensity was increased incrementally across the daily sessions, until the intensity necessary to produce 12-15 dB of TTS at the half-octave frequency was established for each subject individually. Once established, that exposure intensity was used for at least three daily exposure sessions in order to establish a baseline TTS function for each subject. Then, subjects began taking a drug at a dose level and duration of use that was varied across experiments; concentrating on just the extreme aspirin conditions for the moment, subjects took four daily doses of 975 mg each, for a daily total of 3.9 gr for 2-4 days. During that time, the DIHL was determined daily for several test frequencies. On the day scheduled for the exposure, each individual subject also received exactly the same exposure intensity and duration as had been used to establish his

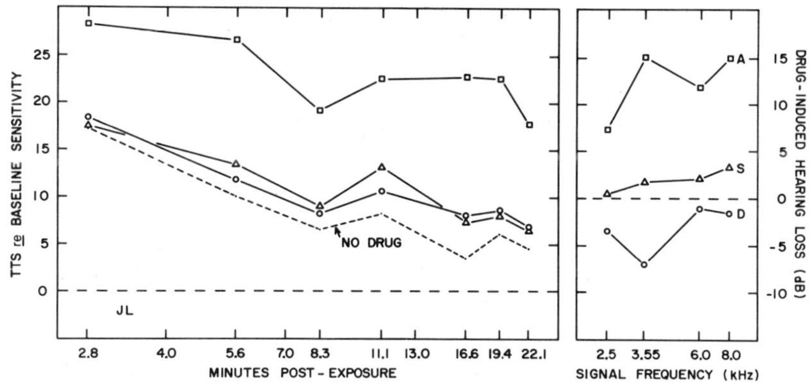

Fig. 1. In the right panel is shown drug-induced hearing loss measured immediately prior to the exposure for a single subject for each of three drugs--A: aspirin, D: diflunisal (Dolobid), and S: sulindac (Clinoril)--each taken for about four days. In the left panel are the post-exposure recovery curves (at 3550 Hz) for that subject for all three drugs and also for a baseline, no-drug condition. Exposure: 10 minutes to a 2500-Hz tone at 96 dB SPL.

own baseline TTS function. The resulting single TTS function obtained on that drug day was then used for comparison with the baseline TTS function. Recovery of hearing from the combination of exposure and aspirin was documented on the days immediately following the final dose and exposure.

In accord with past research, we found that aspirin (acetylsalicylic acid) taken at this dose for two or more days typically caused 5-15 dB of DIHL. More importantly, we found that the combination of aspirin-plus-exposure caused 10-15 dB more total temporary hearing loss than did the same exposure in the absence of the aspirin. Essentially identical outcomes were obtained with sodium salicylate, but the potentiation was minimal or non-existent with two other non-steroidal, anti-inflammatory drugs--sulindac (Clinoril) and diflunisal (Dolobid) [5]. The latter outcome is clearly important, for it reveals that patients in need of non-steroidal anti-inflammatory drugs do have alternatives apparently safer than salicylates. Some typical recovery curves are shown for a single subject in Fig. 1, and in Fig. 2 the results for a subset of our subjects are summarized. In Fig. 3, all our salicylate data are summarized in the form of a correlation space, where the abscissa is the DIHL measured just minutes prior to the exposure, and the ordinate is the increment in EIHL (i.e., the difference between total hearing loss from aspirin-plus-exposure and the baseline TTS established prior to administering any drugs). The product-moment correlation coefficient for all of the data shown in Fig. 3 is r = 0.27, but this correlation should be used for descriptive purposes

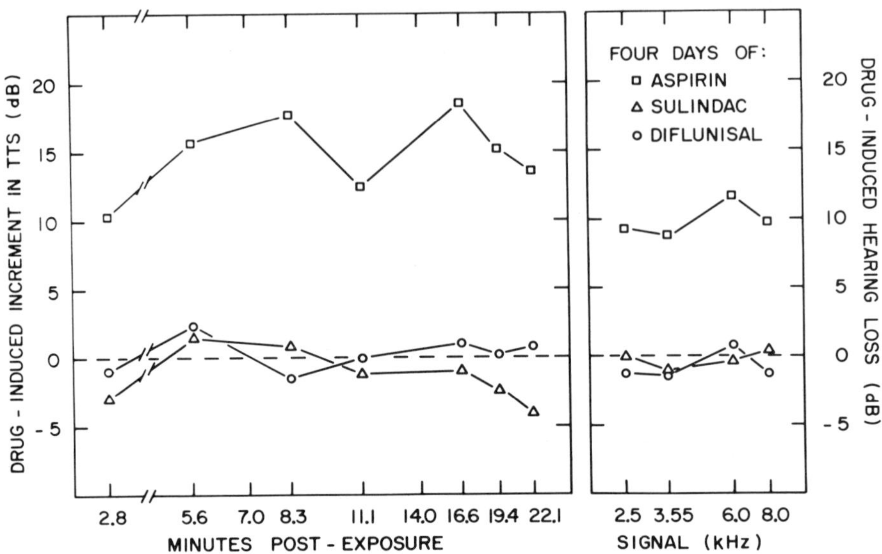

Fig. 2. In the right panel are shown drug-induced hearing losses measured immediately prior to exposure, averaged across 8 subjects for aspirin and 11 subjects for sulindac and diflunisal. In the left panel are shown the average increments between the total hearing losses measured in the drug-plus-exposure conditions and the TTS only in the no-drug condition, for those same subjects. Exposures: 10 minutes to a 2500-Hz tone of 93-108 dB SPL, depending upon the subject.

only since some individual subjects served in more than one condition, which violates this calculation's assumptions about independence. The dashed line in Fig. 3 describes the perfect-additivity case. Visual inspection of the data in Fig. 3 reveals that the effects range from synergism (Outcome 1 above) to less-than-perfect additivity (Outcome 3), with only a few cases clustered around the perfect-additivity line. In comparison with these results, when EIHL is added to a pre-existing PTS, the summation is invariably less than perfect (Outcome 3 above). For example, Ward [6] showed that the TTS produced by a given exposure is less in an ear with PTS than in a normal ear--although the total hearing loss (in terms of the actual sound-pressure level needed for detection) is always greater than normal. Viall and Melnick [7] found the same using an asymptotic threshold shift (ATS) paradigm, and Mills [8] observed a similar effect in chinchillas during the early hours of a long, continuous, but weak exposure.

In addition to potentiating the exposure, aspirin use also alters the course of recovery following exposure. As Fig. 1 reveals, the slope of the recovery curve was reduced in the drug condition; this protracted recovery appears in Fig. 2 as a larger increment in the latter minutes of the recovery session. The data of McCabe and Dey [9] reveal a similar effect. The implications are that under the influence of aspirin, the ear is less able to reverse the adverse consequences of the exposure, and further, that subsequent exposures may be more damaging than otherwise. (Parenthetically, each subject's hearing was back within his own normal range within 24-72 hours after the last dose plus exposure, which is essentially the same time required to reverse the DIHL alone from aspirin.) One gauge of the signi-

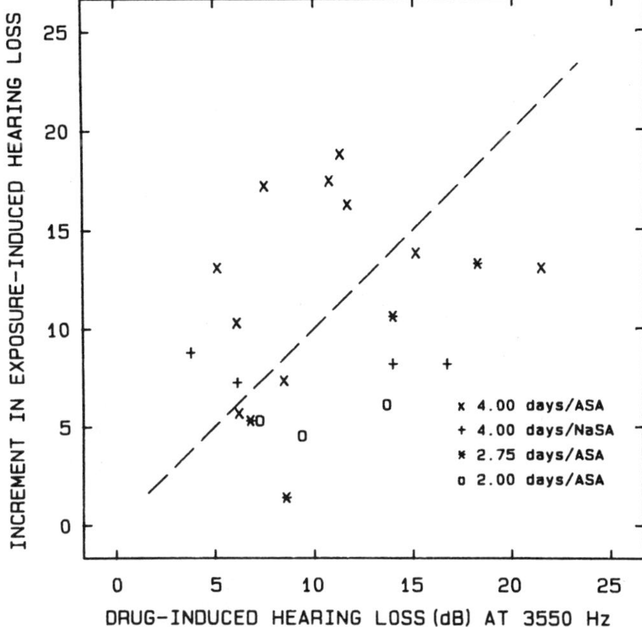

Fig. 3. Correlation space for the drug-induced hearing loss (determined at 3550 Hz immediately prior to the exposure) versus the increment in exposure-induced hearing loss (at 3550 Hz) relative to each subject's own baseline TTS function. The increments were estimated using the first two blocks of trials in the post-exposure sequence, meaning they span about the first 5 minutes post-exposure. The dashed line describes the perfect-additivity case. Different symbols indicate different drugs and different durations of use. ASA: acetylsalicylate acid (aspirin); NaSA: sodium salicylate.

ficance of this 10-15 dB of potentiation is that were it an observed increment in TTS caused by additional exposure in an industrial setting in the USA, it would require a halving of the daily allowable exposure duration (calculations made using the classic figures of Miller [10]).

INTERPRETATION OF RESULTS

Having obtained these aspirin-plus-exposure data, the next obvious question is what they all mean, and that is where some of the old problems mentioned in the introduction arise. A problem that many working on EIHL have struggled with over the years is what pre-exposure baseline to use when calculating the hearing loss produced by a given exposure. That is, if a person enters an exposure session with some pre-existing temporary or permanent hearing loss--owing to a previous exposure--should the hearing loss induced by today's exposure be estimated using today's (shifted) pre-exposure threshold or using a previously determined threshold free from residual, exposure-induced shift, or even a threshold estimate obtained from a control group of some sort? This problem is no less troublesome when the temporary hearing loss measured at the outset of the session is a consequence of drug administration. Above we mentioned work by Ward [6] and others demonstrating that the actual post-exposure SPLs necessary for detection are higher in hearing-impaired listeners than in normals, even though the exposure-induced shift from their resting thresholds (the "TTS") is smaller. Thus, the choice one makes for baseline in such an experiment could determine whether one concludes that a combination of agents constitutes a risk or a prevention; the same is often true in aspirin-plus-exposure experiments. As the data in Fig. 3 show, more than half the time the increment in EIHL was less than the DIHL in our subjects. Thus, the use of the shifted pre-exposure threshold as a baseline would lead one to conclude for these cases that the combination of agents produces less hearing loss than does the exposure alone. It is peculiar to me that this is the calculation apparently favored by Ward [11] and personal communication; for to me, the logical extension of this choice appears to be that aspirin protects the auditory system from exposure in more than half our subjects, and this seems highly unlikely to me.

No matter what the eventual findings about the sites of action of aspirin and the issue of increased PTS and aspirin use, Ward's interpretation of the TTS data disturbs me and I would like to argue against it by analogy with some hypothetical exposure-plus-exposure data. Imagine that Exposure A causes 10 dB of TTS and that Exposure B causes 20 dB of TTS when each are administered separately. Further imagine that when Exposure B immediately follows Exposure A, the total TTS is 20 or 25 dB. Would one now be comfortable with the conclusion that Exposure B only caused 10 or 15 dB of TTS--that is, that the ear received 5 or 10 dB of protection against Exposure B? I don't think so, for in this case we clearly see that had Exposure A not occurred, Exposure B would have produced its typical 20 dB of loss. Now imagine that the total TTS following the combination of exposures is 15 dB. Would one be comfortable with the conclusion that Exposure B was less dangerous than Exposure A because it added only 5 dB to the total hearing loss? Again, I don't think so, and for the same reason. It seems to me that the most logical measure of effect in experiments involving combinations of hearing-reducing agents is the total hearing loss produced relative to some previously-measured baseline (or a population average, when necessary), not the increment produced on the day of exposure. To further emphasize the virtue of this approach, consider a situation in which Agent A improves hearing by 5 dB, and that a subsequent exposure brings hearing to the same sound-pressure level that it had always brought it to. Would one be comfortable concluding that the exposure was more dangerous today than on non-drug days because the increment in hearing loss was greater than the typical TTS produced by the exposure? I would not, for it seems to me that this exposure is having the same absolute effect on the peripheral auditory structures in the drug and non-drug conditions.

To my view, the potential for damage by an agent is likely to be underestimated, perhaps greatly so, by experimenters who calculate the increment in hearing loss relative to a shifted baseline instead of the total hearing loss relative to a previously-determined baseline or population average. In the particular case of drug-plus-exposure experiments, I also believe that total hearing loss is the most prudent way to conceptualize the data until more is known about the consequences of combining various drugs with exposure. In passing, it should be mentioned that McCabe and Dey [9] apparently calculated incremental rather than total hearing loss in their aspirin-plus-exposure conditions; one has to wonder whether they thereby confused even themselves about their outcomes. As a demonstration that this issue is not unique to research on hearing loss, it can be noted that a similar difference of opinion was apparently recently resolved for light adaptation in vision [12]. There, the question was whether to describe the response (physiological or psychophysical) as a function of the total incident light (background plus stimulus increment) or as a function of just the increment intensity relative to the background. With appropriate adjustments, both approaches could be shown to fit certain existing data reasonably well, but Valeton [12] demonstrated that the former approach was superior to the latter in simplicity, generality, and explanatory power. While his conclusions do not transfer directly to the present situation, I cite them because I wish they did. This issue of incremental versus total EIHL is obviously a crucial one for investigators concerned with predicting PTS from TTS in real-world settings.

Now, no matter what calculation one chooses for characterizing the data in a drug-plus-exposure experiment, the over-riding question has to be whether use of the drug does constitute an increased risk of permanent hearing loss. The presence of 10-15 dB more temporary hearing loss would <u>ordinarily</u> imply an equivalent increase in eventual PTS (e.g., Ward [13], and thus, a greater risk of significant hearing loss among aspirin users. The problem in extending this conclusion to our work is that this increment in temporary hearing loss did not arise from a summing of two exposures--which we know would both act at the same physiological sites--but rather, from the combination of an exposure with a drug that logically could have produced this outcome by operating at a different site from the exposure. Thus, the ordinary implication of greater PTS might not apply here, but it is obviously important to find out if it does. In specific reference to our research, it is important to know whether salicylate use will produce greater PTS, not just greater TTS.

Faced with this question, the reader's first inclination might be (as was mine) to check the epidemiological databases on EIHL to see if aspirin use does in fact lead to greater PTS. However, just as early epidemiological researchers on EIHL were plagued by the problem of poor documentation of exposure levels and durations, no EIHL database I have been able to locate contains documentation of chronic or episodic use of drugs, so to date it has been impossible for me to establish from databases whether aspirin, or any other drug, potentiates (or alleviates) noise exposure. Working with indirect evidence is possible, but risky, and ultimately inconclusive; for example, looking at the hearing loss in a noise-exposed sub-population that identifies itself as suffering from (say) arthritis ignores relevant issues such as the severity of the disease, whether aspirin, or some other (or any) drug was taken for the malady, the dose level taken, the dose schedule, the relative timing of the doses and the exposures, etc., and there is always the logical possibility of relevant interactions among different drugs taken by the same person.

Another indirect approach to the question of whether aspirin-plus-exposure might produce more PTS is to try to determine if aspirin affects the same neural elements as exposure does. It is well known that intense sounds alter the cochlear hair cells in various ways (e.g., Liberman and Mulroy [14]). Perhaps if aspirin could be shown to also act at the hair-cell level, the different-sites question might be resolved. (As we shall see, this approach is logically unsound, but let us briefly consider it anyway.) The physiological literature on aspirin does contain a few studies of its effects on the cochlear microphonic (CM), but unfortunately, about half of them indicate that CM is depressed by administration of salicylates while the other half indicate no change in CM [14]; so, no help there. Human electrocochleography (ECOG) uses electrodes in the external meatus and averaging techniques to obtain signals known as summating potentials, which are believed to originate from hair cells. In ECOG experiments (done solely on myself so far), we have shown that aspirin use does diminish the summating potentials--as well as the small CM that was also visible in my averaged response. Spontaneous oto-acoustic emissions (OAEs) are also generally believed to originate from hair cells (e.g., Kemp [15]; we have shown that moderate doses of aspirin abolish spontaneous OAEs [16], which then return at the same frequency and at full strength upon termination of the aspirin. So, two lines of evidence do indicate that aspirin affects the same peripheral location--cochlear hair cells--as is affected by exposure, and a possible conclusion is that combinations of aspirin-plus-exposure will eventually produce more PTS than exposures alone. The logical problem with this approach is that hair cells are complex entities having numerous functional locations, and it is logically possible to alter their response in the same direction via actions at different proximal sites. That is, the sites of action problem exists within a complex entity like a hair cell just as it does across structures composed of those entities. Specifically, aspirin might act in one way to produce a "hearing loss" in the hair cells, and exposure might act there in another way(s), but because the intracellular sites of action are different, the two might not sum to produce greater PTS.

Thus, all of the above procedures for determining whether aspirin-plus-exposure (or any commonly used drug-plus-exposure) does lead to greater PTS are either logically flawed or currently lacking in the necessary data. This state of affairs appears to leave only two possibilities--longitudinal research, with humans or animals. The logistical and ethical difficulties with longitudinal human experiments on PTS are well known, so while such experiments are logically possible sources of information on the question of interest, my expectation is that animal behavioral experiments will ultimately prove to be the primary source of information on this matter. To my view, the best such experiments would involve work-day exposure schedules and dose levels appropriately corrected for the animal's body weight. Unfortunately, I have no such results to report at this point, so I must leave you not knowing whether aspirin-plus-exposure produces more PTS than exposure alone, but I hope to soon begin collaborating on the relevant animal behavioral research.

SUMMARY

In this paper I have tried to combine a brief review of some of our basic findings on the effects of aspirin on the auditory system with a discussion of some new and old problems they raise. One conclusion is that combinations of agents--whether drugs with exposures or exposures with exposures--ought to be evaluated by considering the total induced hearing loss relative to some within-subject baseline, or relative to some population mean, not by considering the increment in hearing loss produced by one of the agents. A second conclusion is that it is extraordinarily difficult to establish from existing data whether exposures combined with use of drugs (of any sort) are more dangerous than exposures without drug use, and the only viable solution to the problem appears to be longitudinal, animal behavioral research. Other effects of aspirin on the auditory system are described in McFadden, Plattsmier, and Pasanen [17].

ACKNOWLEDGMENTS

This work was supported in part by research grants from the National Institute for Neurological and Communicative Disorders and Stroke, and Merck Sharp and Dohme Research Laboratories. Thanks are due Wilson S. Geisler for discussions of these problems and for informing me of the parallel problem in the light adaptation literature.

REFERENCES

1. S. A. Falk, Combined effects of noise and ototoxic drugs, Environ. Health Perspectives, 4:5 (1972).
2. R. P. Hamernik and D. Henderson, The potentiation of noise by other ototraumatic agents, in: "Effects of Noise on Hearing" eds., D. Henderson, R. P. Hamernik, D. S. Dosanjh, and J. H. Mills, Raven Press, New York pp. 291-307 (1976).
3. L. E. Humes, Noise-induced hearing loss as influenced by other agents and by some physical characteristics of the individual, J. Acoust. Soc. Am., 76:1318 (1984).
4. D. McFadden and H. S. Plattsmier, Aspirin can potentiate the temporary hearing loss induced by intense sounds, Hearing Research, 9:295 (1983).
5. D. McFadden, H. S. Plattsmier, and E. G. Pasanen, Temporary hearing loss induced by combinations of intense sounds and nonsteroidal anti-inflammatory drugs, Am. J. Otolaryngol., 5:235 (1984a).
6. W. D. Ward, Auditory fatigue and masking, in: "Modern Developments in Audiology," ed., J. Jerger, Academic Press, New York, pp. 240-286 (1963).
7. J. Viall and W. Melnick, Asymptotic threshold shift in people with sensorineural hearing loss, Trans. Amer. Acad. Ophthalmol. Otolaryngol., 84:459 (1977).
8. J. H. Mills, Threshold shifts produced by exposure to noise in chinchillas with noise-induced hearing losses, J. Speech Hear. Res., 16:700 (1973).
9. P. A. McCabe and F. L. Dey, The effect of aspirin upon auditory sensitivity, Ann. Otol. Rhinol. Laryngol., 74:312 (1965).
10. J. D. Miller, Effects of noise on people, J. Acoust. Soc. Am., 56:729 (1974).
11. W. D. Ward, Noise-induced hearing loss: Research since 1978, Photocopy of talk delivered at 4th International Congress on Noise as a Public Health Hazard, Turin, Italy (1983).
12. J. M. Valeton, Photoreceptor light adaptation models: an evaluation, Vision Research, 23:1549 (1983).
13. W. D. Ward, Adaptation and fatigue, in: "Sensorineural Hearing Processes and Disorders," ed., A. B. Graham, Little Brown, Boston, pp.113-121 (1967).
14. M. C. Liberman and M. J. Mulroy, Acute and chronic effects of acoustic trauma: Cochlear pathology and auditory nerve pathophysiology, in: "New Perspectives on Noise-Induced Hearing Loss" eds., R. P. Hamernik, D. Henderson, and R. Salvi, Raven Press, New York, pp. 105-135 (1982).
15. D. T. Kemp, Stimulated acoustic emissions from within the human auditory system, J. Acoust. Soc. Am., 64:1386 (1978).
16. D. McFadden and H. S. Plattsmier, Aspirin abolishes spontaneous oto-acoustic emissions, J. Acoust. Soc. Am., 76:443 (1984).
17. D. McFadden, H. S. Plattsmier, and E. G. Pasanen, Aspirin-induced hearing loss as a model of sensorineural hearing loss, Hearing Research, 16:251 (1984b).

DISCUSSION

Salvi: What are some of the other psychoacoustic changes you see with aspirin?

McFadden: Just briefly, forward masking is basically unaffected, whereas temporal integration is. The temporal integration function is flattened. The literature you find parallels the effects seen with sensorineural hearing loss. That is, with the amounts of hearing loss that we were able to induce with our drugs, we should not have seen effects on forward masking and we should have seen some effects on temporal integration. As a model for hearing loss, it is a poor model, in the sense that it tends to induce a flat hearing loss whereas noise induced effects obviously can have strong spectral effects.

Salvi: Tinnitus is supposed to be one of the side effects of aspirin. Did you ever do any pitch matching experiments?

McFadden: No. Part of the reason is, I tried to do some of that myself and found it extraordinarily frustrating. Aspirin-induced tinnitus, at least in my ear, is subject to what is known as residual inhibition, i.e., you put in an external sound and you can make tinnitus go away in some ears. My experience was that you put a tone in; you try and match the tinnitus, the tinnitus disappears and you then have to wait for a minute for it to come back again and then you put the tone in again, adjust the oscillator and again the tinnitus disappears. This was extraordinarly inefficient and frustrating so I just quit.

HEARING AND ENDOCRINE FUNCTION

I. Mastrogiacomo, G. Bonanni, V. Colletti*, L. Rossi and P. Zucchetta

University of Padua
Via Ospedale Civile 105,
35100 Padova, Italy

*University of Verona
ENT Department
37134 Verona, Italy

INTRODUCTION

Different systems of the human body are strongly related to each other and the endocrine system is not an exception. At a recent congress held in Verona, Italy, V. Colletti et al. [1] reviewed the relation between internal disease and hearing loss. Similarly, exogenous toxic agents, such as noise and/or vibrations capable of damaging hearing, can also affect other systems of the organism including the endocrine system. For instance, Catapano et al. [2] have shown an increase in all three catecholamine levels in normal healthy subjects following a five minute exposure to road traffic noise.

Catecholamines can be considered hormones and neurotransmitters: hormones because they are produced by adrenal medulla and neurotransmitters because they are produced by neurons. Thus, an increase in the level of plasmatic catecholamine can originate from both systems (adrenal and neural). Therefore, a determination of the relative source is not possible. Borrell et al. [3] found a decrease in encephalic norepinephrine and dopamine in animals exposed to noise. The depletion in the nervous system should bring about a parallel increase in the plasmatic level. As mentioned earlier, in similar experimental conditions, Catapano et al. [2] found an increase in the level of epinephrine. It is known epinephrine is produced almost entirely by adrenal medulla [4]. Therefore, it may be stated than an increase in catecholamine levels is due to complex phenomena, which involve both the endocrine system and the nervous system. Changes in the levels of these hormones may be one of the causes of the increase in systolic and diastolic blood pressure observed during exposure to noise. Changes in the levels of catecholamines are, however, transient. Catapano et al. [2], report that catecholamines return to basal levels 10 minutes after the beginning of noise exposure, even if the exposure to noise persists. The transient increase of this hormone may justify the negative findings of some authors [4,5]. Hence, catecholamines cannot be considered responsible for the persistent hypertension found in people living in noisy environment, reported in some epidemiological studies [6].

Previous reports have shown that noise, mediated by the hypothalamus-hypophysis increases adrenal cortex function. Kraicer et al. [7] found an increase in melanostimulating hormone (MSH) and in adrenocorticotropic hormone (ACTH) in rats. Also, Borrell et al. [3] found an increase in corticosterone in the same species. It is known that corticosterone is the main product of the activity of adrenal cortex in the rat, whereas, in man, the main product is cortisol. A similar increase has been described in men both for 17-hydroxy-corticosteroids and for cortisol. Interestingly, both plasmatic and salivary cortisol levels have been shown to increase [8]. The increase in salivary cortisol level is important since it is an expression of the free, and therefore active, amount of this hormone. As known, protein-bound cortisol does not filter into the saliva. Increases in levels of urinary steroids, resulting from catabolism, and increase in level of cortisol are more persistent than increases in the levels of catecholamines. Thus, steroids can be assessed a few hours after the beginning of the noise exposure. Borrell et al. [3] were able to demonstrate a correlation between cortico-steroids and the amount of depletion of norepinephrine in the brain of rats exposed to sound. This correlation is convincing, since norepinephrine is a neurotransmitter that lowers the production of ACTH and, therefore, of the cortisol. This action takes place at the hypothalamus. Accordingly, Okada et al. [9] have shown that the depletion of norephinephrine, induced by noise, is particularly large in the hypothalamus.

Few reports can be found in the literature concerning the effect of noise exposure on prolactin and the growth hormone. Andren et al. [5] state that noise does not affect either prolactin or growth hormone. However, the assay was performed 20 minutes after the beginning of noise exposure; hence, a transient increase in both hormones in the very early period, similar to the transient changes shown in catecholamines, cannot be excluded.

The above-mentioned studies on catecholamines and adrenal steroids demonstrate that the increase in these hormones is generally temporary. There is a sudden increase at the beginning of the noise exposure followed by a more or less rapid return to normal values, even if exposure to noise persists. In addition, repetitive noise-exposure periods produce progressively lower changes. Contrary to the trends of the previously described studies, noise seems to have a more significant and persistent effect on the gonads.

Zondek et al. [10] found enlargement of the ovaries and irregularity in the estrous cycle, which they attributed to an increase in gonadotrophins, induced by noise. The same authors also reported a significant decrease in fertility in rats exposed to noise. Subsequent studies by Singh et al. [11] confirmed the findings of Zondek et a. [10] partially in that they reported irregularity in the estrous cycle, but disagreed on the ovarian alterations, which they described to be characterized by atrophy. Moreover, a reduction in fertility in animals seems to be confirmed by other authors, who compared animals living near airports to animals living in normal environments [12]. The reduction of fertility observed in animals seems to be present also in humans exposed to noise. Epidemiological studies [13-15] and a single study in men, report hypofertility in workers exposed to noise over a period of years [16].

Beardwood et al. [16] have shown a significant increase in the excretion of urinary gonadotrophins in five men and in two women exposed to tones in the frequency range 4 to 6 kHz at 85-90 dB. Stimuli, lasting one minute, were administered for two hours at intervals of ten minutes, and the same protocol was repeated for three consecutive days. Unfortunately, the measurements did not include radioimmunoassays, a more precise technique. Using radioimmunoassays it is possible to determine separately the levels of FSH and LH, which play different roles in ovarian function. The study by Beardwood et al. [16] lacks data on sexual steroids, and it is therefore impossible to determine if the increase in gonadotrophins is due to gonadic hyperfunction or if it is due to the reduction of sexual steroids, caused by noise. In the latter case, the increase of gonadotrophins would be an expression of a negative feed-back and thus an index of a gonadic hypofunction. These data open a very important issue on the possible toxic effect of noise in the hypothalamus-hypophysis-gonadic axis. Therefore the present research was performed in order to evaluate hypothalamus-hypophysis-gonadic function in a group of workers exposed to noise for many hours a day and for many years.

MATERIALS AND METHODS

Seventy-one male subjects with a mean age of 33 years, workers in a metallurgic mechanic factory, for 8 hours a day, 5 days a week, ranging from 2 to 15 years, were studied. The intensity of the noise during the work had a level ranging from 90 to 99 dBA, with a peak at 125 Hz and a slope of approximately 6 dB per octave. The subjects, during work, were exposed not only to noise, but also to other stressing agents such as heat, intense physical exercise, long periods of orthostatism, etc.

Twenty four normal hearing subjects, matched for age, were studied as controls. A blood sample was collected at the beginning and soon after work (5-6 a.m. and 2 p.m.) from all subjects. The following hormones were assessed by RIA (Biodata): total plasmatic testosterone, free testosterone, follicle stimulating hormone (FSH), luteninizing hormone (LH), 17-beta-estradiol (E2) and prolactin (PRL). This procedure is presently one of the most precise, sensitive and accurate assays that can be done. Sexual-hormone-binding globulin (SHBG) was assessed by radioimmunometric assay (IRMA); this technique uses the presence of a monoclonal antibody anti-SHBG used as tracer in an immunoradiometric assay.

Hearing threshold was evaluated in all workers by means of standard audiometry. Workers were subdivided into two groups, according to their hearing sensitivity. Subjects with normal hearing and subjects with a mild hearing loss formed the first group; subjects with moderate to severe hearing loss formed the second group.

RESULTS

The changes in the levels of the examined hormones are reported in Fig. 1 through 6. Basal prolactin (5-6 a.m.) value was found to be significantly higher in the workers (12 +/- 4.5 vs 7.03 +/- 4.8 ng/ml, with $p < 0.0001$). Prolactin level in the afternoon was equal in both groups (workers and controls). Hence, the 40% decrease in the prolactin level from the basal level was present only in the workers. Thus, it is due to higher level of the hormone in the morning, before starting work in the factory.

Total plasmatic testosterone did not show a significant difference between the workers and the controls. The level in the afternoon, among the workers, was significantly lower than the level in the morning. It must be remembered, however, that the changes, expressed in percentages, of the total testosterone between workers and controls, were not significantly different. The decrease in the level of plasmatic testosterone, however was not accompanied by significant variation in gonadotrophins or in the sexual-hormone-binding globulin (SHBG). Also, 17-beta-estradiol did not show any variation. In contrast to the results for total plasmatic testosterone, the free amount of this hormone, in the afternoon, was significantly lower than in the morning, not only for workers but also for controls, with no variation between the two groups (27.2 +/- 5.4 and 20.6 +/- 5.6 in the workers and 24.3 +/- 7.2 and 19.2 +/- 6.2 pg/ml in controls, with $p < 0.001$). Therefore, this decrease cannot be attributed to factors present during work (noise, heat, vibrations, etc.), but could be due to circadian changes of this hormone. No significant variations were observed for the assessed hormones between the

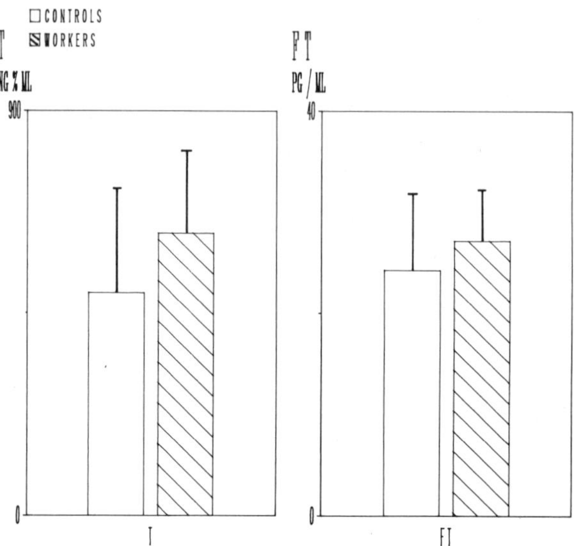

Fig. 1 Basal values (mean +/- SD)of plasmatic total testosterone (T) and free testosterone (FT), in workers and in controls.

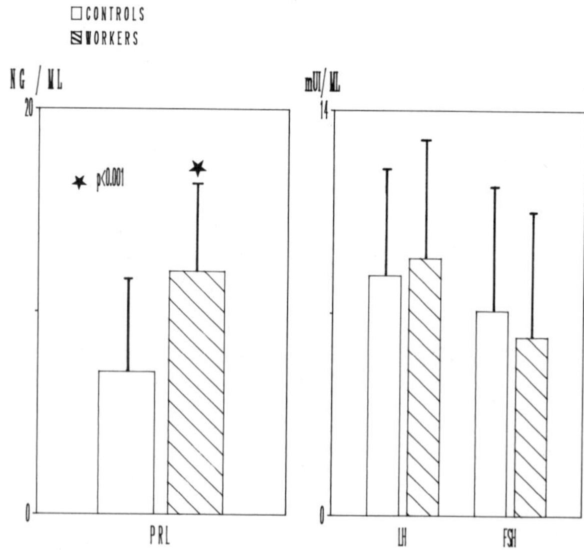

Fig. 2 Basal values (mean +/- SD) of prolactin (PRL), follicle-stimulating hormone (FSH) and luteinizing hormone (LH) in workers and in controls.

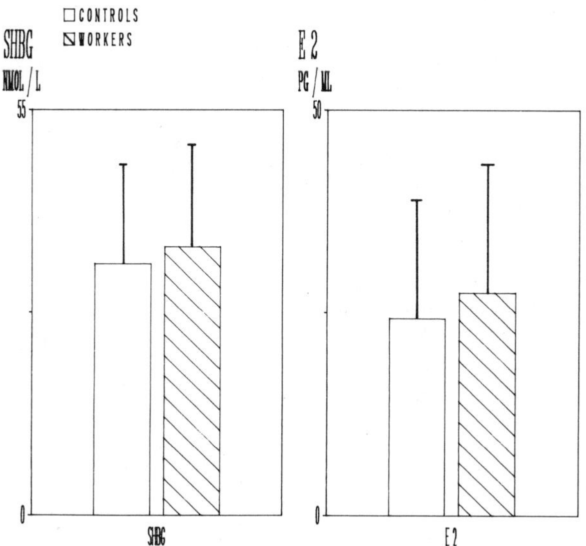

Fig. 3 Basal values (mean +/- SD) of estradiol (E2) and sexual-hormone-binding globulin (SHBG) in workers and in controls.

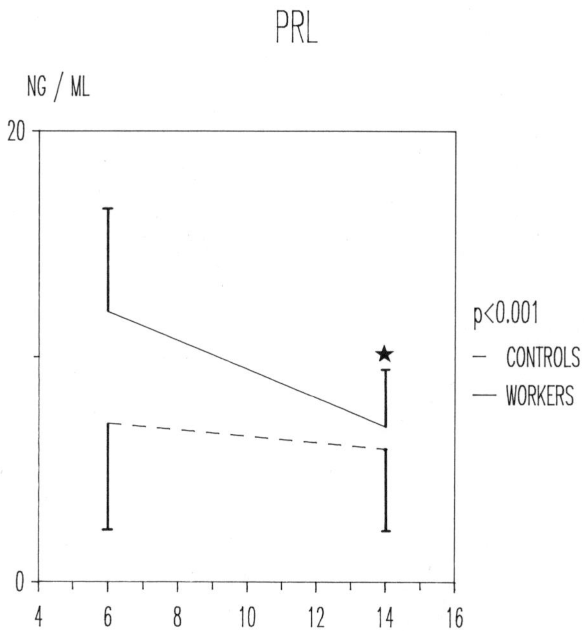

Fig. 4 Level of prolactin (PRL) at 6 a.m. and 2 p.m. (mean +/- SD) in workers and in controls.

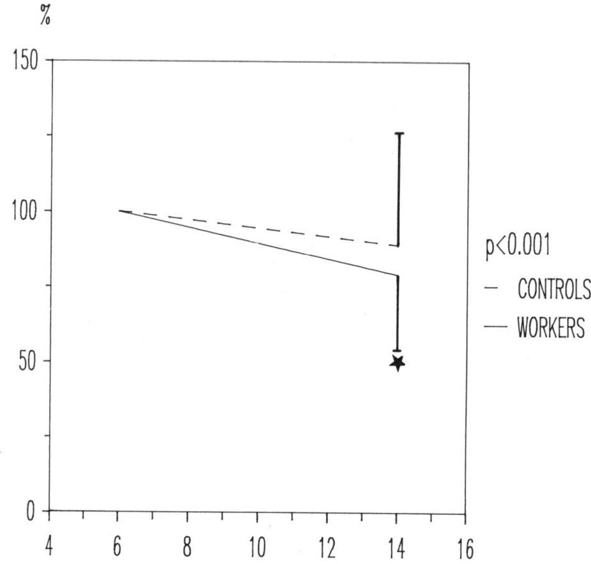

Fig. 5 Changes, expressed in percentages, in testosterone level (T) between morning and afternoon, in workers and in controls (mean +/- SD).

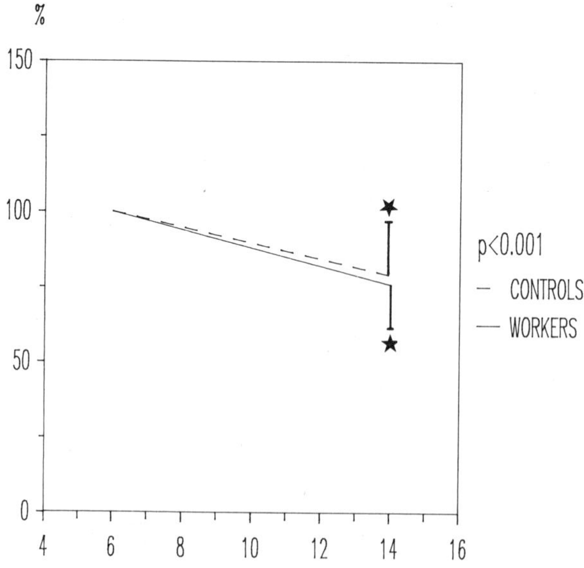

Fig. 6 Changes, expressed in percentages, in free testosterone level (FT) between morning and morning and afternoon, in workers and in controls (mean +/- SD).

two groups of workers. The morning and evening levels of total and free testosterone and prolactin were similar in the two groups (normal and mild hearing loss group and the moderate and severe hearing loss group).

DISCUSSION

The main finding of the present study is the higher value of prolactin, observed in the morning in the two groups of workers. Since, at the end of the day's work, the level of prolactin is equal in both groups (workers and controls), the hyperprolactinemia cannot be attributed to noise exposure. In our opinion, the different behavior in prolactinemia between the two groups, can be ascribed to other factors, such as the stress of starting in the factory or different morning food intake habits. The fact that afternoon plasmatic testosterone level was significantly lower only in the workers, may suggest that noise exposure does, in effect, alter the gonadic function. This finding relates to absolute values, but when the relative changes between morning and afternoon are evaluated, both groups do not differ significantly. In order to explain the observed decrement in the afternoon plasmatic testosterone levels in the workers, it could be hypothesized that noise induces an alteration of the hypothalmus-hypophysis-testis system via the acoustic nerve-brain-hypothalamus-hypophysis-testis. It should be remembered, however, that in our study gonadotrophins did not show any change. This finding indicates, thus, that the decrease in testosterone level cannot be attributed to the above mentioned neuro-endocrine pathway. The decrease in testosterone level could be due to an increased catabolism, but this is unlikely, since SHBG and estradiol were both found to be unchanged in the morning versus the afternoon assays. The more intense muscular activity of the workers may in itself be responsible for the significant decrease in the testosterone level. It is known, that intense physical activity reduces the testosterone level without changes in gonadotrophin levels [17].

The data from the present study indicate that high level noise exposure cannot be considered a toxic agent for the hypothalamus-hypophysis-gonadic axis. Our findings seem to contradict the conclusions of other authors [10,11,13,16]. The quoted results are referred mainly to females and to animals, where changes of volume of ovaries and of estrous cycle has been described. But it is well known that noise is certainly more stressful in animals than in men, who are capable of psychologically controlling noise. On the other hand, it is possible that noise could affect females more than males by acting on the gonadotrophin cyclicity, which is more complex in females. Furthermore, gonadotrophin cyclicity is strongly dependent on central neurotransmitter tone, which is modified by noise exposure.

Epidemiological animal and human investigations would indicate a decrease in fertility. These statements are not strongly convincing, since no detailed information is given whether this decrease is in the males and/ or females. Hypofertility, can also result from other factors. Factors such as noise and/or vibrations, directly involving the external or internal genitalia, have been investigated. Gunther et al. [18] examined testis of guinea pigs exposed to noise and could not observe any significant abnormalities in spermatogenesis. Conversely, Ando et al. [12], demonstrated that women living in high level noise environments presented a significantly lower production of human placental lactogen (HPL) at the end of gestation when compared to women living in normal noise environments. In addition, HPL reduction was consistent with lower weight of newborns. This is certainly a proof that noise and/or vibrations act directly on the internal genitalia (uterus), since HPL is produced by placenta without control of the hypothalamus-hypophysis system. It is thus conceivable that hypofertility might be due to direct effects of vibrations on the uterus, resulting in mucosa alterations or in difficulty for the fertilized oval to implant in the uterus.

The issue of fertility and noise and/or vibrations needs, in our opinion, a clarification which does not imply deeper endocrine investigation but, rather, a determination of number and quality of spermatozoa in males, and in females, mucosal tissue analysis of uterus and placental function.

REFERENCES

1. V. Colletti and S. D. G. Stephens, Disorders with defective hearing, Advances in Audiology, vol. 3, Karger (1985).
2. F. Catapano, P. Portaleone, P. S. Teagno, G. F. Fornaca, F. Bono, G. C. Guiliani, L. Liberali, L. Verdun di Cantogno, Effectti del rumore stradale sulle catecolamine ematiche, sul cAMP e su alcune funzioni cardio-vascolari e metaboliche in un gruppo di soggetti normali, Min. Med. 75:1111 (1984).
3. J. Borrell, A. Torrellas, C. Guaza and S. Borrell, Sound stimulation and its effects on the pituitary-adrenocortical function and brain catecholamines in rats, Neuroendocrinology, 31:53 (1980).
4. G. Brandenberger, M. Follenius and C. Tremolieres, Failure of noise exposure to modify temporal patterns of plasma cortisol in man. Eur. J. Appl. Phys. 36:209 (1977).
5. L. Andren, G. Lindstedt, M. Bjorkman, K. O. Borg and L. Hansson, Effect of noise on blood pressure and stress hormones, Clin. Science 62:137 (1982).
6. A. Jonsson and L. Hansson, Prolonged exposure to a stressful stimulus (noise) as a cause of raised blood pressure in man, Lancet, i, 86-87 (1977).
7. J. Karaicer, G. Beraud, and D. W. Lywood, Pars intermedia ACTH and MSH content: effect of adrenalectormy, gonadectomy and a neurotropic (noise) stress, Neuroendocrinology, 23:352 (1977).
8. K. Yamamura, N. Maehara, T. Sadamoto and I. Harabuchi, Effect of intermittent (traffic) noise in man - temporary threshold shift, and change in urinary 17-OHCS and saliva cortisol levels, Eur. J. Appl. Physiol., 48:303 (1982).
9. A. Okada, M. Ariizumi, and G. Okamoto, Changes in cerebral norepinephrine induced by vibration or noise stress, Eur. J. Appl. Physiol., 52:94 (1983).
10. B. Zondek and I. Tamari, Effect of audiogenic stimulation on genital function and reproduction, Am. J. Obst. Gync., 80(6):1041 (1960).
11. K. B. Singh, Effect of sound on the female reproductive system, Am. J. Obstet. Gynecol. April 1, 981 (1972).
12. Y. Ando and H. Hattori, Effects of noise on human placental lactogen (HPL) levels in maternal plasma, British J. Obstet. Gynecol. 84:115 (1977).
13. Y. Ando and H. Hattori, Journal of the Acoustical Society of America, 47:1128 (1970).
14. Y. Ando and H. Hattori, Statistical studies on the effects of intense noise during human fetal life, J. Sound Vib. 27:101 (1973).
15. L. Carosi and F. Calaro, La prolificata di coniugi operai di industrie rumorose, Folia Medica 51:264 (1968).
16. C. J. Beardwood, C. A. Mundell and W. H. Utian. Gonadotropin excretion in response to audiostimulation of human subjects, Am. J. Obstet. Gynecol. 121, 5:682 (1975).
17. P. Schmid, H. H. Pusch, W. Wolf, E. Pilger, H. Pessenhofer, G. Schwaberger, H. Pristautz and P. Purstner, Serum FSH, LH, and Testosterone in humans after physical exercise, Int. J. Sports Med. 3(2):84 (1982).
18. E. Guenther, Bioassays about effect of stress by noises on male fertility, Andrologia 8, 2:98 (1976).

A PATHWAY FOR THE INTERACTION OF STRESS AND NOISE INFLUENCES ON HEARING

Harold A. Dengerink[1], John W. Wright[1], Joan E. Dengerink[2] and Josef M. Miller[3]

Department of Psychology[1] and Speech[2]
Washington State University
Pullman, WA 99164-4830

Kresge Hearing Research Institute[3]
University of Michigan
Ann Arbor, MI 48109

INTRODUCTION

Threshold shifts following noise exposure, whether temporary or permanent, are frequently described as being variable [1,2]. Such threshold shifts following noise exposure differ markedly from individual to individual. Temporary threshold shifts (TTS) observed for the same individual after repeated exposure to the same noise are also variable. This variability, even with the same listener exposed to sounds with identical physical parameters, implies that noise may interact with other variables to influence hearing acuity. A variety of other variables may be likely candidates for interaction with noise, including environmental and body temperature [3,4], whole body vibration [5], and chemical agents [3,6].

One general theme that has guided research in our laboratory is the possibility that noise interacts with other stressors to influence TTS. The terms stress and stressor are used with markedly differing connotations in the literature. However, one common characteristic of events which are called stressors is alteration in physiological processes mediated by the autonomic nervous and endocrine systems. Thus, events which result in elevated heart rate, increased blood pressure, higher body temperature, peripheral vasoconstriction, etc., may be classified as stressors. Thus, we have chosen to investigate the interaction of noise and a variety of conditions which result in peripheral (cutaneous) vasoconstriction, elevated heart rate and increased blood pressure. Given this definition, noise itself would be classified as a stressor [7,8].

The general finding of this series of studies has been that stressors reduce the magnitude of TTS observed following noise exposure, and that stress-inhibiting conditions increase the magnitude of TTS. For example, in one study, experimental subjects were taught progressive relaxation procedures and permitted to employ these techniques during the noise exposure [9]. These subjects were observed to have lower serum cortisol levels than control subjects (19.5 micro g/100ml vs 23.0 micro g/100ml). The relaxation subjects were also observed to have lower levels of both systolic (Mean 115.0 mmHg) and diastolic (74.0 mmHg) blood pressure than control subjects (Means = 120.6 and 79.0 mmHg respectively). In addition, subjects in the relaxation condition evidenced greater TTS after noise exposure (5 minutes of 105 dB re 20 micro Pa) than the control subjects (11.0 dB vs. 4.0 dB). Thus, persons with low levels of physiological arousal evidenced more TTS than persons with higher levels of physiological arousal.

In other studies we have observed that conditions which result in peripheral vasoconstriction and increased blood pressure result in less TTS than ones which result in vasodilation or smaller amounts of vasoconstriction. Some authors have reported that the magnitude of peripheral vasoconstriction is negatively correlated with the magnitude of TTS [10-12]. Dengerink et al. [10] reported a negative correlation of -0.44 between the last minute of noise exposure and TTS measured at 2 minutes after the exposure. That is, the greater the vasoconstriction in response to noise, the smaller the degree of TTS. Consistent with this negative correlation, we have observed that noise exposure (5 minutes of 110 dB re 20 micro Pa) in cold ambient temperatures (which result in cutaneous vasoconstriction) results in less TTS than noise exposure in hot ambient temperatures [3]. Nicotine consumption and cigarette smoking also result in increased blood pressure and peripheral vasoconstriction. In three different experiments, we have observed that smokers who smoke prior to the noise exposure evidence approximately half the TTS of nonsmokers (See Dengerink and Dengerink [13], for review). Dengerink et al. [3], for example, reported that TTS for smokers was 3.3 dB, while the average for nonsmokers was 8.0 dB. Further, physical exercise, which results in increased blood pressure, appears to facilitate the effect of smoking and to increase the difference in TTS between smokers and nonsmokers [14].

This relationship between TTS and vasoconstriction or blood pressure and TTS appears to be reasonably specific. That is, other indications of physiological arousal do not appear to share the same relationship to TTS. Heart rate has been reported to correlate positively rather than negatively with TTS [3,14]. Further, while both cold temperatures and cigarette smoking both appear to reduce TTS, cold ambient temperatures result in lowered heart rate, but cigarette smoking increases it. Thus, it appears that peripheral vasoconstriction and elevated blood pressure act to reduce TTS, but other measures of physiological arousal may not.

While this relationship appears to be quite consistent, it is not immediately clear why vasoconstriction in the skin or elevated systemic blood pressure should influence TTS. In fact, there may be several possible ways in which stress responses function to reduce TTS. For example, increased levels of circulating catecholamines (which are vasoconstrictors and neurotransmitters) may also alter the threshold for central nervous system transmission. In our research program we have examined the possibility that stress responses such as peripheral vasoconstriction and blood pressure increases may reflect or contribute to increases in cochlear blood flow.

Some previous authors [15] have indicated that threshold shifts may be dependent upon or influenced by blood flow through the cochlea. Blood flow through the cochlea is responsible for maintaining adequate oxygenation, for supplying other nutrients including glucose, and for removing metabolic waste products [16]. Alterations in cochlear blood flow may thus be responsible for variations in TTS by ensuring (or precluding) adequate oxygenation, metabolism, and removal of waste products. Direct examination of the relationship between threshold shifts and cochlear blood flow are very difficult. To do so, one would have to alter cochlear blood flow and examine the resulting magnitude of noise-induced threshold shifts. Further, one would have to do so without altering related phenomena such as blood-borne vasoactive compounds which could conceivably influence TTS independent of cochlear blood flow. The existing technology is not capable of providing such a test.

The strategy we have adopted is a two stage process which provides strong implications for the relationship between physiological stress mechanisms and TTS. The first stage of this strategy is to examine the effect of noise on endogenous physiological agents known to increase blood pressure and peripheral vasoconstriction. The second stage is an examination of the effects that exogenous application of these agents have on cochlear blood flow. If it can be shown that noise increases circulating levels of biochemical agents which increase blood pressure, and that these agents when exogenously administered increase cochlear blood flow, then it can be argued that noise results in increased cochlear blood flow. Variations in the circulating levels of these biochemical agents and therefore in cochlear blood flow, could then be responsible for variations in the magnitude of threshold shifts.

THE EFFECT OF NOISE ON VASOACTIVE AGENTS

The major biochemical agent that we have chosen to examine in this context is Angiotensin II (AII). AII serves an integrative role with regard to cardiovascular function and electrolyte balance (reviewed by Ganong [17]). Most important among angiotensin's effects are its direct ionotropic effect on the heart and its ability to increase vascular resistance. Angiotensin's influence on vascular resistance is a consequence of both direct action on vascular smooth muscle as well as indirect action on the central nervous system, resulting in activation of the sympathetic nervous system and stimulation of vasopressin and catecholamine release. Angiotensin's major water balance effects also involve both central and peripheral actions including increases in thirst, salt appetite, and sodium absorption by the gut, and improved efficiency of water and salt retention by the kidney (reviewed by Johnson [18]). The multiple cardiovascular and body water balance effects, which indirectly influence cardiovascular efficiency, indicate a pivotal role for AII in the regulation of cardiovascular function in general and cochlear blood flow in particular. The potential importance of AII in response to stress has been suggested by Blair et al. [19] who report that renin levels increase with anticipation of adversive events.

One series of studies in our laboratories has been devoted to examining the effects of noise on circulating levels of AII. In the first of these studies [20], rats were tested following a control period or exposure to a variety of stressful conditions. In the control condition, animals were exposed to a low intensity (20 dB re 20 micro Pa) white noise in a normal (21°C) temperature room after 15 minutes of adaptation. In another condition, the subjects were exposed to high intensity (100 dB) white noise for 15 minutes after adaptation. In another, condition the subjects were allowed to adapt to the test room which had been cooled to 5°C and then exposed to the low intensity noise. Following the exposure, a blood sample was taken, the plasma extracted and assayed via a radio-immunoassay procedure [21]. The results indicate that both the cold ambient temperature and the noise exposure resulted in circulating angiotensin elevations. The average (+/-SE) AII for subjects in the control group was 0.26 (+/-0.05 ng/ml). The averages for the cold and the noise condition were 0.56 (+/-0.05) and 0.64 (+/0.03) ng/ml, respectively. The circulating levels AII for subjects exposed to either the cold temperature or to the noise was more than twice that of the control subjects which were exposed only to low intensity noise in a normal temperature room.

In the second of these experiments [22], male human subjects were employed. Half of the subjects were exposed to loud white noise (100 dB re

20 micro Pa) for 15 minutes. Half sat with the earphones on, but did not listen to noise. Thresholds at 4 kHz were measured before and 2 min. after the noise exposure. Blood samples were drawn for measuring AII before the noise and after the second threshold. The initial levels were higher than normal, a finding attributable to the threat (stressor) of having blood samples taken. For subjects not exposed to noise, the AII levels declined significantly from the first to the second sample (Mean change = -0.17 ng/ml). For the subjects exposed to the noise, the second AII measures remained high (Mean change = -0.04 ng/ml). Thus, while noise did not increase the levels of AII, it did arrest a normal decline in AII that was observed for control subjects not exposed to noise. In addition, for subjects in the noise exposure condition, the AII levels prior to and following noise exposure were correlated (-0.35 and -0.24, respectively), with the magnitude of TTS. These correlations are of nearly the same order of magnitude as the negative correlations observed for TTS and cutaneous vasoconstriction [10-12].

In the third experiment in this series [23], guinea pigs were either exposed to the experimental chamber only, or to 120 dB (re 20 micro Pa) white noise in the chamber for 30 minutes. AII assayed in blood samples from animals exposed only to the chamber averaged 0.28 ng/ml. In contrast, animals exposed to the noise evidenced AII levels which averaged 1.08 ng/ml. Thus, in three species, noise appears to elevate circulating levels of AII.

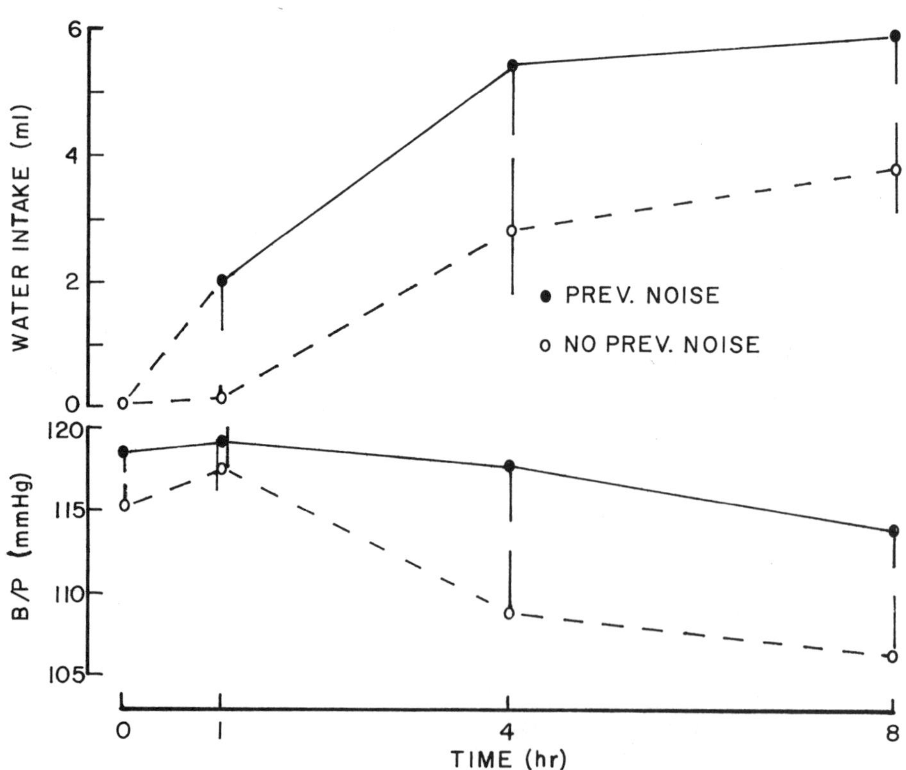

Fig. 1. Mean +/- SE cumulative water consumption and arterial blood pressure for each group on the test day (Morseth et al. [24])

The last experiment in this series [24] assessed the effect of long term impulse noise exposure on some expected consequences of AII elevations, i.e., increase in blood pressure and water consumption. The noise exposure consisted of 0.5 sec bursts of white noise with a peak intensity of 127 dB re 20 micro Pa presented once every 10 sec. Four groups of rats were exposed to this noise for 9 days prior to the test day. The exposure duration for each group was 8 hrs., 4 hrs., 1 hr. or 0 hr. (control). On the test day, this sound exposure was repeated for the previously exposed animals and presented to four additional groups of animals not previously exposed to noise. Blood pressure was measured via an indwelling carotid artery catheter inserted one day before the test. Water consumption was measured for the entire noise exposure period 1 hr. - 8 hrs. or for 1 hr. in the control group.

The results are presented in Fig. 1. As that figure indicates, subjects with a prior history of impulse noise exposure evidenced greater fluid consumption than did those not previously exposed. At the same time, the previously exposed animals evidenced higher levels of blood pressure during the test period than did those not previously exposed.

These findings indicate that long term as well as acute exposure may influence vasoactive processes. They do not, however, demonstrate that these elevations and circulating AII, or other vasoactive agents, influence cochlear blood flow. That is the issue which we address in the next section.

COCHLEAR BLOOD FLOW CHANGES RELATED TO VASOACTIVE AGENTS

Cochlear blood flow is extremely difficult to measure. The vessels are imbedded in bony tissue and follow a tortuous course with many right angles. Further, the vessels are divided into numerous groups serving various structures. No single measure of cochlear blood flow is ideal. All have disadvantages and advantages, depending upon the specific purpose of the investigation. The measure which we chose for assessing the effects of vasoactive agents is the laser Doppler. This measurement technique has the advantage of providing dynamic measures that can assess the rapid changes and demonstrate the time course of the changes in cochlear blood flow resulting from these time-limited agents.

The laser Doppler flowmeter emits a laser-generated monochromatic light which has a wavelength similar to red blood cells. When the light strikes moving particles, the light that is reflected back is shifted slightly in frequency. The amount of shift is proportional to the number of red blood cells in the measurement volume times the velocity of their movement. This product of velocity and mass is referred to as flux. The flowmeter output reflects this difference in frequency and thus the flow through the tissue being assessed. The laser Doppler flowmeters penetrate skin tissue to a depth of approximately 1mm and measure flow in tissue which is approximately 1mm [3]. The depth of penetration in the more dense cochlea is not known, but is assumed to be somewhat less than in the skin. (See Miller et al. [25] for a more thorough discussion of the laser Doppler flowmeter.)

The use of the laser Doppler for measuring cochlear blood flow requires an anesthetized preparation. We employ a combination of Ketamine (100mg/kg) and Xylazine (20mg/kg) to anesthetize guinea pigs and open the bulla using a ventral approach, thus exposing the basal turn of the cochlea. The doppler probe (1.75 mm O.D.) is placed perpendicular to the basal turn over the stria vascularis. We also prepare the animals with a

Table 1. Blood Pressure, Cochlear and Abdominal Skin Flow Changes Following Intra-arterial Injection of Angiotensin II (Values are Means +/- S.E.)

Dosage of AII	Blood Pressure (% of baseline)	Cochlear Flow (% of baseline)	Skin Flow (% of baseline)
0.1 pM/kg Max. Change	+9.6+/-3.5	+3.6+/-0.9	-1.9+/-1.5
1.0 pM/Kg Max. Change	+12.3+/-4.7	+3.7+/-3.1	-4.3+/-2.8
10 pM/kg Max. Change	+32.1+/-4.7	+10.0+/-3.1	-7.2+/-2.3
100 pm/kg Max. Change	+79.2+/-2.5	+20.0+/-2.8	-12.8+/-3.2

carotid cannula which permits monitoring of blood pressure and introduction of the vasoactive substance. A second flowmeter probe is routinely placed on the skin over a shaved portion of the abdomen.

In the first of these experiments [23], we administered AII in varying doses and in random order. The results are summarized in Table 1. As this table indicates, blood pressure and cochlear blood flow increased with increasing doses of AII. In contrast, skin blood flow decreased in a generally dose related fashion. The doses employed (0.1 to 100 pm/kg) bracketed the levels observed when AII was assayed in the plasma of noise-exposed guinea pigs. Thus it appears that the levels of AII which result from noise exposure are capable of causing an increase in cochlear blood flow. The pattern of results further suggests that the changes in cochlear blood flow are secondary to changes in blood pressure. That is, these result do not necessarily indicate that the cochlear vessels themselves are responsive to AII innervation. Rather, the changes in cochlear blood flow may be secondary to systemic changes.

The findings discussed thus far indicate that noise exposure results in elevated AII, and that elevated AII results in increased cochlear blood flow. AII, however, is not the only circulating vasoactive agent which may result from noise exposure or which may be involved in contributing to noise related changes in cochlear blood flow. One set of vasoactive agents that has often been implicated in hearing function are the catecholamines. In a series of papers Muchnik and colleagues [15,26,27] indicated that catecholamines (epinephrine and norepinephrine combined) infused locally (rather than systemically) reduced perilymph Po_2 and cochlear action potentials. When catecholamines were infused systemically, smaller decrements were observed. Given these changes in cochlear function, they inferred that catecholamines cause constriction in the cochlear vasculature which in turn retards cochlear function. They also suggest that systemic catecholamines may increase blood pressure and thus increase cochlear blood flow, which helps to prevent deterioration of cochlear function.

Table 2. Blood Pressure, Cochlear and Abdominal Skin Flow Changes Following Intra-arterial Injection of Saline, Epinephrine and Norepinephrine (Values are Means +/- S.E.)

Drug and Dose	Blood Pressure (% of baseline)	Cochlear Flow (% of baseline)	Skin Flow (% of baseline)
SALINE			
Max. Change	+23.8+/-10.1	+16.2+/-8.3	+2.1+/-5.7
EPINEPHRINE			
0.1 Micro g/Kg			
Max. Change	+22.0+/-8.1	+19.8+/-5.5	-8.8+/-4.8
1.0 Micro g/kg			
Max. Change	+59.8+/-12.0	+34.1+/-6.1	-10.1+/-10.1
10 Micro g/kg			
Max. Change	+140.4+/-15.0	+57.6+/-5.5	-25.1+/-22.1
NOREPINEPHRINE			
0.1 Micro g/Kg			
Max. Change	+34.6+/-5.2	+13.8+/-3.0	-5.8+/-5.3
1.0 Micro g/kg			
Max. Change	+122.4+/-20.0	+22.2+/-12.1	-13.6+/-13.4
10 Micro g/kg			
Max. Change	+119.0+/-32.0	+62.6+/-5.9	-37.2+/-14.5

Our investigations of catecholamines have been limited to systemic infusions and have separately studied the effects of epinephrine and norepinephrine. Using the procedures outlined above for the investigation of AII, we infused several doses of epinephrine and norepinephrine and measured cochlear blood flow with the laser Doppler. The results are summarized in Table 2. As the table indicates, blood pressure and cochlear blood flow increased with infusions of epinephrine and norepinephrine in a dose related fashion. In contrast, skin blood flow decreased with infusion of these substances and did so in a dose related fashion.

These findings indicate that vasoactive substances increase cochlear blood flow. Further, both sets of results indicate that cochlear blood flow, as influenced by these agents may be secondary to changes in blood pressure, as indicated by Snow and Suga [28,29].

The results described here provide a possible explanation for the variability in threshold shifts following noise exposure. These results also suggest a possible pathway by which threshold shifts may be mediated by the interaction of noise and other stressors. If AII and catecholamine elevations do result from noise exposure, then these agents may increase cochlear blood flow and maintain or enhance cochlear function during and following the insult of noise. Further, if AII and catecholamine elevations occur with exposure to other stressors, then these conditions may increase cochlear blood flow and protect the cochlear structures from the fatigue caused by noise insult.

The current results indicate that noise stimulation does result in elevated exogenous levels of plasma AII. They further indicate that both AII and catecholamines administered exogenously increase cochlear blood flow. It should be noted, however, that attempts by other authors to assess the effects of noise on plasma concentrations of catecholamines have been mixed. Some authors [30] have reported that noise elevates plasma catecholamine levels. Others [31] report that catecholamine blocking agents inhibit noise-induced increases in blood pressure. Still, the majority of authors indicate that noise stimulation appears to have no affect on plasma catecholamines [32-34]. This pattern of results may indicate that noise does not result in elevated circulating levels of catecholamines, but that autonomic nervous system activity may increase with noise stimulation and can be inhibited by catecholamine blocking agents. Alternatively, elevations in plasma catecholamines with noise exposure may be delayed or secondary to AII elevations and to sympathetic nervous system activity.

However, even if noise does not increase catecholamine levels, other stressful events do result in increased plasma catecholamines [26]. Since it appears that systemic catecholamines do result in increased cochlear blood flow, these other agents may interact with noise to modify the effect of noise on threshold shifts. Thus, the variability in threshold shifts may be influenced by AII both in response to noise and in response to other stressors. This variability may be influenced by plasma catecholamines only insofar as noise is combined with other stressors.

REFERENCES

1. W. Melnick, Temporary and permanent threshold shifts, in: "Noise and Audiology," D. M. Lipscomb, ed., University Park Press, Baltimore (1978).
2. F. Lindgren and A. Axelsson, Interaction between noise-exposure and other factors assessed by clinical TTS studies. Paper presented at the XVII International Congress of Audiology, Santa Barbara, CA. (1984).
3. H. A. Dengerink, G. W. Trueblood, and J. E. Dengerink, The effects of ambient air temperature and cigarette smoking on noise-induced temporary threshold shifts, Audiology, 23:401 (1984).
4. K. R Henry and R. A. Chole, Hypothermia protects the cochlea from noise damage, Hearing Res., 16:225 (1984).
5. O. Manninen, A review of exposure combinations including noise: The meaning of complex exposures, Proceedings of the Fourth International Congress on Noise as a Public Health Problem: 637 (1983).
6. K. R. Henry, Effects of noise, hypothermia and barbiturate on cochlear electrical activity, Audiology, 19:44 (1980).
7. E. Borg, Tail artery response to sound in the unanesthetized rat, Acta Physiol. Scand., 100:129 (1976).
8. E. Borg, Physiological aspects of the effects of sound on man and animals, Acta Otolaryngol. Suppl., 360:80 (1979).
9. P. Thompson, Noise-induced temporary threshold shifts: The effects of anticipatory stress and coping strategies, Unpublished doctoral dissertation, Washington State University, Pullman, WA. (1983).
10. J. E. Dengerink, H. A. Dengerink, and G. D. Chermak, Personality and vascular responses as predictors of temporary threshold shift, Ear and Hearing., 3:196 (1982).
11. G. Jansen, Effects of noise on physiological state, ASHA Reports, 4:89 (1969).

12. G. Jansen, Relation between temporary threshold shift and peripheral circulatory effects of sound, in: "Physiological Effects of Noise," B. L. Welch and A. M. Welch, eds., Plenum Press, New York (1979).
13. H. A. Dengerink and J. E. Dengerink, The interaction of stress and noise on auditory measures, in: Hearing Research and Theory," J. V. Tobias and E. D. Shubert, eds., Academic Press, New York (1986).
14. J. E. Dengerink, F. Lindgren, A. Axelsson, and H. A. Dengerink, The effects of smoking and exercise on temporary threshold shifts, Paper presented at the meetings of the American Speech and Hearing Association, San Francisco, CA (1984).
15. C. Muchnik, M. Hildesheimer, L. Nedel, and M. Rubenstein, Influence of catecholamines on cochlear action potentials, Arch Otolaryngol., 109:530 (1983).
16. J. E. Hawkins, The role of vasoconstriction in noise-induced hearing loss, Ann. Otorhinolaryngol., 80:903 (1971).
17. W. F. Ganong, The brain renin-angiotensin system, in: "Brain Peptides," D. T. Kreiger, M. J. Brownstein, and J. B. Martin, eds., John Wiley and Sons, New York (1983).
18. A. K. Johnson, Neurobiology of the periventricular tissue surrounding the anteroventral third ventricle (AV3V) and its role in behavior, in: "Circulation, Neurobiology, and Behavior," O. A. Smith, R. A. Galosy, and S. M. Weiss, eds., Elsevier Science Publishing, New York (1982).
19. M. E. Blair, E. O. Feigl, and O. A. Smith, Elevations of plasma serum activity during avoidance performance in baboons, Am. J. Physiol., 231:772 (1976).
20. J. W. Wright. H. A. Dengerink, P. Thompson, and S. Morseth, Plasma angiotensin II changes with noise exposure at three levels of ambient air temperature, J. Acoust. Soc. Am., 70:1353 (1981).
21. M. D. Bailie, F. C. Rector, Jr., and D. W. Seldin, Angiotensin II in arterial and venous plasma and renal lymph in the dog, J. Clin. Invest., 50:119 (1971).
22. H. A. Dengerink, J. W. Wright, P. Thompson, and J. E. Dengerink, Changes in plasma angiotensin II with noise exposure and their relationship to TTS, J. Acoust. Soc. Am., 72:276 (1982).
23. J. W. Wright, H. A. Dengerink, J. M. Miller, and P. C. Goodwin, Potential role of angiotensin II in noise-induced increases in inner ear blood flow, Hearing Res., 17:41 (1985).
24. S. L. Morseth, H. A. Dengerink, and J. W. Wright, Effect of Impulse noise on water consumption and blood pressure in the female rat, Physiol. and Beh., 34:1013 (1985).
25. J. M. Miller, N. J. Marks, and P. C. Goodwin, Laser Doppler measurements of cochlear blood flow, Hearing Res., 11:385 (1985).
26. C. Muchnik, M. Hildesheimer, and M. Rubenstein, Effect of emotional stress on hearing, Arch. Otorhinolaryngol., 228:295 (1980).
27. C. Muchnik, M. Hildesheimer, and M. Rubenstein, Effect of catecholamines on perilymph Po2, Arch. Otolaryngol., 110:518 (1984).
28. J. B. Snow and F. Suga, Control of cochlear blood flow, in: "Vascular Disorders and Hearing Defects," A. J. deLorenzo, ed., University Park Press, Baltimore (1972).
29. F. Suga and J. B. Snow, Cholinergic control of cochlear blood flow, Amer. Otol., 78:1081 (1969).
30. A. Slob, A. Wink, and J. J. Radder, The effect of acute noise exposure on the excretion of corticosteroids, adrenalin and noradrenalin in man, Int. Arch. Arbeitsmed., 31:225 (1973).
31. L. Andren, L. Hansson, R. Eggertsen, T. Hedner, and B. E. Karlberg, Circulatory effects of noise, Acta Med. Scand., 213:31 (1983).

32. L. Andren, G. Lindstedt, M. Bjorkman, K. O. Borg and L. Hansson, Effect of noise on blood pressure and stress hormones, Clin. Sci., 62:137 (1982).
33. B. Metz, G. Brandenberger, and M. Follenius, Endochrine response to acoustic stresses, in: "Environmental Endochrinology," I. Assenmacher, and D. S. Farner, eds., Springer Verlag, New York (1977).
34. M. Follenius, G. Brandenberger, C. Lecornu, M. Simeoni, and B. Reinhardt, Plasma catecholamines and pituitary adrenal hormones in response to noise exposure, Eur. J. Appl. Physiol., 43:253 (1980).

DISCUSSION

Henderson: I know these experiments are in the early stages, but do you have any sense of how long the angiotensin response is maintained for an exposure lasting several days? Do you still get the same kind of elevation?

Dengerink: You are asking about the angiotensin levels associated with long duration noise exposures. The only evidence we have for this is rather indirect since we are not looking specifically at angiotensin. We were looking at blood pressure and at fluid consumption, which as I pointed out at the beginning are the two major effects of angiotensin. In our experiment, we had subjects who were exposed for 9 days prior to the test noise exposure. On the test day, we looked at both the previously exposed subjects and subjects who had not been previously exposed to the noise. We found that subjects who had been previously exposed were showing higher levels of blood pressure and greater fluid consumption than those who were being exposed for the first time. It would appear that there are some long term effects associated with the noise stimulation on angiotensin. Unfortunately, we do not have the angiotensin data here to support that. So with that little bit of data we would suggest, in fact, that there are long term effects apparent in angiotensin rather than just short term quickly adapting kinds of changes.

Manninen: We collected urine samples and measured catecholamine levels and found that the changes, increases induced by noise, are rarely long term effects.

Dengerink: The catecholamine effects that you are seeing, are they a result of the noise exposure alone or is it possible to explain it as a function of the additional stressor like vibration?

Manninen: They are a result of the noise.

Dengerink: If you look at the literature on catecholamines, it is extremely mixed. People have been able to demonstrate, for example, that beta blockers are effective in reducing blood pressure increases following noise exposure. The majority of the literature that I have been able to find indicates that noise exposure does not result in increased plasma catecholamine levels. That does not mean there may not be some increased activity of the autonomic nervous system that perhaps might show up in some of your urine samples.

Alberti: Are you referring to physiological responses, pathological responses, or responses bordering between these? Noise is very much part of everyday life, therefore a number of the responses are physiological.

Dengerink: I should have pointed out that the levels of angiotensin that we were infusing when we were looking at the changes in cochlear blood flow are doses which bracket the levels that we observe after we expose animals to noise. So it appeared the changes we were seeing in cochlear blood flow are responses to the same levels of angiotensin that we observe when we expose the animals to noise. I would suspect that in that case we are certainly working within the physiological range. When we talk about the catecholamine effects on cochlear blood flow, certainly the lower doses are within the physiological range.

Flottorp: I am concerned about what are pathological changes and what is natural physiology. We react as a living mechanism to a lot of stimuli.

Dengerink: Part of what we are suggesting here is that there are some normal physiological processes that occur in response to the noise stimulation. These are in fact appropriate, protective mechanisms that tend to help us deal with noise stimulation. In fact, increases in blood pressure and increases in cochlear blood flow are changes that one would anticipate to be appropriate, protective, kinds of responses. I am not at all suggesting that these are pathological. In fact, I would suggest just the opposite, that there are some normal physiological processes that are important in helping to protect us. Perhaps some of the variations we see in noise exposure studies results from variations in these physiological responses.

THE EFFECTS OF AGE, OTOLOGICAL FACTORS AND OCCUPATIONAL NOISE EXPOSURE ON HEARING THRESHOLD LEVELS OF VARIOUS POPULATIONS

Willy Passchier-Vermeer

TNO Institute of Preventive Health Care
Wassenaarseweg 56, 2333 Al Leiden
The Netherlands

INTRODUCTIONS

In this paper an analysis is presented of two investigations conducted in the Netherlands. One study concerns the effect of age on hearing threshold levels of populations not exposed to noise during working hours. The second investigation deals with the effect of occupational noise exposure on hearing threshold levels. There were about 500 test subjects in the first investigation and 2300 industrial workers in the second one. An analysis of the effects of otological factors on hearing threshold levels, based on both investigations, is given as well.

HEARING THRESHOLD LEVELS OF POPULATIONS NOT EXPOSED TO NOISE DURING WORKING HOURS

Many investigations have shown that hearing threshold levels increase progressively with age, and that this increase is a function of frequency. Spoor [1,2] published his analysis of data on the relation of hearing threshold levels to age. His analysis was mainly based on studies concerning more or less well-screened populations [3-8]. In 1978, Robinson et al. [9] published his analysis of investigations on the relations of hearing threshold levels with age. Based on all available literature - some 40 data sets - he analyzed the hearing threshold levels of three types of populations: (otologically and noise exposure) screened populations (S), otologically-unscreened populations (U) and populations of the mass survey type with public participation (P).

The results of the analysis of the screened populations S were the basis for ISO 7029 [10]. Since the analysis of Spoor [1,2] and that by Robinson [9] were largely based on the data of the same investigations, it was not surprising that it could be shown [11] that minor differences exist between the results presented by Spoor and those given by Robinson. If, in both sets of relations, the median hearing threshold levels at an age of 18 years (H(0,50;18)) are taken as zero, then the mean difference between the results of Spoor and those of Robinson is 0,25 dB for male populations and 0,33 dB female populations. In this respect, differences have been calculated for six frequencies from 500 to 6000 Hz, ages from 20 to 60 years, and percentages of hearing threshold levels from 10 to 90.

According to Robinson, the analysis dealing with unscreened (U or P) populations doses not present data suitable for consideration as the basis of an international standard.

ISO 7029 [10] specifies the median hearing threshold levels and the statistical distribution above and below the median value for audiometric frequencies in the range of 125 to 8000 Hz and for otologically normal persons within the age limits of 18 to 70 years. The data from ISO 7029 were incorporated in ISO/DIS 1999.1 [12] and ISO/DIS 1999.2 [13]. In ISO/ DIS 1999.1, annex A, the data from ISO 7029 [10] are given in data base A and are described in the text as highly screened, otologically normal populations. In addition, ISO/DIS 1999.1 gives an example of a data base, which comprises hearing threshold levels of a typical unscreened population of an industrialized country (data base B). The data for this data base are adapted from the results of a particular U.S.A. survey by the National Center for Health Statistics [14], and some subjects must be assumed to have had unreported occupational or other noise exposure.

Extensive research in the Netherlands industry showed that the hearing of unscreened groups of people, even when exposed to high noise levels during working hours, was in general (much) better than that specified in data base B, especially in he higher frequency range. Therefore, it was concluded that data base B could not be used as a basis for comparing hearing threshold levels of unscreened noise-exposed populations in order to determine the noise-induced part of the hearing loss. Using data base A for the same purpose did not seem correct either, since data base A comprises screened populations. Therefore, it was decided to determine the hearing threshold levels of otologically-unscreened populations. The research was limited to male persons, since in industry mainly males are exposed to high noise levels and the discrepancy for females between data base A and B was much smaller than that for males. After rejection of all persons with relevant noise exposure in present and previous jobs, the analysis of the data was carried out on the hearing threshold levels of nearly 500 test subjects. The test subjects were aged between 18 and 65 years.

Audiometric tests were carried out according to the specifications on ISO 6180 [15], with ambient sound pressure levels in the test room, allowing hearing threshold level measurements from 10 dB HL re ISO 389.

The hearing threshold levels of the test subjects, grouped into classes of 5 year width, were determined as a function of age. The same types of formulae were used as in ISO 7029 [10] for data base A, and the appropriate constants and parameters were determined using a second order regression analysis. As an example, the hearing threshold levels for 3000 Hz are given as a function of age in Fig. 1.

In Figs. 2 to 7, the hearing threshold levels are given as a function of age, together with the data of data base A and B. According to ISO 7029 [10] and Annex A of ISO/DIS 1999.1 [13], for practical purpose the median hearing threshold level at an age of 18 years (A(0,50;18)) may be taken as zero, as specified in ISO 389. In the figures, A(0,60;18) of data base A has therefore been taken equal to zero. However, according to Robinson et al [9], the figures for A(0,50;18 of data base A are not zero but as shown in Table 1. This Table also includes A(0,50;18) for the present research. Other figures of the statistical distribution of the hearing levels at an age of 18 years are also given in the Table. Table 1 touches upon the question of the audiometric zero, as specified in ISO 389. The audiometric zero represents the modal value of the hearing threshold levels of a group of screened people with ages between 18 and 30 years inclusive. This modal value at a mean age of 25 years differs at most a few decibels from the median value at an age of 18 years. According to the TNO-investigation

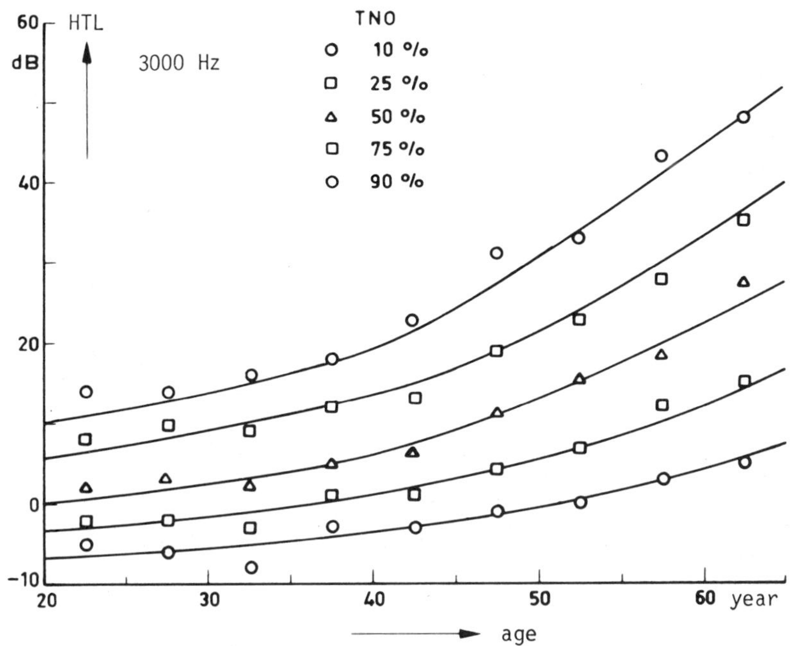

Fig. 1. Hearing threshold levels at 3000 Hz as a function of age. Plotted points are values of subgroups, divided according to age and curves are second regression lines.

Table 1. Hearing threshold levels (in dB) at an age of 18 years according to Robinson and the present TNO investigation

Frequency (Hertz)	Robinson			TNO		
	$A^*_{0,90}$	$A_{0,50}$	$A^*_{0,10}$	$A_{0,90}$	$A_{0,500}$	$A_{0,10}$
500	- 6,1	0,2	8,1	- 4,5	1,7	9,4
1000	- 6,4	- 0,1	7,8	- 5,1	1,2	8,5
2000	- 7,6	- 0,2	9,1	- 7,0	0,2	8,4
3000	- 5,8	2,2	12,2	- 6,8	0,5	10,3
4000	- 5,4	3,1	13,9	- 6,5	1,0	13,1
6000	2,2	11,9	24,1	- 6,5	2,7	12,3

*calculated according to ISO 7029, with $A_{0,50}$ taken as given in this Table.

[16,17], the median values at an age of 18 years are within a few decibels from the audiometric zero, even though the TNO investigation concerns otologically-unscreened populations. The correspondence between the median value of the TNO investigation and audiometric zero, is the first indication that otological screening of subjects does not affect hearing threshold levels to a large degree.

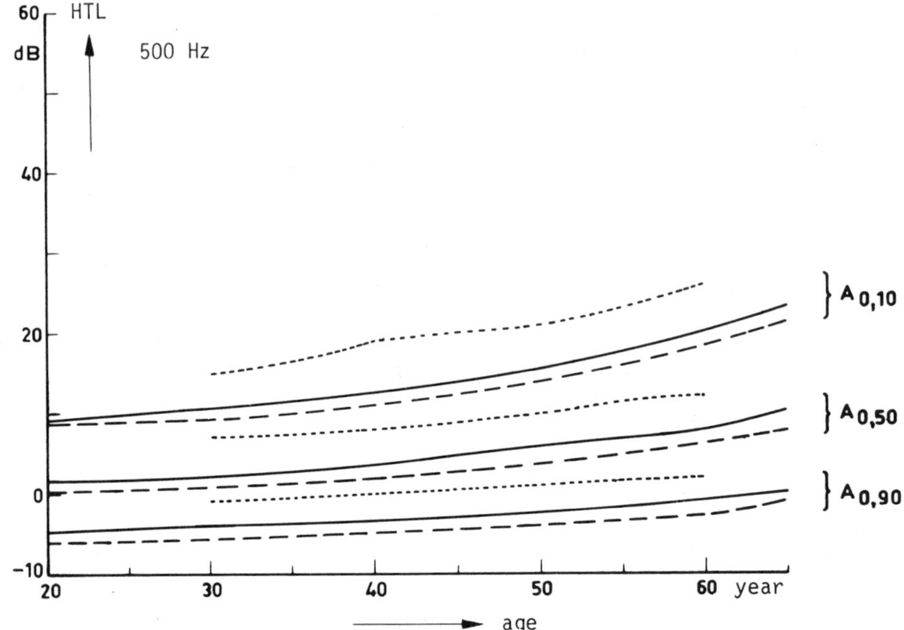

Fig. 2. Hearing threshold levels (A(0,10), A(0,50) and A(0,90) as a function of age according to the present (TNO) investigation (-------) ISO/DIS 1999.1, data base A(-------) and ISO/DIS 1999.1, Example of data base B(......).

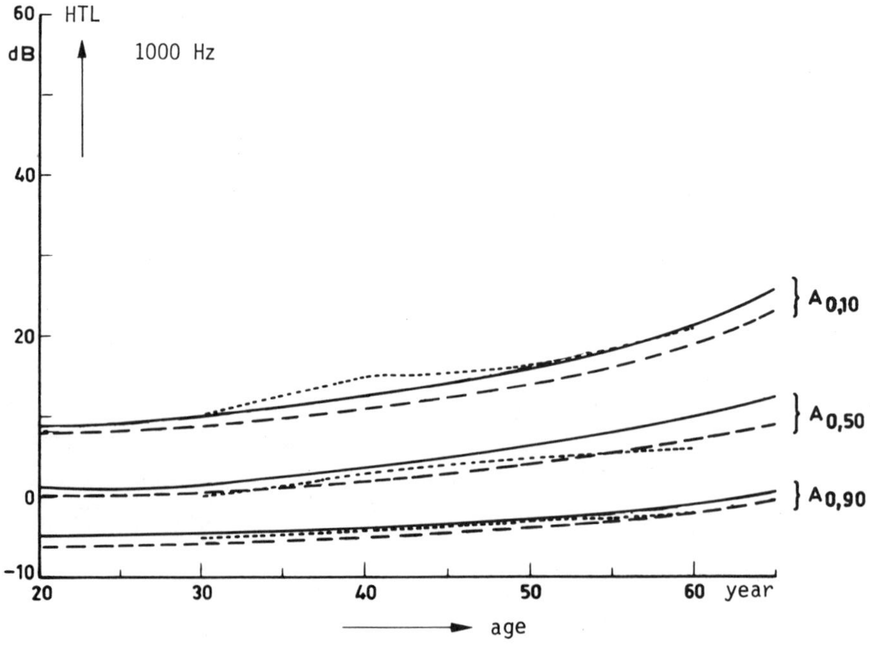

Fig. 3. Hearing threshold levels (A(0,10), A(0,50) and A(0,90)) as a function of age according to the present (TNO) investigation (------) ISO/DIS 1999.1, data base A(------) and ISO/DIS 1999.1, example of data base B(......)

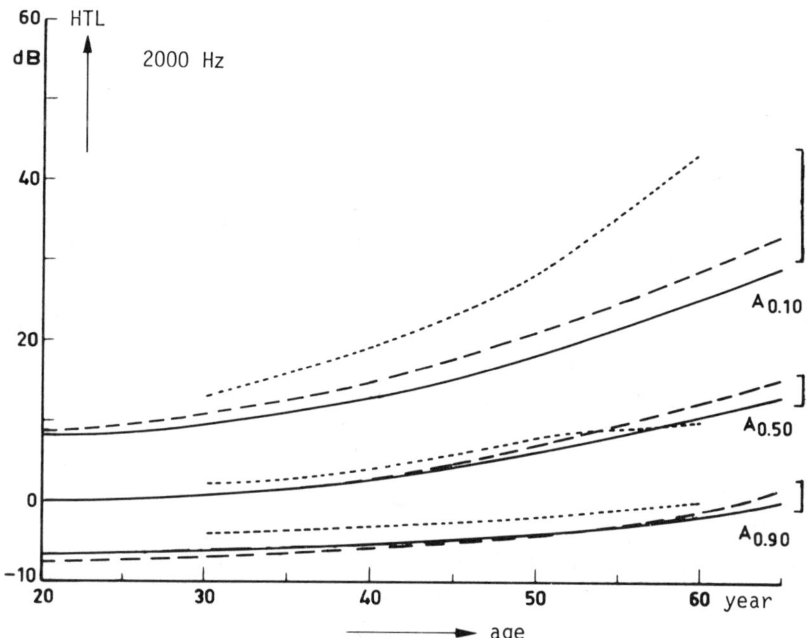

Fig. 4. Hearing threshold levels (A(0,10), A(0,50) and A(0,90) as a function of age according to the present (TNO) investigation (———) ISO/DIS 1999.1, data base A(------) and ISO/DIS 1999.1, example of data base B (......)

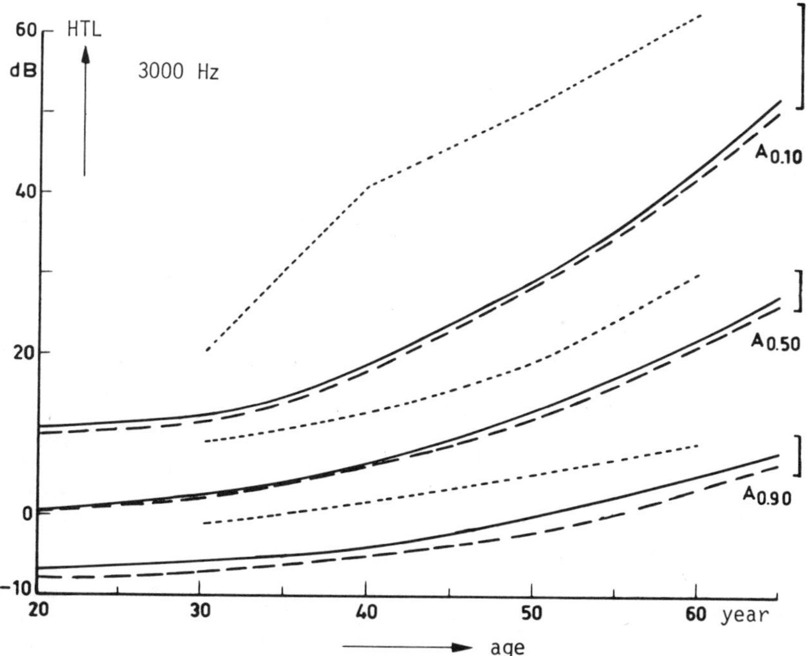

Fig. 5. Hearing threshold levels (A(0,10), A(0,50) and A(0,90)) as a function of age according to the present (TNO) investigation (———) ISO/DIS 1999.1, data base A(------) and ISO/DIS 1999.1, example of data base B(......).

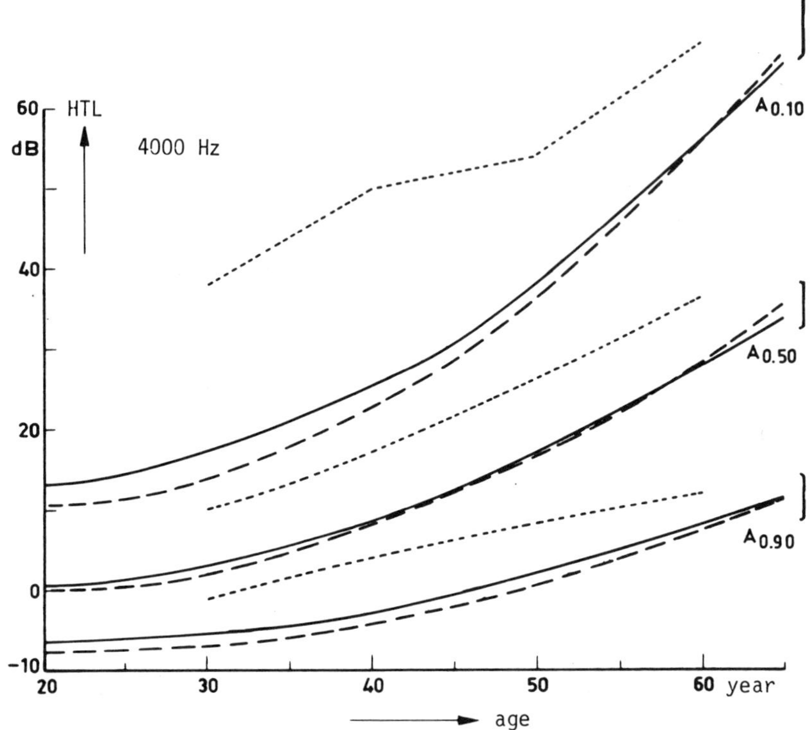

Fig. 6. Hearing threshold levels (A(0,10), A(0,50) and A(0,90)) as a function of age according to the present (TNO) investigation (------) ISO/DIS 1999.1, data base A(------) and ISO/DIS 1999.1, example of data base B(......)

In Figs. 8 and 9, examples of the results of the analysis are given for exposure times of 10 and 40 years and for fractiles of 0,90, 0,50 and 0,10. The N-values according to ISO/DIS 1999.1 are given as well. Comparing the TNO-relations with those from ISO/DIS 1999.1, it is obvious that the curves from the present investigation are less steep than the ISO-curves. At noise exposure levels between 85 and 90 dB(A) there is a rather good agreement between both sets of data.

At the lowest noise exposure levels, the N-values according to the present investigation are less than those according to ISO, at the highest noise exposure levels, the ISO-values exceed those of the present investigation. Possible explanations of the discrepancy between the present investigation and the ISO data on the N-values are:

- temporary threshold shift. Although audiometric tests have been performed only after 20 to 25 minutes after leaving the noisy working environment, a possible effect of TTS can not be excluded. This might explain the small differences between the ISO data and data of the present investigation at the lower noise exposure levels.
- the noise exposure level (L(EX,8h) as the only measure of the noise exposure, besides the exposure time. The N-values according to DIS/ISO 1999.1 were derived from exposures to constant noise. The only parameter of the

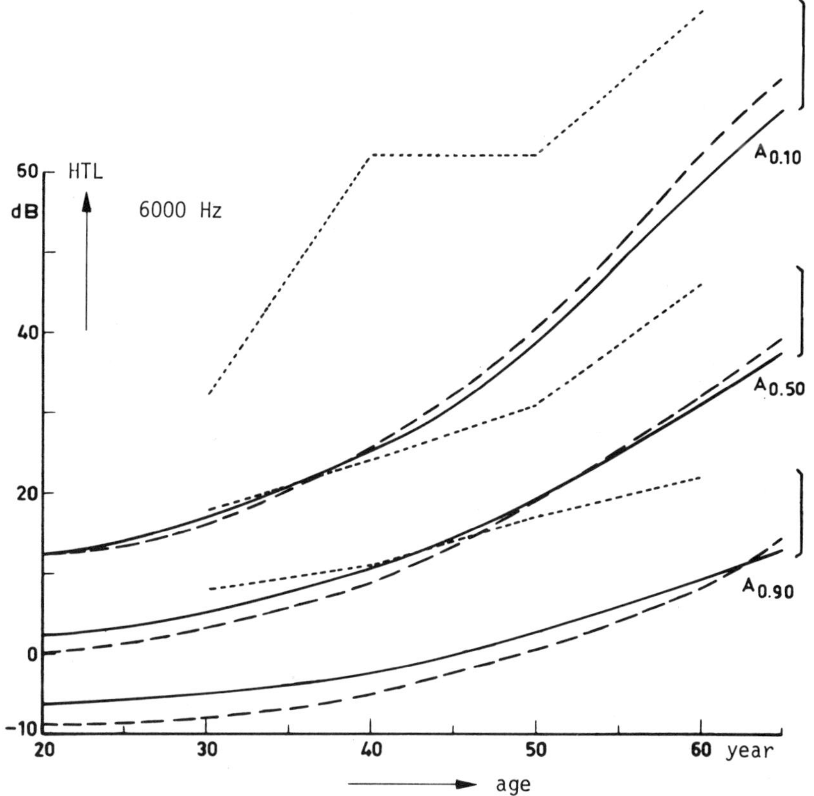

Fig. 7. Hearing threshold levels (A(0,10), A(0,50) and A(0,90)) as a function of age according to the present (TNO) investigation (------) ISO/DIS 1999.1, data base A(------) and ISO/DIS 1999.1, example of data base B(......)

noise exposure is then the measured sound level. The present investigation, however, concerns very divergent types of noise exposures: exposures to intermittent, fluctuating, constant, impulsive noises. If the noise exposure level is not the only parameter which determines noise-induced hearing loss, then the curves could indeed be less steep, which is in agreement with the observed discrepancy.

- the present noise exposure level as an estimation of past noise exposures. A large majority of the people concerned worked in their past in various not exactly known noise situations. Therefore, the noise exposure levels of the workers may have varied considerably during their working career; this phenomenon may indeed explain the discrepancy observed.
- the accuracy of the noise exposure levels determined in the present investigation. Although sound level measurements have been carried out carefully and estimations of exposure times have been made as accurate as possible, the determinations of the noise exposure levels are still based on observations/measurements during a limited time of some days up to some weeks. Therefore, the noise exposure levels, such as determined in the investigation, are only samples and the more complicated the situation, the less accurate the result. This might to some extent explain the discrepancy concerned.

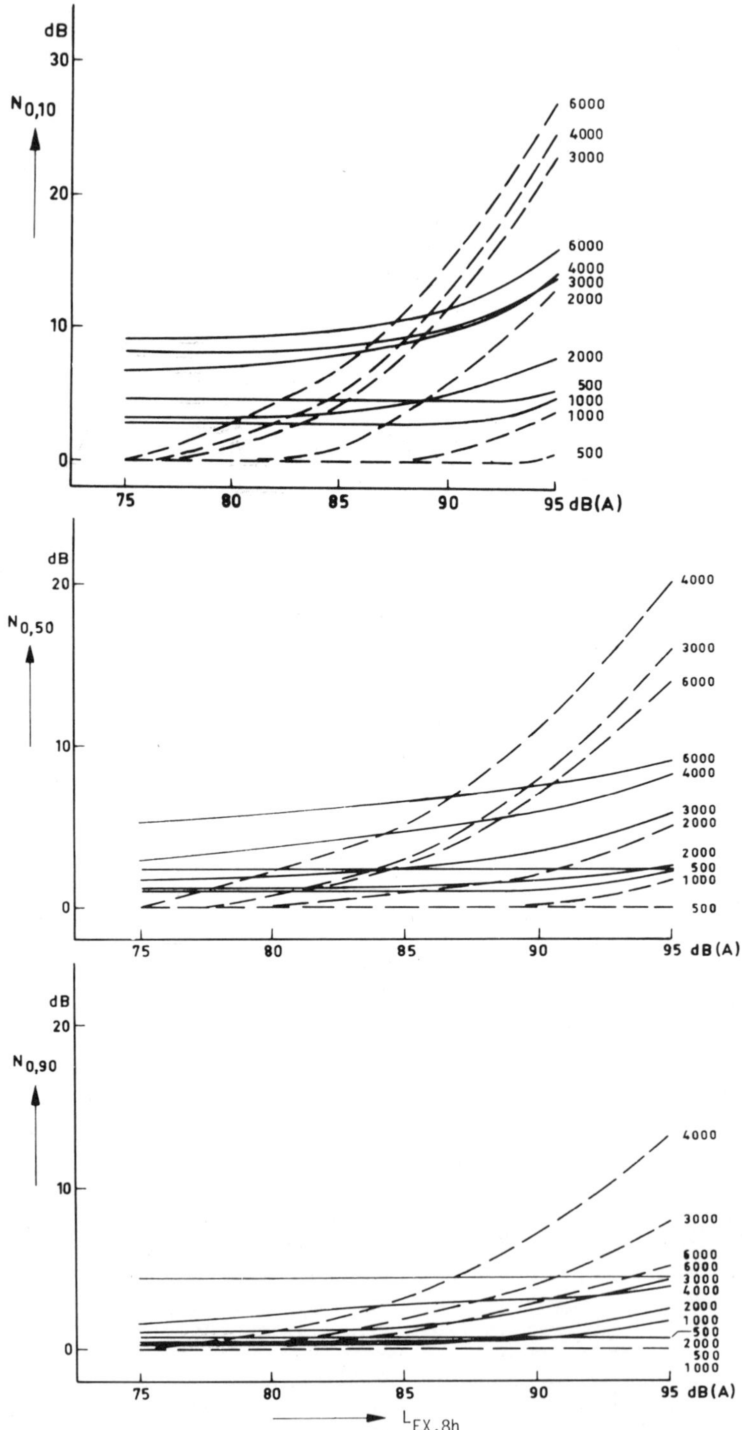

Fig. 8. Noise-induced hearing loss (N) for three fractiles (0,10; 0,50 and 0,90) as a function of noise exposure level (L(EX, 8h)). Plotted curves according to the present TNO investigation. Dotted curves according to ISO/DIS 1999.1 (and .2). Exposure time T: 10 years.

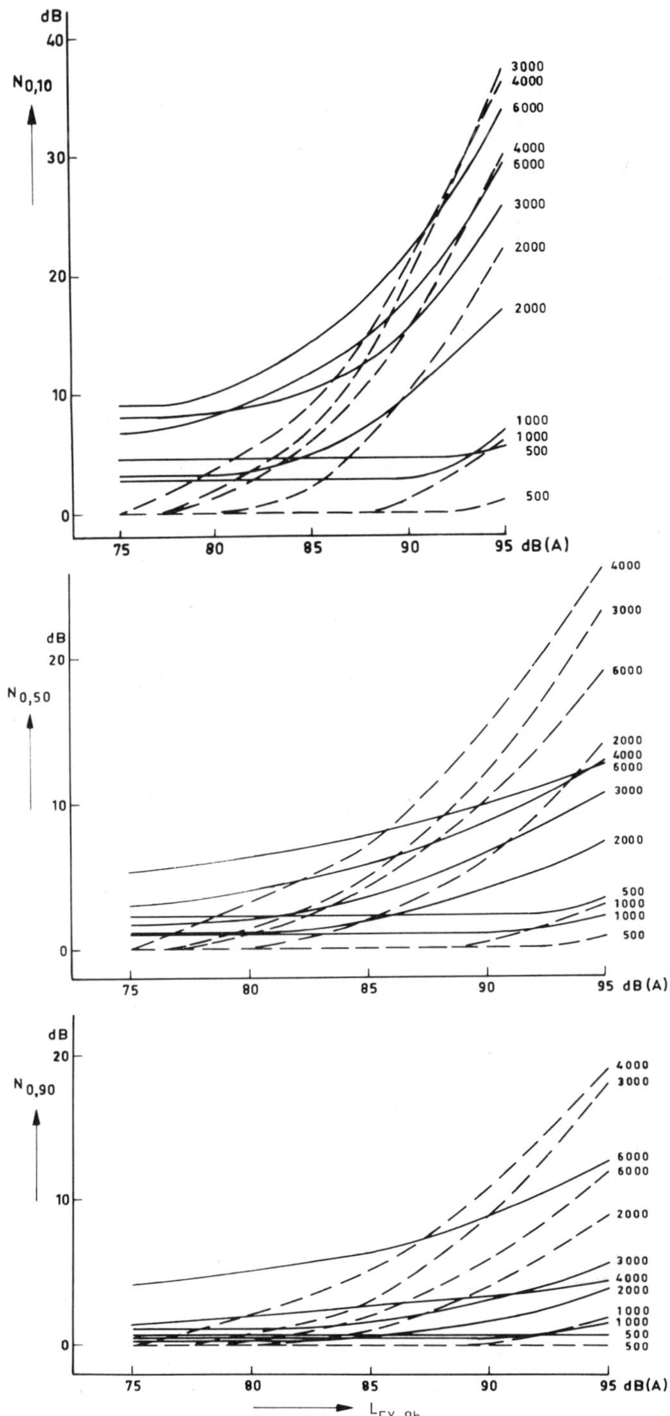

Fig. 9. Noise-induced hearing loss (N) for three fractiles (0,10; 0,50 and 0,10) as a function of noise exposure level (L(EX, 8h)). Plotted curves according to the present TNO investigation. Dotted curves according to ISO/DIS 1999.1 (and .2). Exposure time T: 40 years.

- the relations between noise exposure level and N, presented in ISO/DIS 1999.1, are incorrect.

With these possible explanations of the discrepancy between the ISO data and those of the present investigation in mind, further research data and relevant literature will be analyzed in the future.

Many countries have set limits of acceptable noise levels at workplaces at noise exposure levels in the range of 85 to 90 dB(A). Fortunately, in this range, there is a rather good agreement between the results of the present investigation and the N-data in ISO/DIS 1999.1.

REFERENCES

1. A. Spoor, Presbyacusis values in relation to noise-induced loss, Int. Audiol., 6:48-57 (1967).
2. A. Spoor, and W. Passchier-Vermeer, Spread in hearing levels of non-noise-exposed people at various ages, Int. Audiol., 8:328-336 (1969).
3. K. Jatho and K. H. Heck, Schwellenaudiometrische Untersuchungen uber di Progredienz und Charakteristik der Alterschwerhorigkeit in den verschiedenen Lebensabschnitten, Zeitschr. Laryng. Rhinol. Otol., 38:72-88 (1959).
4. J. F. Corso, Age and sex differences in pure-tone thresholds, Arch. Otolaryngol., 77:385-405 (1938).
5. R. Hinchcliffe, The threshold of hearing as a function of age, Acustica, 9:303-308 (1959).
6. A. Glorig and J. Nixon, Hearing loss as a function of age, Laryngoscope, 72:1596-1610 (1962).
7. A. Glorig, D. Wheeler, R. Quiggle, W. Gringe and A. Summerfield, 1954 Wisconsin State Fair Hearing Survey: Statistical treatment of clinical and audiometric data. Am. Academy of Ophth. and Otolaryngol., Los Angeles (1957).
8. W. C. Beasley, The National Health Survey, 1935-1936, U.S. Public Health Service (1938).
9. D. W. Robinson and G. J. Sutton, A comparative analysis of data on the relation of pure-tone audiometric thresholds to age, NPL Acoustics Report Ac 84 (1978).
10. International Organization for Standardization 7029, Acoustics-Threshold of hearing by air conduction as a function of age and sex for otologically normal persons (1983).
11. W. Passchier-Vermeer, Preventie gehoorschade door lawaai, Voordrachten ter gelegenheid van het 10-jarig jubileum van de NVBA, gehouden op 18 oktober 1985, NIPG-TNO (1985).
12. International Organization for Standardization DIS/ISO 1999.1, (1982).
13. DIS/ISO 1999.2, Acoustics-Determination of occupational noise exposure and estimation of noise-induced hearing impariment (1985).
14. National Center for Health Statistics, Hearing levels of adults by age and sex, United States 1960-72, Vital and Health Statistics, Public Health Service Publication No. 1000, Series 11, No. 11, Washington, D. C., U. S. Government Printing Office (1965).
15. International Organization for Standardization 6189, Acoustics pure tone air conduction threshold audiometry for hearing conservation purposes (1983).
16. W. Passchier-Vermeer, Audiometrie en Anamnese, TNO-rappart B 610 (1984).
17. W. Passchier-Vermeer, Groepsaudiogram en Lawaaiexpositieniveau, TNO-rapport B 626 (1984).

DISCUSSION

Axelsson: What was the screening procedure for Data Base A? Were people with previous military service included or were they taken out of Data Base A? Also, do the industrial workers, working in noise, use ear protection? Were they included or not?

Passchier-Vermeer: Data Base A is comprised of men not working in noisy surroundings in their present and previous jobs. If a person has a noisy job during military service, such as aircraft maintenance, he was excluded from the data base as well, Also, men who occasionally were exposed to gunfire during military service were not excluded from Data Base A.

To determine the relation between noise and noise-induced hearing loss, those industrial workers who wore hearing protection regularly were excluded.

von Gierke: I just want to stress one point. The ISO standard proposal does not include a specific Data Base B. It says Data Base B can be used by any user of the standard by using the unscreened data base of the polulation he is studying, and the standard only includes an example of a Data Base B, which happens to be more or less the Public Health Service Data collected in the USA more than 15 or 20 years ago. But it clearly says this is only an example of a Data Base B, and every investigator or every country or every industrial concern may collect its own representative Data Base B.

Passchier-Vermeer: Being a member of the working group which prepared ISO/DIS 1999.1, I am well aware of the background material and the phrasing of this draft Standard. The main reason why the Public Health Service data were not included in the draft Standard, but were only given as an example of Data Base B in an annex, was the lack of trust in the reliability of the PHS-data. Nevertheless, even as an example in an annex to the draft Standard, the PHS-data is the most serious, since it results in an extreme underestimation of noise-induced hearing loss.

Alberti: I think there is a need for a Data Base C. The Data Base B is Public Health Service, comprised of people not privy to modern audiological health treatment for ear disease. In The Netherlands, a country with good hearing health case, where problems of conductive losses have presumably been eliminated, unscreened populations will contain much less hearing loss. So each country should have its own current standards, because the management of hearing and ear disease varies from country to country, and incidence varies from town to town.

CURRENT PERSPECTIVES ON ISSUES IN PERSONAL HEARING PROTECTION

P. W. Alberti and S. M. Abel

Silverman Hearing Research Laboratory, Department of Otolaryngology, Mount Sinai Hospital Institute and Faculty of Medicine, University of Toronto, Toronto, Ontario, Canada

INTRODUCTION

It remains difficult to obtain a perspective on the role and the potential of hearing protectors in hearing conservation programs because of the wide range of disciplines involved in this work, the diverse publications in which the findings are published and the wish for confidentiality of findings that is equally apparent in industry and the military. At a major meeting held in Toronto in 1980, papers were presented on a wide range of topics encompassing engineering, physiology, epidemiology, and national standards [1]. At that meeting, many of the remaining problems were identified. They included:

1. Significant criticism of current standard methods of measuring the effectiveness of hearing protectors and, in particular, the NRR scales.
2. The lack of an adequate artificial head and ear on which to make standard measurements of protectors, which bear some relationship to real life.
3. The extremely wide range of attenuation provided to the work force by a variety of theoretically appropriate protectors.
4. The discrepancy between attenuation obtained in the laboratory and that found in field tests.
5. The relative paucity of information about the effectiveness of hearing protectors in protecting a noise exposed population from hearing loss.
6. Problems related to communication while wearing ear protectors, including the perception of warning signals.
7. Difficulty related to wearing multiple protectors.

This paper concentrates on three areas:

a) Sex differences in the effectiveness of certain plug-type protectors.
b) Real ear testing technique in high-level noise.
c) Problems related to communication while wearing hearing protectors.

SEX DIFFERENCES IN THE EFFECTIVENESS OF CERTAIN PLUG-TYPE HEARING PROTECTORS

We have been impressed by anecdotal comments that certain hearing protectors may work less effectively in women than in men. There are occasional allusions to this in the literature [2]. That this has not, to our knowledge, been systematically studied previously, may relate to the large number of studies on hearing protector effectiveness initiated by the military, by the overwhelmingly male work force in heavy industry and by the suggestion that women have "tougher" ears and are thus less damaged [3]. We have initiated a study to determine whether the anecdotal evidence is correct and, if so, to find out why.

Preliminary findings are presented here which will be published in detail elsewhere. Three types of plugs were studied: the E A R, the Bilsom soft, and the Willson (Fig.1). The E A R is a foam polymer plug of single size. It is compressed between finger and thumb, placed into the ear canal and allowed to expand to occlude the canal. It is a widely used protective device. The Bilsom soft is a preformed soft plug composed of glass fibre down bulk surrounding a foam core which is enclosed in a thin plastic film. It is soft and easily inserted. It too, comes in one size. The Willson is a double phlanged soft plug with an air filled centre core which comes in standard and small size.

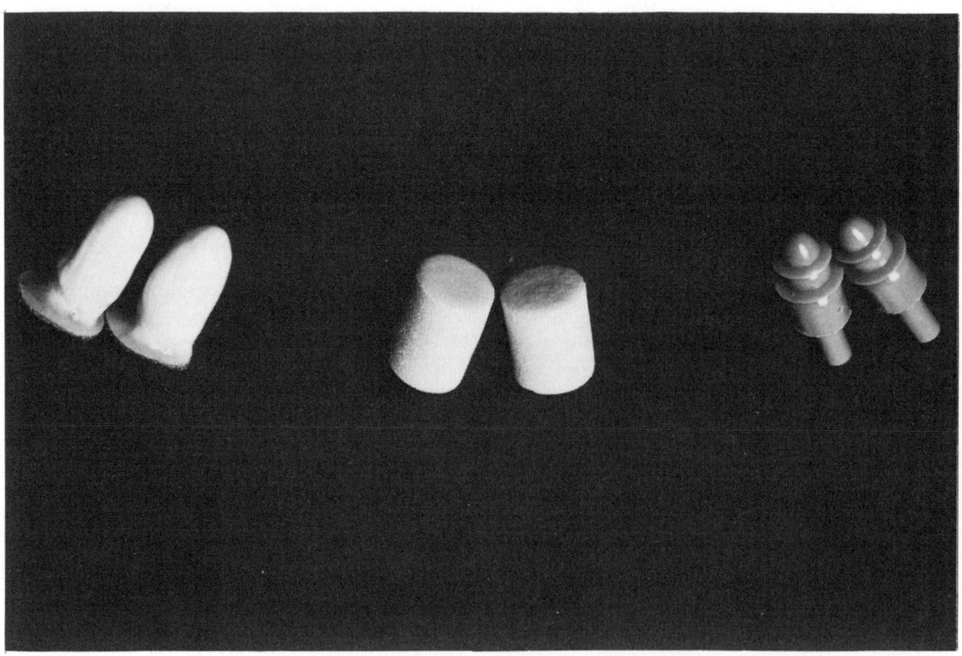

Fig. 1. The 3 types of ear plug used, from left to right, the Willson[R], the E A R[R], and the Bilsom[R] soft.

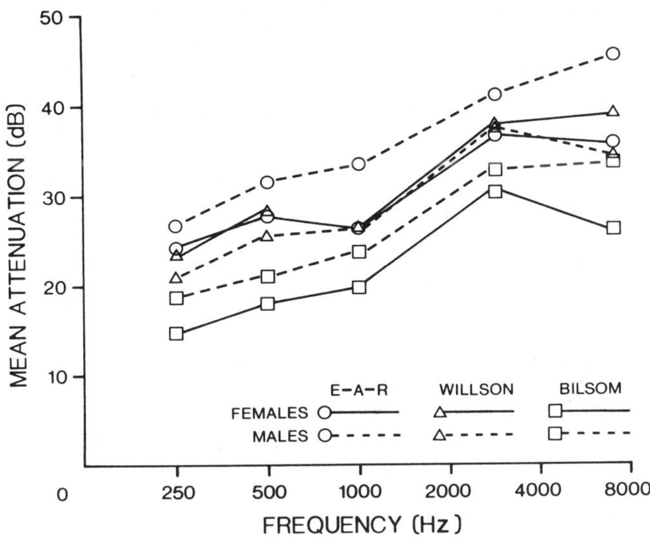

Fig. 2. Attenuation data for 3 types of hearing protector in men and women [9].

While our experiments are still ongoing, they are substantially complete. Studies have been performed on twenty subjects, ten male and ten female in each group, each of whom underwent threshold attenuation tests, under earphones in a sound proof booth (IAC), using one-third octave band noise.

Fig. 2 shows the attenuation for males and females at five frequencies. It can be seen that the mean and range of attenuation for males is significantly greater than for females using the E A R plug. Fig. 2 shows similar results for the Bilsom plug. There is a significant, but less marked difference. There seems to be no real differences between the results utilizing the Willson plug. As far as this small group of subjects is concerned, the anecdotal comments are correct. Confirmation of these findings in the field is required. The explanation is likely to be related to ear canal size, both diameter and length. The E A R plug is fairly firm and of one size only. To be effective, it must be inserted fairly deeply into the ear canal. Women find it less comfortable than men, largely because of the increased pressure of the plug on the smaller diameter ear canal. They also appear to have difficulty in passing it deeply into the canal. Thus, we are currently investigating both shape and size of adult male and adult female ear canals in an attempt to determine the sex variation in ear canal shape and size. We have also started a study of chewing and jaw movement on the attenuation characteristics of protectors. It is theorized that a superficially placed protector is more readily "chewed out" than a deeply placed one. The effectiveness of the Willson plug in women may be related to its initial shorter size and the fact that a smaller diameter is available for people with small ear canals.

MEASURING TECHNIQUES

We have published several papers [4-7] utilizing free-field real-ear threshold techniques to define the attenuation of a variety of hearing protectors. The measurements typically fall below the manufacturer's specifications by 5 to 10 dB on average. There has always been a nagging question whether protectors are as effective in the high levels of sound for which they are intended as they are in threshold measurements obtained in the laboratory. A method of measuring attenuation of protectors in high-level noise is a prerequisite for studying the interaction of hearing protectors and warning signals in the high levels of sound found in industry. Direct measuring techniques utilizing miniature microphones, in the ear canal and outside the protector, have become feasible as a means of testing muff style protectors, but remain inappropriate for testing plugs. My co-author, Sharon Abel, and her colleagues, Hans Kunov and Kathy Fuller and I have devised and tested a Psychoacoustic technique which relies on signal detection theory to measure the attentuation of protectors in high levels of sound.

In brief, the technique consists of a two-interval, forced choice procedure, with events signalled by using a response box. The test is performed using open headphones (Yamaha electrostatic) to provide the signals. In our study, each trial began with a half second warning light followed in succession by two listening periods of 500 milliseconds each. These are shown on the response box by a synchronous light, first on the left and then on the right. A narrow-band signal is used as a stimulus; this occurred during one of the periods of listening either against a quiet or against a noise background. The signal itself had a peak time of 200 milliseconds (rise and fall at each 100 millisecond). The subject had to decide whether the signal occurred in the first or second listening period and indicate which interval by pushing an appropriate button. The response was automatically recorded. Each test consists of a block of 50 trials, the signal occurring randomly in the first or second interval with a probability of 0.5. Across blocks, the level of the signal was varied in order to generate a psychoacoustic function with values for probability of a correct response ranging from 0.50 to 1.00. The details of the procedure have been published previously. It can be seen that this technique allows the study of various signals against various types of background noise.

The procedure can be performed with an open ear canal or wearing ear plugs. In one set of experiments, subjects were asked to detect the signal first in a quiet background without protectors, then in quiet, wearing protectors so that the subjects would be experienced with the signal to be detected and to prevent potential problems with TTS. The results of a normal study are shown in Fig. 4. As the signal intensity is increased to an audible level, the probability of a correct response rises. The 75 percent point is defined as detection threshold, i.e., the detection threshold is the value giving P(C) = 0.75. We subtract the detection thresholds for the open and closed ears to get the attenuation for each frequency. This value is close to that obtained using a standard free-field threshold measurement procedure. It can be seen that in this experiment, in which the listener was wearing an E A R plug, attenuation of a 3 kHz narrow-band signal by the plug is approximately 45 decibels. The experiment was repeated against a background of both steady state and high-level impact noise. Millhouse noise, a steady state noise, and drilling noise, an impact sound, both recorded in Ontario industry were used. When these two sounds were used as background, the detection threshold in a normal hearing subject increased significantly to between 70 and 80 decibels, which corresponds to the levels at which the background sound was presented. Interestingly, in normals, the wearing of protectors lowered the threshold of detectability by about 3 decibels compared to the condition without protectors.

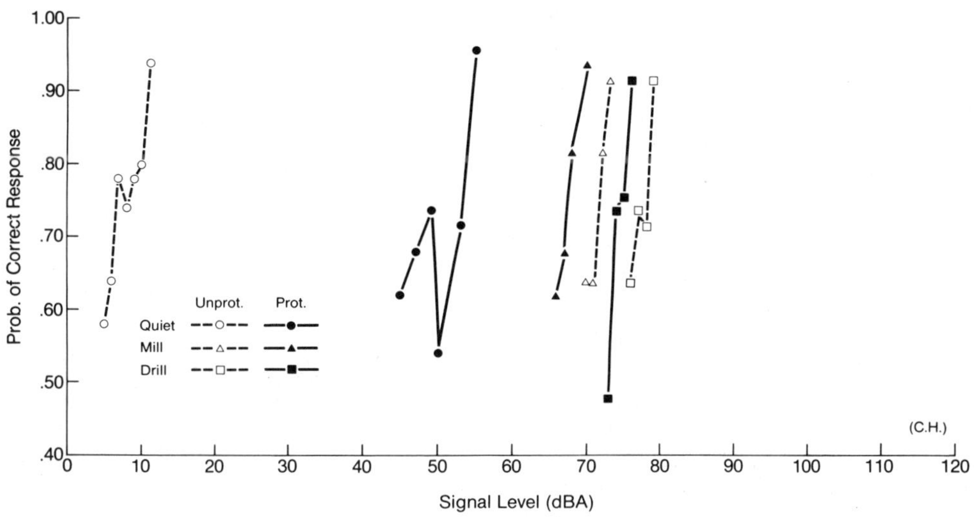

Fig. 3. Detection of a 3 kHz narow-band signal for a subject with normal hearing [9].

The experiment was repeated using a subject with noise-induced hearing loss affecting both 1 and 3 kHz. It is a fairly typical severe loss of a type caused by prolonged exposure to industrial noise. Again, in the signal detection experiment the signals were presented to both ears with and without background noise. The background noise was similar, either mill or drilling noise and the subject wore or did not wear hearing protectors. The pattern of results is very different from that of normals (Fig. 4). The

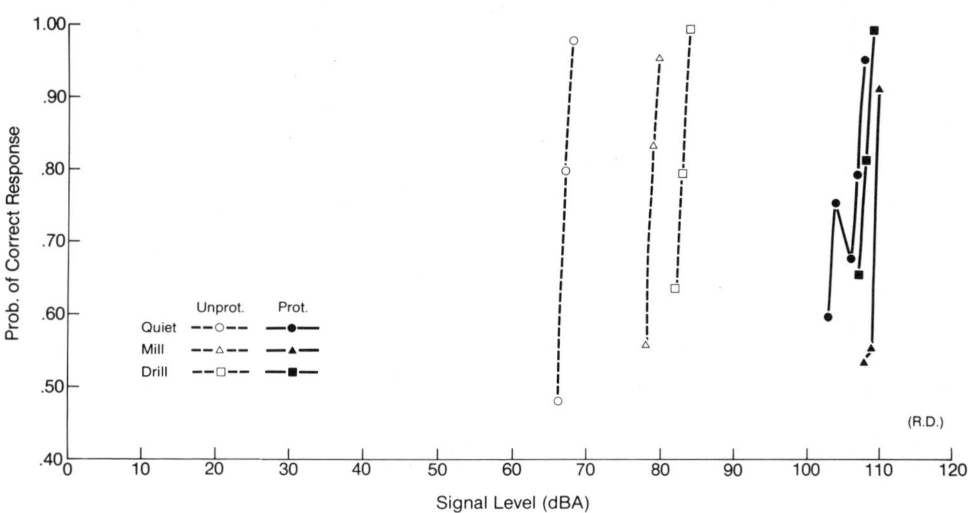

Fig. 4. Detection of a 3 kHz narrow-band signal for a subject with noise induced hearing loss at 1 and 3 kHz [9].

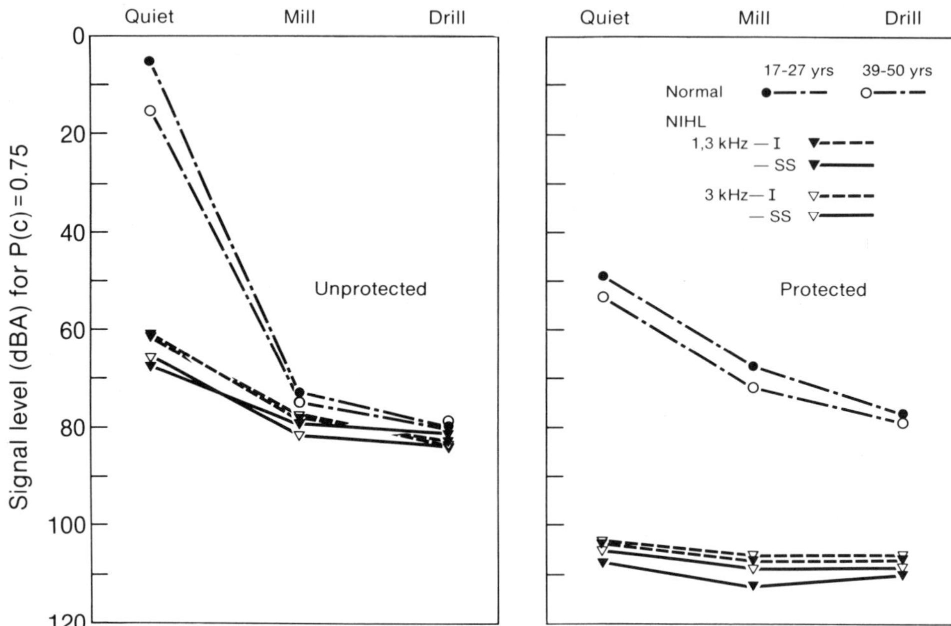

Fig. 5. Group detection of a narrow-band signal centered at 3 kHz [9].

threshold for listening in quiet was raised to 67 dBA and listening in high-level noise shifted the function by less than 20 dB as compared with the shift of 80 dB for the normal listener. Thus, in noise, without protectors, the hearing-impaired person has threshold detection approximately the same as the normal subject. However, when plugs are inserted the detection threshold under all conditions shifted to about 105 dBA. The wearing of protectors thus brings the subject to the limit of hearing as defined audiometrically. Furthermore, the ability to detect a signal, far from being enhanced by use of the protectors, was grossly impaired.

Pooled data from many subjects of two age groups are shown in Fig. 5. The circles indicate normal old and young subjects, and the triangle subjects with hearing losses at 1 kHz and 3 kHz respectively. The detection of signals at 3 kHz is significantly impaired without protection, but is at near normal levels against a background noise. When using protectors, the threshold for signals in quiet is raised, but the ability to detect background noise is improved in the normal listeners whereas wearing protectors grossly interferes with the detection of signals in quiet as well as in noise in the hearing impaired worker. No age differences was detected.

We believe that this technique has considerable application, but needs to be extended to different types and levels of background noise and different signals before broad conclusions can be drawn. However, our results, based on 3 groups (namely workers with high-frequency loss affecting only 3 kHz and above, workers with a loss at both 1 and 3 kHz and normals) using the types and level of noise commonly found in industry and give cause for thought. In general, for those with moderate noise-induced hearing loss, the wearing of protectors did not change the level of signal necessary for threshold detection at the lower frequency of 1 kHz in contrast to the shift noted for 3 kHz. Wearing plugs in quiet increased the detection threshold by roughly 35 decibels, a value equivalent to the manufacturers' specified attenuation for E A R plugs at 1 kHz. Subjects with normal hearing or mild loss at 1 kHz showed neither consistent improvement nor worsening when wearing protectors in noise. In contrast, the 3 kHz thresholds showed a significant decrement in detection in a hearing impaired population. The key factor, we believe, is the additive effect of sensorineural hearing loss and the attenuation produced by protectors; the combination of factors effectively deafens people so that the sense of hearing is globally impaired. Details of these results can be found elsewhere [8,9].

We have developed and tested a model of the preceding findings which is illustrated here [9]. The variables taken into account are the presence and spectrum of background noise, the frequency of the signal, the attenuation of the protector and the configuration of the hearing loss. This allows us to predict the average detection threshold for signals by our subjects. In order to obtain the predicted value of each individual, a simple algorithm was developed. Given the particular narrow-band spectrum and intensity of a signal, the corresponding octave value of background noise is determined. Then the attenuation specified by the manufacturer for the hearing protector under test is subtracted from that value of background noise. If the end sum is greater than the individual's unprotected detection threshold in quiet, then the predicted value is equivalent to the octave noise level of the test frequency. If this value is less than the detection threshold in quiet, then the predicted value is equivalent to the detection threshold in quiet plus the attentuation of the protector. Hopefully, this model will allow one to specify the appropriate attenuation for an individual's hearing loss while working in noise, and maximize signal detection and hearing conservation at the same time.

This raises the whole issue of communication problems in noise. In general terms, a worker may be exposed to verbal instructions and to warning signals. The latter can be divided into two groups: (1) primary warning such as roof noise in a mine or an unusual sound in a machine indicating malfunction and (2) secondary warning, that is, when there is potential or actual danger which triggers specific warning signals, e.g., the noise made by trucks reversing, the whistle of a locomotive, the blare of a fire alarm.

There is concern, and perhaps some confusion, in all three areas. Let us deal first with speech signals. The pioneering work of Kryter [10] showed that in normal hearing listeners, the use of hearing protector did not degrade discrimination of monosyllabic words and indeed there was some advantage. On the other hand, in the industrial situation, Howell and Martin [11] showed that when the speaker as well as listener were wearing hearing protectors, intelligibility was reduced, even though hearing was normal. The explanation was that the speakers reduced their own voice level because of the apparently diminished background sound. There have been several studies of interaction between the wearing of hearing protectors and signal intelligibility in sensorineural hearing impaired subjects [12-16]. Our own work in this area has also taken into account the age of subjects and fluency in the language of the test material, in this instance, English. This latter matter is important because of the mobility of work forces and the ensuing language difficulties that may occur. In our own province, approximately one third of a large sample of compensation claimants spoke neither English nor French (the official Canadian tongues) as their native language [17].

The experimental groups in our study were fluent and non-fluent, hearing-impaired and normal subjects of two age groups. Intelligibility was tested using a list of monosyllabic words in quiet, or in a background of white noise or crowd noise, with and without hearing protectors. Intelligibility varied significantly with hearing configuration, the background noise and fluency. However, there was no interaction between hearing category and fluency; the non-fluent subject had a 10-20 percent decrement in speech intelligibility across all conditions. We also found no age effect. Protectors did make a difference. In normal hearing subjects, they marginally improved intelligibility, thus confirming the initial observations of Kryter. In hearing impaired workers, intelligibility was significantly impaired. The difference between protected and unprotected conditions was determined by attenuation of the hearing protector.

Detection of warning signals by investigators such as Wilkins and Martin [18] and Lambert [19] have given differing results, either showing an elevated threshold or no difference. However, virtually all these studies have been performed with normal hearing subjects. Our own studies of signal detection in noise, as reported earlier, indicate to us the need for careful re-evaluation of warning signal intensity and frequency where this is possible. With primary warning signals such as a malfunctioning machine, this may not be practical.

There are alternative solutions although they are relatively costly. The same problems concern the military. The infantry man, perhaps operating a mobile anti-tank device, requires protection from the noise of his device, but at the same time, he must be able to hear environmental sound. The pilot in his cockpit must be able to hear speech. The solution to both is some form of active hearing protector [20-22] in which quiet sounds are amplified and loud sounds suppressed. In its simplest form, one may think of it as a hearing aid with a significant output limiting circuit and a tight fitting mold producing attenuation. Thus, quiet sounds are amplified, intermediate sounds amplified less, and loud sounds attenuated. There are several variations on this theme including devices which measure the sound level within the protector and use that to regulate the input signal; these are incorporated into helmets and communication sets devised for pilots. (The sound level within the cockpit of modern strike aircraft may well exceed 110 decibels). This type of device has also been recommended for industry as, for example, in mining where noise level may be intermittent and where it is necessary to communicate and hear a variety of mine noises. For example, Durkin has demonstrated that the intelligibility of speech using active protectors in coal miners is significantly increased if wearing the standard passive protector.

CONCLUSIONS

These studies in general emphasize once again the need to listen to the consumer. The workforce in general, particularly the older workforce, has been concerned about the harmful effects of introducing hearing protectors. This is in contrast with new entries who appear to accept them willingly. The difference may well be due to the former already having impaired hearing and the latter having normal hearing. No hearing conservation program based on hearing protectors of which we know takes into account the existing hearing level of the workforce. The "cri de coeur" of the workers is real and based on experience; the hard of hearing worker is deafened by protectors and may have difficulty in hearing speech and detecting warning signals when using them. This philosophy is at last incorporated into one national standard.

The blunderbus approach to hearing protecters should in our opinion be abandoned. More is not always better; appropriate should be the guiding phrase. In relatively low level noise, protectors which provide the greatest attenuation may be neither necessary nor appropriate. With a background noise level of 90 decibels, do we really require a 20 decibel attenuator? These matters should be taken into account when instituting hearing conservation programs. We have no solution to offer for the problems inherent in safety and communication previously described for an existing hard of hearing population to whom a hearing conservation program is introduced. We strongly believe that this is an ignored topic by legislators and we hope at least to draw attention to it.

REFERENCES

1. P. W. Alberti, "Personal Hearing Protection in Industry", Raven Press, New York (1982).
2. S. E. Forshaw and J. I. Cruchley, Protector problems in military operations, in: "Personal Hearing Protection in Industry," P. W. Alberti, ed., Raven Press, New York (1982).
3. L. H. Royster and J. D. Royster, Methods of evaluating hearing conservation program audiometric data bases, in: "Personal Hearing Protection in Industry," P. W. Alberti, ed., Raven Press, New York (1982).
4. S. M. Abel, P. W. Alberti, and K. Riko, User fitting of hearing protectors: attenuation results, in: "Personal Hearing Protection in Industry," Raven Press, New York (1982).
5. P. W. Alberti, Hearing protectors: attenuation in practice and problems, in: "Proceedings of Noise-Con 81," L. H. Royster, F. D. Hart and N. D. Sterwart, eds., New York (1981).
6. P. W. Alberti, S. M. Abel, and K. Riko, Practical aspects of hearing protector use, in: "New Perspectives on Noise-Induced Hearing Loss," R. P. Hamernik, D. Henderson, and R. Salvi, eds., Raven Press, New York (1982).
7. P. W. Alberti, K. Riko, S. M. Abel, and R. Kristensen, The effectiveness of hearing protectors in practice, J. Otol. 8:354 (1979).
8. S. M. Abel, H. Kunov, M. K. Pichora-Fuller, and P. W. Alberti, The effect of hearing protection on narrow band signal detection in industrial noise, J. Otol. 12:83 (1983).
9. S. M. Abel, H. Kunov, M.K. Pichora-Fuller, and P.W. Alberti, Signal detection in industrial noise: effects of noise exposure, history, hearing loss and use of ear protection, Scand. Audiol. Suppl. (In Press)
10. K. D. Kryter, Effects of ear protective devices on the intelligibility of speech in noise, J. Acoust. Soc. Am. 18:413 (1946).
11. K. Howell and A. M. Martin, An investigation of the effects of hearing protectors on vocal communication in noise, J. Sound Vib. 41:181, (1975).
12. E. H. Berger, The effects of hearing protectors on auditory communications, EARlog #3, E-A-R Division, Cabot Corporation, (1979).
13. A. H. Suter, The ability of mildly hearing impaired individuals to discriminate speech in noise, Aerospace Medical Research Lab., Wright-Patterson Air Force Base, Ohio (1978).
14. T. L. Rink, Hearing protection and speech discrimination in hearing impaired persons, Sound and Vib. 13:22, (1979).

15. D. Y. Chung and R. P. Gannon, The effect of ear protectors on word discrimination in subjects with normal hearing and subjects with noise-induced hearing loss, J. Amer. Aud. Soc. 5:11,(1979).
16. S. M. Abel and C. A. Haythornthwaite, The progression of noise induced hearing loss - survey of workers in selected canadian industries, J. Otol. Suppl. 13, (1984).
17. P. W. Alberti and R. B. Blair, Occupational hearing loss, Laryngoscope 92:535 (1982).
18. P. A. Wilkins and A. M. Martin, The effects of hearing protection on the perception of warning sounds, in: "Personal Hearing Protection in Industry, P. W. Alberti, ed., Raven Press, New York (1982).
19. D. R. Lambert, Effects of hearing protectors on thresholds of machinery cues in noise, (Experiment 1: Naive Subjects), Technical Paper, Naval Ocean Systems Center, San Diego, Calif (1980).
20. J. Durkin, Effective electronic hearing protectors on speech intelligibility, Report of an Investigation 83580, United States Department of the Interior Bureau of Mines, (1979).
21. P. D. Wheeler, A. Howard, and S. G. Halliday, An active noise reduction system for air crew helmets, AGARD Conf. 311, paper 22, (1981).
22. D. W. Maxwell, C. E. William, R. M. Ritson, G. P. Thomas, Evaluation of two active hearing protective devices, J. Acoust. Soc. of Am. Suppl. 1, 76S44, (1984).

DISCUSSION

Borchgrevink: We have had a problem with the hearing of helicopter pilots in the Norwegian Armed Forces because the low frequency content of the noise in the helicopter is insufficiently damped by headsets. We introduced ear plugs on the inside, so that they wore plugs plus the headset. The subjects were requested to be certain that their speech perception was good. Our results are very much like yours. Young people with normal hearing, jumped to the solution immediately. The older people found they had trouble. So I think your point is very well take. If we could ever have a flat attenuation device, not only for moderate, but also for high level dampling, the situation would be greatly improved.

Van der Venne Marcel: Regarding the efficiency and attenuation of protectors in high noise levels, I am sure you are aware of the existence of a French method which has been standardized. The procedure which, by using bone conduction, allows the subjective determination of attenuation in rather high noise levels. They are using levels around 100 dBA background noise. This method has been compared with the standard ISO method. The attenuation factors were determined for the same protectors, the same conditions and the same subjects. To my knowledge, it is the first time that this has been done. The results are that there is a small, but statistically significant difference around 3-5 dB less attenuation measured by the French standardized method than with the ISO method.

HEARING CONSERVATION AND IMPULSE NOISE IN THE BRITISH ARMY

M. R. Forrest

Army Personnel Research Establishment
c/o Royal Aircraft Establishment
Farnborough, Hants, GU 14 6 TD, UK

INTRODUCTION

Army service has always presented a risk to hearing from impulse noise in addition to noise from small arms, with a typical peak pressure of 160 dB at the user's ear; a number of weapon systems in current service give peak pressures up to 185 dB (35 kPa) in crew positions. To an increasing extent, soldiers are also exposed to continuous noise in vehicles or in workshops; these levels can exceed 100 dBA at the ear, even where hearing protection is used. The problem is becoming more acute, since the quest for more power from equipment of reduced size and weight tends to increase noise at the user's position. At the same time, interest in hearing conservation measures is increasing, not only because of the greater risk of hearing loss, but also because awareness of the effects of noise is increasing as the use of monitoring audiometry becomes more widespread. It is therefore becoming vital to be able to predict the risk of hearing loss and the resulting disability from measurements (or, in the case of equipment still at the design stage, from predictions) of the noise exposure.

HEARING CONSERVATION MEASURES IN THE BRITISH ARMY

Hearing conservation measures were first introduced in the British Army in 1966, following findings of widespread high-tone hearing loss in Infantry soldiers [1]. The principal means of protection was a soft plastic ear plug of the V-51R pattern; an ear muff was also available to specialist users exposed to very intense noise. Both the ear plug and the ear muff were shown to be effec- tive protectors when used as intended; despite this, high-tone hearing loss continued to occur. The main problem was that some soldiers were not fully convinced of the need to conserve hearing, despite the introduction of a training film and other material; hearing loss was not seen as a handicap. It was evident that individuals with severe noise-induced hearing loss were continuing in service, so that the motivation to conserve hearing was reduced.

The hearing protectors available to the Army also had serious shortcomings; in particular, the V-51R pattern ear plug needed careful placement in the ear canal if it were to be effective, and it was obvious that it was not always placed with care; also, since it was available in a number of different sizes (initially three, but the need for an extra small and an extra large size soon became apparent), there was a possibility of the wrong size being used. In theory, the correct size was selected by the unit's medical officer, but this did not always happen in practice. Some users complained of discomfort, to the extent of their being unwilling to use it, or of selecting too small a size. The ear muffs were fragile, the liquid-filled seals being a frequent source of failure, and were incompatible with any form of helmet.

A survey carried out in 1979 [2] showed that, despite efforts made up to that date, noise-induced hearing loss was still prevalent; it was therefore necessary to pursue an Army Hearing Conservation Programme with increased vigor. The essential parts of this programme are: a. measurement and evaluation of noise hazards; b. provision of improved individual hearing protection and indication of the areas where its use is required; c. screening audiometry of new entrants, and regular monitoring audiometry of all personnel (at 2 year intervals in most cases); d. health education. For monitoring audiometry, the sums of hearing levels at low frequencies (0.5, 1, 2 kHz) and high frequencies (3, 4 and 6 kHz) are used to make the assessment, as follows:

Degree	Sum of hearing levels at low frequencies	Sum of hearing levels at high frequencies
H1	not more than 45 dB	not more than 45 dB
H2	" " " 84	" " " 123
H3	" " " 150	" " " 210
H4 or H8	more than 150	more than 210

Each ear is assessed separately, and an overall grading assigned on the result from the worse ear. H3 may lead to career restrictions, H4 will not permit front-line service, H8 requires medical discharge. The distinction between H4 and H8 is made by an ENT (ear-nose-throat) specialist, factors in addition to audiometric threshold being considered. Any downgrading to H3 or below requires referral to an ENT specialist. Entry to the Army requires a grade of H1 or H2.

The plastic ear plug is being replaced by a robust ear muff designed to be compatible with the ballistic helmet; a disposable foam ear plug has been introduced for those situations where an ear plug is still required. In addition, an ear muff giving a very good noise attenuation, at the expense of compatibility with other headgear, is available for those situations that require it. A variety of special-purpose protectors are available for use in armored vehicles and by Artillery personnel; one ear muff used by the Artillery incorporates an electro-acoustic transmission system, with an externally mounted microphone, which allows voice communication while protecting against the noise from the gun. Despite all this, we are aware that the totally satisfactory hearing protector has yet to be designed, so that we are interested in the development of new and improved protectors.

LIMITS FOR IMPULSE NOISE EXPOSURE

Ideally, it should be possible to consider impulse and continuous noise together, rating both types of noise by a common method. Unfortunately, standards for evaluating continuous noise, such as BS 5330:1976 [3] find it necessary to place a restriction on the maximum peak level such that they cannot be used to rate weapon noise.

A number of different specifications have therefore been developed for impulse-noise exposure in military practice [4-11]. The specification for maximum exposure within the UK is given in Defence Standard 00-27/1 [4]; this standard is based on the work of Coles, Garinther, Hodge and Rice [5] and CHABA [6], together with some more recent experience. It is similar, but not identical, to the impulse-noise specifications in US MIL-STD-1474B [7]. In common with many other standards, the limits to exposure in Defence Standard 00-27/1 are specified in terms of peak (maximum instantaneous departure from ambient) pressure and duration of the impulse, and the number of impulses. A correction (normally 20 dB, exceptionally 25 dB) is made for the use of hearing protection. Two limits are specified: a preferred limit which should be observed wherever possible, and a maximum limit which must not be exceeded under any peacetime circumstances. These limits, and the definitions of peak pressure and duration, are illustrated in Figs. 1, 2, 3 and 4.

RECENT SURVEYS OF NOISE-INDUCED HEARING LOSS

The prevalence of high-tone hearing loss in Army populations has been demonstrated by a large number of surveys carried out in a number of different national armies. However, these surveys leave many questions unanswered. Firstly, the noise exposure (which typically consists of both impulse and continuous noise) is generally known only very approximately, so that the relation between noise exposure and hearing loss is uncertain. Secondly, the use of hearing protection is unsatisfactory and intermittent, and the extent of its use unrecorded, adding further uncertainty. Finally, all surveys show that the magnitude of the noise-induced hearing loss varies between individuals, even when the noise exposures are apparently similar, to the extent that some show almost normal hearing while others show very large losses. At present, we have no means of forecasting which individuals are susceptible to the effects of noise.

Some indication of the effect of impulse noise on hearing is given by a survey carried out by Brown [12] on hearing levels in British Infantry following Operation Corporate (the Falklands conflict). The survey, which was carried out from APRE, illustrates a number of important points and will therefore be described in some detail. It differed from many other surveys in that the noise exposure consisted almost entirely of impulse noise, and was reasonably well defined and of relatively short duration; and also in that pre-exposure audiograms were available from routine medical screening for many of the subjects. The hearing loss was chiefly at the higher frequencies, the mean hearing level of 3, 4 and 6 kHz, taken as an average for all personnel, increasing by 5.5 dB in the left ear and by 5.1 dB in the right. However, the loss varied considerably between different groups, and those soldiers firing 81 mm mortar suffered, on average, a change in mean hearing level at these frequencies of 12.2 dB and 7.8 dB in the left and right ears respectively.

It is, however, obvious from the results given by Brown [12] that the average hearing loss for a number of individuals is, by itself, a very inadequate descriptor of the effect of the noise on hearing. The distribution of hearing losses shows clearly that there are very large differences between individuals, the majority showing either no hearing loss or a relatively small loss. However, a small proportion of personnel show very large losses which cannot be explained by differences in noise exposure. Hearing protection did not confer any obvious benefit. It is probable that actual (as opposed to reported) usage of protection was very low.

Many surveys (including the pre-exposure hearing levels reported by Brown [12]) have demonstrated a high incidence of hearing loss in soldiers

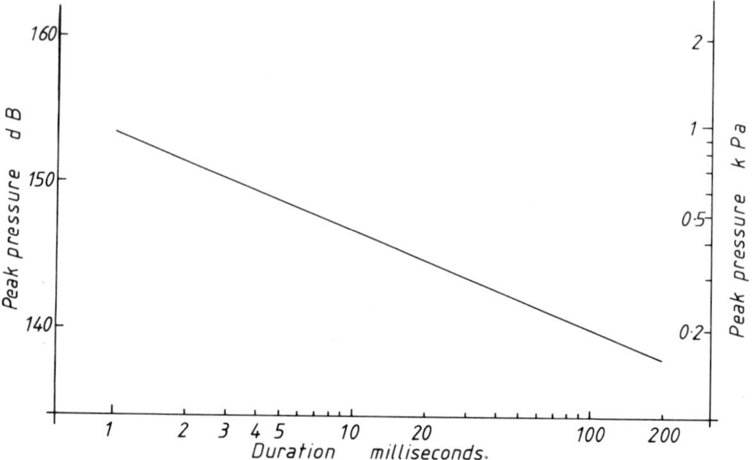

Fig. 1. Preferred limit of Defence Standard 00-27/1 [4].

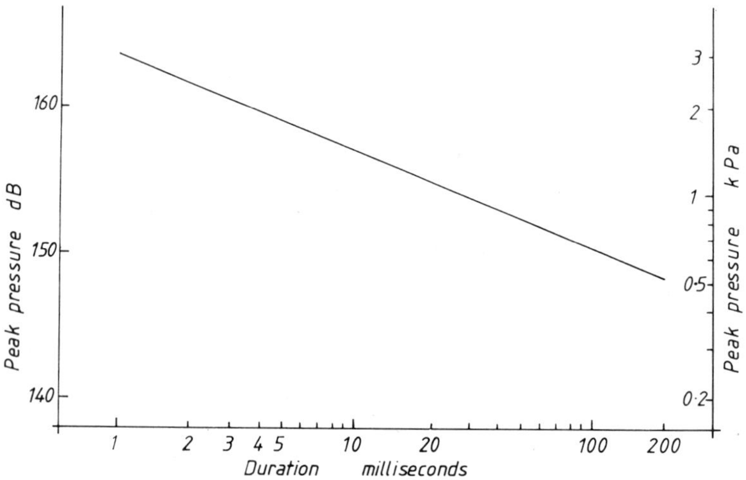

Fig. 2. Maximum limit of Defence Standard 00-27/1.

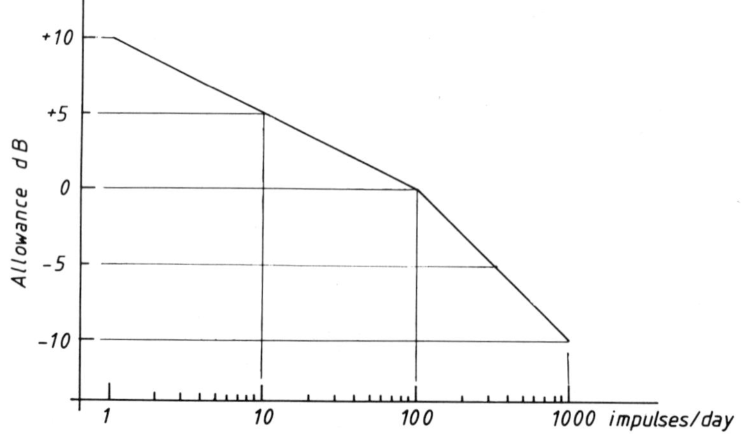

Fig. 3. Allowance for number of impulses (rounds).

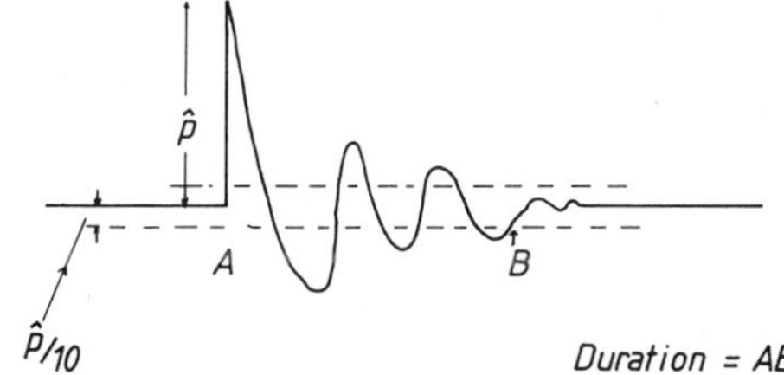

Fig. 4. Definition of peak pressure, p, and duration, following Defence Standard 00-27/1 [4].

exposed to noise only during training. In order to investigate the effect of noise exposure (principally from small arms fire) during basic training, hearing levels were measured in 1000 Infantry recruits at the start of training, and again at the conclusion of training. Analysis of results is not yet complete, but it is evident that the incidence of hearing loss is very low, indicating essentially no hazard [13]. Hearing protectors were used during all exposures to potentially damaging noise.

HEARING PROTECTION

The ideal means of hearing conservation is always to reduce the noise at source; unfortunately, it is often difficult or impossible to reduce the noise sufficiently, and the use of some form of personal hearing protection - ear muffs, ear plugs or a noise-excluding helmet - becomes necessary. Noise reduction is especially difficult with impulse noise from gunfire, where substantial reduction would reduce the effectiveness of the gun or increase its size and weight.

The use of hearing protection therefore assumes critical importance in an Army hearing conservation program. There are two problems: firstly, ensuring that the protectors can attenuate the noise sufficiently; and secondly, ensuring that the protectors are sufficiently robust for military use, that they do not interfere with military tasks or military equipment (such as ballistic helmets or sights), that any adverse effect on communication is minimized, and that the soldier is prepared to use them effectively on all occasions of noise exposure [14,15]. The second of these tasks is by far the more difficult; its importance is emphasized by the results of the surveys described above.

There are a number of means whereby the attenuation of the protectors can be determined [16,17]. The accepted standard methods based on real-ear attenuation at threshold, such as ISO 4869 [18], are not very helpful, since the attenuation is measured as a function of frequency and the results therefore cannot be used unless the noise is also analyzed in terms of frequency; also, the results can be used only if the attenuation is assumed to be independent of pressure [19]. Results from measurements using artificial heads can give useful information on the mechanism by which the protector operates, but artificial heads can not, at their present stage of development, be used to give a quantitative assessment of the attenuation expected in practical use. Three other methods are available and have been used to estimate attenuation:

a. The noise outside the protector, and the noise reaching the ear beneath the protector, can be measured using miniature microphones [16-20]. The measurements can be performed using a number of test subjects, so that the standard deviation as well as the mean value of the attenuation can be estimated. The technique is relatively simple with ear muffs or noise-excluding helmets, although much more difficult with ear plugs! Fig. 5 shows a typical result, using noise from a small howitzer, for a measurement on one subject wearing an ear muff. It can be seen that the noise is very much altered by the ear muff; the higher frequencies in the noise are attenuated much more than the lower frequencies, leaving a predominantly low-frequency impulse noise of increased duration.

b. The risk to hearing in personnel using hearing protectors can be estimated by measurements of temporary hearing threshold shift. This is useful mainly to show that the exposure is "acceptable," although comparisons with conventional limits to unprotected noise exposure can be used to generate a nominal value for hearing protector attenuation for the noise in question. The technique is a difficult one, dominated by the need for consistently accurate audiometry and by the requirement to ensure that the shifts are small enough to be genuinely temporary. Patterson [21] has given an especially elegant demonstration of the technique in the context of noise from a medium howitzer and from an anti-tank weapon.

c. Where a known and potentially hazardous noise exposure occurs, hearing levels can be monitored to determine whether any hearing protection used is adequate. Of course, the noise exposures and the choice of hearing protection are outside the experimenter's control. An example of this approach is given by Forrest, Forshaw and Crabtree [22], showing effective protection by an ear muff against a very intense noise exposure from 81 mm mortar. This agrees with the result of the survey, mentioned earlier, on hearing levels in recruits. In general, it appears that little or no hearing loss is found if a satisfactory form of hearing protection is always used correctly, while careless or occasional use confers little benefit.

These methods yield broadly similar results; in particular, they agree that the way a protector is used is of greater importance than its maximum potential attenuation under ideal conditions. This is especially true of ear plugs, which tend to show a greater variation in attenuation than do ear muffs, depending on how well the device is fitted.

DISCUSSION

Although this paper is primarily concerned with experience of impulse noise within the British Army, it also highlights a number of general points which will be relevant to this workshop. Our experience is consistent with that of other national forces, and also with experience in civil industry, in that hearing conservation measures need to be pursued vigorously if they are to have any effect, and that a monitoring audiometry program is vital. If the individual at risk is not fully aware of the effect of noise on his hearing, and on his subsequent career, he is unlikely to take effective action to safeguard either. Hearing protection must not only be used, but used effectively on all occasions of exposure; this implies that the protection supplied must not only give sufficient attenuation, but must also be robust and compatible with other items of equipment. These points have been made previously by many authors, but are of such fundamental importance that they will bear repetition.

The limits to impulse-noise exposure described in Defence Standard 00-27/1 [4] are, like all other limits used by other national forces, intended as a practical guide rather than as an exact definition of hazard. There is general agreement that more precise limits should be possible, but very little agreement on what form the improved limits should take! A discussion of these issues is given by Dancer and Franke [23]. The use of

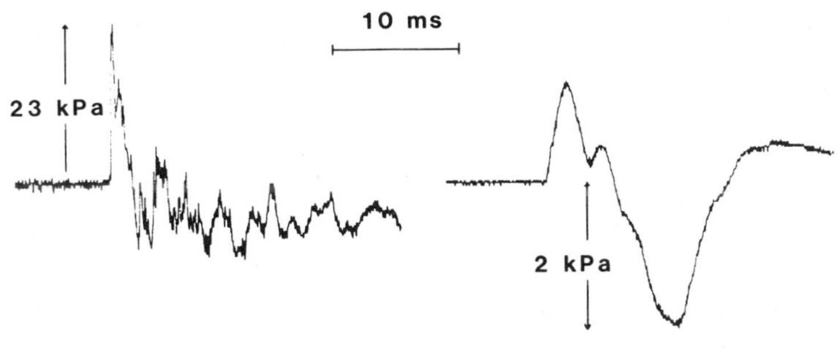

Fig. 5. Gunfire noise measured a) outside, and b) inside, an ear muff.

some form of frequency-dependent weighting, such as the A-weighting, has been widely advocated [24], as has the concept of the "critical level," above which the risk is greatly increased [25]. In my own view, we do not at present have sufficient data to make a definite choice as to which of the many options is most nearly correct. The development of a model of the response of the cochlea to impulse noise is likely to be helpful in this respect.

Limits to impulse noise exposure also depend on the risk of hearing loss considered "acceptable." Broadly speaking, the limits in current use specify a risk (generally in terms of conventional pure-tone audiometry) comparable with, or less than, that assumed for industrial practice for continuous noise. The assumed risk has, of course, a critical effect on the limits to noise exposure. Ideally, the risk should be defined in terms of effect on military efficiency, as well as in terms of social disability. Unfortunately, this issue has been relatively little studied. Many sounds of interest to ground forces, such as the proverbial snapping twig or the noise of a footfall on gravel, have much of their energy at high frequencies where hearing loss tends to be greatest; it is therefore reasonable to assume that a small high-tone hearing loss which would have relatively little effect on the hearing of speech could (depending on circumstances, such as the level of ambient masking noise) have an adverse effect on military performance [26,27]. At present, there is insufficient evidence for a quantitative relation between hearing loss (measured by conventional audiometry) and effectiveness of ground troops.

There is an obvious need for an authoritative and generally applicable limit for impulse-noise exposure. Unfortunately, we are still some way from being able to formulate such a limit in terms which would command general acceptance. Meanwhile, in the author's view, any attempt to alter existing limits to exposure on the basis of insufficient information should be resisted, since such alterations serve only to generate confusion; the probable result would be that the limits would be ignored altogether.

REFERENCES

1. B. Livesey, Acoustic trauma as an occupational hazard in Infantrymen. Journal of the Royal Army Medical Corps, 111:188 (1965).
2. D. H. Coombe, The implications of the Army's audiometric screening programme; Part 1: Acoustic trauma among serving Infantry personnel, Journal of the Royal Army Medical Corps, 126:18 (1980).

3. British Standards Institution, Method of test for estimating the risk of hearing handicap due to noise exposure, BS 5330:1976 (1976).
4. Ministry of Defence, Acceptable limits for exposure to impulse noise from military weapons, explosives and pyrotechnics, Defence Standard 00-27/Issue 1 (1985).
5. R. R. A. Coles, G. R. Garinther, D.C. Hodge, and C. G. Rice, Hazardous exposure to impulse noise, J. Acoust. Soc. Am., 43:336 (1968).
6. CHABA (National Academy of Sciences, National Research Council, Committee on Hearing, Bioacoustics and Biomechanics), Proposed damage-risk criterion for impulse noise (gunfire), W. D. Ward ed., Report of Working Group 57 (1968).
7. U.S.A. Department of Defense, Military Standard - Noise Limits for Army Material, MIL-STD-1474B(M1) (1979).
8. F. Pfander, Das Knalltrauma, Springer-Verlag (1975).
9. F. Pfander, H. Bongartz, H. Brinkmann, and H. Kietz, Danger of auditory impairment from impulse noise, J. Acoust. Soc. Am., 67:628 (1980).
10. G. F. Smoorenburg, Damage risk criteria for impulse noise, in: "New perspectives on noise-induced hearing loss," R. Hamernik, D. Henderson, and R. Salvi, eds., Raven Press, New York (1982).
11. Ministere de la Defense, Groupe de coordination technique "Facteurs Humains et Ergonomie," Comite "Bruits d Armes," Recommandation relative a l'evaluation physioacoustique du pouvoir lesionnel des bruits, also available as: Recommendation on evaluating the possible harmful effects of noise on hearing, DTAT Traduction AT-83/27/28 (May 1983).
12. J. R. Brown, Noise-induced hearing loss sustained during land operations in the Falklands Islands campaign 1982, J. Soc. Occup. Med., 35:44 (1985).
13. A. G. Harwood, personal communication, 1985.
14. S. E. Forshaw, Hearing protection practice in the Canadian Forces, Scand. Audiol., Suppl. 16:53 (1982).
15. G. F. Smoorenburg, and A. M. Mimpen, Assessment of personal hearing protection in practice, Scand. Audiol., Suppl. 16:13 (1982).
16. M. R. Forrest, Protecting hearing in a military environment, Scand. Audiol., Suppl. 16:7 (1982).
17. M. R. Forrest, The efficiency of hearing protection to impulse noise, Scand. Audiol., Suppl. 12:186 (1980).
18. International Organization for Standardization (ISO), Acoustics - Measurement of sound attenuation of hearing protectors - Subjective method, ISO 4869-1981 (1981).
19. A. M. Martin, Dependence of acoustic attenuation of hearing protectors on incident sound level. Br. J. Ind. Med., 36:1 (1979).
20. H. Brinkmann, Effectiveness of ear protection against impulse noise, Scand. Audiol., Suppl. 16:23 (1982).
21. J. H. Patterson, Direct determination of the adequacy of hearing protection for use with the Viper missile and the M198 howitzer, in: "Technical proceedings of the blast overpressure workshop," The Technical Cooperation Program, Technical Panel W-2 (1982).
22. M. R. Forrest, S. E. Forshaw, and R. B. Crabtree, Investigation of hearing loss from exposure to noise from 81 mm mortar. Department of National Defence - Canada, DCIEM Report No. 81-R-09 (1981).
23. A. Dancer and R. Franke, Effects of weapon-noise on hearing, in NATO Advanced Study Workshop "Noise-induced hearing loss - Basic and applied aspects," Lucca (September 1985).
24. H. E. von Gierke, D. W. Robinson, S. J. Karmy, Results of the workshop on impulse noise and auditory hazard, J. Sound Vib., 83:579 (1982).
25. G. R. Price, Mechanisms of loss for intense sound exposures, in: "Hearing and Other Senses; Presentations in Honor of E. G. Wever," R. R. Fay and G. Gourevitch, eds., Amphora Press (1983).

26. G. R. Price, and D. C. Hodge, Combat sound detection: 1. Monaural listening in quiet, US Army Human Engineering Laboratory, Technical Memorandum 35-76.
27. M. W. Savill, unpublished Ministry of Defence memorandum (1985).

DISCUSSION

Borchgrevink: For the H-1 group, do you have problems of having a 15 dB mean cutoff because of background noise in the test booth?

Forrest: I think the answer is probably yes. You saw some data earlier that showed hearing levels at 500 hz which were not very good; this is probably an effect of background noise. It only seems to have an effect at 500 Hz.

Borchgrevink: In Norway we have a 20 dB mean instead of a 15 dB mean for the best category. We find that works out much better than the 15 dB would have. My next point; you do not count 8,000 Hz. That means you would not discriminate between the loss you would allow if a person had an early presybcusis or a similar audiogram.

Forrest: The 8 kHz information could be important, but I am not going to pretend that our limits are the last word. They are not a research tool, but rather just a practical means of finding out if a man is fit for army service and in what capacity.

Borchgrevink: Do you allow H3 to have service in noise?

Forrest: I think it is basically a question not for the medical services, but for the military commander. So it would be for the director of infantry possibly to say whether a particular grade was suitable for infantry service. It depends, in other words, on what you want to do.

Borchgrevink: So it is an operative criterion?

Forrest: Yes, It is up to the army to say whether they will accept these various grades. In general, H1 and H2 are suitable for any occupation. H4 would not permit front line service; H8 would demand a medical discharge. I think it is open for the army to say what they would do with H3 individuals of whom there are, in fact, quite a large number.

Borchgrevink: What do you do with the people with a mid frequency loss who would not reach the criterion either in the high or the low criterion? We find a number of people with a mid frequency hereditary loss who, if they began to obtain an NI PTS, would have very poor hearing and very quickly.

Forrest: I do not think this is a problem we have really met. My reading of the problem is very much that we are working at noise-induced loss almost entirely and not at hereditary loss.

MATHEMATICAL SIMULATION OF THE COCHLEAR MECHANISM APPLIED TO DAMAGE-RISK CRITERIA FOR IMPULSE NOISE

Guy O. Stevin

Laboratory for Acoustics
Technical Services of the Army STFT/CT
Quartier Housiau - B-1801 Brussels (Peutie) - Belgium

SUMMARY

A mathematical simulation of the human hearing mechanism, involving the non-linear effect of the middle ear, has been used to compute the risk of impairment for hearing produced by impulse noise. This model provides, therefore, a reference method which can be used for evaluating the loudness of any kind of acoustical noise. The results of impulse noise analysis obtained from different damage-risk criteria can then be compared with the results of the theoretical model, allowing for evaluation of the respective merits of these criteria.

The main conclusion of this study is that the A-weighted sound exposure level L_{AE} appears to be the best damage-risk criterion for impulse noise. The spectral sensitivity of the human hearing mechanism might then be approximated by the A-weighting filter. These elements emphasize the possibility of using a unique damage-risk criterion applicable for any kind of noise, including continuous and fluctuating noises as well as industrial and gunfire impulse noises. This criterion would be applicable for the high peak pressure levels up to 170 dB, which can be experimentally encountered for gunfire. The damage level for a daily exposure of eight hours would be around 130 dB, corresponding to a steady state pressure level equal to 85 dB. This conclusion is in full agreement with the most recent results on impulse noise obtained by psychoacoustical experiments in the U.S., Germany, the Netherlands, and Japan.

INTRODUCTION

The human hearing mechanism can be impaired by noise exposure. The degree of impairment depends on the level, the duration and the frequency content of the noise, as well as on the sensitivity of the individual. Organizations concerned with ear protection should be able to forecast the risk which noise, particularly impulse noise, can cause to hearing.

There is no uniformity in the present rating methods. Continuous noise is rated by its A-weighted sound pressure level or by octave band analysis, according to ISO 1999; industrial sound impulses are rated by special methods which may or may not use the A-weighting network. Impulses from gunfire are covered by other damage-risk criteria (DRC) based on peak pressure and impulse duration.

The method for assessing the risk to hearing by noise described in ISO 1999 is only applicable for continuous noises. This limitation is due to the technology of the present sound level meters (IEC 651), which are appropriate only for this kind of sound. The basic circuity of the sound level meter is a square-law detector which computes the root mean-square (rms) value of the pressure signal (filtered or not) for a period to which is referred to as the "time constant" of the meter. The standard values for T_o are in the range of the seconds.

Damage-risk criteria for impulse noise do not presently take the spectrum of the impulse into account; however, it is known that the human auditory system is spectrally tuned. A few years ago, when impulse criteria were proposed, the spectrum of impulsive signals was difficult and time-consuming to analyze. Because of this technical problem, spectral analysis was not included in the criteria. This problem can now be solved by digital processors using the fast Fourier transform. We now have the ability for spectral analysis of impulse signals, but we still need a spectral criterion. Recent work in this area [1] shows that the spectral sensitivity of the ear to impulses can be described by curves similar to the A-weighting curve. However, the numerical values of the critical level are missing. Such information is required before this kind of method can be applied as a damage-risk criterion. For these reasons, a new approach seems to be necessary to eliminate the imperfections of the present measuring techniques and the subsequent disparity in hearing conservation methods.

GENERALIZATION OF CONTINUOUS NOISE RATING METHODS FOR IMPULSE NOISE

The Sound Exposure Level as Hazard Parameter

The concept of noise dose combines in a single parameter the sound pressure level and the duration of exposure to the noise. The best way to determine the noise dose is found in the definition of the sound exposure, that is, the time integral of the squared sound pressure p(t) over a stated time period τ, according to Eq. (1):

$$E = \int_0^{\tau} p^2(t)dt \qquad (1)$$

A convenient unit for sound exposure is 1 Pa^2s. From Eq. (1), one can say that the sound exposure is an estimate of the sound energy associated with the noise over the time τ. The sound exposure level (abbreviated SEL) is the expression in decibels of the ratio of the weighted sound exposure to the reference sound exposure. The reference sound exposure is equal to the product of the squared reference sound pressure (p_o = 20 μPa) and the reference duration (t_o = 1 s). The symbol is L_{AE} when A-weighting is used.

$$L_{AE} = 10 \log_{10}\left(\int_0^{\tau} p^2(t)dt/p^2{}_o t_o\right) \qquad (2)$$

First take an A-weighted sound pressure level of 85 dB for a daily duration of 8 h. This exposure can be regarded as a realistic DRC for continuous noise. The corresponding sound exposure level is 130 dB. The correction is 45 dB and comes from the expression in decibels of the ratio of the 8-h duration (=28,800 s), to the reference duration (1 s).

Let us now consider the noise impulse for which the damage-risk level, according to Pfander [2], is reached for a single impulse per day. This impulse has a peak pressure level (flat weighted) equal to 160 dB and its effective duration is 1 ms. Assuming this peak pressure level is held during the complete duration of the impulse, one obtains an approximate sound exposure level equal to 130 dB. Because both continuous and impulse noise DRC lead to equivalent numerical values for the sound exposure level, it would seem reasonable to consider the sound exposure level as an acceptable hazard parameter, applicable to all kinds of noise.

It must be noted that this statement implicitly involves the linearity of the hearing damage mechanism, better known as the "energy rule." However, there is a limit to the application of this rule. This limit can be estimated to lie at 170 dB (flat-peak level) because the risk of damage to the ear drum begins at this level.

The Weighted SEL for Rating Impulse Noise by use of the "Integrating Sound Level Meter"

Considering the previously-mentioned properties of the sound exposure level with regard to damage-risk to hearing, one can use this parameter for rating the risk of impulse noise to hearing, provided Eq. (1) is correctly evaluated. This is not possible with a standard "precision sound level meter" as defined in IEC 651, for the reasons previously explained.

The use of an integrating sound level meter seems to be the best way to measure the SEL. This is certainly the case for impulse noise, but such a device can also be used for continuous noise and other types of fluctuating noises. The definition of the sound exposure level permits the combination of exposures to different kinds of noise in the same daily duration.

Frequency Analysis by Octave Band

Using Parseval's identity, the sound exposure can be expressed in the frequency domain by using the Fourier pressure spectrum F(f) of the sound signal:

$$E = \int_{-\infty}^{+\infty} p^2(t)dt = \int_{-\infty}^{+\infty} |F|^2 df = 2\int_{0}^{\infty} |F|^2 df \qquad (3)$$

The final form of Eq. (3) permits use of positive frequency only. It follows from this identity that the square of the Fourier transform of a pressure signal has dimensions of pressure squared by time per unit frequency. When a band filter (f_1-f_2) is used, the band sound exposure level is equal to

$$L_{E12} = 10 \log_{10} \left(2\int_{f_1}^{f_2} \frac{|F|^2}{p_o^2 \; t_o} df\right) \qquad (4)$$

This can be called the integrated octave band sound exposure level. The rating method for impulse noise is derived from ISO 1999; the shape of the hearing curves is obtained by inverting and shifting the A-weighting curve. The octave band for which the damage-risk to hearing is greatest can be found by determining the band for which the octave band SEL is maximum, after correction for A-weighting. For high level noise, the octave band with maximum corrected SEL indicates the band for which the risk of impairment for hearing is the greatest.

Measurement of the Octave Band SEL for Impulsive Noises

Because impulsive noises are single events with a very short duration, octave band measurements for such signals by means of integrating sound level meter can only be made when at least seven integrating channels are simultaneously available, each of them being equipped with a different octave band filter. Another technique is now available using digital Fourier analyzers. The spectral transformation implemented in these analyzers is based on the definitions of the discrete Fourier transform and is computed with the fast Fourier algorithm (FFT) [3]. The main difficulty of spectral analysis is the scale factor converting the relative decibels measurements into absolute acoustical decibels. The easiest way to solve this problem is by a calibration procedure. Another advantage of calibration is that it involves all parts of measuring chain in the calibration process, not only the analyzer but also the pressure transducer, preamplifiers, and attenuating devices which contribute to the overall scale factor. The Fourier analyzer does not permit the analysis of slowly fluctuating noise or nonsteady combinations of continuous noise and impulses.

For this general case, the seven-channel integrating sound level meter seems to be the best way to achieve the octave band analyses. Unfortunately, such equipment is not currently available in a compact form and one is obliged to use seven different nonsynchronized, integrating sound level meters to perform this kind of measurement, which is a costly and difficult procedure.

Comments

The generalization made in the previous paragraphs consists simply of replacing the sound pressure level by the concept of noise dose expressed by the sound exposure level over a standard 8-h daily period. Assuming the human hearing mechanism to be a linear system allows these modified rating methods to be extrapolated in order to obtain a damage-risk criterion by fixing the maximum allowed sound exposure level.

THEORETICAL EVALUATION OF THE PROPOSED METHODS FOR IMPULSE NOISE

Modeling the Risk of Impairment

The loudness of noise can be regarded as a subjective measurement of the electrical energy transmitted along the auditory nerve to the brain. The electrical signals in the nerve are related to the motion of the basilar membrane; the hair cells play the role of mechanical-to-electrical transducers. It can be assumed that the electrical energy is proportional to the mechanical energy introduced in the inner ear, through the middle ear and the outer ear, by the acoustical stimulus, as illustrated in the simplified diagram of Fig. 1. This energy can be computed when the motion of the basilar membrane is known.

A bi-dimensional model of the movement of this membrane can be used, similar to the model given by Flanagan [4]. We use the following notation: $y(x,t)$ is the displacement versus longitudinal position x along the membrane; $B(f)$, $G(f)$, $H(f)$ are, respectively, the transfer functions of the outer ear, the middle ear, and the inner ears; $F(f)$ is the Fourier pressure spectrum of the acoustical stimulus $p(t)$; and K is a constant with dimensions kg/ms^3. The mechanical energy by unit length $E_y(x)$ is then:

$$E_y(x) = K \int_{\mathcal{T}} y^2(x,t)dt$$

$$= 2K \int_0^{\infty} |FBGH_x|^2 \; df \tag{5}$$

The time range $\mathcal{T}$ can be determined by introducing in a simplified manner the recovery rate of the human hearing mechanism. Using the same assumption as Pfander [2], we compute the energy accumulation during a daily exposure of 8 h, assuming that the normal rest period is sufficient for complete recovery, even if it takes much longer than one day. The total mechanical energy (E_L) expressed by Eq. (6) can be used for a theoretical computation of the loudness of the sound stimuli.

$$E_L = \int_0^L E_y(x)dx \tag{6}$$

In order to evaluate the risk of impairment to the hair cells, it would be more appropriate to compute the highest mechanical energy (E_{DRC}) dissipated in group of hair cells corresponding to the characteristic frequency band:

$$E_{DRC} = \max\,[k.E_y(x)] \tag{7}$$

In so doing, we neglect the contributions of other locations to the total energy. This can be done because the filter effect of the inner ear is rather selective.

For computation of Eqs. (6) and (7), we choose Flanagan's equations [4] (Eq. 4.1 for Hx and Eq. 4.3 for G). The resonance effect of the outer ear is obtained by introducing a resonance of about 14 dB at 3 kHz. Numerical adjustment of the constants appearing in Eqs. (6) and (7) has been made for a 1-kHz pure tone stimulus with sound exposure level equal to 130 dB, so that the total mechanical energy is expressed in decibels by the numerical value of 0 dB. In so doing, we refer all results for the simulated hearing mechanism to an arbitrary but realistic damage-risk threshold level.

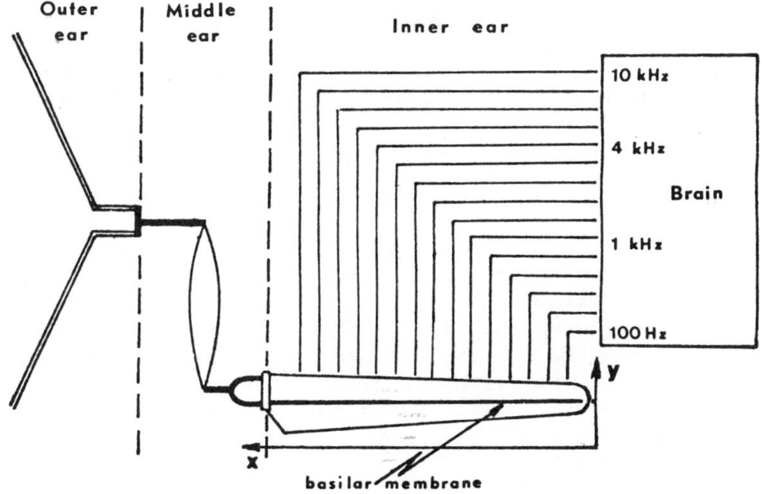

Fig. 1. Functional diagram of the human hearing mechanism

Assessment of the Extended Spectral Methods

On one hand, the set of possible rating methods for noise, developed in the previous section is available. On the other hand, a theoretical procedure is given by Eqs. (6) and (7) to compute the reference loudness of the damage-risk level which this noise produces in the human hearing mechanism. Comparing the results of the first methods with the reference ones provided by the second, and doing so for various impulse signals, allows us to judge the respective merits of the different rating methods, or DRC.

This comparison has been made with 46 sound impulses which were mathematically generated using attenuated cosines with and without reflections and some N waves to simulate sonic booms. All of these models are fitted with a flat-weighted peak pressure level (PPL) equal to 160 dB. Their durations lie between 0.25 and 64 ms. The 46 impulses were analyzed according to the 14 rating methods detailed in Table I. The mechanical energy in the inner ear was also computed according to Eq. (7) as reference damage-risk prediction. We thus obtain 15 arrays, each of them containing 46 elements, one for each of the 46 sound impulses simulated. The first 14 arrays can be considered as approximations of the 15th, which is the reference one. Subtracting the 15th array from the other 14 provides 14 error arrays, which represent the statistics of error for the studied rating methods.

The standard deviation can be regarded as a measure of the spectral spread of the method concerned, that is, a measure of its spectral accuracy. For this reason, this parameter has been chosen as the figure of merit to rank order the different rating methods for impulse noise as listed in Table I. The smaller the standard deviation, the more spectrally accurate is the rating method with regard to the ear simulation.

It must be noted that this kind of trial must be carefully prepared because the statistical results are only valid for the set of impulses tested. In defining this set, we tried to assemble representative gunfire impulses. We also tried to use representative samples of broadband spectra, that is, spectra with a high cutoff frequency going from 300-400 Hz up to 5 kHz.

Another important point should be emphasized. The spectrum of white noise is sometimes used to define acoustical continuous noise. This spectrum is the spectrum of the mathematical ideal impulse [Dirac (t) function]. This impulse is only different from zero at a single point (for t=0), where it is infinite. The equivalence between continuous noise and impulse noise from a spectral point of view permits us to extend the results of an impulse simulation to all kinds of noise signals, which have similar spectra. Continuous noise is therefore included in this study.

Results of the Simulation

The results of the statistical trial are listed in Table I. From a statistical point of view, a standard deviation equal to 2.5 dB means that 65% of the errors between the tested method and the reference hearing mechanism are within the 2.5 dB, 87% are within the 5 dB, and 95% are within the 7.5 dB, of the average error. It is thus evident that a perfect rating method does not exist. For the A-SEL, which is the best of the studied methods, there are still 5% of the noises which are incorrectly analyzed, giving an error greater than 7.5 dB. If the separation between acceptable and nonacceptable methods is arbitrarily fixed at 2.5 dB for the standard deviation, then the conclusions are very clear:

There is only ONE acceptable method for impulse noise: the A-weighted sound exposure level L_{AE}.

All other methods, the CHABA criterion for A-waves excepted, are too inaccurate and should therefore be disregarded. The excellent results of the CHABA method are unfortunately restricted to A-impulses (pure blast waves in open field): this means for less than 10% of impulse noises encountered in real cases.

Other general comments according to Table I are:

- The mean DRC error of the Pfander impulse DRC and that of the A-SEL are no more than 1 dB. Because this criterion is supported by much experimental evidence, it can be concluded that gunfire impulses up to 170 dB (flat-PPL) are well covered by the linear ear model.

- The ear simulation gives evidence that the CHABA criterion is more restrictive by about 6 dB than Pfander's and 5 dB more than Smoorenburg's criterion. These differences are in full agreement with recent comparative trials made by Pfander et al. [7]. This is due mainly to the different methods of measuring the effective duration of the impulse for both criteria; it generally results in a longer duration for CHABA.

- Finally, it seems evident that the ear model used can be regarded as an additional procedure which would provide a reference damage-risk prediction for any kind of acoustical noise. Computation of the hearing equations according to Eqs. (6) and (7) requires large memory computer facilities.

Modeling the Hearing Mechanism

The results presented in Table I are slightly different from those published earlier [8]: the standard deviations are now much greater. This is due to the model for the OUTER and MIDDLE ears which was too sharply tuned by 6 dB in the previous study. The consequences of this change are that frequency analysis and resonant methods like D-weighting are now dropped from the recommended methods.

The present model includes the acoustical reflex of the middle ear. This reflex has no influence on the impulse simulation because its latency is too long compared with the short duration of the impulses analyzed.

We also tried a more sharply tuned model (+10 dB) for the INNER EAR, according to results published by Rhode [9]. This change has no significant effects on the risk for hearing. So it appears clearly that the INNER EAR mechanism is not critical for modeling the risk of impairment, but that the main factor is the frequency response of the OUTER and MIDDLE EAR. This conclusion is in full agreement with recent works in this area [10,11].

CONCLUSIONS

Evaluation of loudness as well as hazard to hearing produced by impulse noise was derived from the noise dose principle which is widely applied to continuous noise. The sound exposure level has been recognized as the most appropriate quantity for this purpose when associated with the A-weighting. This weighting filter appears to be best for analysis of the spectral sensitivity of the human hearing mechanism.

These important results are supported by a mathematical simulation of the hearing mechanism, which permits loudness and damage-risk to hearing

Table I. Rank order and results of the impulse simulation

Rank	Method	Loudness Mean Error (dB)	DRC Mean Error (dB)	Standard Deviation (dB)
1	CHABA-A [5]	-	+ 6.0	2.0
2	A-SEL(L_{AE})	- 0.5	+ 2.0	2.5
3	A-Octave	- 4.0	1.5	3.5
	D-SEL(L_{BE})	+ 5.0	+ 7.5	3.5
	B-SEL(L_{BE})	+ 9.0	+ 11.5	3.5
	CHABA[5]	-	+ 7.0	3.5
4	A-1/3 Octave	- 1.5	+ 0.5	4.0
	US-MIL-STD-1474	-	+ 8.0	4.0
5	Pfander [2]	-	+ 1.0	4.5
	Smoorenburg [6]	-	+ 2.0	4.5
	D-Octave	+ 1.0	+ 3.5	4.5
	D-1/3 Octave	+ 4.0	+ 6.0	4.5
	Flat SEL(L_E)	+ 3.5	+ 6.0	4.5
6	C-SEL(L_{CE})	+ 2.5	+ 5.0	5.0

produced by composite noises to be computed from a single formula. This model provides, therefore, a reference method which can be used for evaluating the loudness of any kind of acoustical noise.

These elements emphasize the possibility of using a unique damage-risk criterion applicable for any kind of noise, including continuous and fluctuating noises as well as industrial and gunfire impulse noises. This criterion would be applicable for high peak pressure levels up to 170 dB which are experimentally encountered with gunfire. The proposal for this universal damage-risk criterion is obtained by fixing the threshold of the A-weighted sound exposure level at 130 dB for a daily duration of 8 h. This proposal is supported by different authors [6,12] in recent publications. Measurement of the sound exposure level for impulse noises requires new equipment such as the integrating sound level meter or the digital Fourier analyzers. This improved equipment is presently available; standardization of these measurement techniques is imperative to support future work on impulse noise control procedures.

REFERENCES

1. G. R. Price, Loss of auditory sensitivity following exposure to spectrally narrow impulses, J. Acoust. Soc. Am. 66:456 (1979).
2. F. Pfander, "Das Knalltrauma," Springer-Verlag, Berlin (1975).
3. E. O. Brigham, "The Fast Fourier Transform," Prentice Hall, New York (1974).

4. J. L. Flanagan, "Speech Analysis, Synthesis and Perception," Springer-Verlag, Berlin (1965).
5. W. D. Ward, Proposed damage-risk criterion for impulse noise (gunfire), Report of Working Group 57, National Academy of Sciences - National Research Council, Committee on Hearing, Bioacoustics and Biomechanics (CHABA), Washington DC (1968).
6. G. F. Smoorenburg, Damage-risk criteria for impulse noise, in: "New Perpectives on Noise-Induced Hearing Loss," R. Hamernik, D. Henderson and R. Salvi (eds), Raven Press, New York, (1982).
7. F. Pfander, H. Bongartz, H. Brinkmann and H. Kietz, Danger of auditory impairment from impulse noise: A comparative study of the CHABA damage-risk criteria and those of the Federal Republic of Germany, J. Acoust. Soc. Am. 67:628 (1980).
8. G. O. Stevin, Spectral analysis of impulse noise for hearing conservation purposes, J. Acoust. Soc. Am. 72 :1945 (1982).
9. W. S. Rhode, Observation of the vibration of the basilar membrane on squirrel monkeys using the Mossbauer technique, J. Acoust. Soc. Am. 49:1218 (1971).
10. G. R. Price, "Practical application of basic research on impulse noise hazard," U.S. Army Human Engineering Laboratory no 1/85 (1985).
11. D. W. Robinson, The spectral factor in noise-induced hearing loss: a case for retaining the A-weighting, J. of Sound and Vibr. 90:103 (1983).
12. S. Kuwano, S. Namba, Y. Nakajima, On the noisiness of steady state and intermittent noises, J. of Sound and Vibr. 72:87 (1980).

DISCUSSION

Forrest: What you have done is to correlate the various methods you displayed against the theoretical results from your considerations. Is there anywhere, in your modeling, any comparison with permanent or temporary threshold shift data from impulse noise exposures?

Stevins: This is a purely theoretical study, without any experiments. Naturally the validity of these conclusions are related to the validity of the hearing model used. But I think that the conclusions are strengthened by the fact that the hearing model that was used here does have an experimental basis.

Forrest: From the data we have seen at the symposium, I would hesitate to say that an A-weighted model or any other model is really a full simulation of the way the hearing mechanism works. In other words, we still need experimental data, especially data on PTS.

Price: We did see data presented in which A-weighted energy did not appear to rate hazard very accurately, i.e., the projected hazard was 40 dB less than the measured loss. It is the only data I know of where we actually have permanent hearing loss or temporary hearing loss to low frequency impulses. Also, the transfer functions for the middle and external ear of man and cat are not significantly different; just shifted upwards perhaps by 1/2 octave. So there is not a major difference between the and external middle ears of man and cat. The losses were produced by impulses from a primer fired alone; no shell, just a primer, from a rifle and from 105 mm howitzer.

ACOUSTIC REFLEX AND EXCHANGE RATE FOR WHITE NOISE SHORT STIMULI

G. Rossi

Institute of Audiology, Turin University
Via Genova, 3 - 10126 Torino, Italy

INTRODUCTION

The "equal energy principle" has been proposed as the basis of a damage risk criterion to set the limits for daily exposure to on-going noise for periods shorter or longer than 8 hours and to fluctuating, intermittent and impulse noise. The principle, supported by the studies of Elred et al. [1] and Kylin [2], was primarily validated by Burns and Robinson [3] for exposure to steady-state noise and then extended to other types of noise, including impulse exposure [4-8].

The "equal energy principle" assumes that noise-induced hearing loss is proportional to the amount of acoustic energy absorbed by the ear during the working day, irrespective of the type of noise and its physical parameters. The inner ear is thus seen as an "integrator of energy" that responds to a constant noise dose in the environment by developing a constant hearing loss, apart from the spatial or temporal distribution of the noise itself [9]. The time/intensity relationship allows a 3 dB increase in sound pressure level for each halving of the duration to create the equal risk of hearing loss (3 dB exchange rate).

The "equal energy principle", coined on a mathematical ground, ignores not only the individual susceptibility, but also the part played by the middle ear in determining how much acoustic energy in the external environment actually reaches Corti's organ [9].

Those who argue against the "equal energy principle" recommend a 5-dB reduction for each doubling of the noise duration (5 dB exchange rate). From studies of Ward [10], the 5 dB rule appears to be the more appropriate DRC in the cases of intermittent noise exposure.

The 3 dB and the 5 dB exchange rates have been incorporated in legislations of regulations of particular countries. Among 49 laws, proposals and recommendations examined, the 3 dB exchange rate was incorporated in 25 of them. Another 22 documents accepted a 5 dB exchange rate, while two other documents put forward respectively the 4 dB [11], as first proposed by Pfander [12], and a 6 dB exchange rate [13] (all references from [14]). Thus, there is no common agreement with regard to the time/intensity relationship.

The behavior of the acoustic reflex could have important implications about the validity of the various exchange rates proposed. In fact, once the reflex threshold is surpassed, the strength of muscle contraction, as expressed by the concomitant middle ear impedance change, increases over an approximately 30 dB range, above which it levels off. Maximally active muscles can produce reductions in middle ear transmission up to 20-30 dB at low frequencies [15].

AIM OF THE RESEARCH

The behavior of the acoustic reflex amplitude in response to various kinds of protracted noise with the same energy content administered with different temporal patterns, was investigated in a previous research [16]. The objest of concern in the present study was to check the exchange rate to maintain constant acoustic reflex amplitude for WN short stimuli. Given that the amplitude of acoustic reflex is proportional to the stimulus intensity [17], it was especially interesting to assess the acoustic reflex amplitude in relation to some other parameter patterns.

MATERIAL AND METHOD

Four males and six females were chosen from 32 subjects aged 18-23 yrs. with normal bilateral hearing (threshold for airborne pure tones $\leq$ 10 dB HTL for frequencies between 250 and 8000 Hz). Starting from 80 dB SPL and with subsequent 1 dB increments to 90 dB SPL, they also displayed the minimum stimulus intensity capable of provoking a distinct, baseline deflection of the trace of the oscilloscope connected to the signal generator (Visual Detection Thresholds [18]) in five successive stimulations with WN 125 msec bursts (rise/fall time: 1 msec; frequency: 0.2/sec).

Since there was an imprecise area of about 10 dB at the threshold level of the input-output function curve for amplitude and intensity [17], the test was commenced with 100 dB SPL stimuli. With this stimulus intensity, these 10 subjects displayed an acoustic reflex with an amplitude of 2.20 to 2.60 uV in 10 preliminary tests with WN bursts (rise/fall time: 1 msec; duration: 500 msec; frequency 0.2/sec). The uV is the arbitrary parameter adopted for evaluation of the reflex amplitude when working with the instruments employed in this study.

Signal generation and evaluation of the data were done with an Amplaid MK VI coupled to a Teksys 9000 and linked to a 702 Amplaid impedance meter via an Amplaid A.R.I. interface. A 220 Hz probe tone was used. The electrical hysteresis of the instrument was 45 msec. The computer acquisition parameters were: pass band 0.01-10 Hz; analysis 2 sec, with 500 msec preanalysis; sensitivity 5 uV, with automatic rejection of artifacts (interpreted as 100% of the input).

Each subject was exposed to 5 stimuli lasting 500, 250 and 125 msec ten times on ten different days (WN bursts: rise/fall time: 1 msec; frequency: 0.2/sec). Their spectrum (Fig. 1) was evaluated with a Revox M 3500 microphone located at the headset level. Starting from 100 dB SPL and 500 msec, each halving of the duration was accompanied by intensity increases of 3, 4, 5 and 6 dB SPL respectively (exchange rates: 3, 4, 5, 6 dB SPL).

Five subjects received the stimuli in the right ear and five in the left through a TDH 39 headset. The observations were made on the contralateral ear in a faradized silent chamber.

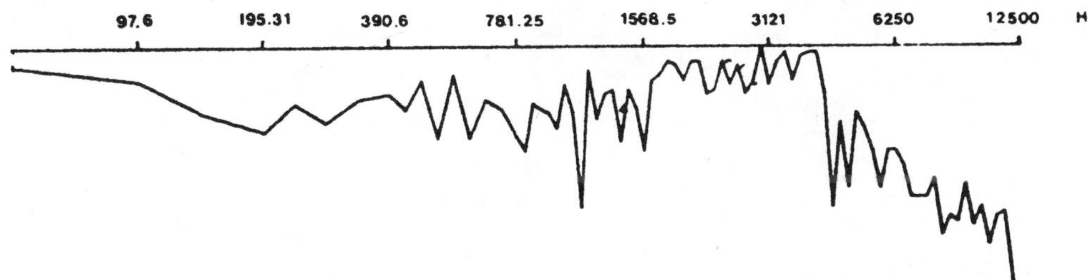

Fig. 1. Headset signal spectrum (log scale FFA).

The computer supplied an average curve for 5 stimuli in succession to reduce the margin of error. A 2-min. pause, during which the pressure status of the outer and middle ear was rechecked, was inserted between each set of signals at different exchange rates.

Each subject was examined five times starting from the longer and less intense stimuli, and then five times starting from the shorter and more intense stimuli, to offset possible sequence-induced differences in response. The four exchange rates were used in a random order.

The computer provided a mean for the 500 findings for the three parameters examined with reference to each type of stimulus:

1) reflex latency: interval in msec between start of stimulus and start of reflex;

2) reflex amplitude: difference in uV between the value recorded by the computer at the start of contraction and at maximum contraction;

3) reflex recruitment time: interval in msec between start of contraction and maximum contraction.

The electrical hysteresis of the instrument was substracted when calculating parameter 1). The latency was also deduced in the case of parameter 3).

RESULTS

The results can be summarized as follows:

1) reflex latency (Table I, Fig. 2): this appeared to be solely tied to the reflex threshold. Once this level was exceeded, the latency was constant, irrespective of the intensity and duration of the stimulus;

2) reflex amplitude (Table II, Fig. 3): this was only constant at 5 dB SPL exchange rate. With 3 and 4 dB SPL there was a statistically significant reduction compared with 5 dB SPL, whereas the difference between 5 and 6 dB SPL were not significant;

3) reflex recruitment time (Table III, Fig. 4): The maximum contraction amplitude was always reached before the end of the stimulus. The per cent ratio between reflex recruitment time and stimulus duration did not change significantly when the stimulus parameter was altered (Table IV, Fig. 5).

Table I

REFLEX LATENCY (msec)				
Stimulus duration (msec)				
500	17.55 ± 3.48			
	Exchange rate			
	3 dB SPL	**4 dB SPL**	**5 dB SPL**	**6 dB SPL**
250	17.40 ± 3.85	16.40 ± 3.59	17.40 ± 4.02	16.00 ± 3.58
125	18.00 ± 3.50	17.60 ± 3.34	16.81 ± 3.96	17.15 ± 3.23

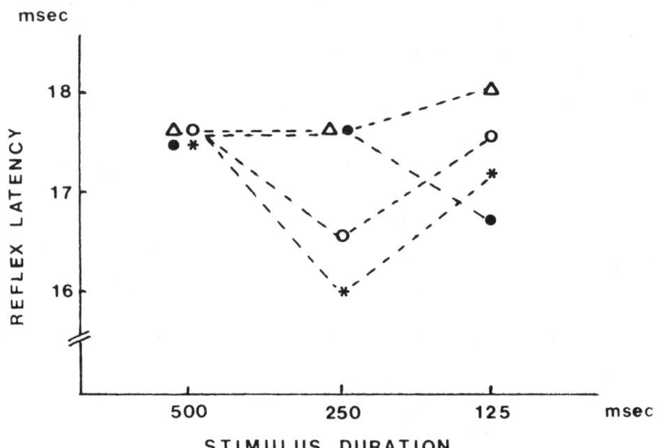

Fig. 2. Reflex latency

DISCUSSION AND CONCLUSIONS

When assessing the protective effect of the acoustic reflex on Corti's organ, it must be remembered that the amplitude of a muscle response is the result of the ratio linking the two main components of the stimulus: intensity and duration. This amplitude is dependent on the number of motor units the stimulus is able to activate, as determined by their characteristics,* i.e., different motor units or different groups of motor units possess a different threshold level [19].

In this experiment the previous ratio between duration and intensity constantly activating the same number of motor units was only reestablished at the CNS level with 5 dB SPL exchange rate: with this exchange rate the amplitude of the reflex remained constant, whereas it fell with 3 and 4 dB SPL.

The difference in amplitude between 5 dB and 6 dB exchange rate was not significant. This means that no further increases in amplitude are obtained from rates above 5 dB SPL. Probably at this rate a ratio between intensity and duration capable of activating all the existing motor units, even those with a highest threshold, was created.

* A motor unit consists of a motor neuron, its nerve fiber and the muscle fibers related to the latter.

Table II.

REFLEX AMPLITUDE (μV)				
Stimulus duration (msec) 500	2.34 ± 0.10			
	Exchange rate			
	3 dB SPL	4 dB SPL	5 dB SPL	6 dB SPL
250	a 2.04 ± 0.09	c 2.06 ± 0.10	e 2.36 ± 0.08	g 2.41 ± 0.11
125	b 1.92 ± 0.11	d 2.00 ± 0.11	f 2.35 ± 0.10	h 2.40 ± 0.13
«t» test				
a ↔ c : $p < 0.3$	c ↔ e : $p < 0.001$	e ↔ g : $p < 0.2$		
b ↔ d : $p < 0.1$	d ↔ f ; $p < 0.001$	f ↔ h : $p < 0.2$		

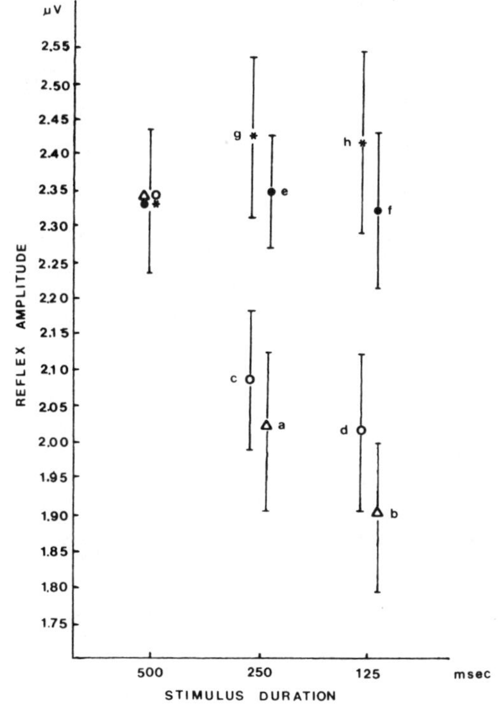

Fig. 3. Reflex amplitude

Table III.

REFLEX RECRUITMENT TIME (msec)				
Stimulus duration (msec) 500	449.00 ± 15.48			
	Exchange rate			
	3 dB SPL	4 dB SPL	5 dB SPL	6 dB SPL
250	223.72 ± 12.09	220.40 ± 11.82	219.01 ± 9.81	217.61 ± 10.95
125	109.80 ± 6.37	111.60 ± 6.03	109.20 ± 5.87	109.23 ± 6.09

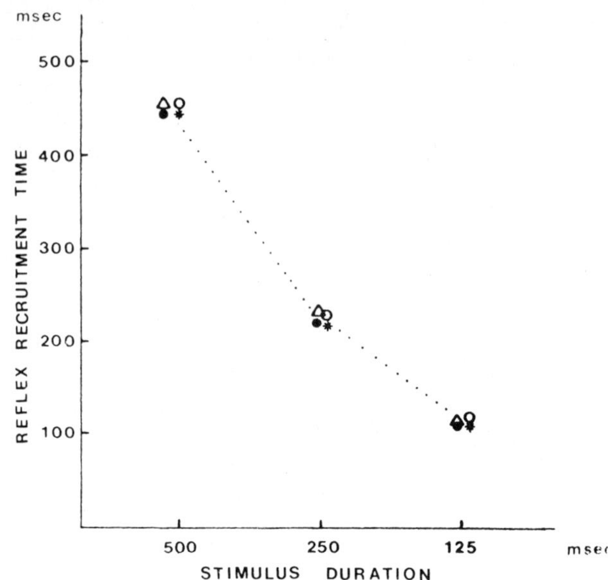

Fig. 4. Reflex recruitment time.

Table 4.

PER CENT RELATIONSHIP BETWEEN REFLEX RECRUITMENT TIME AND STIMULUS DURATION				
Stimulus duration (msec)				
500	89.80 ± 3.10			
	Exchange rate			
	3 dB SPL	4 dB SPL	5 dB SPL	6 dB SPL
250	89.49 ± 3.23	88.16 ± 4.73	87.60 ± 3.92	87.04 ± 4.38
125	87.20 ± 5.97	89.28 ± 4.82	87.36 ± 4.70	87.38 ± 4.87

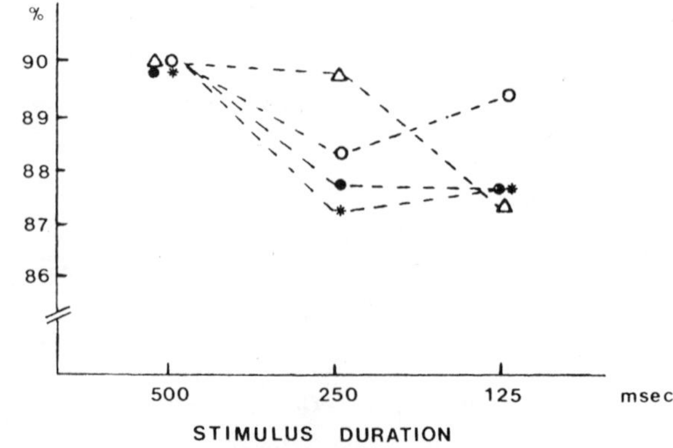

Fig. 5. Percent relationship between reflex recruitment time and stimulu duration.

The latency values observed did not alter with changes in intensity and duration, as previously reported for pure tones [9] and WN bursts [20]. This is also in agreement with those obtained with masking noise in man, evaluated by Fisch and Schulthess [21] with electromyographical method.

This finding further underscores the importance of the acoustic reflex amplitude in altering middle ear impedance and causing (albeit not to the same degree at all frequencies) a reduction in the amount of the acoustic energy reaching Corti's organ.

Since the percent ratio between recruitment time and duration of the stimulus was virtually constant, the active part of the reflex was always finished by the time the stimulus had acted for about 9/10 of its duration.

The reflex fall time has not been taken into consideration, because it did not provide information of importance in relation to the purpose of this research.

ACKNOWLEDGMENTS

Prof. G. Sacerdote and Prof. W. Sulkowski are gratefully acknowledged for their technical and scientific assistance. This research was supported by a grant from Assessorato alla Sanita ed alla Sicurezza Sociale della Regione Piemonte (Deliberazione G.R. 6 luglio 1982; n. 98-17320).

REFERENCES

1. F. E. Eldred, W. J. Gannon, and H. von Gierke, Criteria for short time exposure of personnel to high intensity jet aircraft noise, WADC-TN-355, Aerospace Medical Laboratory, Wright Patterson AFB, Ohio (1955).
2. B. Kylin, Temporary threshold shift and auditory trauma following exposure to study-state noise. An experimental and field study. _Acta Otolaryng., Suppl._, 152 (1960).
3. W. Burns and D. W. Robinson, Hearing and noise in industry, Her Majesty's Stationary Office, London (1970).
4. G. R. C. Atherley and A. M. Martin, Equivalent continuous noise level as a measure of injury from impact and impulse noise, _Ann. Occup. Hyg._, 14:11 (1971).
5. E. Guberan, J. Fernandez, J. Gardiner, and G. Terrier, Hazardous exposure to industrial impact noise: persistent effect on hearing, _Ann. Occup. Hyg._, 14:345 (1971).
6. A. M. Martin, The assessment of occupational noise exposure, _Ann. Occup. Hyg._, 16:353 (1973).
7. C. G. Rice and A. M. Martin, Impulse noise damage risk criteria, _Ann. Occup. Hyg._, 28:359 (1973).
8. A. Martin, The equal energy concept applied to impulse noise, _in_: "Effects of Noise on Hearing," D. Henderson, R. P. Hamernik, D. S. Dosanjh and J. Mills eds., Raven Press, New York (1976).
9. G. Rossi, Characteristics of the acoustic reflex elicited by pure tones and white noise bursts with different overall acoustic energy, _in_: "Relationships between Ambient Acoustic Energy and Inner Ear," G. Rossi ed., _Acta Otolaryng., Suppl._ 387 (1982).
10. W. D. Ward, Temporary threshold shift and damage-risk criteria for intermittent noise exposure, _J. Acoust. Soc. Amer._, 48, No. 2 (Part 2):561 (1970).

11. U.S. Department of Air Force, Hazardous noise exposure, Air Force Regulation 161-35, Washington, D.C. (1973).
12. F. Pfander, Uber die Toleranzgrenze bei akustischen Einwirkung, HNO (Berlin), 13:27 (1965).
13. U.S. Department of Health, Education and Welfare, Occupational exposure to noise, HSM 73-11001 (2nd ed.) Washington, D.C. (1972).
14. G. Rossi, G., Il danno uditivo da trauma acustico cronico: aspetti generali e problemi specifici, Collana di monografie sulle malattie professionali No. 5, Edizioni I.N.A.I.L., Roma (1984).
15. P. Dallos, "The Auditory Periphery: Biophysics and Physiology," Academic Press, New York (1973).
16. G. Rossi, Acoustic reflex amplitude in response to continuous noise and impulse noise with the same energy content, in: "Proceedings of the Fourth International Congress on Noise as a Public Health Problem," G. Rossi ed., Edizioni Tecniche a cura del Centro Ricerche Studi Amplifon, Milano (1983).
17. V. Colletti, Impedenzometria, Edizioni Tecniche a cura del Centro Ricerche e Studi Amplifon, Milano (1984).
18. J. Jerger, L. Mauldin, and N. Lewis, Temporal summation of the acoustic reflex, Audiology, 16:177 (1977).
19. G. Moruzzi, Fisiologia della vita di relazione, 2nd ed., U.T.E.T., Torino (1981).
20. G. Rossi, P. Solero, and M. Rolando, Relationships between acoustic reflex patterns elicited by unfiltered white noise and narrow band noise stimuli of different duration but of the same intensity, J. Laryng., (1985) (in press).
21. U. Fish and G. von Schulthess, Electromyographic studies on the human stapedial muscle, Acta Otolaryng., 56:287 (1963).

THE PROPOSED ISO STANDARD DETERMINATION OF OCCUPATIONAL NOISE EXPOSURE AND ESTIMATION OF NOISE-INDUCED HEARING IMPAIRMENT

H. E. von Gierke

Harry G. Armstrong Aerospace Medical Research Laboratory
Wright-Patterson AFB, Ohio 45433, USA

INTRODUCTION

Research on the relationship between noise exposure and noise-induced hearing loss has been very intense over the last 30 years, and steady progress has been made in spite of many remaining questions and unresolved problems regarding the mechanism. For the time being, avoidance of excessive noise exposure is the only way to prevent noise-induced hearing loss; this is the reason why governments, industry, workers and their representatives have been looking for scientific exposure criteria and guidelines to prevent hazardous noise exposure as part of comprehensive hearing conservation programs. Although it was clear from the beginning that noise-induced hearing loss in a population with exactly defined noise exposure would exhibit a statistical distribution due to differences in biological susceptibility, the epidemiological statistical data were not available to describe quantitatively the difference between the percentage of people with impaired hearing in a noise exposed group and the percentage of people in a non-noise-exposed group, i.e., the risk of noise-induced hearing impairment. All data suffered from inherent inaccuracies in the noise as well as exposure time measurement and from the limited knowledge and differences in opinion on what to define as "normal," non-noise-exposed hearing. Early Damage Risk Criteria such as the U. S. National Academy of Sciences (CHABA) [1] recommendations of 1966 and their subsequent adoption, simplification and modification by various individuals and agencies relied on the postulated relationship between temporary threshold shift (TTS) and permanent threshold shift (PTS) produced by a specific noise and on the assumption that exposures that produce equal TTS are equally hazardous. When, in the 1960's, international agreement on a method to estimate the risk of noise-induced hearing loss became desirable, the working group of ISO tackling this problem for many years had only very limited epidemiological data at their disposal. Important data used by this group were unfortunately only published much later [2]. The ISO Recommendation resulting from this effort in 1971 (later converted into the technically equivalent ISO Standard 1999) [3] presented a simple method to calculate the equivalent continuous sound level for a work-weeks' exposure from sound measurements and to estimate for equivalent continuous sound levels between 80 and 115 dB(A) and exposure times from 0 to 45 years the risk of impaired hearing or the total percentage of a population with impaired hearing. Hearing was considered to be impaired, according to compensation rules used in some countries, if the arithmetic average of the permanent threshold hearing level of the subject at 500, 1000 and 2000 Hz is shifted 25 dB or more compared with the corresponding average of the normal population defined by the ISO Standard for pure-tone audiometers.

Between 1968 and 1973, landmark epidemiological industrial studies [2,4-8] were published and analyzed by Johnson [9,10]. This analysis provided the necessary data base to describe noise-induced hearing loss in exact statistical terms, gave new data on the normal non-noise-exposed hearing threshold of populations as a function of age [11,12] and allowed new comparison of the much debated relationship between the effects of steady noise compared to intermittent and varying noise exposure [13]. The concepts of "effective quiet" and asymptotic TTS [14] were much discussed and the latter shed serious doubt on the hypothesis of the quantitative relationship between TTS and PTS. In addition, increasing awareness of the importance of frequencies above 2000 Hz for speech intelligibility and of communication difficulties in noise environments, particularly for older individuals, made it desirable to reanalyze the previous definition of "impairment for conversational speech" and the 25 dB "fence" [15] In summary, as soon as the first ISO Standard was finally agreed upon and published, it was time to start on its revision. A new ISO working group was decided upon in 1977 and started working in 1978 and provided a ISO/DIS 1999 for vote in 1982 [16]. Although 20 countries approved the DIS versus seven disapprovals and two absentees, it was decided to revise the text of the DIS taking into account as many of the comments (which were frequently not of a technical nature) as possible. The circulation of this second DIS will take place in 1985 and it is believed that it constitutes the best possible compromise for an International Standard at the present time, and that it will be accepted with still wider approval. ISO 1999 constitutes the basis for legislation in many countries and therefore a revised ISO Standard is urgently needed. In the following, the basic philosophy and specific features of the new proposed standard are briefly reviewed and its applications explained.

OUTLINE OF THE NEW STANDARD

The new DIS coming up for vote this year has the designation "ISO/DIS 1999.2 - Acoustics - Determination of Occupational Noise Exposure and Estimation of Noise-Induced Hearing Impairment". After the introductory sections (Scope, References and Definitions), Section 4 of the proposed standard deals with the description and measurement of noise exposure; Section 5 with the prediction of the effects of noise on hearing threshold and Section 6 with assessment of risk of noise-induced hearing impairment and handicap. Five Annexes, which are not part of the standard, and a bibliography conclude the document. Annex A describes the calculation of the age-related threshold level of a normal, "highly screened" population according to the new Standard ISO 7029 [17]. Annex B gives an example of a data base for an unscreened non-noise-exposed population. Annex C provides as a bridge to the 1975 ISO 1999 [3], data for an unscreened population, which when used with the new standard, results in the risk tables of the 1975 standard. Annex D gives an example of the new procedure and Annex E contains tables with numerical data calculated according to the formulas in the body of the proposed standard.

Section 4 on description and measurement of the noise exposure solves several dilemmas of present noise exposure evaluations: how to describe daily non-standard workday exposure and how to evaluate noise environments with intermittent, irregular and impulsive character or pure tone components. All exposures during an average workday are to be energy-averaged and expressed in terms of the A-weighted sound exposure

$$E_T = \int_0^T P_A^2(t)\,dt \quad \text{in Pascal}^2\ \text{seconds} \tag{1}$$

$P_A(t)$ is the instantaneous A-weighted sound pressure and the period T is chosen to cover a whole day's occupational exposure, commonly eight hours (28.8 ks). A footnote, much debated because of its potential legal implications, advices that E_T might be extended to include the daily nonoccupational leisure time exposure. The noise exposure level is

$$L_{EX,T} = 10 \log \frac{E_T}{E_0} \text{ in decibels, where} \tag{2}$$

E_0 has been chosen to be $1.15\ 10^{-5}\ Pa^2s$, so that L_{EX} for an eight hour exposure is numerically equal to the widely used equivalent, continuous A-weighted sound pressure level L_{Aeq}.

$$L_{EX,T} = L_{Aeq,T} + 10 \log \left(\frac{T}{To}\right) \tag{3}$$

where the reference duration To is eight hours. In the concept presented, the integration period applies to a working day or working week, but an extension of the integration period over a working lifetime (noise-immission) is not included.

To relate noise-induced hearing loss directly to the A-weighted sound energy of the exposure and to extend this concept even to impulse noise, was not strictly the result of simplicity and convenience. As several recent analyses have shown [18,19], taking all available data into account, no other measure of noise exposure has been generally accepted to result in a better relationship. With respect to various types of varying and intermittent noises, Passchier-Vermeer [13] had selected from approximately 200 studies 20 sets of data, of which she compared after age correction and normalization to a 15 year exposure time the median noise-induced permanent threshold shift (NIPTS) values for the intermittent noises, with the values predicted by the more generally accepted steady-state broad band exposure studies. Recently this important study was revisited and the data renormalized according to the functions proposed in the standard under discussion [20]. The result is presented in Fig. 1. The curves show good agreement for the exposure frequencies where maximum hearing loss occurs (2000 to 4000 Hz) and a systematic deviation is only evident at 6000 Hz. The curves calculated according to DIS 1999 are solid lines only for L <100 dB, since the proposed standard states that "extrapolations to higher levels are not supported by quantitative data."

To include impulse noise in the noise exposure level had been proposed by several investigators [21] and was finally endorsed by a special workshop on impulse noise and auditory hazard convened in 1981 to analyze available data. Among the conclusions of this workshop [22], attended by most researchers actively pursuing this problem, one reads: "There is no convincing evidence not to accept A-weighting for all practical applications as the method of evaluating all types of noises having different frequency spectra (10 - 20000 Hz) and time functions with respect to their permanent threshold shift-inducing hazard as long as their unweighted instantaneous peak sound pressure level does not exceed approximately 145 dB." The proposed standard recommends that the peak instantaneous sound pressure level should not exceed 200 Pa, i.e., 140 dB relative to 20 uPa.

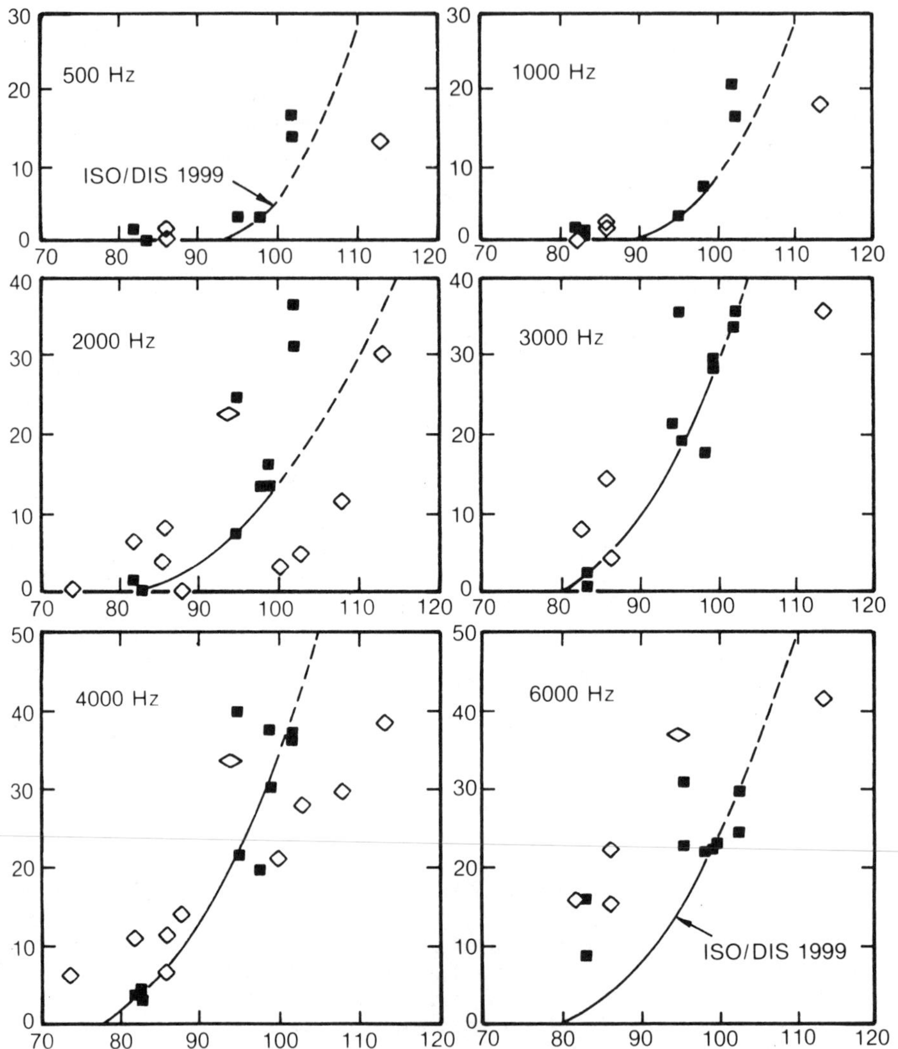

Fig. 1. NIPTS FROM INTERMITTENT NOISES COMPARED TO ISO/DIS 1999: Comparison of noise-induced hearing loss at various test frequencies due to intermittent and varying noise exposure. (intermittent: differences between highest and lowest sound levels at least 20 dB. Intermediate levels negligible. Varying: intermediate levels present for considerable fraction of time. "Long" > 5 minutes. 1 minutes < "short" < 5 minutes.) The data represent the analysis by Passchier-Vermeer [13] updated and compared to ISO/DIS 1999-1982 by Shaw [20].

The fact that this limitation of it's applicability requires for impulsive type noises with peak levels expected in this range, a sound measurement instrument with peak or overload indication at 140 dB is a minor shortcoming of the new method. However, integrating sound level instruments which are commercially available, and for which standards are in preparation [23], can address this problem. The 140 dB limit is not a practical limitation for industrial occupational exposure: since all hearing conservation programs require the wearing of personal hearing protectors at levels above 85 to 95 dB, the 140 dB peak exposure of the ear translates at least to 150 dB or higher outside of the ear protector, a level very seldom exceeded in industry. For those rare situations, special attention to more effective ear protection and application of the impulse/blast criteria developed for military exposures is recommended.

The method proposed has the great advantage that all noises from steady state to impulse are included in the exposure measure, and can be measured with an integrating-averaging sound level meter or a personally worn noise dosimeter. The standard recommends methods for direct and indirect determination of the exposure level and discusses sampling methods.

To summarize Section 4, the energy-averaged daily exposure over the years of exposure/employment is the only environmental measure needed to calculate hearing impairment or risk of hearing handicap, as long as the following conditions are met: maximum instantaneous sound pressure level less than 140 dB, average 8-hour daily exposure does not exceed 100 dB(A) (after accounting for personal hearing protectors) and the maximum individual daily exposure is not more than 10 dB above the average of all daily exposures.

The following Section 5 presents the method for predicting the effects of the noise exposure on hearing. It avoids the difficult value judgement, social and economic decision of what amount of noise-induced hearing loss constitutes a hearing handicap, impairment of hearing for conversational speech or risk of hearing handicap. These medico-legal decisions are left up to the user of the standard, governments or administrative bodies. The standard does not assume a fixed "fence," since it is obvious that no agreement on this quantity could be reached nor should be expected from the various users because the "fence" is to a large degree an administrative-economical-social decision and not a scientifically determined quantity. Nor does the new standard assume a specific combination of hearing threshold levels at specified frequencies to calculate the hearing handicap for conversational speech. It lists eight frequency combinations presently in use and/or advocated in various countries, but realizes that these combinations might be subject to change and might be different for different languages and cultures. All these not strictly scientific decisions are left up to the user.

What the standard provides is a simple practical method to calculate, based on available epidemiological data, the hearing threshold level (HTL) of a noise-exposed population by the formula

$$H = A + N - \frac{AN}{120} \qquad (4)$$

where H is the HTL

A is the age-related hearing threshold level (ARTL)

N is the potential noise-induced permanent threshold shift (NIPTS)

For risk calculations it is accurate enough to simplify this formula to

$$H = A + N \qquad (5)$$

since the term $\frac{AN}{120}$ starts to modify the result significantly only when A+N is above approximately 40 dB, i.e., well above any practical fence. Equations 4 and 5 apply to all corresponding fractile values of H, A and N.

The difficulty of defining a "normal," non-noise-exposed population as a function of age and sex and of deciding to what degree diseases, effects of ototoxic drugs and unknown non-occupational noise exposures should be included as part of the normal aging process led to the following compromise: the standard permits two data bases (A and B) to be used for ARTL. Data base A is the threshold distribution of the ideal "highly screened" population free of all signs of ear disease, obstructing wax and without undue history of noise exposure. This normal threshold of hearing as a function of age and sex has recently been standardized in ISO 7029 [17], and the applicable formulas are given in Annex A. As data base B, any carefully collected data base covering an occupationally non-noise-exposed population considered to be a valid control for the noise-exposed population, is permissible. Every country, industry or researcher can select the subpopulation most appropriate for its analysis. As an example, for data base B, Annex B gives the data from the US Public Health Service surveys [24]. Which data base, A or B, is more appropriate depends entirely on the questions to be answered. It is obvious that the accuracy of HTL in equations (4) or (5) depends critically on the accuracy of the data base, i.e., ARTL. For the user of the ISO Standard, it must be emphasized that the only accurate data bases available, given as A and as example for B, are based on populations in European and North American countries.

For the calculation of the NIPTS, values for the frequencies from 500 to 6000 Hz formulas are presented valid for exposure times between 0 and 40 years and average daily noise exposure levels $L_{EX,T}$ between 75 and 100 dB. The statistical distribution of the calculated potential NIPTS (the same for both sexes) is considered a reliable approximation to the experimental data for the .05 to the .95 fractiles.

With the noise-induced permanent threshold shift established for all frequencies, the user can now calculate the hearing handicap or the risk of hearing handicap according to the formula selected from Section 6 or according to the one prescribed or customary in the respective country.

Although the data base which formed the basis for ISO 1999 - 1975 was incomplete and inaccurate compared to the new data, as explained in the introduction, it appeared desirable to list in Annex C selected ARTL values, which, when used with the new procedure, result in the same hearing risk as predicted by Annex B of the 1975 procedure. Since ISO 1999 is the basis for legislation in many countries, inclusion of this example for data base B, although scientifically outdated, appeared desirable to facilitate acceptance of and transition to the new standard.

APPLICATION OF THE PROPOSED NEW STANDARD

The practical use of the new standard and the insight it allows into the dependence on the various parameters is illustrated by an example in Annex D. For a male population, 50 years of age exposed to $L_{EX,8h}$ = 90 dB daily for 30 years (8 hours/day, 5 days/week, 50 weeks/year) the ARTL, NIPTS and HTL are calculated. For handicap assessment, the frequency combination 1, 2 and 4 KHz is assumed. The risk of handicap due to age and noise is easily derived from the graphical presentation of the results (Fig. 2), and the importance of the height of the fence or the dependence on the frequency combination is obvious. It is also easy to see how much higher the risk of hearing handicap would be in an unscreened population compared to the screened population assumed in the illustration.

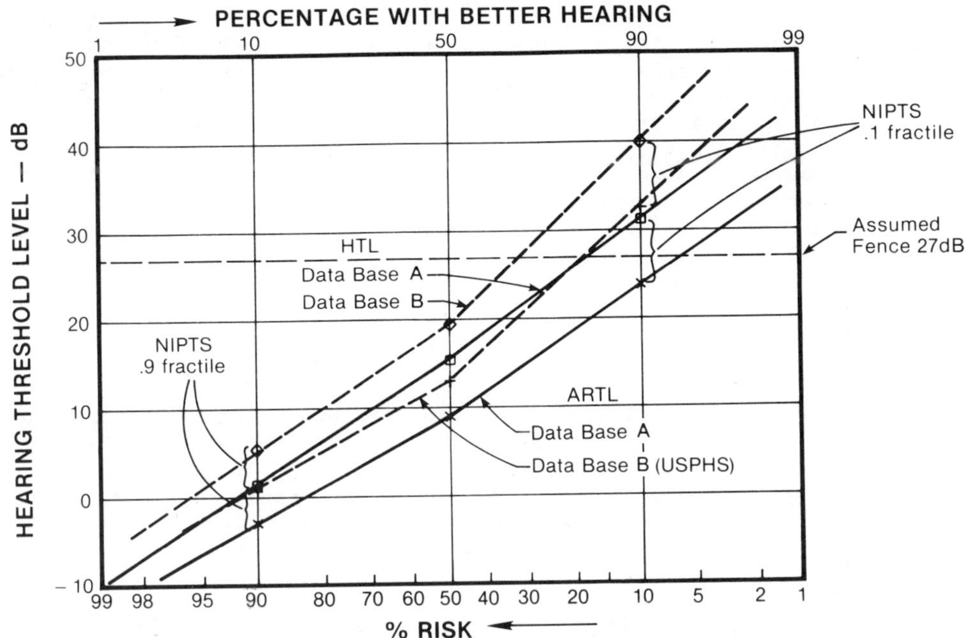

Fig. 2. Example for hearing impairment and hearing risk assessment from ISO/DIS 1999-1982. Noise exposure level $L_{EX,8h}$ = 90 dB for 30 years with ARTL data from data base A [16].

CONCLUSIONS

The proposed revision of ISO 1999 is an important step forward in standardizing in a practical procedure, the scientific findings of the past 20 years. It should be a useful tool for governments and industries alike, to estimate noise-induced hearing loss and risk of hearing handicap according to a uniform procedure, leaving important parameters to the users' judgement or local rules. It must be emphasized that the NIPTS predictions are based on statistical data and should therefore not be used to predict or justify hearing impairment in individual persons. The standard constitutes an important international agreement regarding noise measurement and monitoring at the workplace, particularly with respect to including impulse noise (below 140 dB unweighted instantaneous peak levels) in the total noise exposure. Adoption of the standard should support more realistic and effective hearing conservation programs.

In the future, once we have experience with the new procedure, and new research results become available, revisions of the standard will undoubtedly be indicated. Several areas would profit from additional data and an estimate of the uncertainty associated with the procedure would be desirable. Similarly, extension of the validity of the procedure to situations when the maximum observed eight hour exposure level exceeds the average eight hour equivalent exposure level by more than 10 dB is of practical interest, and the inclusion of non-occupational leisure time exposure deserves further consideration. Verification of the assumptions regarding impulse noise and perhaps specification of the maximum instantaneous sound pressure level in dB(A) should be addressed. However, in spite of these potential improvements with new data, the present draft standard appears to represent today the best compromise and practical application of generally accepted research results. It is hoped that it will be accepted by a large majority vote of ISO member countries, because a revision of the old standard is urgently needed.

REFERENCES

1. K. D. Kryter, W. D. Ward, J. D. Miller and D. H. Eldredge, Hazardous exposure to intermittent and steady-state noise, J. Acoust. Soc. Am. 39:451 (1966).
2. W. L. Baughn, Relation between daily noise exposure and hearing loss based on the evaluation of 6835 noise exposure cases, AMRL-TR-73-53, National Technical Information Service, Springfield Virginia, USA (1973).
3. ISO 1999, Acoustics - assessment of occupational noise exposure for hearing conservation purposes, (Identical with ISO Recommendation R1999-1971), International Organization for Standardization, Geneva, Switzerland (1975).
4. W. Passchier-Vermeer, Hearing loss due to exposure to steady state broadband noise, Institut Voorgesondheidtechniek (Netherland) Report 35 (1968). See also "Hearing Loss Due to Continuous Exposure to Steady-State Broadband Noise," J. Acoust. Soc. Am. 56:1585 (1974).
5. D. W. Robinson, The relationship between hearing loss and noise, National Physical Laboratory Aero Report Ae32 (Teddington, Middx., England) (1968).
6. D. W. Robinson, Estimating the risk of hearing loss due to exposure to continuous noise, in: "Occupational Hearing Loss," British Acoustical Society Special Volume No. 1, Academic Press, New York (1971).
7. D. W. Robinson, Characteristics of occupational noise-induced hearing loss, in: "Effects of Noise on Hearing," D. Henderson, R. P. Hammernik, D. S. Dosanijh and J. H. Mills eds. Raven Press, New York (1976).
8. W. Burns and D. W. Robinson, Hearing and noise in industry, (HM Stationery Office, London) (1970).
9. D. L. Johnson, Prediction of NIPTS due to continuous noise exposure, Aerospace Medical Research Laboratory Report AMRL-TR-73-91. (National Technical Information Service, Springfield, Virginia, USA.) (1973).
10. D. L. Johnson, Derivation of presbyacousis and noise-induced permanent threshold shift (NIPTS) to be used for the basis of a standard on the effects of noise on hearing, AMRL-TR-78-128. (National Technical Information Service, Springfield, Virginia, USA.) (1978).
11. A. Spoor, Presbycusis Values in Relation to Noise Induced Hearing Loss, Int. Audiol. 6:48 (1967).
12. A. Spoor and W. Passchier-Vermeer, Spread in hearing levels of non-noise exposed people at various ages, Int. Audiol. 8, (1969).
13. W. Passchier-Vermeer, Noise-induced hearing loss from exposure to intermittent and varying noise, in: "Proc. Int. Cong. on Noise as a Public Health Problem," Dubrovnik (U.S. Environmental Protection Agency, Washington, D. C.) (1973).

14. AGARD, Effects of long duration noise exposure on hearing and health, M. A. Whitcomb ed., AGARD Conf. Proceedings No. 171, AGARD, Neuilly-sur-Seine, France (1975).
15. A. H. Suter, The ability of mildly hearing-impaired individuals to discriminate speech in noise, EPA 550/9-78-100 and AMRL-TR-78-4, National Technical Information Service, Springfield, Virginia, USA (1978).
16. ISO/DIS 1999, Acoustics - determination of occupational noise exposure and estimation of noise-induced hearing impairment, International Organization for Standardization, Geneva, Switzerland (1982).
17. ISO/DIS 7029, Normal threshold of hearing by air conduction as a function of age and sex, International Organization for Standardization, Geneva, Switzerland (1982).
18. EPA, Information on levels of environmental noise requisite to protect public health and welfare with an adequate margin of safety, U.S. Environmental Protection Agency Report 550/9-74-004 (Washington, D. C.) (1974).
19. World Health Organization, Environmental health criteria 12, Noise, Geneva, Switzerland (1980).
20. E. A. G. Shaw, Draft Report of the Scientific Advisor to the Special Advisory Committee on the Ontario Noise Regulation, (Second Draft), National Research Council, Ottawa, Canada (1984).
21. G. R. C. Atherley and A. M. Martin, Equivalent continuous noise level as a measure of injury from impact and impulse noise, Ann. Occup. Hyg., 14:11 (1971).
22. H. E. von Gierke, D. W. Robinson and S. J. Karmy, Results of the Workshop on Impulse Noise and Auditory Hazard, Memorandum 618, Institute of Sound and Vibration Research (University of Southampton, England) (1881).
23. IEC Draft Proposal, Integrating-averaging sound level meters, SC29C - International Electromechnical Commission, Geneva, Switzerland (1983).
24. USPHS, National Center for Health Statistics, Hearing Levels of Adults by Age and Sex, United States, 1960-62, Vital and Health Statistics, Public Health Service Publication No. 1000, Series 11, No. 11, U.S. Government Printing Office, Washington, D.C (1965).

DISCUSSION

Smoorenburg: I have a question which I think is of a very fundamental nature and has to do with the problem of additivity of presbycusis and NIHL. We do not know the correlation between the susceptability for presbycusis and the susceptability to noise-induced hearing loss, thus, it is probably correct to add to two phenomena in the population, but it is not adviseable for the individual.

von Gierke: It is quite clear the standard cannot and should not be applied to the individual case. It is based on statistical data and it can give you only statistical results. It is obvious that the danger is that in some compensation cases it will be argued the subject has such and such probability of getting a such and such noise-induced hearing loss. This is not the way the data should be interpreted and can be interpreted. I think this is clearly indicated in the standard.

Alberti: Is this standard valid for odd type exposure intervals? For example, individuals in the petro-chemical industry work three 12 hour days then take 4 days off. The oil drilling rigs are 12 hours on 12 hours off for 10 days at a time and then 10 days off. Does this standard risk table cover that type of odd exposure?

von Gierke: I think yes, it does not cover it with the same degree of accuracy as it covers a 5 day work week. I would still go to the noise exposure per week and calculate from this noise-induced hearing loss.

Stevins: I think this proposal for a new ISO standard is a very positive step in the direction I defended earlier, but I think there remains one main limitation for applying this standard to impulse noise, and that is the evaluation of levels over 145 dB peak SPL. To be specific, my concern is that it may be possible to show that one single series of impulses, in one day, with peak intensities over 165 dB, but having an A-weighted level equal to 85 dB remains covered by the same rules.

PRESIDENT FAREWELL ADDRESS

G. Rossi

Institute of Audiology, Turin University
Via Genova, 3 - 10126 Torino

Dear friends and colleagues, ladies and gentlemen,

Our International Workshop on Basic and Applied Research on Noise-Induced Hearing Loss is over. The time has therefore come to draw up an albeit no more than provisional initial balance sheet and then allow time to show how far our first impressions were sound.

As president of this Workshop, it is my task to put the question: "What has been the significance of this meeting at the international level?".

The first conclusion to emerge from this meeting, I feel, is that it has shown the extent of the commitment devoted to the question of noise-induced hearing loss in all parts of the world where this problem is encountered. Furthermore, the scientific involvement of a large number of researchers is accompanied by an equally significant commitment on the part of the international organisations that gave their patronage to our workshop.

N.A.T.O., for example, has again proved that its purposes and aims do not stop at the defence of the nations of which its membership is composed, but also extend to matters of a strictly civilian nature concerned with living conditions in the world of today.

The Commission of the European Communities, too, through its General Management V, has provided further evidence of the commitment and sensitivity with which it attends to both the scientific and the practical aspects of problems associated with working conditions and the work environment, and especially those related to noise.

The extent to which these two great international organisations devote their attention to every aspect of noise-induced hearing loss underscores the importance of a problem that Europe, too, is now examining through investigation of each of its many facets.

The current position in Italy with respect to noise-induced hearing loss does not fully emerge, perhaps, from the Workshop programme. There has, however, been a particular awakening of interest in the subject in Italy recently, though attention has perhaps been directed more to the epidemiological and medicolegal aspects of the subject rather than its theoretical side and the questions thus posed. One should, indeed, not lose sight of the fact that noise-induced hearing loss constitutes about 60% of the cases of occupational disease recognised and indemnified each year by INAIL, the Italian National Work Accident Insurance Agency.

It is clearly impossible for me to consider at this stage all the individual aspects of the topics that were dealt with, the doubts that were resolved, the solutions put forward, and the problems for which a solution appears to lie on a very distant horizon.

Noise-induced hearing loss, indeed, is such a vast topic that each of its many aspects deserves considered and deliberate assessment.

As time passes, we shall undoubtedly feel the need to weigh up the various features of the subject, not so much with regard to their specific and particular meaning as in relation to an overall vision of the problem. Our effects, in fact, cannot be confined to the simple recognition and awareness of a particular situation, but must set out to supply mankind, whose work involves exposure to noise, with increasingly improved living conditions.

For this reason, I feel sure that what has emerged during these five days will soon be able to be judged within a perspective that is no longer sectorial, in other words in the context of a comprehensive vision, wherein both mathematical theory and biological reality will find their boundaries, which sometimes appear distinct and clear-cut, more subtly intermingled, so that a practical solution can be offered for a problem that both claims and demands it by its very nature.

May I also express the hope that the memory of these days spent in a tranquillity that was in itself an invitation to study and meditation will not remain an end, but will engender in the heart of each participant a desire - unconscious, perhaps, at first - to renew these meetings from time to time.

Progress in our field follows a long and difficult path, one along which we must march with a critical mind but a confident step, in the assurance that tomorrow's successes are perhaps born at the very moment when are led to doubt ourselves and the usefulness of all that we have done so far.

Morphologie des cils des cellules ciliées à la suite d'un traumatisme sonore

B. Engstrom et E. Borg, Stockholm, Suède

Les stéréocils des cellules ciliées de l'organe de Corti sont indispensables à la transduction des signaux acoustiques en signaux électriques. Lorsque l'oreille est sur-stimulée par le bruit, les stéréocils sont lésés de façon pratiquement systématique. Ils peuvent fusionner, se casser ou disparaître de la surface cellulaire tandis que le reste de la cellule ciliée peut ne pas être modifié. Lorsqu'il y a fusion, celle-ci affecte les cils en partie ou en totalité. La rupture des stéréocils survient juste au dessus de leur point d'ancrage dans la membrane cuticulaire et entraîne l'inclinaison ou la disparition des stéréocils ainsi que des fusions avec les stéréocils adjacents.

Les lésions apparaissent au niveau des stéréocils de façon différente au niveau des cellules ciliées internes et externes selon l'emplacement considéré le long de la cloison cochléaire et selon les conditions d'exposition.

Chez le lapin l'exposition à un bruit de large bande (2-7kHz, 115dB, 15 minutes) produit des dommages importants au niveau des cellules ciliées internes tandis que les cellules ciliées externes ne présentent que peu ou pas de lésions.

Les lésions des stéréocils au niveau des cellules ciliées internes correspondent à des fusions ou à des inclinaisons ciliaires mais rarement à la disparition des cils. De plus si l'examen est effectué plusieurs mois après l'exposition au bruit, on peut observer des cils géants. Ces cils géants sont présents lorsque la plupart ou tous les cils d'une cellule sont anormaux. En microscopie électronique à transmission, les cils originels ne sont souvent pas reconnaissables parmi les cils géants nouvellement formés.

Sur les cellules ciliées externes on observe souvent des cils qui ont disparu tandis que d'autres semblent fusionnés et/ou normaux. Dans le tour apical, les cils fusionnés peuvent former des cils géants. De plus, il semble que l'écart entre une cellule ciliée externe lésée et une cellule ciliée externe morte est ténu dans le reste de la cochlée du lapin.

Les lésions décrites ci-dessus se rencontrent également chez l'homme, le rat, le singe et le cobaye mais elles peuvent atteindre selon des proportions différentes les cellules ciliées externes et internes. Nous avons également découvert qu'il est possible d'augmenter la proportion des cellules ciliées externes lésées chez le lapin en délivrant l'énergie acoustique de façon différente (faible niveau: 85dB et durée d'exposition importante: 512 heures).

En conclusion on peut dire que l'aspect morphologique des lésions des stéréocils après une sur-stimulation acoustique est assez reproductible mais que l'étendue et la répartition des lésions varient considérablement en fonction de l'espèce, de l'emplacement et de l'exposition sonore.

Modifications mécaniques des stéréocils à la suite d'un traumatisme sonore: observations, mécanismes possibles

J.C. Saunders et B. Canlon, Université de Pennsylvanie, USA
A. Flock, Karolinska Institut, Suède

Les descriptions anatomiques de la pathologie des stéréocils à la suite de l'exposition à des sons intenses ainsi que la démonstration récente des relations entre cette pathologie et les modifications fonctionnelles dans le système auditif seront résumées. Ces relations sont intéressantes et importantes mais elles ne constituent au mieux que des corrélations et non une relation évidente de cause à effet. Il y a peu de doute que des modifications structurales drastiques peuvent survenir sur les pinceaux de cils aussi bien que sur des cils isolés, cependant les implications fonctionnelles de ces lésions en termes de micromécanique des stéréocils ne sont pas connues. De plus il existe une confusion considérable en ce qui concerne la possibilité ou non pour les stéréocils de récupérer les lésions subies pendant la stimulation.

Sur des préparations de cochlées de cobayes isolées on présentera une démonstration expérimentale montrant le développement et de la récupération d'un déficit auditif à partir de la micromécanique des stéréocils, à la suite d'une exposition à une stimulation intense. Ces résultats montrent clairement qu'une sur-stimulation produit une réduction de la raideur du faisceau de stéréocils et que cette altération peut se réduire avec le temps. Une démontration supplémentaire selon laquelle la récupération de la raideur des stéréocils dépend de la présence de cellules ciliées normales et en bonne santé sera présentée. Lorsque les cellules ciliées sont bloquées métaboliquement soit par refroidissement soit par empoisonnement avec du NaCN, aucune récupération de la raideur mécanique n'a pu être détectée à la suite de la stimulation. Les différentes modifications structurales qui pourraient être à l'origine de la perte de la raideur des stéréocils aussi bien que les mécanismes cellulaires conduisant à la récupération de ces lésions seront développées. Enfin la relation possible entre les modifications physiologiques de la micromécanique des stéréocils et les altérations de la fonction auditive seront discutées.

Morphologie des stéréocils et de leurs liaisons en relation avec les dommages dûs au bruit

J.O. Pickles, M.P. Osborne et S.D. Comis, Université de Birmingham, Grande-Bretagne

La morphologie des stéréocils et de leurs liaisons a été étudiée chez des cobayes normaux ainsi que chez des cobayes exposés au bruit, immédiatement après la fin de l'exposition. Les cochlées furent fixées sans tetroxyde d'osmium, soit au glutaraldéhyde seul soit au glutaraldéhyde/picrate. Elles furent examinées en microscopie à transmission et à balayage.

Chez les cobayes normaux les stéréocils sont liés latéralement par un faisceau étendu de liaisons croisées qui sont concentrées dans une région située vers le sommet des stéréocils. Les liaisons semblent se poursuivre à l'intérieur de renforcements desmosomiques dans les parois des stéréocils, avec une augmentation de densité des membranes des deux stéréocils, et dans le faisceau filamenteux central sous jacent. De ce fait les liaisons possèdent des caractéristiques morphologiques suggérant qu'elles forment des connections solides entre les stéréocils. Les liaisons qui partent du sommet des stéréocils courts, liaisons dont on a pensé qu'elles jouaient un rôle dans les processus de transduction, s'insèrent également dans les stéréocils au niveau de zones denses et spécialisées et se projettent dans le noyau filamenteux du stéréocil.

Dans des cochlées lésées par le bruit, les stéréocils furent examinés à partir des régions où les dommages étaient modérés en bordure des zones plus lourdement atteintes. Les signes de lésion comprennent des modifications de la texture de la membrane des stéréocils et des courbures de ces derniers. Les courbures sont concentrées dans les régions où les stéréocils ne sont liés que de manière lâche aux stéréocils adjacents; les zones centrales des stéréocils qui sont plus fortement attachées tendent à maintenir leur organisation spatiale. De plus, il est encore possible d'observer quelques liaisons, correspondant à celles supposées importantes pour la transduction, dans des faisceaux de stéréocils qui montrent d'autres signes lésionnels.

Les résultats suggèrent que les liaisons latérales entre les stéréocils sont importantes pour le maintien de l'intégrité spatiale des pinceaux durant la sur-stimulation. De plus, au moins quelques unes des structures supposées importantes pour la transduction peuvent résister à des niveaux de sur-stimulation qui produisent des arrachements sur les stéréocils.

Innervation de l'organe de Corti: Morphologie des différents types de synapses, neurotransmetteurs putatifs, implications physio-pathologiques

R. Pujol, M. Eybalin et M. Lenoir, INSERM U254, Montpellier, France

Les fibres nerveuses dans l'organe de Corti sont classiquement divisées en deux grandes catégories: afférentes et efférentes. Deux systèmes afférents sont bien connus. Les dendrites des gros neurones myélinisés du ganglion spiral (95% de la population totale) sont connectés radialement avec les cellules ciliées internes (CCI) dont elles reçoivent le message auditif. Les dendrites des petits neurones sont connectées avec les cellules ciliées externes (CCE): 1 neurone est en contact avec un grand nombre de CCE des 3 rangées; la signification fonctionnelle de ce système n'est pas claire. De la même façon, les efférences ont été récemment subdivisées en deux systèmes. Le latéral provient essentiellement de l'olive supérieure ipsilatérale et se termine sous les CCI en formant des synapses avec les dendrites afférentes. Le système médian provient essentiellement du corps trapézoïdal controlatéral et effectue des synapses axo-somatiques avec la base des CCE.

Ce chapitre a pour but de décrire les synapses que chacun de ces 4 systèmes forme dans l'organe de Corti. Leur ultrastructure est précisée, en faisant appel aux données ontogénétiques lorsqu'elles permettent de mieux comprendre l'organisation de type adulte. Des indications morphologiques sur les neurotransmetteurs putatifs sont commentées. Enfin les implications d'une telle organisation synaptique sur la physiopathologie cochléaire liée au trauma acoustique sont discutées.

Morphologie de la membrane cellulaire normale et pathologique et des structures de jonction dans la cochlée

A. Forge, Institut de Laryngologie et d'Otologie, Londres, Grande-Bretagne

Le fonctionnement de la cochlée dépend du maintien et de la modulation de différences de concentrations ioniques et de potentiels électriques entre des compartiments séparés. De telles caractéristiques sont vraisemblablement reliées à des spécialisations dans la structure et la fonction des membranes cellulaires. On sait aussi que quelques agents ototoxiques peuvent affecter les propriétés des membranes cellulaires. L'examen détaillé des membranes cellulaires dans la cochlée est ainsi d'une grande importance. La technique de fracture après congélation permet l'étude ultrastructurale des membranes par observation directe. Il est possible d'identifier les traits d'organisation des membranes et des jonctions intercellulaires. Aussi bien les "tight junctions" (TJ) qui se comportent comme des "obturateurs" empêchant la diffusion des ions dans les espaces intercellulaires que les "gap junctions" (GJ) qui permettent des communications intercellulaires directes, peuvent être examinées en détail. Une amélioration complémentaire de la méthode est possible en employant des sondes spécifiques de certains composants des membranes cellulaires. Les plus employées visent à localiser le cholestérol membranaire. On présentera dans ce texte une revue des résultats de l'application des techniques de fracture après congélation aux tissus cochléaires normaux ainsi qu'à ceux endommagés par les ototoxiques.

Dans les tissus normaux, cette technique a mis en évidence les caractéristiques des membranes de la plupart des différents types cellulaires. La distribution des jonctions intercellulaires a également été déterminée. Les TJ sont présentes entre toutes les cellules qui bordent l'espace endolymphatique. Elles sont aussi présentes entre les cellules basales de la strie vasculaire. Les TJ entre les cellules basales et celles de la lame réticulaire de l'organe de Corti sont remarquablement étendues. Les GJ sont présentes entre les cellules de soutien de l'organe de Corti ainsi qu'entre les cellules du ligament spiral. Dans la strie vasculaire elles sont associée de façon prépondérante avec les cellules basales. Les cellules basales de la strie vasculaire forment des GJ avec les autres cellules basales, avec les autres types cellulaires de la strie et avec les cellules du ligament spiral.

Dans les tissus cochléaires d'animaux qui ont reçu un ototoxique, des altérations des régions membranaires comportant des jonctions aussi bien que de celles qui n'en comportent pas ont été notées, particulièrement dans la strie. Après administration chronique de gentamycine, les TJ des cellules marginales apparaissaient désorganisées et les GJ montraient des altérations morphologiques variées. Immédiatement après la fin du traitement des particularités de la membrane latérale des cellules marginales furent observées. Avec des diurétiques des altérations significatives des GJ et des membranes des cellules intermédiaires furent notées alors que il n'y avait que très peu d'autres indications d'effets ototoxiques. Les changements dans les membranes des cellules intermédiaires furent particulièrement mis en évidence grâce aux sondes de cholestérol membranaire. Ces résultats indiquent que les études de fracture après congélation peuvent être utiles pour détecter les effets précoces d'agents lésionnels sur les tissus cochléaires.

Modifications morphologiques induites mécaniquement dans l'organe de Corti

R.P. Hamernik, M. Roberto et G. Turrentine, Université de Dallas, USA

Les modifications anatomiques de l'organe de Corti à la suite de l'exposition à des bruits intenses et en particulier à des bruits impulsionnels ou à des ondes de choc peuvent être considérables. A l'aide de préparations en microscopie optique et en microscopie à balayage, nous avons suivi la séquence des altérations qui surviennent sur les différentes cellules épithéliales du canal cochléaire à la suite d'une exposition à des bruits impulsionnels de niveau élevé (160dB). Les expériences ont été réalisées sur le chinchilla.

Très tôt après l'exposition on observe des décollements d'origine mécanique étendus des structures de soutien et des structures sensorielles sur la membrane basilaire, c'est à dire la déchirure des liaisons cellulaires qui assurent l'intégrité structurale de l'organe de Corti aussi bien que des déchirures étendues des liaisons des cellules épithéliales à la membrane basilaire. Le résultat est que 7 mm ou plus de l'organe de Corti sont détachés de la membrane basilaire. On peut montrer que ces lésions se développent à partir d'une série de très petites déchirures localisées à l'origine au niveau de la fixation des cellules de Hensen. La réaction immédiate des cellules épithéliales demeurant sur la membrane basilaire consiste en une prolifération de la membrane cellulaire dans le but de ré-épithélialiser la membrane basilaire. De plus une population dense de microvilli qui est le mieux observable sur les cellules du sillon interne se développe sur la plupart des cellules restantes. Les cellules du sillon interne semblent être activement impliquées dans l'endocytose des débris cellulaires. Cette réaction de la surface cellulaire est maximale environ 10 jours après l'exposition et se poursuit au moins jusqu'au trentième jour. L'état des cellules ciliées internes est variable et dépend largement de la nature et de l'étendue des lésions mécaniques. La persistance d'un grand nombre de cellules ciliées internes dans les zones lésées qui sont complètement dépourvues de cellules ciliées externes peut expliquer la limite supérieure des déficits auditifs de 40dB qui est fréquemment rencontrée chez les animaux exposés à de tels stimulus.

Application des principes de morphométrie et de stéréoscopie aux tissus épithéliaux: considérations théoriques et pratiques

F. H. White, Université de Sheffield, Grande-Bretagne

Les techniques morphométriques et, en particulier, stéréoscopiques permettent d'obtenir des informations quantitatives relatives à la structure des tissus biologiques. La morphométrie se limite essentiellement à des mesures faites en une ou deux dimensions telles que le nombre, la longueur et la surface, tandis que les mesures stéréoscopiques peuvent fournir une dimension supplémentaire et apporter des résultats plus significatifs en termes biologiques.

Des informations quantitatives peuvent être obtenues sur des échantillons représentatifs de cellules ou de tissus à partir d'un certain nombre de techniques relativement simples. Diverses techniques de mesures peuvent être utilisées pour obtenir des résultats soit directement à partir de coupes soit indirectement à partir de clichés réalisés en microscopie optique ou en microscopie électronique. Ces résultats de base caractérisent les composants structuraux d'après leur longueur leur nombre ou leur surface; de tels résultats peuvent être convertis en informations plus évoluées se rapportant à des caractéristiques plus particulièrement intéressantes à l'aide de formules simples. On obtient ainsi des estimations de densité; par exemple le volume d'organites cytoplasmiques comme les mitochondries peut être exprimé par rapport au volume unitaire du cytoplasme cellulaire tandis que des caractéristiques relatives aux surfaces cellulaires comme le nombre ou la surface des jonctions intercellulaires peuvent être reliées à l'unité de surface de membrane plasmatique sur laquelle elles sont observées. Au niveau histologique des paramètres analogues peuvent être fournis, par exemple le volume d'un type particulier de cellules par rapport au volume unitaire de l'organe qui les contient. Ces estimations de densité peuvent être converties en résultats encore plus élaborés si les volumes absolus ou les surfaces de référence peuvent être déterminés. En utilisant la combinaison de mesures directes et de procédés stéréoscopiques, il est possible d'obtenir des valeurs absolues, par exemple, du volume total de mitochondries dans une cellule "moyenne", de la surface totale de la membrane plasmatique formant une jonction intercellulaire particulière dans une cellule spécialisée "moyenne" ou du volume total de cellules d'un type donné à l'intérieur d'un organe.

Les procédés qui permettent l'application pratique des principes morphométriques et stéréoscopiques sont décrits. Des exemples illustrent la façon dont ces techniques peuvent être utilisées tant au niveau histologique qu'au niveau ultrastructural en biologie expérimentale des épithéliums, à partir d'un modèle d'évaluation des effets d'aggressions chimiques sur un épithélium squameux stratifié. Au plan histologique, je décrirai comment le système vasculaire est affecté, en fonction du temps, dans les tissus connectifs de la muqueuse orale soumise à un traitement prolongé par l'hydrocarbure cancérigène DMBA. Au niveau ultrastructural, en utilisant une méthode expérimentale analogue, les effets du DMBA sur quelques composants des tissus connectifs épithéliaux seront examinés en fonction des modifications histopathologiques induites plutôt que par rapport à la durée du traitement. Ces résultats montreront comment l'information quantitative structurale, qui est à la fois fiable et objective, peut être obtenue en biologie expérimentale des épithéliums à l'aide de techniques ne nécessitant qu'un minimum d'équipement spécialisé. De plus l'amélioration de l'objectivité et de la sensibilité de l'analyse apportée par la quantification structurale peut révéler l'extension d'altérations structurales suspectées aussi bien que détecter des modifications non prévues. Les analyses morphologiques quantitatives apportent ainsi une dimension nouvelle aux études morphologiques des structures épithéliales normales et anormales.

Evaluation de la microvascularisation cochléaire à l'aide de méthodes morphométriques

L.C. Shaddock, Université du Michigan, USA

Plusieurs méthodes d'analyse quantitative de la microvascularisation cochléaire ont été décrites dans la littérature. La technique de préparation de spécimens de surface souples d'Axelsson s'accompagne de la quantification de 20 paramètres vasculaires; pour chaque demi tour de cochlée une valeur numérique est enregistrée pour chaque paramètre sur tous les vaisseaux cochléaires. Cette technique a été appliquée à l'étude des effets des bruits sur la vascularisation cochléaire. Santi a quantifié la densité volumique des cellules marginales, intermédiaires et basales et des capillaires de la strie vasculaire en utilisant des techniques stéréoscopiques standards adaptées à ce type de tissu. En utilisant cette méthode, Santi a décrit la morphologie normale de la strie vasculaire et les changements morphologiques qui suivent l'administration de bumetanide. Smith a utilisé un système d'analyse d'image par ordinateur pour mesurer la densité vasculaire et la distribution en érythrocytes dans la strie vasculaire de cobayes normaux, de cobayes exposés au bruit et de cobayes traités à la quinine.

Notre technique comprend une analyse d'image assistée par ordinateur de tous les vaisseaux du mur latéral. Les vaisseaux sont divisés en trois groupes en fonction de leurs relations avec la strie vasculaire, le ligament spiral et la proéminence spirale, et 7 variables vasculaires sont quantifiées. Cette méthode a été utilisée pour décrire la pathologie vasculaire causée par la rupture de la membrane de Reissner. Du fait de la variabilité de la disposition des vaisseaux d'un animal à l'autre et de la nature subtile des variations pathologiques des vaisseaux, l'analyse statistique est une nécessité indispensable pour toutes les méthodes quantitatives. Toutes les méthodes histologiques ont le désavantage de présenter une image statique d'un processus dynamique; les techniques de sacrifice et d'anesthésie sont très importantes et des groupes de contrôle importants sont essentiels pour valider les résultats.

Conséquences mécaniques du traumatisme sonore sur les vibrations de la membrane basilaire

R. Patuzzi, Université de Western Australia, Australie

Des observations récentes des vibrations de la cloison cochléaire chez le chat (Science 215: 305-306, 1982), le cobaye (J. Acoust. Soc. Am., 72: 131-141, 1982) et le chinchilla (J. Acoust. Soc. Am., 76: S35, 1984) ont confirmé et complété les travaux de Rhode (J. Acoust. Soc. Am., 49, 1218-1231, 1971) chez le singe écureuil. Ces études ont montré que chez l'animal normal de nombreuses caractéristiques des réponses électriques des cellules ciliées internes (et par là même des fibres afférentes qui les innervent) peuvent être expliquées en termes de déplacements de la cloison cochléaire.

Ces déplacements, observés dans le tour basal de la cochlée du cobaye normal, seront résumés et leur rôle dans l'origine du décalage d'une demie octave de la fatigue auditive sera discuté. De plus, les modifications des vibrations de la cloison cochléaire observées à la suite d'un traumatisme chirurgical ou de l'exposition au bruit suggèrent qu'au moins une partie des déficits auditifs peuvent être attribués à une altération de ces vibrations. En comparant les vibrations de la cloison cochléaire en fonction de la fréquence avec les réponses nerveuses et les réponses électriques des cellules ciliées internes sur des cochlées intactes et des cochlées traumatisées par le bruit, il est possible d'évaluer jusqu'à quel point les altérations des vibrations de la cloison cochléaire contribuent aux déficits auditifs induits par le bruit. De telles comparaisons montrent que la réduction des vibrations de la cloison cochléaire ne peut rendre compte de tous les déficits auditifs mais elles suggèrent que, pour les faibles durées d'exposition, la diminution de sensibilité mécanique correspond à la majeure partie des élévations de seuil. Ces modes de vibration normaux et anormaux de la cloison cochléaire seront replacés dans le contexte de l'action possible de mécanismes non linéaires d'éléments à rétroaction positive et les directions futures de recherche seront discutées.

Seuils d'audition, fatigue auditive et mécanique cochléaire

A. Dancer et R. Franke, Institut franco-allemand de recherches de Saint-Louis, France,
P. Campo, INRS, Nancy, France

Selon Dallos (1973), Zwislocki (1975) et Dancer (1983), l'allure de la courbe des seuils de sensibilité auditive en fonction de la fréquence est déterminée par celle de la fonction de transfert qui relie le signal acoustique en champ libre au signal acoustique d'entrée de la cochlée (pression acoustique à la base de la rampe vestibulaire). Pour un signal d'entrée de la cochlée constant, le seuil serait lui constant. A partir de résultats théoriques (modèles) et expérimentaux (mesures de pression acoustique intracochléaire, de déplacement de membrane basilaire, de courbes d'accord...) il semble que le seuil de réponse d'une fibre nerveuse survienne toujours pour la même vitesse de déplacement de la membrane basilaire.

Connaissant le paramètre des mouvements de la membrane basilaire responsable de l'initiation des réponses au seuil, nous avons étudié l'influence de ce paramètre (c'est à dire de la vitesse de la membrane basilaire) sur les déficits auditifs.

Nous avons appliqué à la cochlée du cobaye des sons purs de fréquence comprise entre 2 et 11,3 kHz (par pas d'une demie octave) d'énergie acoustique constante. Cette dose était ajustée à l'aide d'une procédure basée sur l'enregistrement du potentiel microphonique cochléaire. Vingt minutes après la fin de l'exposition, nous avons mesuré les déficits auditifs par électrocochléographie entre 2 et 32 kHz (par pas d'une demie octave).

a) Pour d'obtenir des déficits auditifs maximums constants de 10 dB et/ou de 25 dB, le niveau de la stimulation acoustique à l'entrée de la cochlée devait être diminué de 4 dB par octave.

b) Des déficits auditifs constants de 8 dB à 16 kHz et de 12 dB à 22,6 kHz étaient obtenus (pour un son fatigant de fréquence inférieure) lorsque le niveau de la stimulation acoustique à l'entrée de la cochlée décroissait de 10 dB par octave environ.

Pour un signal d'entrée cochléaire d'amplitude constante nous avons pu montrer que:

l'amplitude des déplacements de la membrane basilaire à la base est constant pour les fréquences inférieures à la meilleure fréquence et que par conséquent la vitesse de la membrane basilaire double avec la fréquence,

l'amplitude des déplacements de la membrane basilaire près de la meilleure fréquence double chaque fois que la fréquence est divisée par deux et que par conséquent la vitesse de la membrane basilaire demeure constante tout au long de la cochlée.

A partir de ces observations il est permis de penser que la différence de pente en fonction de la fréquence, différence qui est relative au niveau de la stimulation entre les cas a) et b) (c'est à dire 6 dB par octave), montre que la vitesse de la membrane basilaire joue un rôle significatif dans l'apparition des déficits auditifs.

Réponse des cellules ciliées de la cochlée des mammifères à une sur-stimulation acoustique

A.R. Cody et I.J. Russell, Université du Sussex, Grande-Bretagne

Les modifications de sensibilité et de sélectivité en fréquence des fibres afférentes du premier neurone auditif après exposition à une sur-stimulation acoustique dépendent des modifications des réponses des cellules ciliées qu'elles innervent. Nous avons enregistré les potentiels continus de récepteur des cellules ciliées internes dans le tour basal de la cochlée du cobaye et nous avons trouvé qu'à la fois la sensibilité et les caractéristiques de la courbe d'accord de la cellule sont réduites à la suite de l'exposition à des sons intenses (110dB SPL, 225 ms) de fréquence inférieure d'une demie octave (12,5kHz) à la meilleure fréquence des cellules (CF: 16-20kHz). La perte de potentiel continu de récepteur de la cellule ciliée interne dans la zone voisine de CF est particulièrement importante puisque ce potentiel est essentiel à la détection des sons de haute fréquence par les fibres nerveuses afférentes du premier neurone. Ce composant du potentiel récepteur a vraisemblablement pour origine une conductance assymétrique du transducteur qui induit un flux net de courant vers l'intérieur de la cellule, flux qui est filtré passe bas par les propriétés électriques de la membrane cellulaire. Bien qu'il ne soit pas possible de contrôler, aux fréquences élevées de stimulation, les variations de conductance dans la cellule ciliée à la suite de la sur-stimulation acoustique, ces variations peuvent être enregistrées pour des sons correspondant à la zone basse fréquence de la courbe d'accord. Dans ce cas l'amplitude crête-à-crête du potentiel de récepteur est réduite à la suite du son intense et ce potentiel devient davantage symétrique ce qui réduit l'amplitude de la composante continue.

Des enregistrements intracellulaires dans les cellules ciliées externes montrent qu'aux basses fréquences ces cellules produisent aussi des potentiels de récepteur assymétriques à des intensités de stimulation modérées (<90 dB SPL), mais contrairement aux cellules ciliées internes l'assymétrie se situe dans la phase d'hyperpolarisation. De plus il existe une petite composante continue dans le potentiel de récepteur indépendamment de la fréquence de stimulation. Après le son intense l'assymétrie d'hyperpolarisation n'existe plus et il y a une réduction de l'amplitude du potentiel de récepteur. Les cellules ciliées externes présentent également une dépolarisation additionnelle et cumulative de la cellule après chaque exposition. A la fin du son intense la repolarisation de la cellule ciliée externe suit la récupération de l'amplitude et de l'assymétrie des potentiels récepteurs des cellules ciliées internes et externes. Cette repolarisation récupère de la même façon que la sensibilité cochléaire comme on peut le voir à partir de l'enregistrement du potentiel d'action global en réponse à des bouffées de sons purs. Au vu de ces résultats nous proposons l'hypothèse selon laquelle la dépolarisation soutenue des cellules ciliées externes et la repolarisation qui lui fait suite peuvent refléter ou sous-tendre les modifications mécaniques dans l'organe de Corti qui se traduisent dans les réponses aux sons des cellules ciliées et de leur innervation afférente. Les cellules ciliées externes pourraient par conséquent jouer un rôle essentiel dans la localisation des déficits auditifs induits par le bruit et dans leur mécanisme.

Corrélations structure-fonction dans les oreilles lésées par le bruit Etude par microscopie optique et électronique

M.C. Liberman, L.W. Dodds et D.A. Learson,
Eaton-Peabody Laboratory, Boston, USA.

L'étude des réponses nerveuses de cochlées lésées par le bruit a apporté un aperçu des mécanismes normaux de la transduction cochléaire ainsi que des informations au sujet des modifications de structure correspondant aux déficits auditifs temporaires ou chroniques induits par le bruit. Puisque chaque fibre nerveuse auditive de type I contacte une seule cellule ciliée interne (IHC), l'enregistrement unitaire donne une vue fonctionnelle d'une région bien précise de l'organe de Corti. En utilisant des techniques de marquage des fibres unitaires, nous pouvons identifier précisément la cellule ciliée interne qui a produit une réponse nerveuse donnée et établir des corrélations structure-fonction détaillées au niveau unitaire.

Dans le cas de dommages permanents induits par le bruit, la cause la plus importante des déficits auditifs, indépendamment des pertes de cellules sensorielles, semble être les dommages survenus aux stéréocils. Les stéréocils des cellules ciliées internes semblent plus vulnérables que ceux des cellules ciliées externes. Au niveau des cellules ciliées externes, les touffes de cils de la première rangée semblent les plus fragiles. La microscopie optique montre que les anomalies des stéréocils correspondent à des déplacements latéraux, à des inclinaisons au niveau de la base, à des fusions avec les cils voisins, ou à leur disparition totale. La perte des stéréocils des cellules ciliées internes est invariablement corrélée avec la chute des taux de décharge spontanée et tout autre dommage causé à ces stéreocils tend à élever la partie basses fréquences des courbes d'accord enregistrées sur les neurones correspondants. D'autre part, les dommages causés aux cils des cellules externes sont associés à une élévation de la pointe des courbes d'accord. La première rangée des cellules ciliées externes apparait comme étant la plus sensible à cet égard. Quand les dommages aux cellules externes ne s'accompagne pas de dommages aux cellules internes, la partie basse fréquence des courbes d'accord est hypersensible. Les implications de ces corrélations pour les mécanismes normaux de transduction seront discutées.

Les corrélations structure-fonction dans des oreilles atteintes de façon définitive par le bruit sont suffisamment constantes pour qu'il soit possible de prédire, à partir de l'ensemble des réponses nerveuses physio-pathologiques unitaires, la nature, le degré et l'étendue des dommages cellulaires. Quoique la pathologie cellulaire soit toujours corrélée à des déficits auditifs significatifs dans les neurones correspondant, il demeure certains types de déficits auditifs qui ne peuvent pas, en microscopie optique, être reliés à une lésion cellulaire. Ainsi, dans des cas précis, une analyse par microscopie électronique à transmission a été réalisée. Cette analyse n'a pas encore mis en évidence de pathologie ultrastructurale autre que celle suggérée par l'observation en microscopie optique. Il ne semble pas exister de pathologie ultrastructurale dans les corps cellulaires, dans les terminaisons nerveuses ou dans les synapses et ce, même chez des cellules présentant des lésions significatives des stéréocils. De plus, la plupart des anomalies ultrastructurales des stéréocils sont associées à des modifications visibles en microscopie optique. Les stéréocils qui apparaissent normaux (posture, insertion) semblent également normaux au niveau ultrastructal. Une pathologie ultrastructurale telle que la dépolymérisation des filaments d'actine se limite aux stéréocils qui sont nettement incurvés et/ou fusionnés. La fracture des racines ciliaires à la surface de la cuticule correspond à la pathologie ultrastructurale la plus commune mais cet état est associé à un déplacement latéral des stéréocils qui est visible en microscopie optique.

Les modifications structurales correspondant à des déficits auditifs aigus sont totalement différentes. Des oreilles présentant des déficits auditifs de 40 à 60 dB mesurés 8 à 16 heures après l'exposition peuvent ne montrer aucune pathologie en microscopie optique, bien qu'une vacuolisation des dendrites des fibres radiales soit visible dans certains cas. A partir des résultats limités dont nous disposons, il semble que le gonflement des terminaisons nerveuses apparaisse seulement après des expositions à des sons purs. Dans un cas d'exposition à un bruit de large bande, nous avons analysé l'ultrastructure des stéréocils à l'aide de coupes sériées. Nous n'avons trouvé aucune évidence de dépolymérisation des fibres d'actine ou de rupture de racine. Il semble que les racines des stéréocils dans la zone de cochlée affectée par l'exposition soient quelque peu raccourcies mais des études supplémentaires sont nécessaires. Il semble à l'heure actuelle évident que les mécanismes des déficits auditifs temporaires et permanents sont significativement différents.

Aspects psychophysiques et physiologiques du traitement temporel du signal sonore chez les animaux normaux et chez les animaux exposés au bruit

R.J. Salvi, S.S. Saunders, W. Ahroon, B. Shivapuja et S. Arehole,
Université du Texas, Dallas, USA

Des sujets qui présentent des déficits auditifs ont souvent des troubles de perception de la parole. Des techniques analytiques visant à comprendre ces troubles se sont dirigées sur des problèmes de codage en fréquence. Il n'est pas surprenant de constater que les pertes auditives influencent également la capacité du système auditif à apprécier la résolution temporelle.

Cet article passera en revue différents tests du traitement temporel du signal sonore (méthodes psychophysiques) qui ont été utilisés pour évaluer cette fonction chez des sujets présentant des pertes auditives (détection d'intervalle, seuils de modulation d'amplitude, masque préalable). Les résultats de ces études montrent que la résolution temporelle se détériore lorsque les pertes auditives dépassent environ 25 dB. De plus, la détérioration est plus prononcée lorsque les pertes se situent aux fréquences élevées. Récemment des enregistrements de fibres nerveuses unitaires aussi bien que des mesures de potentiels auditifs ont apporté une perspective nouvelle sur les modifications du traitement temporel du signal sonore qui sont induites par le bruit. La plupart de ces études ont utilisé un schéma de stimulation avec masque préalable pour mesurer la récupération de la sensibilité auditive à la fois chez l'animal normal et chez l'animal exsposé au bruit. Aussi bien les potentiels unitaires que les potentiels évoqués suivent un schéma de récupération exponentiel qui peut être caractérisé par une constante de temps. Les résultats obtenus à partir de chinchillas présentant des pertes auditives montrent que les constantes de temps relatives aux réponses unitaires et aux réponses évoquées sont parfois supérieures à celles mesurées chez l'animal normal. Le type de relation existant entre les résultats physiologiques et les résultats comportementaux sera discuté.

Accroissement de la sensibilité auditive au niveau central pendant la stimulation par des sons continus ou à la suite de perte auditive

G.M. Gerken, R. Simhadri-Sumithra et K.H.V. Bhat, Université du Texas, USA

La perte auditive a souvent été représentée comme une réduction de la qualité et de la quantité du signal d'entrée des centres. Dans ce modèle, les centres sont supposés traiter le signal d'entrée de la même façon que chez l'individu normal. Récemment des études en provenance de divers laboratoires ont commencé à montrer une variété de modifications centrales concomittantes à la perte auditive. Ce rapport résume quelques unes de ces études et présente de nouveaux résultats. Quatre phénomènes reliés aux mécanismes auditifs centraux sont décrits. Deux de ces effets surviennent chroniquement chez des chats éveillés présentant des pertes auditives. Les deux autres surviennent chez des animaux éveillés ayant une audition normale seulement pendant la présentation d'un son continu.

1) Le premier effet concerne les seuils de détection mesurés par une technique comportementale et obtenus à l'aide de stimulus électriques appliqués par l'intermédiaire d'électrodes chroniques implantées dans les noyaux auditifs du tronc cérébral. Les seuils de stimulation étaient en particulier nettement diminués (hypersensitivité à la stimulation) par la perte auditive produite par un son intense ou par un dommage mécanique à la cochlée.

2) L'hypersensibilité à la stimulation survenait également chez des animaux d'audition normale si les seuils de détection de la stimulation électrique étaient mesurés pendant la présentation d'un stimulus tonal d'intensité modérée.

3) Chez le chat présentant des déficits auditifs, les réponses évoquées auditives enregistrées directement dans le colliculus inférieur peuvent être considérablement plus importantes que les réponses enregistrées dans la même zone avant l'installation du déficit auditif. Cet effet n'a pas été rencontré dans les réponses enregistrées à partir du noyau cochléaire ce qui suggère la mise en jeu d'un mécanisme plus central.

4) Le quatrième effet, et le principal sujet de cet article, se rapporte également à une augmentation substantielle de l'amplitude des réponses évoquées auditives. L'accroissement d'amplitude était obtenu chez des animaux d'audition normale en présence d'un son continu d'intensité modérée (amélioration de la réponse évoquée). Cette amélioration était observée à des étages supérieurs du système auditif (c'est à dire dans les corps genouillés médians et sur les réponses évoquées corticales) mais pas dans les réponses précoces du tronc cérébral. De plus, l'amélioration était grandement diminuée ou même absente chez l'animal anesthésié.

La première variable indépendante: la perte auditive, affecte de façon permanente deux variables dépendantes: l'amplitude des réponses évoquées et le seuil de stimulation électrique. Ces deux variables sont importantes pour le traitement central de l'information. La seconde variable indépendante, le son continu, affecte les deux variables dépendantes d'une façon analogue mais transitoire. Si tant est que l'on puisse assigner un emplacement aux variations de la réponse évoquée auditive, il semblerait qu'il soit plus central (thalamus, cortex). Nous avons proposé ailleurs que l'hypersensibilité à la stimulation soit due également à des modifications centrales plutôt que périphériques. Les quatre phénomènes sont plus complexes que l'on ne peut l'expliciter dans ce bref résumé mais, sur la base de relations parallèles entre les deux variables indépendantes, nous suspectons un mécanisme central commun. Quelques unes des conséquences d'un tel mécanisme seront discutées.

Période critique pour la sensibilité au traumatisme acoustique

M. Lenoir, R. Pujol, INSERM U254, Montpellier, France
G. Bock, CIBA Foundation, Londres

Une période critique de sensibilité au trauma acoustique pendant le développement a été découverte, en physiologie, chez le chat, le hamster et la souris. Elle a aussi été suggérée, en histologie, chez le cobaye, et elle pourrait intéresser les nouveaux-nés humains.

Nous avons expérimenté sur le jeune rat et trouvé qu'une exposition (120dB/30minutes) à un bruit blanc provoquait des pertes auditives importantes et permanentes lorsqu'elle était réalisée entre le 16ième et le 40ième jour postnatal. Le maximum de pertes était enregistré avec une exposition au bruit réalisée le 22ième jour. Des observations en microscopie électronique réalisées 7 jours après l'exposition révèlent d'importantes lésions cytologiques dans les cellules ciliées et les fibres nerveuses. Un mois après l'exposition l'organe de Corti a complètement dégénéré à la base de la cochlée. Cela suggère une fragilité métabolique des structures neuro-sensorielles de la cochlée durant la période critique.

La période de sensibilité maximale est bien corrélée avec la fin de la maturation structurale et physiologique de la cochlée qui se situe aux environs du 20ième jour postnatal chez le rat. Un chevauchement avec l'hypersensibilité aux antibiotiques se réalise ainsi plaçant la cochlée qui achève sa maturation dans une période à très haut risque.

Réflexe acoustique et bruit d'impact industriel

ıR. Nilsson, Göteborg, Suède

Le rôle potentiel du réflexe acoustique (RA) dans la protection de l'oreille interne contre les pertes auditives induites par le bruit a depuis longtemps été le sujet d'études et de spéculations. Il est certain que son activation aux niveaux sonores modérément élevés et que sa nette capacité à élever l'impédance de l'oreille moyenne en réduisant ainsi la transmission acoustique sont en faveur d'un tel rôle protecteur.

Nous pensons à l'heure actuelle que le besoin le plus important est d'étendre notre connaissance de base des caractéristiques du RA et de sa fonction dans l'environnement industriel c'est à dire là où le bruit induit réellement des pertes auditives.

Plusieurs études furent conduites avec des bruits de chantier naval représentant une exposition typique à un bruit industriel. Les deux premières études concernaient la fatigabilité du réflexe et les deux autres l'action protectrice du réflexe vis à vis de la fatigue et des pertes auditives.

Dans la première étude des sujets d'audition normale étaient exposés sur une seule oreille à une séquence de 30 minutes de bruit de chantier naval.

La seconde étude était une étude réalisée sur le terrain et se rapportait à la fatigabilité du réflexe chez des individus présentant une audition normale après une journée normale de travail dans le chantier. Les résultats de ces deux études montrent que le réflexe n'est en moyenne que peu fatigable.

Dans la troisième étude, la fatigue auditive après exposition à un bruit de chantier naval enregistré était déterminée chez 10 sujets qui présentaient une paralysie faciale unilatérale aiguë. La fatigue auditive maximale était supérieure sur les oreilles privées du fonctionnement du muscle stapédien. La fréquence du TTS maximum se déplaçait de la zone 4 kHz vers la zone conversationnelle (2kHz) et les TTS étaient plus prononcés avec une extension principalement vers les plus basses fréquences. La surface totale des TTS était significativement supérieure sur les oreilles privées de réflexe acoustique.

Le rôle du réflexe acoustique au niveau des pertes auditives fut également étudié chez le lapin. Chez l'un des animaux, le muscle stapédien était énervé tandis que chez tous les autres animaux les muscles de l'oreille moyenne étaient désactivés par une anesthésie générale. L'oreille normale par rapport à l'oreille désactivée fut exposée au bruit de chantier naval. Dans tous les cas les pertes auditives étaient plus faibles sur les oreilles présentant un réflexe normal.

Sur la base de ces expériences, nous pensons que les arguments contre le réflexe acoustique en tant que mécanisme protecteur pour les bruits industriels sont largement battus en brèche. Ces résultats suggèrent également que les variations individuelles des caractéristiques du réflexe acoustique représentent une explication de la grande variabilité interindividuelle des déficits auditifs résultant de l'exposition aux mêmes environnements bruyants. En se basant sur ces résultats, il semble que la mesure des caractéristiques individuelles du réflexe acoustique puisse être intéressante pour prédire la susceptibilité au bruit.

Le réflexe acoustique correspond à un des aspects de la susceptibilité individuelle; les caractéristiques du réflexe acoustique et de la fatigabilité de ce réflexe peuvent servir de lignes directrices pour un travail "d'ergonomie du bruit" en effet, les effets nocifs du bruit pourraient être considérablement diminués si la faculté de protection du réflexe acoustique était prise en compte dans les efforts faits pour contrôler l'émission du bruit. Les enregistrements du réflexe peuvent aussi en eux-mêmes fournir une information sur la fatigue auditive et sur les dommages subis par l'oreille interne.

Simulation du réflexe acoustique appliquée au risque lésionnel des bruits d'armes pour l'audition

G.O. Stevin, Bruxelles, Belgique

Le réflexe acoustique peut être décrit comme un mécanisme de rétroaction qui réduit la transmission acoustique de l'oreille moyenne lorsque le niveau détecté dans le cerveau est trop élevé. L'effet de ce réflexe est d'augmenter la raideur du muscle stapédien produisant ainsi une modification de la réponse de l'étrier. Le processus de contraction du stapédien conduit à une réduction de la transmission des sons par l'oreille moyenne mais aussi à une augmentation de la résonance et de la fréquence de coupure de l'oreille moyenne. Ces deux effets, comme le prévoit le modèle, semblent être analogues à ceux observés chez les animaux et à ceux estimés chez l'homme. Le modèle est complété par un mécanisme de rétroaction ayant son siège dans le cerveau où un détecteur de seuil élabore la commande de contraction et la renvoie au muscle stapédien à travers un filtre passe-bas.

Le modèle fonctionnant sur ordinateur a été appliqué à la prévision de la sonie de bruits impulsionnels produits par des armes. Les normes actuelles d'exposition aux bruits impulsionnels précisent que seul le premier coup d'une rafale doit être pris en compte pour l'évaluation des risques lésionnels pour l'audition. Ceci signifie que les impulsions produites par les autres coups de la rafale sont suffisamment atténuées par le réflexe acoustique; elles sont ainsi négligées par les normes. Le modèle confirme sur une base théorique cette règle pratique mais seulement pour des armes classiques ayant une cadence de tir inférieure à 600 par minute.

Pour des armes de cadence supérieure, le nombre de coups survenant pendant les 100 millisecondes qui suivent le premier semble représenter un paramètre important pour le risque auditif. Ceci est principalement dû aux composantes spectrales de 2 et 3 kHz qui ne sont pas atténuées mais amplifiées par le réflexe acoustique. Les critères actuels d'évaluation des bruits impulsionnels conduisent à sous estimer le risque pour l'audition lors de cadences de tir élevées.

L'étrange décalage d'une demie octave en fréquence des déficits auditifs

D. McFadden, Université d'Austin, Texas, USA

Le décalage d'une demie octave des déficits auditifs est probablement la conséquence la plus largement connue de l'exposition au bruit, cependant les mécanismes qui sous-tendent cet effet n'ont fait l'objet que de peu d'attention tant sur le plan théorique que sur le plan expérimental. Il n'existe pas d'explication généralement reconnue de cet effet pas plus qu'il n'existe d'hypothèses concurrentes soutenues par différentes équipes permettant de l'expliquer.

Le premier objectif de cet article est de démontrer que les décalages d'une demie octave peuvent se rencontrer dans une très grande variété d'expériences psychophysiques et physiologiques et non pas seulement dans celles correspondant à l'exposition à un son intense. Un certain nombre de mécanismes possibles seront proposés et soumis à la critique. Parmi ces propositions on trouve des modifications possibles de la mécanique de la cloison cochléaire ainsi qu'un déplacement possible du maximum de l'enveloppe de l'onde propagée avec l'augmentation du niveau de la stimulation. Des résultats psychophysiques et physiologiques se rapportant à chacune de ces explications seront présentés.

Expériences relatives aux effets du bruit sur l'homme utilisant un modèle de fatigue auditive

F. Lindgren et A. Axelsson, Hôpital Sahlgrens, Göteborg, Suède

Nous avons développé un modèle expérimental basé sur la fatigue auditive pour étudier de possibles diminutions de sensibilité auditive dues à des facteurs aggravants tels que le tabac, l'aspirine, les vasodilatateurs, la charge de travail etc... .

Les principales étapes de cette méthode sont les suivantes:

a) utilisation d'une procédure standardisée au cours de laquelle les sons test aussi bien que les bruits sont appliqués au sujet par un écouteur TDH-39 connecté à un speculum. L'écouteur et le speculum sont montés sur un serre-tête pour permettre l'insertion correcte du speculum au niveau du conduit auditif externe. Cette procédure réduit les causes d'erreur dues aux variations de position de l'écouteur (lorsqu'il est fixé dans un casque) par rapport à l'oreille et ce, aussi bien lors de l'exposition aux bruits qu'aux sons test.

b) utilisation d'un audiomètre informatisé à balayage en fréquences de type Békésy qui calcule, à partir des audiogrammes pré et post-exposition, les TTS à des fréquences discrètes ainsi que la surface totale des TTS sur toute la gamme des fréquences.

c) expositions multiples de sujets normaux. Les sujets sélectionnés pour une étude particulière sont en général exposés, de façon aléatoire, 5 fois au bruit seul et 5 fois au bruit en combinaison avec un possible facteur aggravant (par exemple l'aspirine).

d) Récupération des TTS. Les seuils de sensibilité auditive sont mesurés dans la gamme de fréquences touchée par les TTS pendant une heure après l'audiométrie post-exposition avec un intervalle de 6 minutes entre chaque test.

Le principal avantage de ce modèle est la fiabilité bien supérieure des mesures de TTS au niveau individuel qui permet de ne provoquer que des TTS limités et qui permet également de distinguer de petites différences de TTS.

Le modèle sera discuté et les résultats de différentes études seront présentés.

Relation entre des mesures psychoacoustiques et la réception de la parole avec des pertes auditives

R.S. Tyler, Université de l'Iowa, USA

On sait que l'exposition au bruit a une influence sur la performance à de nombreux tests psychoacoustiques tels que la détection au seuil, l'intégration temporelle, la croissance de la sonie, la discrimination en intensité et en fréquence, la résolution en fréquence et la détection des intervalles. Ces mêmes mesures sont cependant également influencées par d'autres types de pertes auditives neurosensorielles.

J'examinerai tout d'abord sur la base de tests psychoacoustiques si les sujets présentant des pertes auditives induites par le bruit présentent un profil de réponse différent de ceux ayant des pertes auditives d'origine neurosensorielle. La réduction de la performance aux divers tests psychoacoustiques influence vraisemblablement de diverses façons la reconnaissance de la parole. Un schéma théorique relatif à la manière selon laquelle chaque anomalie psychoacoustique peut agir sur la perception de la parole sera décrit et ses suggestions seront testées à l'aide de quelques résultats anciens et récents.

Perception de parole synthétique dans le bruit

C.W. Nixon, T.R. Anderson et T.J. Moore, Dayton, Ohio, USA

Parmi les nombreuses applications de la parole synthétique se trouve l'usage potentiel qui pourrait en être fait pour fournir des informations ou des mises en garde dans de nombreux environnements contaminés par le bruit. Plusieurs des possibles avantages de tels signaux pourraient être perdus si le signal de parole synthétique était plus susceptible au masquage par le bruit que la parole normale ou d'autres signaux d'alarme.

Cette étude a comparé, dans le bruit, la perception de la parole naturelle à celle de signaux de parole synthétique d'une qualité allant de faible à très bonne. Le critère de mesure pour la perception était l'intelligibilité du mot sous la forme du Test de Rhyme Modifié. Des listes de mots de ce test étaient produites par un locuteur, par trois différents synthétiseurs texte-parole et par trois différents vocoders. Ces échantillons de parole étaient présentés, par l'intermédiaire d'un système de communication à dix canaux d'un rapport signal de parole sur bruit de -6 à +18dB, à un groupe de 10 sujets entraînés. Le système de communication fonctionnait dans un mode large bande et les sujets portaient des écouteurs de haute qualité. Les résultats ont été analysés en termes de pourcentage moyen de réponses correctes aux différents signaux de parole naturels et synthétiques présentés dans des conditions bruyantes. Dans cet article on discutera la perception relative de la parole naturelle et de la parole synthétique dans le bruit.

Perception de la parole chez des sujets ayant des pertes auditives induites par le bruit

G.F. Smoorenburg, TNO Soesterberg, Pays-Bas

Dans de nombreuses publications et même dans des normes il est proclamé que les fréquences importantes pour la perception de la parole sont les fréquences de 1/2, 1 et 2 kHz. Ceci impliquerait que les pertes auditives dues au bruit, qui sont maximales aux environs de 4 kHz, n'auraient que peu d'effet sur la perception de la parole.

Cependant nos études, réalisées sur 400 oreilles présentant différents niveaux de pertes auditives dues au bruit, montrent que de telles pertes peuvent entraîner un handicap sérieux pour la perception de la parole et ce particulièrement dans le bruit. Les seuils de réception de la parole furent déterminés en ambiance silencieuse ainsi qu'en présence de bruits de 35, 50, 65 et 80 dB(A). L'analyse de ces résultats et des audiogrammes tonaux montrent que les seuils de réception de la parole dans le bruit peuvent être efficacement prédits à partir de l'audiogramme tonal sur la simple base des pertes auditives à 2 et 4 kHz. Le coefficient de corrélation est de 0,82 alors que si l'on tient compte de l'erreur de mesure, la plus haute valeur possible de ce coefficient est de 0,91. On n'observe pratiquement pas d'amélioration de la valeur de ce coefficient (0,82) si l'on augmente le nombre de fréquences audiométriques utilisées pour prédire le seuil de réception de la parole. D'autres mesures psychoacoustiques fondées sur le masquage et en particulier sur le rapport critique et l'étendue supérieure du masquage ne contribuent pas à une meilleure prédiction du seuil de réception de la parole. La relation entre le seuil de réception de la parole dans le bruit et l'audiogramme tonal suggère qu'une perte auditive moyenne supérieure à 30 dB sur les fréquences 2 et 4 kHz représente un handicap pour la perception de la parole. Cette perte auditive de 30 dB correspond à une valeur d'environ 11,5 dB lorsque l'on considère la moyenne sur les fréquences 1/2, 1 et 2 kHz. La valeur de 11,5 dB est considérablement plus faible que la limite de 25 dB proposée par l'AAOO pour le début du handicap auditif. A mon avis, la limite de l'AAOO est trop élevée du fait que l'AAOO ne tient pas compte de la perception de la parole dans des conditions bruyantes.

Compréhension de la langue maternelle et d'une seconde langue dans le bruit

H.M. Borchgrevink, Oslo, Norvège

Des phrases simples et usuelles de norvégien (10) et d'anglais (10) ont été lues par un adulte bilingue puis enregistrées et présentées à des sujets adultes dont le norvégien (13) ou l'anglais (13) était la langue maternelle et qui possédaient un bon niveau dans l'autre langue (niveau universitaire). Chaque phrase d'un niveau de 65 dB SPL était tout d'abord présentée dans un bruit de fond USASI si élevé qu'elle ne pouvait être perçue puis la phrase était répétée dans des niveaux de bruit progressivement décroissants (par pas de 2 dB) jusqu'à ce qu'elle puisse être correctement répétée par le sujet. Les sujets présentaient tous une audition normale avant le test.

Les résultats montrent pour chaque groupe de sujets que les phrases en langue maternelle étaient correctement répétées après un plus petit nombre de présentations, c'est à dire avec un rapport signal sur bruit de 3 dB environ inférieur à celui nécessaire pour la compréhension des phrases présentées dans l'autre langue. Les différences de seuil entre la langue maternelle et l'autre langue étaient statistiquement significatifs pour chaque groupe ($p<0,001$ en appliquant le test en t au nombre moyen de présentations nécessaires à la répétition correcte des phrases). Le même résultat était obtenu lorsque on utilisait un critère qui tolérait une erreur lexicale ou deux erreurs grammaticales.

Etant donné que les phrases a-grammaticales, sans signification, sont plus difficiles à "suivre" que les phrases possédant un sens (Miller et Isard, 1963), la répétition d'un schéma sonore sans signification nécessitera un meilleur rapport signal sur bruit que celui nécessaire à la répétition de phrases ayant une signification. Si l'on augmente le rapport signal sur bruit d'une phrase inconnue en commençant à un niveau inintelligible comme dans cette expérience, le seuil de compréhension de la phrase sera atteint avant le seuil de répétition du son sans signification. En conséquence la répétition d'une phrase représente la compréhension de celle-ci dans notre schéma expérimental.

Les résultats ont montré que les sujets ont besoin de moins d'indices acoustiques pour comprendre même des phrases simples et usuelles présentées dans leur langue maternelle que les phrases correspondantes dans l'autre langue et ce, même lorsqu'ils possèdent une bonne connaissance de cette autre langue. Présenté d'une autre façon on peut dire que la capacité du sujet à "remplir", deviner ou synthétiser ce qui est caché dans le bruit de fond et parvenir à un message vraisemblable et significatif est meilleure dans la langue maternelle qui est acquise avec l'apprentissage des concepts et le développement cognitif dans la petite enfance.

Les mêmes stimulus étaient présentés aux mêmes sujets dans les mêmes conditions.

La perception de la parole doit ainsi être considérée comme un processus actif qui dépend largement des aspects cognitifs et de concepts de référence et de cohérence. Le phénomène peut influencer la compréhension du message et ainsi avoir une effet négatif sur les conditions d'apprentissage par exemple, il peut influencer les opérations de contrôle et de sécurité qui sont basées sur la communication verbale spécialement lorsque des messages complexes ou inattendus sont fournis à des sujets étrangers dans des conditions de communication qui sont juste suffisantes pour des sujets de même langue maternelle (par exemple dans le cas du trafic aérien).

Evaluation paramétrique du principe d'isoénergie

D. Henderson, R.P. Hamernik et R.J. Salvi, Université du Texas, Dallas, USA

Le principe d'isoénergie est basé sur l'hypothèse selon laquelle le risque pour l'audition associé à une exposition au bruit est une fonction croissante de l'énergie acoustique totale reçue par un sujet. Bien que l'on s'accorde pour dire que ce principe représente une bonne approximation pour certaines expositions à des bruits continus, il n'est pas sûr qu'il puisse être valable pour des bruits impulsionnels ou des bruits d'impact.

On présentera une série d'expériences au cours desquelles le principe d'isoénergie a été testé pour des bruits d'impact de niveau compris entre 107 et 143 dB à des cadences de 4/s à 1/16s et de durées d'exposition totale allant de 20 jours à 1,8 minute. Toutes les conditions d'exposition contenaient la même énergie acoustique; ainsi, si l'amplitude des pertes auditives est déterminée par cette quantité, tous les groupes devraient présenter les mêmes effets. Plusieurs tendances apparaissent:

(i) aux niveaux compris entre 107 et 119 dB tous les groupes présentent essentiellement la même fatigue auditive, les mêmes pertes auditives et les mêmes destructions cellulaires,

(ii) les dommages audiologiques et histologiques augmentent très fortement pour les niveaux supérieurs à 119 dB,

(iii) pour des niveaux identiques, l'amplitude des dommages croît lorsque le rythme de répétition décroit (c'est à dire de 1/4 s à 4/s),

(iv) pour ce spectre d'impact étendu, les principaux effets surviennent entre 2 et 4 kHz.

Ces résultats montrent que le principe d'isoénergie décrit les résultats aux niveaux d'exposition les plus faibles et pour les cadences lentes, mais qu'il ne prédit pas les lésions rencontrées chez les groupes exposés à 125 dB ou plus.

Risque dû à l'exposition aux bruits impulsionnels en fonction de leur niveau et de leur composition spectrale

G.R. Price, Aberdeen Proving Ground, USA

Un niveau critique fonction de la fréquence a été proposé comme explication au comportement de l'oreille lors de l'exposition à des sons intenses (Price, 1981, J. Acoust. Soc. Am., 69: 171-177). Il semble très probable que les dommages survenant à la cochlée sont d'origine essentiellement mécanique à partir du moment où le niveau de la stimulation est suffisamment élevé pour qu'une contrainte mécanique critique soit obtenue dans l'oreille interne.

On a donc suposé qu'en ce qui concerne les bruits d'armes, ceux contenant de l'énergie aux basses fréquences seraient moins dangereux ayant une même surpression de crête mais contenant de l'énergie aux fréquences moyennes (qui correspondent à celles auxquelles l'oreille est la plus sensible). Cette hypothèse est contraire à tous les critères d'exposition existants. Dans une série d'expériences réalisées chez le chat, à l'aide de mesures électrophysiologiques de la sensibilité auditive, les animaux ont été exposés à 50 bruits de canon, de fusil ou d'amorce (maximum spectral respectivement à 100, 800 et 4000 Hz) à un niveau fonction du type de bruit (140 à 166 dB crête). Les pertes auditives furent mesurées le jour de l'exposition et deux mois plus tard. Les résultats vont dans le sens de l'hypothèse présentée plus haut et montrent que des pertes auditives peuvent être engendrées par des énergies acoustiques bien inférieures à 1J/m2 (Leq <75dB) et ce spécialement lorsque le niveau est élevé et que l'énergie est localisée sur les fréquences où l'oreille est la plus sensible. De plus, la fréquence correspondant à la perte auditive maximale pour tous les bruits impulsionels était de 4kHz et l'observation histologique réalisée sur certaines oreilles confirme ce résultat. Ceci suggère que l'ajustement de l'oreille est plus aigu que celui du spectre dans le milieu aérien.

Etudes expérimentales relatives aux effets des bruits impulsionnels

P. Nilsson, D.E. Dunn, J. Grenner, S. Rydmarker et B.S. Katbamna, Suède

Des groupes de cobayes furent systématiquement exposés à différentes énergies acoustiques présentées soit sous forme de bruit impulsionnel soit sous forme de bruit continu ayant une répartition spectrale identique. Le seuil du potentiel d'action était différent pour chaque type de bruit. En accord avec Ward et coll. (JASA 1979) un niveau critique défini comme la zone de transition entre l'absence de dommages et des dommages croissants en fonction de l'augmentation de l'énergie acoustique fut mise en évidence avec l'exposition au bruit continu. Les expositions aux bruit impulsionnel ont montré des dommages aussi à des niveaux d'énergie plus faibles. Le niveau critique pour les expositions aux bruits impulsionnels fut par conséquent défini comme une modification de la fonction entrée-sortie.

Des comparaisons furent faites entre deux groupes d'animaux exposés à la même énergie acoustique totale, un groupe avec des bruits impulsionnels et l'autre avec des bruits continus, présentant des pertes auditives comparables. La microscopie stéréoscopique à balayage électronique a mis en évidence des types de dommages différents et a permis en particulier d'observer significativement plus de lésions au niveau des cellules ciliées internes et externes dans le groupe exposé au bruit continu.

Rôle du niveau de crête dans la détermination du risque dû à l'exposition aux bruits impulsionnels

J.H. Patterson, I.M. Lomba-Gautier et D.L. Curd, Fort Rucker, USA
R.P. Hamernik, R.J. Salvi, C.E. Hargett et G. Turrentine,
Université du Texas, Dallas, USA

Les critères d'exposition aux bruits impulsionnels les plus courants sont rédigés en fonction du niveau de crête qui représente l'indice principal du pouvoir lésionnel ou du risque associé à l'exposition au bruit impulsionnel. Puisque le niveau de crête n'est que l'un des nombreux paramètres d'un bruit impulsionnel la question se pose de savoir si une norme basée sur ce niveau de crête peut représenter efficacement le risque que constituent les bruits impulsionnels pour l'audition.

Les expériences décrites dans ce rapport ont pour but de savoir si le niveau de crête est un paramètre adéquat pour caractériser un critère d'exposition aux bruits impulsionnels. L'approche générale fut de produire deux types de bruits impulsionnels ayant le même spectre mais des niveaux de crête différents. Ceci a permis de comparer les pertes et les lésions dues à des impulsions ayant la même énergie acoustique totale distribuée de la même façon en fonction de la fréquence, mais ayant des niveaux de crête différents. Nous avons aussi pu comparer les lésions entraînées par des impulsions de même niveau de crête et de différentes énergies. 36 animaux furent divisés en 6 groupes (6 animaux par groupe). Les groupes 1 et 2 furent exposés à des impulsions ayant environ la même énergie mais de niveaux de crête qui différaient de 8 dB. De la même façon les groupes 3 et 4 et les groupes 5 et 6 formaient des paires à l'intérieur desquelles l'énergie était équivalente mais où le niveau de crête différait de 8 dB. D'un autre côté les groupes 2 et 3 reçurent des expositions dans lesquelles le niveau de crête était identique mais où l'énergie différait de 8dB. Les déficits auditifs furent mesurés 30 jours après la fin de l'exposition et les lésions cochléaires furent observées à l'aide de préparations de surface de la membrane basilaire. Les déficits auditifs mesurés durant les premières heures après l'exposition présentent une variation systématique avec la pression de crête et l'énergie. Les pertes auditives mesurées 20 à 30 jours après l'exposition ainsi que les lésions cellulaires dépendent fortement de l'énergie mais moins du niveau de crête. Ces résultats indiquent que le niveau de crête n'est pas un indicateur suffisant du risque que représentent les bruits impulsionnels pour l'audition; cependant l'énergie acoustique seule ne constitue pas non plus un indicateur suffisant.

Effets des bruits d'armes sur l'audition

A. Dancer, Institut franco-allemand de recherches de Saint-Louis, France

Les bruits d'armes diffèrent généralement des bruits industriels ou des bruits de l'environnement par leur surpression de crête (qui peut atteindre 100kPa) et leur durée (généralement une fraction de milliseconde ou, au plus, quelques millisecondes).

Ces caractéristiques particulières ont plusieurs conséquences en ce qui concerne les effets de ces bruits sur l'audition ainsi que les méthodes d'évaluation de ces effets.

Dans certaines conditions d'exposition aux bruits d'armes les lésions cochléaires peuvent survenir presque instantanément par effet mécanique direct du stimulus acoustique sur les structures sensorielles de l'organe de Corti; dans d'autres conditions, les lésions apparaissent plus progressivement comme dans le cas des bruits industriels. La transition entre ces deux processus se produirait pour un certain "niveau critique" au delà duquel les déficits auditifs augmenteraient très rapidement. L'existence d'un tel niveau critique restreint le domaine d'application des méthodes générales d'évaluation des effets lésionnels des bruits d'armes.

L'évaluation des risques d'exposition aux bruits d'armes est rendue également difficile du fait de l'interaction probable existant entre les composantes basses et hautes fréquences des bruits impulsionnels au niveau de l'oreille moyenne et/ou de l'oreille interne. On a pu montrer, sur deux espèces animales différentes, que des ondes de choc de niveau de surpression de crête donné et de durée de première phase positive longue provoquaient moins de déficits auditifs que des ondes de choc analogues mais ayant une durée de première phase positive courte alors que les premières contiennent au moins autant d'énergie acoustique que les secondes quelle que soit la fréquence considérée (en fait, beaucoup plus pour les basses fréquences).

De tels problèmes nous interdisent d'utiliser de façon générale (pour toutes les conditions d'exposition) les méthodes simples d'évaluation des effets lésionnels des bruits d'armes dont on dispose actuellement.

Niveau critique relatif au risque d'exposition au bruit impulsionnel: pertes auditives chez des groupes de militaires exposés à des bruits impulsionnels variant de façon connue

H.M. Borchgrevink, O. Woxen et G. Oftedal, Norvège

Entre 1982 à 1983 (nouvelles recrues) le groupe d'apparat de la garde royale norvégienne modifia sur sa propre initiative la position de tir du fusil: de l'horizontale à la verticale et utilisa des munitions à blanc plus puissantes durant le tir des salves que ce groupe exécute sans protection auditive à l'issue des quelques 20 cérémonies officielles qui ont lieu pendant une période de 3 mois. Les pertes auditives dans le groupe 1983 furent notablement augmentées. Le reste de l'entraînement n'avait pas été modifié. Ceci nous a fourni l'occasion unique de réaliser une étude définie rétrospectivement ! et contrôlée des effets de la position des armes et de leur bruit sur les pertes auditives, chez l'homme, en faisant tirer sous surveillance audiométrique le groupe 1984 avec la munition de1982 et avec la position de 1983.Les mesures audiométriques ont montré que dans le groupe 1984 les pertes auditives étaient aussi rares que dans le groupe 1982; l'effet de la position de tir semble donc négligeable.

Des mesures de bruit furent réalisées sur le terrain de cérémonie standard qui est recouvert d'asphalte et ces bruits furent analysés par FFT. En quelques millisecondes, les impulsions atteignaient l'oreille sous la forme d'une succession rapide de pics isolés conduisant à une augmentation de la durée du bruit impulsionnel mais avec des niveaux de crête correspondant à celui d'un bruit isolé: pour la munition 1982: ≤ 160dB et pour la munition 1983: ≤ 170 dB crête.

L'examen des signaux de pression ne montre aucune différence ni au niveau du temps de montée ni à celui des durées A, B, C ou D qui pourrait rendre compte des différences de risque potentiel entre les deux types de munitions.

Du fait du petit nombre d'expositions à des niveaux plus élevés (≈ 20) distribuées au hasard sur une longue période (3 mois), le degré élevé des pertes auditives observées sur le groupe 1983 est difficilement compatible avec le concept d'isoénergie mais milite plutôt en faveur de l'existence d'un niveau critique pour l'exposition aux bruits impulsionnels, niveau au delà duquel les lésions de l'oreille interne seraient très étendues même après des expositions courtes et peu fréquentes.

A notre avis les résultats ci-dessus indiquent que c'est le niveau de crête d'environ 170 dB qui est responsable des pertes auditives substantielles observées sur le groupe 1983 et que ceci signifie qu'un niveau critique existe chez l'homme entre 160 et 170 dB crête au moins pour des bruits impulsionnels de mêmes composition spectrale, temps de montée et durée.

Les TTS peuvent-ils servir d'indicateur de la susceptibilité aux PTS

K. Buck et R. Franke, Institut franco-allemand de recherches de Saint-Louis, France

Afin de savoir si les TTS ou certains paramètres qui y sont associés peuvent être utilisés en tant qu'indicateur de la susceptibilité aux PTS, des cobayes furent exposés à un bruit de bande (1/3 d'octave centré sur 8 kHz) de 103 dB pendant 5 minutes. Les TTS induits par l'exposition furent mesurés par électrocochléographie (électrode chronique sur la fenêtre ronde) jusqu'à récupération complète (généralement 1 à 2 jours). Une semaine plus tard les mêmes animaux furent exposés à un deuxième bruit de même composition spectrale mais d'énergie supérieure (110dB pendant 30 minutes). Ceci provoqua un PTS qui se stabilisa au bout de 15 jours. Les PTS et les TTS étaient comparables à ceux décrits dans la littérature (TTS maximum de 25 dB à 16 kHz; PTS maximum de 15 dB à 8 kHz). Cependant nous n'avons pu trouver aucune corrélation au niveau individuel entre les TTS (ou d'autres paramètres associés) et les PTS.

Ainsi il semble que les tests de susceptibilité individuelle ne peuvent être basés sur des mesures de TTS. Le fait que le PTS maximum apparaisse à une fréquence inférieure à celle du TTS maximum indique que des mécanismes différents pourraient être responsables des TTS et des PTS.

Etude sur le terrain de tir d'une garnison des bruits impulsionnels au plan de l'environnement

ıH. Brinkman, BWB Coblence, République Fédérale d'Allemagne

Le bruit produit par les armes a une importance toujours plus grande en tant que nuisance pour l'environnement et ce spécialement dans un pays à population dense comme la République Fédérale d'Allemagne. A la fin des années 60 et au début des années 70, des mesures furent effectuées avec des armes portatives en champ libre, sur un terrain de tir militaire. Ces mesures ont été maintenant complétées par d'autres réalisées dans un champ de tir de garnison possédant des écrans isolants. Ces mesures récentes furent réalisées au cours de 5 périodes en 1983 et 1984 pour déterminer les effets des conditions météorologiques pendant les différentes saisons de l'année. Les résultats de cette étude de terrain sont présentées. Ces résultats ont servi de base au développement d'un modèle prédictif d'émission sur les champs de tir. Ce modèle est également présenté.

Résultats d'études à long terme des traumatismes sonores dûs aux bruits impulsionnels chez des militaires: relation entre la fatigue auditive et les pertes auditives

ıF. Pfander, Brème, République Fédérale d'Allemagne

Des études à long terme montrent que la fatigue auditive résultant d'expositions quotidiennes à des bruits impulsionnels intenses augmente. La durée de récupération s'allonge également. Les observations effectuées sur des soldats de carrière qui sont fréquemment exposés aux traumatismes des bruits impulsionnels montrent qu'en dépit de la protection auditive, des expositions continuelles peuvent faire passer progressivement de la fatigue aux pertes auditives. D'un autre côté il est évident qu'en dépit de l'accroissement de la durée de la récupération, celle-ci est encore possible même après plusieurs mois. L'expérience selon laquelle le dommage auditif causé par un seul traumatisme sonore tend à récupérer ou à demeurer constant durant la période qui y fait suite, s'applique à l'évidence également aux dommages qui se développent progressivement du fait d'aggressions multiples causées par les bruits impulsionnels. Du fait du port, aujourd'hui obligatoire, des protecteurs d'oreille, le pourcentage de personnes menacées est tombé à environ 5%. Mais même ces sujets ont une chance de récupérer après quelques mois si l'exposition est stoppée. Ceci est important pour l'évaluation de l'invalidité.

Effets des ondes de choc sur les tissus épithéliaux non auditifs

J. B. Moe, C.B. Clifford et D.D. Sharpnack, Walter Reed Institut, Washington, USA

Les lésions des tissus épithéliaux représentent un des effets primaires de l'exposition aux ondes de choc. L'expression morphologique de ces lésions varie selon l'organe. Dans le parenchyme pulmonaire, l'hémorragie qui survient à la suite de l'exposition au blast noie les alvéoles, masquant ainsi les lésions directes de l'épithélium alvéolaire et provoquant une menace réelle de suffocation. Chez les animaux sévèrement lésés par le blast, les lésions épithéliales du parenchyme pulmonaire se manifestent principalement par la rupture des septums alvéolaires. Dans le larynx, la trachée et les bronches d'animaux lésés on observe fréquemment des zones d'épithélium mises à nu. Le mécanisme fondamental de ce décapage épithélial n'est pas clairement établi mais il représente probablement un effet direct de l'onde de choc car il survient fréquemment en l'absence de toute autre manifestation lésionnelle localisée.

Dans une expérience récente, des trachées de rats exposés à des ondes de choc répétées furent examinées par microscopie à balayage pour rechercher la présence de ce décapage épithélial. Le seuil d'exposition qui produit ce décapage est d'environ 10 psi (20 coups) et 100% des animaux sont atteints à 22,5 psi (20 coups). Dans le même groupe de rats le seuil d'hémorragie pulmonaire était d'environ 16 psi (20 coups). L'examen microscopique des tissus gastrointestinaux lésés suggère que la rupture épithéliale survient à la suite de la lésion vasculaire.

Quoique les implications biologiques des lésions du parenchyme pulmonaire, des voies aériennes supérieures et du tractus gastrointestinal soient incomplètement connues, il semble qu'il existe d'importantes possibilités de complications pendant la période de récupération. Les réponses des tissus des espèces de mammifères de grande taille à différents types d'ondes de choc de différents niveaux seront également discutées.

Effets extra-auditifs d'expositions répétées à des bruits impulsionnels intenses

Y.Y. Phillips, Walter Reed Institut, Washington, USA
A. Dancer, I.S.L., France
D.R. Richmond, Los Alamos, USA

L'exposition aux bruits impulsionnels intenses peut entraîner des lésions de toutes les structures de l'organisme qui contiennent de l'air. Bien que l'oreille soit l'organe le plus sensible, le tractus respiratoire (URT), les poumons, et les intestins peuvent être lésés par le blast aérien. Ces lésions extra-auditives ont été étudiées dans le cadre des effets des bruits d'armes. Le développement de systèmes d'artillerie légers et à grande portée ainsi que d'armes d'épaule puissantes a conduit à l'élévation du niveau des bruits impulsionnels auxquels les soldats sont exposés. Les lésions auditives sont reconnues comme un cas d'invalidité d'origine militaire et l'arrivée d'armes plus bruyantes a fait craindre que les lésions extra-auditives puissent constituer un problème pour l'établissement de limites de sécurité.

La recherche animale fut entreprise en Europe et aux USA afin de préciser ce nouveau risque. Des moutons et des porcs ont été autopsiés après exposition à divers types d'exposition à des impulsions. Il fut rapidement mis en évidence que lors d'expositions répétées, les lésions extra-auditives pouvaient se développer à des niveaux de pression relativement faibles. Dans une série d'expériences, des groupes de 6 animaux furent exposés à 20 blasts de même niveau de crête (P; 69 kPa) mais de différentes valeurs d'impulsion de première phase positive (I; 63, 110, 145, 184 et 222 kPa.ms). Dans une étude complémentaire des groupes de même taille furent exposés à 20 blasts d'impulsion analogue (140 kPa.ms) mais de niveau de crête variable (26,48,69,115,126 et 262 kPa). Ces expériences ont montré que les lésions survenaient dans l'URT, les intestins et les poumons avec une fréquence et une sévérité de plus en plus élevées lorsque I était augmentée, avec un niveau de crête constant, ou lorsque que ce niveau de crête était augmenté alors que I restait constante. L'URT était le système le plus sensible avec au moins des pétéchies laryngées chaque fois qu'il y avait lésion des intestins ou des poumons. Les lésions de l'URT surviennent souvent en l'absence de toute autre lésion organique. Les lésions extra-auditives entraînées par les ondes de choc produites en champ libre sont fonction du nombre d'expositions, du niveau de crête et de l'impulsion.

Les pétéchies observées au niveau du tractus respiratoire supérieur (URT) constituent la première manifestation apparente de lésion et peuvent être utilisées pour définir des conditions limites d'exposition.

Etudes analytiques et expérimentales des effets des ondes de choc sur les principaux systèmes de l'organisme

J.H. Stuhmiller, San Diego, USA

Le fait qu'il apparaisse des lésions extra-auditives aiguës chez l'animal à la suite de l'exposition à des ondes de choc intenses et la possibilité d'apparition de lésions chroniques chez les servants d'armes conventionnelles a fait apparaître la nécessité de modèles biomécaniques détaillés pour aider l'US Army à définir des critères d'exposition chez l'homme. La méthodologie utilise des modèles mathématiques et des codes de calcul pour établir des relations causales et vérifiables entre le blast extérieur et les contraintes locales dans les tissus. L'observation directe, in vitro, des processus lésionnels ainsi que la mesure de la résistance des tissus conduit à la détermination de seuils critiques lésionnels qui définissent ainsi les conditions mécaniques qui produisent la lésion.

La distribution de la pression sur un modèle de torse exposé à des ondes de choc de 3 à 30 psi de niveau de crête fut utilisée pour valider les calculs de mécanique des fluides relatifs à l'interaction onde-volume corporel et pour développer une relation préliminaire de charge due au blast. Un modèle à éléments finis d'une section transversale de thorax de mouton a été mis au point et des calculs paramétriques faisant varier ses propriétés mécaniques ont montré que les seules quantités importantes sont la densité et la compressibilité du parenchyme pulmonaire ainsi que le module de cisaillement de la cavité thoracique. Toutes les propriétés du matériel pulmonaire nécessaires pour le modèle de thorax ont été mesurées sur différentes espèces et la capacité du parenchyme pulmonaire à supporter une onde de compression de faible vitesse a été directement mesurée. La comparaison des prédictions du modèle et des résultats disponibles chez l'animal en ce qui concerne les pressions intra-thoraciques a été satisfaisante; la variation de la pression intrathoracique sous des conditions d'iso-impulsion correspond bien aux résultats expérimentaux. Une technique de perfusion a été développée qui permet une investigation in vitro des origines mécaniques des lésions du tractus gastrointestinal. Les résultats indiquent clairement le rôle joué par les bulles de gaz dans les sections d'intestin, bulles qui induisent des mouvements amples et des contraintes dans les parois intestinales adjacentes et qui provoquent éventuellement des lésions.

Audition chez les gardes côtiers et les pêcheurs

A. Axelsson, I. Arvidsson et T. Jerson, Göteborg, Suède

Les pêcheurs et les gardes côtiers ont une organisation du travail très différente de celle d'un travailleur normal dans l'industrie. Au lieu de 8 heures de travail suivies de 16 heures de repos, 5 jours par semaine, les pêcheurs et les gardes côtiers travaillent fréquemment plusieurs jours d'affilée en étant exposés continuellement au bruit. Même pendant leur sommeil ils sont exposés à de hauts niveaux sonores du fait du moteur du bateau. De plus ils sont exposés à d'autres facteurs d'environnement défavorables comme la houle, les vibrations sur l'ensemble de l'organisme, de rapides variations climatiques, la privation de sommeil, le travail de nuit,... . Il est parfaitement possible que le bruit soit plus dangereux pour l'audition dans des conditions défavorables.

L'examen de l'audition d'un grand nombre de pêcheurs et de gardes côtiers a montré une mauvaise audition particulièrement chez les jeunes. On suppose que l'origine majeure de ce mauvais état de l'audition est l'exposition au bruit pendant le travail peut-être en interaction avec d'autres facteurs ototraumatiques. Dans les périodes de repos, des activités de tir chez 24 et 28% des pêcheurs et des gardes côtiers respectivement semblent avoir contribué à cet état de mauvaise audition. Des contrôles annuels répétés, une protection améliorée de l'oreille, et des diminutions de bruit à bord des bateaux pourraient améliorer considérablement l'audition des personnes exerçant ces professions.

Interactions entre différents types de bruit

O.J. Manninen, Université de Tampere, Finlande

Ce rapport concerne les modifications de la fatigue auditive mesurée deux minutes après la fin de l'exposition (TTS2), de la pression sanguine systolique (SBP), de la pression sanguine diastolique (DBP), du rythme cardiaque (HR) et de l'index hémodynamique (HDI) qui se produisirent lors de l'exposition de nos sujets à différents bruits stables.

Dans chacune des quatre expériences le niveau sonore était de 90dB et les fréquences de coupure de 1 et 2kHz, 1 et 4 kHz, 1 et 8kHz, 2 et 4 kHz, 4 et 6 kHz, 4 et 8 kHz ou 0,2 et 16 kHz. Afin d'examiner la fiabilité des effets du bruit et de déterminer la signification d'autres facteurs de l'environnement les sujets furent exposés aux bruits décrits plus haut et (en même temps ou séparément) à des vibrations de basse fréquence (fréquences de 5 Hz ou de 2,8 à 11 Hz, accélération efficace 2,12m/s2) appliquées à tout le corps (axe Z) à deux températures différentes (20° et 30°C). Pendant les expositions les groupes de sujets, 13, 14, 70 ou 108 étudiants volontaires masculins jeunes et en bonne santé, durent réaliser un travail intellectuel ou physique astreignant. Les expériences ont été réalisées dans une cabine d'exposition de conception spéciale. Une expérience sur un individu durait 1h45min. L'expérience était divisée en: une période de contrôle de 30 minutes, trois périodes successives d'exposition de 16 minutes, une pause de 4 minutes pour les mesures et une période de récupération de 15 minutes. Les résultats montrent que lorsque les sujets réalisaient à leur guise un simple travail de contrôle à 20°C, l'augmentation des valeurs de TTS2 était maximale à 4 kHz s'ils étaient seulement exposés à un bruit de fréquences de coupure de 2 et 4 kHz, 1 et 4 kHz, 1 et 8 kHz ou 0,2 et 16 kHz. Dans des conditions similaires l'accroissement des valeurs de TTS2 à 6 kHz était maximale avec les bruits de fréquences de coupure de 4 et 6 kHz, 4 et 8 kHz ou 1 et 4 kHz, 1 et 8 kHz ou 0,2 et 16 kHz. D'une façon générale, les effets des bruits sur les TTS2 à 8 kHz étaient nettement plus faibles que sur les TTS2 à 4 et 6 kHz. Les valeurs de TTS2 à 4, 6 et 8 kHz furent moins affectées par le bruit de fréquences de coupure de 1 et 2 kHz. Durant une exposition combinée à un bruit de bande large (fréquences de coupure 0,2 et 16 kHz) et à une vibration sinusoïdale de 5 Hz, les valeurs de TTS2 à 4 kHz étaient 1,2 à 1,5 fois plus grandes que celles entraînées par le bruit seul. Une température de 30°C et un stress du type "compétition mentale" accéléraient l'augmentation des TTS2 à 4 et 6 kHz lorsque les sujets étaient exposés à un bruit de large bande ou, simultanément, à ce bruit et à une vibration verticale. Une vibration large bande (gamme de fréquences: 2, 8 à 11,2 Hz) accélérait l'augmentation des TTS2 légèrement plus que la vibration sinusoïdale de 5 Hz lorsque le niveau de bruit était de 90dB, la température de 30°C et que les sujets réalisaient leur test. Les effets d'un travail musculaire intense (charge de travail 8 W) étaient opposés à ceux de la situation compétitive c'est à dire que ce type de travail semble diminuer les TTS2 lorsque les sujets sont exposés au bruit et à la vibration à 20° ou 30°C. Les valeurs de HR, SBP, DBP et HDI reflètent les diverses combinaisons d'exposition et sont corrélées avec les TTS2. Le stress de type compétition mentale accélère particulièrement l'augmentation des TTS2 et des valeurs de HR et de SBP lorsque les sujets sont exposés au bruit ou à une combinaison bruit-vibration.

Interactions entre les ototoxiques et l'exposition à un son intense

D. McFadden, Université du Texas, Austin, USA

On fera le point des connaissances actuelles relatives aux interactions entre les médicaments et le bruit. Des études aussi bien physiologiques que psychophysiques seront passées en revue. Les différentes façons selon lesquelles les drogues peuvent interagir avec l'exposition au bruit seront discutées et des distinctions seront établies entre les drogues qui produisent par elles-mêmes des pertes auditives et celles qui ne le font pas. Les difficultés d'interprétation des expériences passées ainsi que les difficultés de ce type de recherches chez l'homme seront mises en évidence. Le sujet principal concernera nos résultats selon lesquels des doses modérées de salicylates prises pendant deux jours ou plus peuvent augmenter temporairement les seuils d'audition de 10 à 15 dB tandis que d'autres anti-inflammatoires non stéroïdiens ne potentialisent pas l'exposition au bruit.

Une voie d'interaction entre les effets du stress et du bruit sur l'audition

H.A. Dengerink, J.W. Wright, J.E. Dengerink et J.M. Miller, USA

Bien qu'elle soit très difficile à mesurer, l'irrigation de la cochlée est supposée jouer un rôle dans les effets lésionnels du bruit. Il est aussi bien connu que l'irrigation varie avec les activités homéostatiques de l'organisme, avec l'activité physique et avec le stress. Etant donné que l'irrigation cochléaire est un agent important des pertes auditives induites par le bruit et que les conditions de circulation varient avec le stress, on peut imaginer que le bruit (qui est lui-même un agent stressant) puisse interagir avec d'autres agents stressant pour influencer l'importance des déficits auditifs consécutifs à une exposition sonore. Si les réponses physiologiques au stress augmentent l'irrigation cochléaire alors on peut suggérer que de tels processus pourraient réduire les effets lésionnels du bruit. L'effet des réponses physiologiques au stress sur l'irrigation cochléaire n'est pas bien compris. Cet article résume nos recherches qui concernent ces interactions.

L'angiotensine est un puissant agent de contrôle de la pression sanguine et de l'irrigation vasculaire, il s'agit d'un peptide circulatoire qui est converti à partir de l'angiotensinogène par la rénine. Les effets primaires de l'angiotensine sont la vasoconstriction, l'augmentation de l'absorption de liquides et la faim de sel, et la libération de vasopressine. Quelques auteurs ont indiqué que les taux d'angiotensine sont augmentés en anticipation ou en réponse à des stress. Un autre système majeur de réponse au stress qui agit sur la pression sanguine et l'irrigation locale est le système catécholaminergique.

Une de nos stratégies de recherche a été d'évaluer les effets du bruit sur les taux d'angiotensine. A la fois chez l'homme et chez l'animal nous avons observé des augmentations des taux plasmatiques d'angiotensine à la suite d'une exposition de courte durée au bruit. Nous avons également observé une consommation accrue de liquides, due probablement à l'angiotensine, lors d'expositions de longue durée.

Une seconde stratégie de recherche a été la mesure du flux sanguin cochléaire à l'aide d'un système laser Doppler. Le laser Doppler permet une évaluation dynamique du flux sanguin dans de petites zones tissulaires sans sacrifier l'animal. En utilisant ce système nous avons mesuré le flux sanguin cochléaire pendant la perfusion d'angiotensine et de catécholamines dans la carotide de cobayes. L'angiotensine, l'épinéphrine et la norépinéphrine élèvent la pression sanguine systémique et accroissent le flux sanguin. Le flux sanguin au niveau de la peau décroit lors de l'administration de ces substances.

Ces résultats suggèrent que le flux sanguin varie, en partie, à la suite de modifications de la pression sanguine systémique. De plus, étant donné que les taux d'angiotensine et de catécholamines sont augmentés sous l'action du stress, l'irrigation cochléaire doit l'être aussi. Cet effet des réponses au stress physiologique sur l'irrigation cochléaire indique une voie d'interaction possible entre le bruit et le stress sur les pertes auditives induites par le bruit.

Effets de l'âge et de l'exposition au bruit sur les seuils de sensibilité auditive de diverses populations

W. Passchier-Vermeer, TNO Leiden, Pays-Bas

On présente l'analyse de deux études réalisées aux Pays-Bas. La première étude concerne l'effet de l'âge sur les seuils de sensibilité auditive de populations non exposées au bruit au cours de leur vie professionnelle passée et présente. 500 sujets masculins furent testés. De cette étude les conclusions suivantes ont été tirées:

Dans un but pratique les résultats base A des normes ISO 7029 et ISO/DIS 1999/1 peuvent être utilisés comme population de référence pour des populations blanches non contrôlées otologiquement, si les sujets ne sont pas exposés au bruit dans leur travail (passé ou présent). Selon Driscoll et coll. pour des populations noires d'autres bases pourraient être plus appropriées.

Les résultats base B (de l'ISO/DIS 1999/1, Annex B) ne peuvent de façon générale pas servir de base pour des populations otologiquement non contrôlées et non exposées au bruit.

La deuxième étude, relative à environ 2000 ouvriers exposés au bruit dans 28 usines, se rapporte aux effets de l'exposition au bruit sur les seuils de sensibilité auditive de populations exposées pendant les heures de travail. Dans cette analyse, les pertes auditives (N) causées par l'exposition au bruit (calculées comme la différence entre les seuils d'audition mesurés et les seuils selon les résultats de la base A) étaient calculés pour différents pourcentages (0,90 - 0,10). Les courbes les mieux ajustées furent déterminées selon le type de formules données dans la norme ISO/DIS 1999/1. On montre qu'un bon accord, au niveau de 85 dB(A), existe entre les valeurs N données dans la norme ISO/DIS 1999/1 et celles de cette étude. Aux niveaux d'exposition inférieurs et supérieurs une différence existe cependant entre les deux groupes de résultats.

Les valeurs N0,50- (et les N0,10-) des 30 groupes d'ouvriers (au total environ 1000 personnes), exposés à des niveaux compris entre 85 et 90 dB(A) montrent une variation considérable. On a pu mettre en évidence que 11 des 30 valeurs N0,50- étaient supérieures à celles que l'on pouvait attendre de l'analyse statistique. Ces valeurs N supérieures pourraient être dues à l'exposition au bruit impulsionnel puisque tous les 11 groupes avaient subi une exposition aux bruits impulsionnels considérable dans le travail du métal ou du bois par exemple. Cependant la même remarque peut s'appliquer à quelques uns des 19 autres groupes. De ce fait les résultats seront analysés plus avant.

Etat actuel des solutions de protection individuelle de l'audition

P.W. Alberti et S.M. Abel, Université de Toronto, Canada

La protection auditive est maintenant largement acceptée comme une partie importante des programmes de lutte contre le bruit. Néanmoins il existe de grandes difficultés dans ce domaine. Les techniques d'évaluation des protecteurs auditifs sont largement subjectives en ce sens qu'elles mesurent habituellement la protection au seuil d'audition et dans le silence. Des résultats récents incluent le développement de méthodes psychoacoustiques pour évaluer l'atténuation dans les forts niveaux de bruit dans lesquels les dispositifs de protection sont utilisés. Une confiance de plus en plus grande a été placée sur les têtes artificielles munies de microphones pour mesurer l'atténuation réelle sous des casques. Il existe aussi une recherche continuelle de protecteurs actifs c'est à dire de protecteurs qui permettent aux faibles niveaux de bruit de passer sans être atténués mais qui éliminent les forts niveaux. Un tel protecteur a des avantages évidents pour la communication. Ces développements ont principalement été le fait des militaires. Un problème permanent relatif aux bouchons d'oreille est la difficulté de placer et de sceller un dispositif dans les contours irréguliers et cachés du conduit auditif. Cet article passera en revue les tentatives récentes faites pour résoudre ces problèmes. Une tentative sera faite pour évaluer l'efficacité de protecteurs auditifs personnels en tant qu'élément d'un programme de lutte contre le bruit évaluant les techniques utilisées pour tester le degré d'efficacité des protecteurs.

Surveillance de l'audition et bruit impulsionnel dans l'armée britannique

M.R. Forrest, Farnborough, Grande-Bretagne

Le service militaire a toujours représenté un risque pour l'audition du fait des bruits impulsionnels; de plus au bruit des armes légères, d'une pression de crête d'environ 160dB, s'ajoute le bruit de certains systèmes d'armes d'usage courant qui produisent des niveaux de crête allant jusqu'à 185dB (35kPa). Enfin un nombre toujours croissant de soldats est exposé à des bruits intenses.

Quoique la protection auditive individuelle ait été introduite en 1966, un certain nombre d'études qui y ont fait suite ont montré une incidence toujours importante des pertes auditives induites par le bruit. Récemment l'audiométrie de contrôle a été introduite dans les tests médicaux de routine; ceci combiné à la mise à disposition de protecteurs auditifs améliorés et à une plus grande prise de conscience des effets des bruits sur l'audition devrait réduire l'importance des pertes auditives. L'efficacité des mesures de conservation de l'audition est montrée par les résultats d'une étude sur des recrues pendant l'entraînement. Des détails de cette étude sont fournis avec les résultats relatifs aux changements du niveau d'audition à la suite de l'exposition aux bruits impulsionnels pendant des opérations militaires.

Les niveaux d'exposition maximums au bruit sont données dans le standard UK 00-27/1; comme tous les standards équivalents l'exposition au bruit doit être définie en termes simples et directs de telle sorte qu'elle puisse être utilisée lors de la conception de l'équipement militaire. Avec la majorité des systèmes d'armes, l'utilisation de ces standards montre qu'une protection auditive est nécessaire, cependant l'efficacité de la protection est limitée auusi bien par des facteurs pratiques comme la compatibilité avec d'autres équipements, que par ses propriétés acoustiques.

Les mesures de sauvegarde de l'audition dans l'armée sont d'une importance particulière car les soldats ont besoin d'une bonne ouïe pour accomplir leur mission correctement. Des pertes d'audition aux hautes fréquences peuvent en particulier conduire à ne pas détecter des indices acoustiques d'importance vitale. Le besoin d'une audition correcte dans l'armée est plus grand que dans la vie civile.

Simulation mathématique des mécanismes cochléaires, application aux critères d'exposition aux bruits impulsionnels

G.O. Stevin, Bruxelles, Belgique

Les critères d'exposition au bruit impulsionnel ne prennent pas actuellement en compte le spectre des bruits impulsionnels; cependant on sait que le système auditif humain est spectralement accordé. Le présent article milite en faveur de l'extension au bruit impulsionnel du concept de dose de bruit largement utilisé pour les bruits continus. Cette approche est basée sur la mesure de l'exposition sonore plutôt que sur celle de la pression sonore: l'exposition sonore inclut en fait en un seul paramètre le niveau et la durée de l'exposition.

ıUne simulation mathématique des mécanismes de l'audition humaine prenant en compte l'effet non linéaire de l'oreille moyenne a été utilisée pour calculer le risque lésionnel dû aux bruits impulsionnels. Ce modèle fournit, ainsi, une méthode de référence qui peut être utilisée pour évaluer la sonie de n'importe quel bruit. Les résultats de l'analyse des bruits impulsionnels obtenus à partir de différents critères peuvent alors être comparés à l'aide du modèle théorique qui permet d'évaluer les mérites respectifs de ces critères.

La principale conclusion de cette étude est que le niveau d'exposition pondéré A semble être le meilleur critère pour le bruit impulsionnel. La sensibilité spectrale des mécanismes de l'audition humaine pourraient ainsi être approchés par le filtre de pondération A. D'autres techniques proposées pour les bruits impulsionnels sont dérivées de l'analyse par bande d'octave.

Ces éléments mettent en évidence la possibilité d'utiliser un critère unique applicable pour tous les types de bruits y compris les bruits continus et fluctuants aussi bien dans l'industrie qu'en ce qui concerne les bruits d'armes à feu. Ce critère serait applicable aux niveaux de pression élevés jusqu'à 170dB, niveau qui peut être rencontré pour les bruits d'armes. Le niveau lésionnel pour une exposition de 8 heures serait aux alentours de 130dB ce qui correspondrait à un niveau continu équivalent de 85dB. Cette conclusion est en plein accord avec les expériences les plus récentes sur les bruits impulsionnels réalisées par des études psychoacoustiques en Allemagne, aux Pays-Bas et au Japon.

L'équipement nécessaire à la mesure du niveau d'exposition produit par des bruits impulsionnels doit être plus sophistiqué que l'équipement standard utilisé pour mesurer le niveau de pression du bruit continu. Au minimum on doit utiliser un sonomètre intégrateur avec la pondération A. Une analyse bande d'octave du bruit impulsionnel nécessite un processeur digital pour l'analyse de Fourier avec une conversion bande d'octave ou un sonomètre intégrateur à 7 canaux. La standardisation de ces nouvelles techniques de mesure est absolument nécessaire pour permettre le travail futur de simplification des procédures de contrôle de bruit.

Réflexe acoustique et rythme d'échange pour des stimulus WN courts

G. Rossi et M. Rolando, Université de Turin, Italie

La recherche est relative à 10 sujets (4 hommes et 6 femmes) agés de 10 à 23 ans ayant des seuils d'audition meilleurs que 15dB dans la gamme de 125 à 8000Hz. Tous les sujets présentaient un réflexe acoustique net pour des stimulus de 90 dB SPL de 500 millisecondes de durée. Une impédancemètre Amplifon 702 fut utilisé en relation avec un microphone Amplaid MK VI pour produire les signaux et traiter les résultats. On a utilisé un son test de 220Hz. L'ordinateur a fourni une moyenne de 500 valeurs pour chaque type de stimulus (WN bursts de 500, 250 et 125 ms). En démarrant avec 100dB SPL chaque sujet recevait 10 jours de suite 5 cycles de stimulus (temps de montée et de descente: 1ms, fréquence 0,2 par seconde). Chaque division par deux de la durée du stimulus était accompagnée respectivement par des augmentations d'intensité de 3,4,5 et 6dB SPL. Cette recherche démontre que l'amplitude du réflexe acoustique et que son action protectrice sont toujours les mêmes seulement lorsque la division par deux de la durée du stimulus correspond à un accroissement de 5 dB SPL en intensité. Nous pensons que le processus temporel de sommation survenant dans le système nerveux central donne naissance à ce comportement du réflexe acoustique. Cette recherche ne concerne pas ce qui survient lorsque des stimulus de plus de 500 ms sont utilisés.

Standard ISO pour l'exposition au bruit

H.E. von Gierke, Ohio, USA

Une modification substantielle du standard ISO établi en 1975 (ISO 1999 "Acoustics-Assessement of occupational noise exposure from hearing conservation purpose" est en cours depuis 1978 et a produit un protocole international ISO/DIS 1999 "Acoustics- Determination of Occupational Noise Exposure and estimation of Noise induced Hearing Impairment". Ce document qui représente le meilleur compromis possible entre différentes approches, ainsi que les résultats et les avis vont être soumis au vote dans le but d'établir un standard international en 1985. Puisque l'ISO 1999 constitue la base de la législation dans de nombreux pays et qu'une approche uniforme du problème des effets du bruit est hautement désirable, l'adoption d'un standard ISO pour des buts pratiques et opérationnels de conservation de l'audition est urgente. Ce rapport résume l'approche adoptée par ce standard pour mesurer l'exposition à des bruits continus, intermittents, fluctuants et impulsionnels et discute la méthode proposée pour l'évaluation du handicap auditif selon la formule désirée ou prescrite dans un pays donné ainsi que la définition des expositions maximales tolérables ou permises selon le risque accepté.

CONTRIBUTORS

S. M. Abel, Mount Sinai Hospital, Suite 405, 600 University Ave., Toronto, Ontario M5G 1X5, Canada

W. Ahroon, University of Texas at Dallas, Callier Center for Communication Disorders, 1966 Inwood Rd., Dallas, Tx 75235, U.S.A.

P. Alberti, Mount Sinai Hospital, Suite 405, 600 University Ave., Toronto, Ontario M5G 1X5, Canada

T. R. Anderson, Harry G. Armstrong Aerospace Medical Research Laboratory, Wright-Patterson AFB, OH 45433, U.S.A.

A. Arehole, University of Texas at Dallas, Callier Center for Communication Disorders, 1966 Inwood Rd., Dallas, Tx 75235, U.S.A.

I. Arvidsson, Sahlgrenska Sjukhuset, Dept. of Audiology and Occupational Medicine Center, Goteborg, S413 45, Sweden

A. Axelsson, Sahlgrenska Sjukhuset, Dept. of Audiology and Occupational Medicine Center, Goteborg, S413 45, Sweden

M. J. Bauman, Otological Research Laboratories, Henry Ford Hospital, Detroit, Michigan 48202, U.S.A.

K. H. V. Bhat, University of Texas at Dallas, Callier Center for Communication Disorders, 1966 Inwood Rd., Dallas, Tx 75235, U.S.A.

G. R. Bock, The Ciba Foundation, London, England

G. Bonanni, Via Ospedale Civile 105, 35100 Padova, Italy

H. Borchgrevink, Joint Medical Service of the Norwegian Armed Forces, FSAN Oslo mil/Huseby, Oslo 1, Norway

D. K. Brandt, Otological Research Laboratories, Henry Ford Hospital, Detroit, Michigan 48202, U.S.A.

H. Brinkmann, BWB/AFB-FE IV, Erpobungsstelle der Bundeswehr, 4470 Meppen, West Germany

K. Buck, 12 rue de l'Industrie, P.O. Box 301, 68301 St. Louis, France

P. Campo, Institut National de Recherche et de Securite, P. O. Box 27, 54501 Vandoeuvre Cedex, France

B. Canlon, Department of Physiology II, Karolinska Institute, Stockholm, S-104 01, Sweden

L. Carlisle, Kresge Hearing Research Institute, University of Michigan, Ann Arbor, MI 48109, U.S.A.

C. B. Clifford, Div. of Pathology, Walter Reed Army Institute of Research, Walter Reed Army Medical Center, Washington, D.C. 20307-5100, U.S.A.

A. R. Cody, The University of Sussex, M. R. C. Neurophysiology Group, School of Biological Sciences, Brighton, BN1 9QG, England

V. Colletti, ENT Department, University of Verona, 37134 Verona, Italy

S. D. Comis, University of Birmingham, Birmingham, B15 2TJ, England

D. L. Curd, Sensory Research Division, U. S. Army Aeromedical Research Laboratory, P.O. Box 577, Ft. Rucker, AL 36362-5000, U.S.A.

A. Dancer, French-German Research Insitute of Saint Louis, 12 rue de l'Industrie, 68301 St. Louis, France

H. A. Dengerink, Department of Psychology, Washington State Univ. Pullman, WA 99164-4830, U.S.A.

J. E. Dengerink, Department of Speech, Washington State Univ. Pullman, WA 99164-4830, U.S.A.

L. W. Dodds, Massachusetts Eye and Ear Infirmary, 243 Charles St. Boston, MA 02114, U.S.A.

D. E. Dunn, Department of Experimental Research, University of Lund, Malmo General Hospital, Sweden

B. Engstrom, University Hospital, Uppsala, S751.85, Sweden

M. Eybalin, INSERM-U.254, Laboratoire de Neurobiologie de l'Audition, CHR Hopital St. Charles, 34059, Montpellier Cedex, France

T. Fiorino, Universita di Verona, Policlinico Borgo Roma, Verona, 37100, Italy

A. Flock, Department of Physiology II, Karolinska Institute, Stockholm, S-104 01, Sweden

A. Forge, Institute of Laryngology and Otology, 330-332 Gray's Inn Road London, WCIX 8EE, England

M. Forrest, Army Personnel Research Establishment, c/o Royal Aircraft Establishment, Farnborough Hants, GU14-6TD, England

R. Franke, French-German Research Insitute of Saint Louis, 12 rue de l'Industrie, 68301 St. Louis, France

G. Gerken, University of Texas at Dallas, Callier Center for Communication Disorders, 1966 Inwood Rd., Dallas, TX 75235, U.S.A.

J. Grenner, Department of Experimental Research, University of Lund, Malmo General Hospital, Sweden

R. P. Hamernik, University of Texas at Dallas, Callier Center for Communication Disorders, 1966 Inwood Rd., Dallas, TX 75235, U.S.A.

C. E. Hargett, Jr., University of Texas at Dallas, Callier Center for Communication Disorders, 1966 Inwood Rd., Dallas, TX 75235, U.S.A.

D. Henderson, University of Texas at Dallas, Callier Center for Communication Disorders, 1966 Inwood Rd., Dallas, TX 75235, U.S.A.

T. Jerson, Sahlgrenska Sjukhuset, Dept. of Audiology and Occupational Medicine Center., Goteborg, S413 45, Sweden

B. J. Katbamna, Department of Experimental Research, University of Lund, Malmo General Hospital, Sweden

D. A. Learson, Massachusetts Eye and Ear Infirmary, 243 Charles St., Boston, MA, 02114, U.S.A.

M. Lenoir, INSERM-U.254, Laboratoire de Neurobiologie de l'Audition, CHR Hopital St. Charles, 34059, Montpellier Cedex, France

M. C. Liberman, Department of Physiology, Harvard Medical School, Boston, MA 02115, U.S.A.

F. Lindgren, Department of Audiology, Sahlgrenska Sjukhuset, S-413 45, Goteborg, Sweden

I. M. Lomba-Gautier, Sensory Research Division, U. S. Army Aeromedical Research Laboratory, P.O. Box 577, Ft. Rucker, AL 36362-5000, U.S.A.

D. McFadden, University of Texas, Mezes Hall 330, Austin, TX 78712, U.S.A.

O. J. Manninen, The Academy of Finland, Department of Public Health, Faculty of Medicine, University of Tampere, Box 607, SF - 33101 Tampere, Finland

I. Mastrogiacomo, Universita di Padua, Padua, Italy

J. M. Miller, Kresge Hearing Research Institute, University of Michigan, Ann Arbor, MI 48109, U.S.A.

Lt. Col. J. Moe, Div. of Pathology, Walter Reed Army Institute of Research, Walter Reed Army Medical Center, Washington, D.C. 20307-5100, U.S.A.

T. J. Moore, Harry G. Armstrong Aerospace Medical Research Laboratory, Wright-Patterson AFB, OH 45433, U.S.A.

D. W. Nielsen, Otological Research Laboratories, Henry Ford Hospital, Detroit, Michigan 48202, U.S.A.

P. O. L. Nilsson, Department of Occupational Audiology, University of, Goteburg, Sahlgrenska Sjukhuset and Department of Department of Otolaryngology, Goteburg, S413 45, Sweden

R. Nilsson, Research Department, Projekt Lindholmen, P.O. Box 8714, S-402 75 Goteborg, Sweden

C. W. Nixon, Harry G. Armstrong Aerospace Medical Research Laboratory Wright-Patterson AFB, OH 45433, U.S.A.

G. Oftedal, ELAB, NTH, 7000 Trondheim, Norway

M. P. Osborne, University of Birmingham, Birmingham, B15 2TJ, England

W. Passchier-Vermeer, TNO Institute of Preventive Health Care, Wassenaarseweg 56, 2333 Al Leiden, The Netherlands

R. Patuzzi, University of Western Australia, Physiology Department Perth, Western Australia, 6009, Australia

J. H. Patterson, Jr., Sensory Research Division, U. S. Army Aeromedical Research Laboratory, P.O. Box 577, Ft. Rucker, AL 36362-5000, U.S.A.

F. Pfander, St. Joseph - Stift Bermen, Schwachhauser Heerstr. 163a 28 Bremen, West Germany

Maj. Y. Y. Phillips, Division of Medicine, Walter Reed Army Inst. of Res., Washington, D.C. 20307, U.S.A.

J. O. Pickles, University of Birmingham, Birmingham, B15 2TJ, England

G. R. Price, U. S. Army Human Engineering Lab, Aberdeen Proving Grounds, MD 21005-5001, U.S.A.

R. Pujol, INSERM-U.254, Laboratoire de Neurobiologie de l'Audition, CHR Hopital St. Charles, 34059 , Montpellier Cedex, France

D. R. Richmond, Life Science Division, Los Alamos National Laboratory, Los Alamos, NM 87545, U.S.A.

M. Roberto, Universita di Bari, Bari, 70124, Italy

G. Rossi, Via Genova 3, Torino, 10126, Italy

I. J. Russell, The University of Sussex, M. R. C. Neurophysiology Group, School of Biological Sciences, Brighton, BN1 9QG, England

S. Rydmarker, Department of Experimental Research, University of Lund, Malmo, General Hospital, Sweden

R. Salvi, University of Texas at Dallas, Callier Center for Communication Disorders, 1966 Inwood Rd., Dallas, Texas 75235, U.S.A.

J. Saunders, Department of Otorhinolaryngology and Human Communication University of Pennsylvania, Philadelphia, PA 19104, U.S.A.

S. S. Saunders, University of Texas at Dallas, Callier Center for Communication Disorders, 1966 Inwood Rd., Dallas, Tx 75235, U.S.A.

D. D. Sharpnack, Div. of Pathology, Walter Reed Army Institute of Research, Walter Reed Army Medical Center, Washington, D.C. 20307-5100, U.S.A.

I. Sherban, Cardiology Department, University of Verona, 37134 Verona, Italy

B. Shivapuja, University of Texas at Dallas, Callier Center for Communication Disorders, 1966 Inwood Rd, Dallas, Tx 75235, U.S.A.

R. Simhadri-Sumithra, University of Texas at Dallas, Callier Center for Communication Disorders, 1966 Inwood Rd., Dallas, TX 75235, U.S.A.

W. Sittoni, ENT Department, University of Verona, Policlinico, Borga Roma, 37134 Verona, Italy

G. Smoorenburg, Institute for Perception TNO, Post Box 23, 3769 ZG Soesterberg, The Netherlands

G. O. Stevins, Laboratory for Acoustics, Technical Services of the Army, STFT/CT, Quartier Housiau - B-1801, Brussels (Peutie), Belgium

J. M. Stuhmiller, Fluid Dynamics Division, JAYCOR, P. O. Box 85154, San Diego, CA 92138, U.S.A.

O. Tech, BWB/AFB-FE IV, Erpobungsstelle der Bundeswehr, 4470 Meppen, West Germany

G. Turrentine, University of Texas at Dallas, Callier Center for Communication Disorders, 1966 Inwood Rd., Dallas, TX 75235, U.S.A.

N. Tye-Murrary, Dept. of Speech Pathology and Audiology, University of Iowa, Iowa City, IA 52242, U.S.A.

R. S. Tyler, Dept. of Otolaryngology, Head and Neck Surgery, The University of Iowa, Iowa City, IA 52242, U.S.A.

H. E. Von Gierke, Harry G. Armstrong Aerospace Medical Research Laboratory Wright-Patterson AFB, Ohio 45433, U.S.A.

F. H. White, University of Sheffield, Department of Anatomy and Cell Biology, Sheffield, S10 2TN, England

O. Woxen, Professor, Joint Medical Service of the Norwegian, Armed Forces, FSAN, Oslo mil/Huseby, Oslo 1, Norway

J. W. Wright, Department of Psychology, Washington State Univ., Pullman, WA 99164-4830, U.S.A.

P. Zucchetta, Via Ospedale Civile 105, 35100 Padova, Italy

INDEX